# SMALL ANIMAL
# Endoscopy

# SMALL ANIMAL
# Endoscopy

### Second Edition

## Todd R. Tams, DVM

Diplomate, ACVIM

Chief Medical Officer
Veterinary Centers of America, Inc.
Santa Monica, California

Staff Internist
VCA West Los Angeles Animal Hospital
West Los Angeles, California

*with 1130 illustrations, including 880 in color*

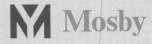

St. Louis  Baltimore  Boston  Carlsbad  Chicago  Minneapolis  New York  Philadelphia  Portland
London  Milan  Sydney  Tokyo  Toronto

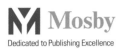
**Mosby**
Dedicated to Publishing Excellence

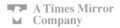
A Times Mirror
Company

*Publisher:* John A. Schrefer
*Executive Editor:* Linda L. Duncan
*Senior Developmental Editor:* Teri Merchant
*Editorial Assistant:* Amy Shehi
*Project Manager:* Linda McKinley
*Senior Production Editor:* Catherine Comer
*Manuscript Editor:* Barrett M. Schroeder
*Design:* Elizabeth Young
*Design Coordinator:* Renée Duenow
*Manufacturing Manager:* Karen Boehme

**Second Edition**

**Copyright © 1999 by Mosby, Inc.**

Previous editions copyrighted 1990

Composition by Graphic World, Inc.
Lithography/color film by Graphic World, Inc.
Printing/binding by Walsworth Publishing Co.

Mosby, Inc.
11830 Westline Industrial Drive
St. Louis, Missouri 63146

International Standard Book Number 0-8151-8743-2

98  99  00  01  02  /  9  8  7  6  5  4  3  2  1

# Contributors

**Colin F. Burrows, BvetMed, PhD, MRCVS**
Diplomate, ACVIM,
Professor and Chair,
Department of Small Animal Clinical Sciences,
University of Florida,
College of Veterinary Medicine,
Gainesville, Florida

**Christopher J. Chamness, DVM**
General Manager,
Karl Storz Veterinary Endoscopy–America, Inc.
Goleta, California

**Gregory Grauer, DVM**
Diplomate, ACVIM,
Professor, Department of Clinical Sciences,
Colorado State University,
College of Veterinary Medicine,
Fort Collins, Colorado

**Darryl J. Heard, BSc, BVMS, PhD**
Diplomate, ACZM,
Assistant Professor,
Wildlife and Zoological Medicine,
Department of Small Animal Clinical Sciences,
College of Veterinary Medicine,
University of Florida,
Gainesville, Florida

**Albert E. Jergens, DVM, MS**
Diplomate, ACVIM,
Assistant Professor,
Veterinary Clinical Sciences,
Iowa State University,
College of Veterinary Medicine,
Ames, Iowa

**Hans Joachim Lunemann**
Director of Documentation,
Karl Storz GMBH and Company,
Tuttlingen, Germany

**Susan E. Johnson, DVM, MS**
Diplomate, ACVIM,
Associate Professor,
Veterinary Clinical Sciences,
The Ohio State University,
Columbus, Ohio

**Michael L. Magne, DVM, MS**
Diplomate, ACVIM,
Assistant Clinical Professor,
Department of Surgery and Radiology,
University of California,
Davis, California;
Staff Internist,
Internal Medicine,
Animal Care Center,
Rohnert Park, California

**Brendan C. McKiernan, DVM**
Diplomate, ACVIM,
Professor of Medicine,
University of Illinois,
College of Veterinary Medicine,
Urbana, Illinois

**Frances M. Moore, DVM**
Diplomate, ACVP,
Veterinary Pathologist and Section Head,
Veterinary Division,
Marshfield Laboratories,
Marshfield, Wisconsin

**Philip A. Padrid, DVM**
Assistant Professor of Medicine,
Pulmonary and Critical Care Medicine,
University of Chicago,
Chicago, Illinois

**Keith Richter, DVM**
Diplomate, ACVIM,
Internal Medicine Staff,
Veterinary Specialty Hospital of San Diego,
Rancho Santa Fe, California

**David F. Senior, BVSc**
Diplomate, ACVIM,
Professor and Head,
Veterinary Clinical Sciences,
School of Veterinary Medicine,
Louisiana State University,
Baton Rouge, Louisiana

**Robert G. Sherding, DVM**
Diplomate, ACVIM,
Professor and Department Chair,
Department of Veterinary Clinical Sciences,
The Ohio State University,
Columbus, Ohio

**Michael Taylor, DVM**
Service Chief,
Avian and Exotic Animals,
Small Animal Clinic,
Ontario Veterinary College,
University of Guelph,
Guelph, Ontario, Canada

**Robert A. Taylor, DVM, MS**
Diplomate, ACVS,
Alameda East Veterinary Clinic,
Denver, Colorado

**David C. Twedt, DVM**
Diplomate, ACVIM,
Professor,
Department of Clinical Sciences,
Colorado State University,
College of Veterinary Medicine,
Fort Collins, Colorado

**Ronald S. Walton, DVM, MS**
Diplomate, ACVIM,
Diplomate, ACVECC,
Fort Leavenworth, Kansas

**Michael D. Willard, DVM**
Diplomate, ACVIM,
Professor,
Small Animal Medicine and Surgery,
Texas A&M University,
College Station, Texas

*To my wife, Sazzy*

*For knowing what I'm saying even when I'm not talking*
*For teaching me the value of listening*
*For the small, daily, nameless acts of love and kindness that go (almost) unnoticed*
   *but that weave and nurture the fabric of our family*

*To my 8-year-old son, "Snapper," who needs me*

*To run*
*To wrestle*
*To laugh*
*To catch*
*To throw*

*To applaud and console*
*With equal measure*

*To hug, to hold*
*To listen with my heart*

*To treasure the moment*
*To cherish the time*

*To my parents, Margaret and Roland*

*Whose love, understanding, and encouragement have meant so much to me*
   *over all the years*

# Preface

The second edition of *Small Animal Endoscopy* meets the original goal of the first edition—it provides a comprehensive standard reference work for veterinarians that encompasses all aspects of endoscopic examination of canine, feline, and avian patients. The text of this edition has been expanded, so *Small Animal Endoscopy* remains the most complete reference work on endoscopy in veterinary medicine. The text is directed toward interns, residents, and specialists who are interested in improving their skills and also toward veterinarians in private practice who wish to utilize endoscopic equipment to its fullest capabilities. In the 8 years since the first edition was published, interest in endoscopy has increased tremendously among specialists and generalists alike. The majority of the procedures described in this text can be readily performed in most private practice settings. All that is required is dedication to achieve needed skills, recognition of the many indications for endoscopy in practice, and utilization of appropriate instrumentation. I encourage veterinarians interested in improving their endoscopy skills to review text chapters of interest in detail, partake in laboratory training sessions as needed, and use new knowledge for the benefit of their patients and their patients' owners.

Endoscopy is one of the most diagnostically useful tools available in small animal medicine. It affords the clinician a minimally invasive method to examine much of the gastrointestinal tract, upper and lower airways, postuterine and lower urinary tracts, abdominal cavity (laparoscopy), thoracic cavity (thoracoscopy), and joint spaces (arthroscopy). Few technological advances in medicine have come along that are as affordable for the general practitioner, diagnostically versatile, and professionally rewarding. Indeed, many practitioners with whom I have spoken over the years have described the great sense of satisfaction and enjoyment they experienced in their practices once endoscopy capabilities began being utilized. Much can be accomplished through the use of endoscopic techniques.

## ORGANIZATION

The primary goal of *Small Animal Endoscopy* is to *teach*. The text uses a systematic approach to viewing the inside of the body while providing practical information about the role of endoscopy in the overall diagnostic scheme of various disorders. Relevant chapters include detailed descriptions of techniques and a color atlas of both normal and abnormal examination findings that may be encountered during a procedure. *Small Animal Endoscopy* is a clinically oriented composite of many years of clinical experience in endoscopic observation and documentation by leading specialists.

More than 850 color photographs provide a large range of appearances from which to learn and with which to compare findings, which helps less experienced endoscopists gain confidence. This represents an increase of more than 100 photographs from the first edition. In addition, some of the photographs from the first edition have been replaced with better examples of the lesions being described. Instrumentation, examination, and recommended sample procurement techniques are described in detail.

Chapters are organized according to the specific area of the body being discussed (e.g., esophagus, stomach, small intestine, abdominal cavity, urethra and urinary bladder). Each chapter provides information on indications for endoscopy, instrumentation, examination technique, descriptions of endoscopic findings pertaining to various disorders, and limitations of the procedures. Many of the chapters include an atlas section at the end. The atlas sections begin with a series of photographs of normal appearances. The order of these illustrations reflects the order in which the endoscopic examination is being performed. When possible, abnormal findings have been grouped by type of disorder (e.g., inflammatory, motility, neoplastic). A table of contents at the beginning of each atlas section provides a quick reference for the reader. The contributors and I have made every effort to be as thorough as possible in preparing this collection of photographs but are well aware that no atlas can ever be fully comprehensive. Certain rarities have likely been omitted that may be of special interest to the reader.

## FEATURES OF THE SECOND EDITION

Significant additions have been made to the second edition, such as discussions of newer techniques and a more dedicated discussion of topics that were only briefly discussed in the first edition. Changes include the following:

- A new chapter on flexible endoscopy in exotic animal species
- A new chapter dedicated to detailing recommendations on endoscopic biopsy specimen collection, clinical utility of brush cytology in gastrointestinal endoscopy, and important histopathologic considerations
- An expanded chapter on percutaneous endoscopic gastrostomy tube placement
- Expanded chapters on rhinoscopy and tracheobronchoscopy
- An expanded chapter on urethroscopy and cystoscopy
- An expanded chapter on rigid endoscopy of avian and reptilian species
- A new chapter on canine arthroscopy
- A new chapter on thoracoscopy

All of these changes and additions reflect exciting advances in the field of endoscopy as described by recognized experts.

## ACKNOWLEDGMENTS

I am indebted to the authors who contributed to this book. They are highly experienced clinicians who have demonstrated expertise in either private or academic practices. I thank each of them for their efforts and willingness to share their knowledge and experience with others. They all share the common thread of being excellent teachers. I have the greatest respect for their contributions to our profession.

I offer a special thanks to Dr. Sazzy Borden, who graciously spent countless hours assisting with manuscript review, taking photographs, preparing diagrams, and offering moral support during work on both the first and second editions. Carreen Schuller, Vicky Powers, Michelle Briggs, Sue Jenkins, and Kris Huber, my technical assistants over the years, have been exceptionally caring while assisting me with many of the endoscopy procedures done on the patients presented in my chapters. Charlie Kerlee of Colorado State University provided expert advice regarding endoscopic photographic technique. Dr. Christopher Chamness of the Karl Storz Veterinary Endoscopy–America Company provided many instrument photographs for inclusion in the text. I found the staff at Mosby–Year Book to be extremely knowledgeable, helpful, and patient as we worked together to prepare the second edition. I especially thank my developmental editors—Linda Duncan and Amy Shehi—and the production editing staff—Cathy Comer, Barrett Schroeder, René Spencer, and Linda McKinley—for the quality of their work and their professionalism.

**Todd R. Tams**

# Contents

# Chapter 1

# Endoscopic Instrumentation

## Christopher J. Chamness

Until recently endoscopic instrumentation was designed by manufacturers with an almost exclusive interest in human applications. Similarly, the overwhelming majority of available references on endoscopy cater to the needs of internists and surgeons in various specialties of human medicine. To best serve the needs of veterinary practitioners, this chapter presents a general and practical overview of the abundance of currently available instrumentation—its proper care, economic implications, and possible applications in veterinary medicine.

## ENDOSCOPE SYSTEM

The modern endoscope system has at least three components: (1) the endoscope (rigid or flexible), (2) a light source, and (3) a light-transmitting cable (which carries light from the source to the endoscope). With most flexible endoscopes, the light-transmitting cable is permanently attached to the endoscope and has a section that plugs directly into the light source. Numerous accessories and ancillary instruments may be added to the basic endoscope system. This equipment enhances functionality, diagnostic or therapeutic capability, and communications. Accessories can include various sheaths and instruments for biopsy, grasping, aspiration, cytology, electrosurgery, and laser surgery; pumps for suction, insufflation, and irrigation, and attachable video cameras for monitor viewing, videotaping, printing, and digital storage or transmission.

## FLEXIBLE ENDOSCOPES

The two basic flexible endoscopes are the fiberscope and the videoendoscope. The difference between the two relates to the systems for sensing and transmitting images. In a fiberoptic endoscope the image is carried from the subject being examined to the eyepiece via bundles of optical glass fibers. In a *true* videoendoscope the image is transmitted electronically to a video monitor from the distal tip of the endoscope where it is "sensed" by a charge coupled device (CCD) chip. Fiberoptic images can also be transmitted to video monitors and accessories by attaching a CCD camera to the eyepiece of the endoscope. Although fiberoptic image quality cannot match that of the CCD sensor, the fiberoptic systems have considerable cost advantages. The features of fiberscopes and videoendoscopes are compared in Table 1-1.

Flexible endoscopes are available in diameters ranging from 14 mm to less than 1 mm. Most larger flexible scopes (greater than 2 mm in diameter) are equipped with an accessory channel and a deflectable tip. Currently the most popular endoscope in small animal practice is the gastroscope, which has a four-way deflecting tip. The tip's two-plane deflection capability (up, down, left, right) is crucial to the successful navigation of the gastrointestinal tract, particularly in the most challenging maneuvers through the pylorus and ileocolic orifice.

Because most gastroscopes have an outer diameter of 7.8 mm or greater, they cannot be used in smaller patients for such procedures as bronchoscopy, rhinoscopy, and urethrocystoscopy. Consequently, the second most popular flexible endoscope in small animal practice is a

**Table 1-1**    Features of Fiberscopes and Videoscopes

| Feature | Fiberscope | Videoscope |
| --- | --- | --- |
| Image quality | Good | Excellent |
| Portability | Excellent | Poor |
| Cost | Moderate | High |
| Diameters available | Wide range available | Smaller diameters not available* |
| Video capability | Requires attachable CCD camera | Integral |

*Due to limitations on chip miniaturization.

small-diameter fiberscope that is used primarily for endoscopy of the airways and urinary tract. This fiberscope generally has limited tip deflection capability (one way or two way) and a considerably smaller working channel. The working channel is the section of the endoscope through which ancillary instruments are advanced into the patient.

## Fiberscopes

### The Optical System

The image- and light-transmitting components of a fiberscope consist of bundles of optical fibers. Each fiber, typically 8 to 12 $\mu$m in diameter, has a core of optical-quality glass. This core is surrounded by glass cladding that must have a lower refractive index than the core. The differential in refractive indices results in a state of nearly total internal reflection, which allows the fiber to transmit light with only negligible losses.

Because each fiber is only capable of transmitting a spot of uniform color and brightness, several thousand fibers must be arranged in a coherent order to transmit an image. *Coherent bundles* are formed by fusing the individual fiber faces of each end of the bundle in exactly the same pattern (Figure 1-1). Broken fibers are seen as black spots on the image viewed through the eyepiece (see Figure 3-4). The resolution and size of a fiberoptic image is determined in part by the number and size of individual fibers. A typical image bundle, also called an *image guide* (IG), contains from as few as 3000 to as many as 40,000 individual fibers. The diameter of an IG bundle is commonly in the range of 0.5 to 3 mm. Naturally, the possible size of an image bundle is limited in smaller diameter fiberscopes; consequently, image size is reduced in these models. The optical benefits of reducing

individual fiber diameter are also limited. With a reduction in fiber diameter, the ratio of cladding to core glass increases, resulting in reduced light transmission and a prominent honeycomb pattern that is more easily seen by the viewer.

In addition to the IG bundle, a fiberscope typically contains one or two light guide (LG) bundles that transmit light from the light source to the distal tip of the fiberscope to illuminate the area being visualized. Although the fibers in the LG bundles may be similar to those in the IG bundles, they are not arranged in any particular pattern because they do not need to transmit an image. These fiber bundles are called *incoherent bundles* (see Figure 1-1).

The lens systems in an endoscope, which are located at each end of the fiber bundles, also contribute significantly to image quality. The *objective lenses* are at the distal tip and serve to focus the image of the mucosa on the distal face of the IG bundle. The focal point of this lens system determines the *depth of field*, which is the range of distances over which the image is in focus. Modern fiberscopes commonly have a depth of field from about 3 to 100 mm. The *ocular lenses* are in the eyepiece of a fiberscope. Their basic purpose is to magnify the image transmitted to the proximal face of the IG bundle so that it can be comfortably seen by the viewer. Several factors contribute to the overall magnification of structures seen through an endoscope, but perhaps the most important one is the distance between the tip of the endoscope and the subject. *Illumination lenses* at each end of the LG bundles maximize the amount of light carried to the object being illuminated. The development of higher quality illumination lens systems and improvements in fiberoptic technology have been crucial in providing adequate brightness in the newer endoscopes with smaller diameters and greater fields of view.

### Basic Construction and Handling

The gastrointestinal fiberscope has three major sections (Figure 1-2, *A*): the insertion tube, the hand piece, and the umbilical cord. Construction of the insertion tube is the most complex and technically challenging aspect of fiberscope design, because this portion of the instrument contains IG and LG fiberoptic bundles; channels for suction, irrigation, and insufflation; four deflection cables; and several layers of protective materials along the entire length of the tube. All of these components must be contained within an insertion tube that has the smallest possible diameter, largest possible accessory channel, and maximal tip deflection capabilities. Because of the complexity of construction and the fragile nature of some components, damage to the insertion tube is the most expen-

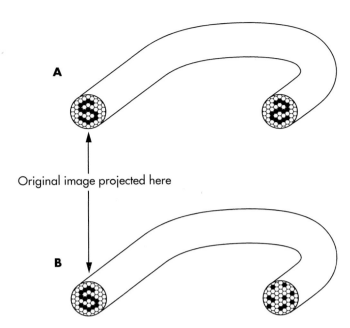

A

Original image projected here

B

**Figure 1-1 A,** Coherent fiber bundle, the image is transmitted perfectly from one end of the fiber bundle to the other. **B,** Incoherent fiber bundle. The image projected on one face of fiber bundle is lost at the other end because of the random order of fibers. (Courtesy Karl Storz Veterinary Endoscopy–America, Inc., Goleta, Calif.)

sive type of repair performed on fiberscopes. Most insertion tube damage can be prevented by observing the following:

1. *Always* handle the insertion tube carefully; avoid sharp bends, tight coiling, or accidental striking of the tube against hard surfaces.
2. *Always* use a mouth speculum when passing the tube through the oral cavity of anesthetized patients.
3. *Never* force instruments or pass foreign objects through the accessory channel. If these rules are *consistently* followed, the life span of an endoscope can be *significantly prolonged* and repairs can be minimized.

The last several centimeters of a fiberscope with tip deflection capability is called the *bending section*. Controlled by the deflection knob(s) in the hand piece, this portion of the insertion tube may be deflected in one or two planes. Deflection in a single plane (*one-way* or *two-way angulation*) is common in small-diameter endoscopes used for procedures such as bronchoscopy and urethroscopy. However, endoscopes designed for gastrointestinal use are equipped with *four-way angulation* (up, down, left, right), which allows the endoscopist to deflect the tip in any direction by coordinating the simultaneous movement of the up/down and left/right control

knobs. Two-plane deflection capability is essential to a thorough endoscopic examination of the gastrointestinal tract. The degree of tip deflection varies among models, but complete retroflection (180 degrees or greater) in at least one direction is desirable in a multipurpose endoscope. Many of the newer endoscopes are capable of 210-degree tip deflection in at least one direction.

A close-up inspection of the distal tip of an insertion tube shows the cross-sectional location of several of the internal structures (see Figure 1-2, *A*). The insufflation channel allows room air to be blown into the gastrointestinal tract, distending the viscus and enabling examination of the mucosa. The water jet exiting the irrigation channel is directed over the distal lens of the IG to remove debris and mucus when necessary. The accessory channel is used for mucus suction and the passage of instruments such as biopsy forceps, grasping forceps, and cytology brushes.

The hand piece contains the eyepiece with its diopter adjustment ring, air/water and suction valves, deflection control knobs and locks, and the opening to the accessory channel. The hand piece is designed to be held in the left hand (Figure 1-2, *B*). The index finger controls suction by fully depressing the first (front) valve. The air/water valve can be controlled by the index or middle finger. Insufflation is activated by placing the fingertip over the hole in the top of the valve, and irrigation is activated by fully depressing the valve. The thumb of the left hand is used to control the up/down deflection knob. The right hand controls the left/right deflection knob, inserts channel accessories, and advances the insertion tube, applying rotational torque when necessary. Excessive torque should *not* be applied to the insertion tube, and care should be taken to ensure that deflection locks are in the *unlocked* position before deflection knobs are used. (More information on the handling and maneuvering of gastrointestinal fiberscopes is provided in Chapter 3.)

The umbilical cord contains the portion of the fiberscope that connects to the light source, including connectors for insufflation and irrigation in gastrointestinal scopes. Although the umbilical cord is not nearly as fragile as the insertion tube, it contains light-carrying fiber bundles and therefore should be handled with caution. Light sources for gastrointestinal fiberscopes generally contain an integral air pump that provides air for insufflation and air pressure for forcing water from an attached bottle through the irrigation channel. A separate connector for suction allows a tube to be attached to an independent suction pump. A pressure compensation valve in this region prevents damage from external pressure changes that may occur during ethylene oxide (ETO) sterilization or shipping by air. A manometer-type pressure tester attached to this valve is used to check for

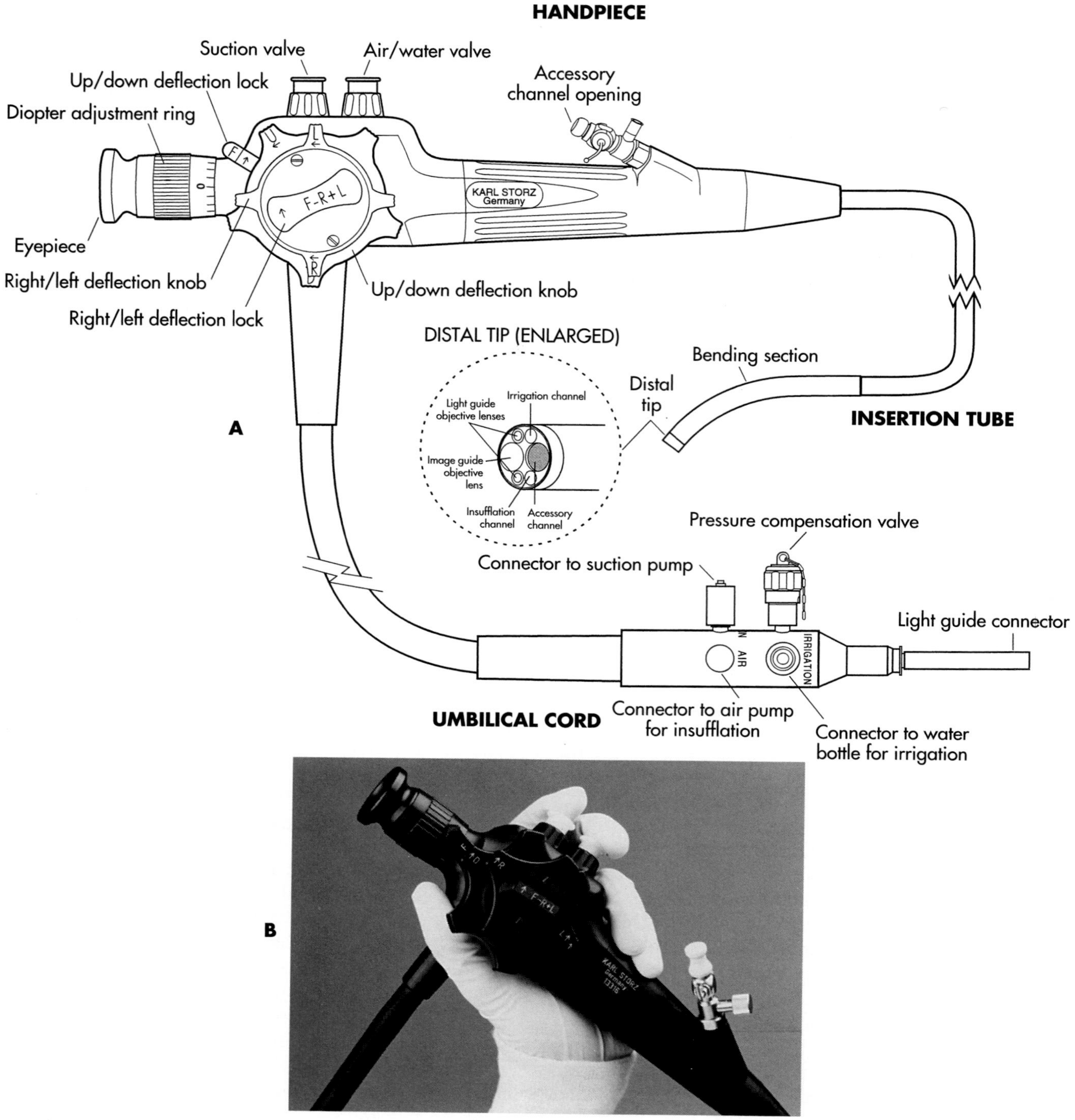

**Figure 1-2 A,** Typical gastrointestinal fiberscope **B,** Position in which the fiberscope is held. (Courtesy Karl Storz Veterinary Endoscopy–America, Inc., Goleta, Calif.)

internal leaks before and after each use. When the pressure tester is attached (Figure 1-3), the endoscopist simply squeezes the bulb until the desired pressure is reached according to manufacturer's specifications. The needle of the pressure gauge should remain stable if the system is free of leaks. Pressure testing is quick and easy and should be done as a matter of routine after each procedure. *Early* detection of leaks may prevent *costly* water damage to the internal components of a fiberscope.

## Videoendoscopes

The mechanical functions of a videoendoscope are similar to those of a fiberscope. The primary difference lies

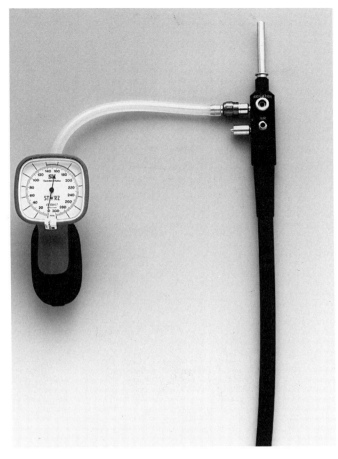

**Figure 1-3** Leakage tester connected to fiberscope. (Courtesy Karl Storz Veterinary Endoscopy–America, Inc., Goleta, Calif.)

in the way the image is produced. Instead of a fiberoptic image, the videoendoscope produces an electronic image that is sensed by a CCD chip at the distal tip of the insertion tube just behind the objective lens. A CCD is a semiconductor capable of converting an optical image (photons) into an electrical signal (electrons) that is then carried via wires along the length of the videoendoscope to a processor. The processor converts this electronic information into a standard video signal that can be distributed to devices such as monitors, videocasette recorders (VCRs), and printers.

Video systems offer distinct advantages in terms of client relations, teaching, and documentation. The ability to view the endoscopic image on a video monitor and record or print this information is not unique to videoendoscopes. *Indirect* videoendoscopy can be accomplished by attaching an endoscopic video camera to the eyepiece of a fiberscope (see Endoscopic Video Cameras and Accessories in this chapter).

Higher image quality is the primary advantage of videoendoscopes over fiberscopes. The resolution of a fiberoptic image cannot approach that of an electronically produced image. Furthermore, because the image is

not dependent on individual glass fibers, image defects (commonly seen as small black spots in a fiberoptic image) are not a problem.

However, in some settings economic concerns may preclude the purchase of a videoendoscope, which is significantly more expensive than a fiberscope. Furthermore, the versatility of attachable video cameras is attractive to veterinary practitioners who are looking for video capabilities compatible with a variety of endoscopes. Until the technologic limitations on the miniaturization of CCD chips are overcome, the production of smaller diameter videoendoscopes is not possible.

## Flexible Instruments

A variety of flexible instruments are available for use with endoscopes that have an accessory channel (Figure 1-4). Both flexible and rigid endoscopes may accommodate the passage of flexible instruments, depending on their design. The most widely used instruments are for biopsy and foreign body retrieval. Other popular flexible instruments include cytology brushes, aspiration tubing, injection/aspiration needles, polypectomy snares, and coagulating electrodes. A vast number of styles and sizes is available; user preference and experience generally dictate which models work best.

Most flexible instruments are classified as either "reusable" or "disposable" (i.e., designed for single use). Reusable instruments are more expensive and durable, although veterinarians frequently reuse disposable instruments. Caution should be used when selecting instrumentation made by a manufacturer other than that of the endoscope itself. It is *not uncommon* to damage the working channel of an endoscope by using "more economic" disposable instruments that are *not compatible* with a particular scope.

To prevent costly damage to the accessory channel of a flexible endoscope, the endoscopist should observe the following general recommendations:

1. The instrument diameter should not exceed that recommended by the manufacturer.
2. The instrument should never be forced through the channel when resistance is met.
3. Foreign objects should not be retrieved through the accessory channel; instead, the entire endoscope should be removed from the patient once the object has been firmly grasped.
4. Before passing instruments through a deflected tip, the manufacturer's recommendations should be reviewed.

## RIGID AND SEMIRIGID ENDOSCOPES

The original rigid endoscope was simply a hollow tube through which light was directed into a body cavity. The

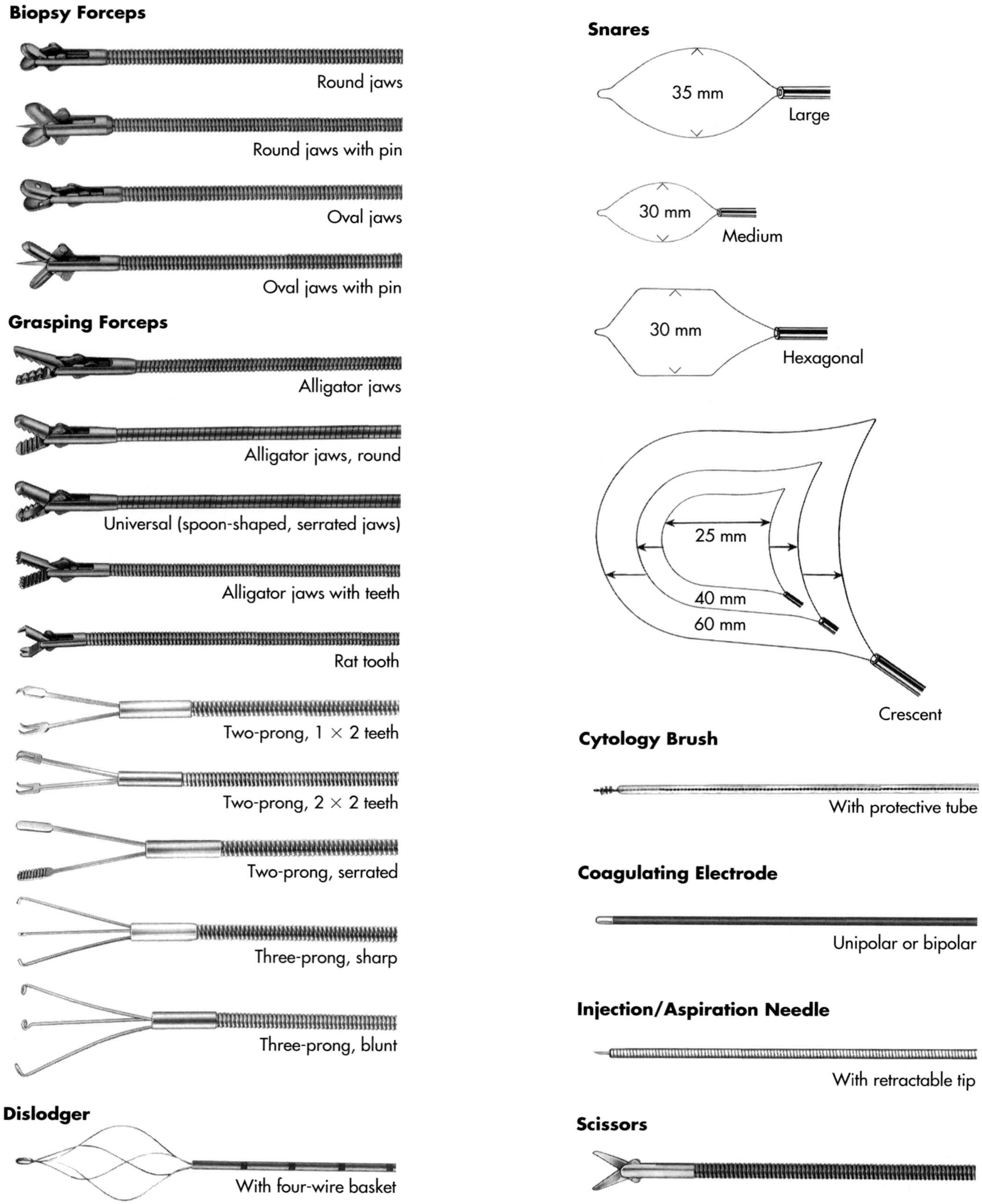

**Biopsy Forceps**

Round jaws

Round jaws with pin

Oval jaws

Oval jaws with pin

**Grasping Forceps**

Alligator jaws

Alligator jaws, round

Universal (spoon-shaped, serrated jaws)

Alligator jaws with teeth

Rat tooth

Two-prong, 1 × 2 teeth

Two-prong, 2 × 2 teeth

Two-prong, serrated

Three-prong, sharp

Three-prong, blunt

**Dislodger**

With four-wire basket

**Snares**

35 mm
Large

30 mm
Medium

30 mm
Hexagonal

25 mm
40 mm
60 mm
Crescent

**Cytology Brush**

With protective tube

**Coagulating Electrode**

Unipolar or bipolar

**Injection/Aspiration Needle**

With retractable tip

**Scissors**

**Figure 1-4** Flexible instruments for use with endoscopes that have an accessory channel. (Courtesy Karl Storz Veterinary Endoscopy–America, Inc., Goleta, Calif.)

conventional telescope lens system (Figure 1-5, *A*) was first developed by Nitze in 1879. The next crucial breakthrough occurred in 1966, when Hopkins invented the rod-lens system (Figure 1-5, *B*), which is still recognized as the gold standard of the industry. Modern optical systems offer several significant improvements in image quality, including better light transmission, higher resolution and contrast, greater magnification, and a wider field of view. The variety of available rigid endoscopes and the visualization afforded by even the smallest models open up an

enormous new field of minimally invasive diagnostic and therapeutic possibilities to veterinary practitioners. As a profession, veterinary medicine is beginning to more actively explore applications for these rigid instruments in the diagnosis and management of animal diseases.

Rigid and semirigid endoscopes have outer diameters ranging from about 1 to 10 mm. Larger scopes have greater light-carrying capacity and larger image size. Smaller scopes are less invasive and fit into smaller areas (e.g., nasal passages, urethras, joints). Some of the more common applications of rigid endoscopy in small animal medicine include laparoscopy, thoracoscopy, urethrocystoscopy, rhinoscopy, arthroscopy, vaginoscopy, and avian endoscopy. As with flexible endoscopes, no one size of rigid or semirigid endoscope is suitable for all procedures in all patients. The appropriate-sized telescope should be selected based on the procedures most commonly performed (Table 1-2). Although smaller telescopes tend to be more versatile, illumination is limited when these scopes are used in larger, more light-absorptive cavities.

The *viewing angle* of a telescope is an important consideration because it affects both orientation and visualization (Figure 1-6). Forward-viewing telescopes (0 degrees) provide the simplest orientation but the most limited viewing field. A 25- or 30-degree viewing angle allows the endoscopist to view a larger area by simply rotating the telescope on its longitudinal axis. Spatial orientation becomes more challenging with an oblique-viewing scope. Some telescopes are available in even more acute angles of view (e.g., 70, 90, 120 degrees), but

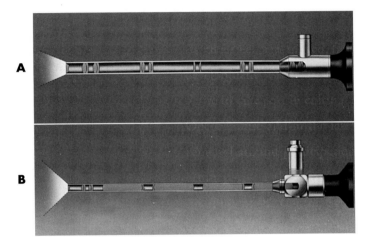

**Figure 1-5** **A,** Traditional telescope optical system. **B,** Hopkins rod lens system. (Courtesy Karl Storz Veterinary Endoscopy–America, Inc., Goleta, Calif.)

**Table 1-2** Recommended Canine Applications of Common Telescopes by Diameter*

| Telescope diameter (mm) | Procedure | | | | | |
|---|---|---|---|---|---|---|
| | **Laparoscopy** | **Thoracoscopy** | **Urethrocystoscopy†** | **Rhinoscopy** | **Arthroscopy** | **Avian** |
| 2.7 | + | + | + + + (In females weighing 5 to 45 lb) | + + + | + + + | + + + |
| 4 | + + | + + + | + + + (In females weighing more than 15 lb) | — | — | — |
| 5 | + + + | + + + | Percutaneous cystoscopy only | — | — | — |
| 10 | + + + | + + | — | — | — | — |

+ , Fair; + + , good; + + + , excellent.
* These recommendations are based on the most common adult patient sizes seen in small animal practice. The ratings of excellent, good, and fair are based on the best compromise between maximal visualization and minimal invasiveness, given the assumed patient population. Individual and breed variations exist.
† Transurethral cystoscopy using rigid endoscopes is only possible in females. A percutaneous approach (prepubic, transabdominal) to the bladder can be used in males; this approach can be used in females which a scope is too large to pass transurethrally. A small-diameter flexible endoscope is required for complete endoscopic examination of the male canine urethra.

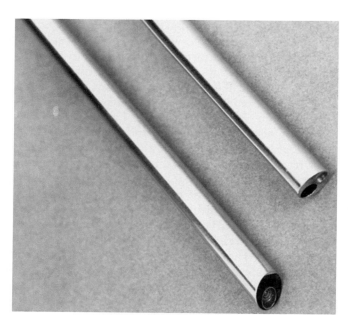

**Figure 1-6** Telescope viewing angles: 30 degrees and 0 degree. (Courtesy Karl Storz Veterinary Endoscopy–America, Inc., Goleta, Calif.)

these instruments are rarely used in veterinary practice. The choice of telescope largely depends on the procedure being performed and the experience of the endoscopist.

Perhaps the most popular telescope used today in small animal practice is the 2.7-mm telescope. Frequently referred to as an *arthroscope*, this versatile telescope is ideally suited for many procedures including urethrocystoscopy, rhinoscopy, otoscopy, and avian endoscopy. A popular sheath system for this telescope (originally designed for human pediatric urethrocystoscopy) accommodates flexible instruments and allows the introduction of fluids or gas (Figure 1-7). A variety of sheaths and cannulas are available for telescopes of every size. These accessories are designed to suit the anatomy and functional requirements of various procedures.

Larger telescopes (5 to 10 mm in diameter) are better suited for endoscopic examination of larger cavities such as the abdomen and thorax of most dogs and cats. Although smaller scopes can also be used for these procedures, illumination and image size are limited. The vast array of ancillary instrumentation available for performing minimally invasive surgery goes beyond the scope of this chapter. Examples of recommended instruments for performing laparoscopy include not only the telescope, light source, light-transmitting cable, and video camera (optional) but also cannulas with trocars, hand instruments, a Veress needle, and an insufflator. (Complete discussions of the instrumentation required for laparoscopy and thoracoscopy can be found in Chapters 14 and 20 respectively.)

Rod lens telescopes are generally not available in diameters less than approximately 1.9 mm. However, recent developments have led to the introduction of very small-diameter endoscopes, which are generally classified as semirigid, because their flexibility falls between that of completely rigid endoscopes and flexible scopes. These tiny scopes rely on fused silica bundles to transmit an image. Although the optical quality cannot match that of the rod lens or even traditional fiberoptic systems, these semirigid scopes enable practitioners to examine anatomic structures previously unavailable for endoscopic evaluation and to develop new less invasive techniques that may further reduce the morbidity of current procedures. Fused–silica-bundle technology is also significantly less expensive than traditional endoscopic technologies.

## LIGHT SOURCES

Historically, endoscopic illumination was achieved by placing a fragile, heat-emitting incandescent bulb at the distal tip of the endoscope. In 1960, Dr. Karl Storz discovered that a fiber optic light cable could transmit light from a remote light source through an endoscope to the examination site. This discovery heralded the birth of *cold light endoscopy*, which is the basis for the design of all modern endoscopic light sources. Although the light is not actually "cold," the technology represents a marked reduction in the incidence of thermal injury during endoscopic procedures.

Factors that contribute to the illumination or brightness of an endoscopic image include the technology type and power of the light source, the number of hours clocked on bulbs of certain types, and the diameter of the endoscope being used. Other important factors are the length of the illumination chain, the light-carrying capacity and condition of any LGs and lenses in the chain, the cleanliness of any lens surfaces or other interfaces through which light must pass, and the size of the cavity being examined. If a video camera is being used, the light sensitivity of the camera is a contributing factor.

### Power and Type

The array of light sources currently available for endoscopic applications can be categorized by two parameters: the *power* of the source (usually expressed in watts) and the *type* of illumination technology. The three common types of endoscopic light sources are xenon, metal-halide, and tungsten-halogen. They range in power from 25 to 500 W.

The *power* of a light source is a rough measure of its brightness in that the higher the wattage, the brighter the

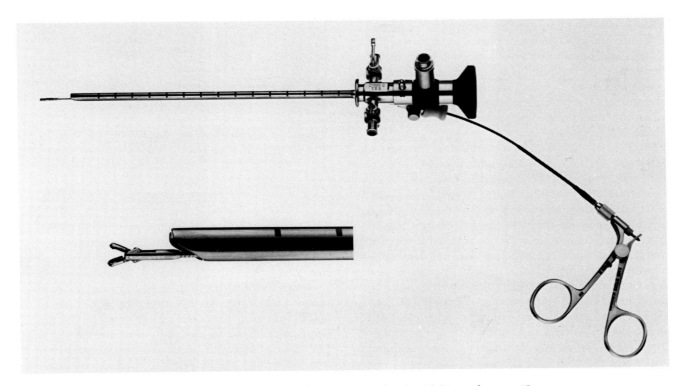

**Figure 1-7** A 2.7-mm telescope in a urethrocystoscopy sheath with biopsy forceps. (Courtesy Karl Storz Veterinary Endoscopy–America, Inc., Goleta, Calif.)

illumination. This measure is generally accurate for comparing light sources of the same type but is not always valid for comparing light sources of different types. Naturally, a common, household lightbulb of 100 W is brighter than one of 40 W. However, the *power rating* of a lightbulb or light source is actually the measure of how much power it *consumes,* not how much light power it *produces.* The 40-W lightbulb consumes 40 W of electrical power but does not produce 40 W of light; in fact, this incandescent bulb produces mostly heat. A 40 W fluorescent lamp, on the other hand, produces much more light than the incandescent bulb while consuming the same 40 W of electrical power. Furthermore, the fluorescent bulb produces a different-colored light than the incandescent bulb. These two characteristics (wattage and color variation) are also true of endoscopic light sources.

Xenon light sources offer excellent color reproduction for video endoscopy. They have become the standard in endoscopy primarily because their quality of light most closely approximates that of pure sunlight. A 150- to 300-W xenon light source is recommended for general-purpose veterinary endoscopy when the examination is being videotaped. Xenon light sources provide adequate illumination for the endoscopes used in veterinary practice. In addition, they often have sophisticated features such as automatic exposure control and flash generator

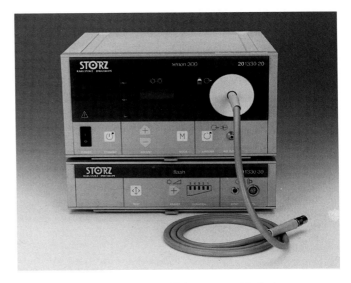

**Figure 1-8** A 300-watt xenon light source with flash generator attached. (Courtesy Karl Storz Veterinary Endoscopy–America, Inc., Goleta, Calif.)

capabilities for still photography (Figure 1-8). Because the spectral intensity of the output is relatively continuous, all of the colors in the visible spectrum are reproduced. A xenon lamp burns for 400 to 1000 hours before it must be replaced.

Before xenon light sources were introduced, metal halide was the light source of choice for endoscopy. The spectral-light output from this type of lamp is not continuous but has "spikes" at a few wavelengths. Consequently, illuminated objects appear slightly more gray or less colorful. A metal halide lamp usually burns for 200 to 250 hours before needing replacement. The lamp produces a bluish light.

Tungsten-halogen lamps are similar in intensity and color to household incandescent lightbulbs. The color they produce is toward the red/yellow end of the color spectrum. These light sources are relatively inexpensive and are frequently used in veterinary practice. Although they do not provide the same quality of light as xenon lamps, halogen light sources can be acceptable when light intensity and color reproduction are not critical. The bulbs on halogen light sources must be changed regularly because they lose much of their intensity after only a fraction of the estimated life span (approximately 100 hours).

Important factors in the selection of a light source for flexible gastrointestinal endoscopy include the availability of a pump for insufflation and irrigation and the style of attachment to the light connector. The compatibility of the light source and the endoscope must be considered. If the two are not compatible, the availability of an adapter to connect them becomes a crucial issue.

## Light-Transmitting Cables

Once a light source with acceptable color and brightness has been selected, a vehicle is needed to transmit this light to the endoscope or directly to the examination site. As discussed previously, the advent of fiber optics has made this possible. Although LGs are frequently built into the umbilical cord of flexible endoscopes, they are also available as separate detachable cables for use with some models and with rigid endoscopes. Thousands of fibers ranging in size from 30 $\mu$m to several hundred microns are bundled together, surrounded by a protective jacket (Figure 1-9), and equipped with metal end fittings in order to make an endoscopic light-transmitting cable. The cable is typically inserted into the light source at one end and attached to the LG post of the endoscope at the other end.

Some cables transmit light through a fluid-filled medium. Although fluid-filled cables are capable of carrying a greater amount of light, they are less flexible and much more expensive. As a result of recent technologic innovations, fiberoptic cables can now carry almost as much light as fluid-filled cables, at a much lower cost.

Light-transmitting cables are available in different diameters. The correct diameter depends on the size of the endoscope that is being used. Matching the right cable to the right scope prevents overheating or under illumination. Generally speaking, a smaller scope requires a smaller LG cable.

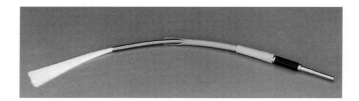

**Figure 1-9** Light-transmitting cable in which the fibers are bundled together and surrounded by a protective jacket. (Courtesy Karl Storz Veterinary Endoscopy–America, Inc., Goleta, Calif.)

The construction of light-transmitting cables also varies from manufacturer to manufacturer. A cable with additional armouring lasts longer than one without this protection. Handling a light cable with care prolongs its life span and keeps it in top condition for use in endoscopy. An LG degrades over time by discoloration and breakage. Discoloration changes the color appearance of the light that comes out of the LG. An operator can check for discoloration by holding one end of the cable to a lightbulb or fluorescent lamp and looking at the other end. If the LG cable is discolored, it probably looks considerably more yellow than the source light. Breakage of individual fibers is the other type of degradation. Using the same viewing arrangement, the finding of small black dots indicates that the cable has broken fibers. A few broken fibers does not necessarily affect the transmission of light, but when one third of the fibers are broken, it is time to replace the light cable.

## ENDOSCOPIC VIDEO CAMERAS AND ACCESSORIES

Video is perhaps the most significant new endoscopic technology. When the endoscopic image is displayed on a video monitor, the endoscopist is able to work more comfortably and share information during a procedure with any number of observers. Other advantages include the ability to document procedures in many forms (e.g., print, slide, videotape), which can be enormously useful for client relations; medical records; and referral, teaching, or consulting purposes.

The basic endoscopic video camera system consists of the endoscopic adapter, camera head, camera control unit (CCU), and monitor (Figure 1-10). Depending on the design, the endoscopic adapter and camera head may be individual units joined by a threaded connector, or they may be permanently attached.

The endoscopic adaptor on the camera head connects to the endoscope eyepiece where it focuses and magnifies the endoscopic image onto the imaging sensor of the camera head. The amount of magnification depends on

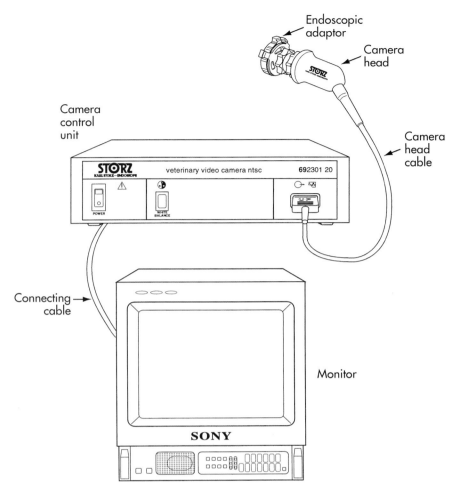

**Figure 1-10** Basic endoscopic video camera system. (Courtesy Karl Storz Veterinary Endoscopy–America, Inc., Goleta, Calif.)

the focal length of the adaptor, with higher focal lengths corresponding to higher magnification. Lenses with different focal lengths (25 to 40 mm) are available for use in different situations. If a variety of focal lengths is desired, a camera with a built-in variable focal-length zoom adaptor should be purchased. This zoom adaptor enables the surgeon to vary the magnification and consequently the image size at any point throughout the procedure without the inconvenience of changing lenses.

The camera head contains the semiconductor (CCD) that transforms the optical image into an electronic signal. This signal can then be transmitted down the head cable to the CCU (Figure 1-11). The optical image is projected onto the CCD surface, which has an area of about 20 to 35 mm$^2$. This surface is subdivided into approximately half a million individual picture elements referred to as *pixels*. The continuous optical image should be reproduced as faithfully as possible. This can be done by maximizing the number of pixels. The greater the number of pixels, the higher the resolving power of the CCD.

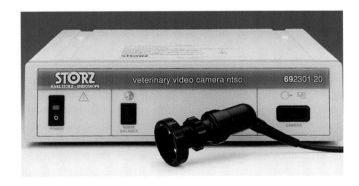

**Figure 1-11** Endoscopic video camera, consisting of a camera control unit and camera head. (Courtesy Karl Storz Veterinary Endoscopy–America, Inc., Goleta, Calif.)

Two basic camera types are available: single-chip cameras, which use one CCD and three-chip cameras, which use three CCDs. The camera types differ in their horizontal resolution, a factor that affects detail recognition, color, and price. Most single-chip cameras use a mosaic filter pattern to reproduce color. One of four different-colored filters is placed over each pixel. This filter array requires an electronic process to reconstruct the colors and detail of the original image. Because every color is not available at each pixel, the reconstructive process does not fully recover all of the color and detail information that was present in the original optical image. Therefore single-chip cameras theoretically have lower resolution and less accurate color reproduction than three-chip cameras. However, current state-of-the-art single-chip technology produces images that are very close to those obtained with three-chip cameras.

Three-chip cameras use a prism to separate light into the three primary colors: red, green, and blue [RGB]. Each of the three sensors transmits one color to the video monitor. Because no electronic process is required for color conversion, the colors are more accurate. In addition, all information available for resolution is used solely for that purpose. However, a three-chip camera costs approximately $4000 more than one with a single chip.

The electronic image information is transmitted via the camera cable to a connector that fastens the cable to the processor or CCU. The CCU houses the power supply and electronics that decode the information from the sensor and convert the picture information into a standard video signal. This signal can then be distributed to monitors, VCRs, and printers.

The CCU also contains the electronics for functions such as white balance and automatic exposure control. *White balancing* is the process by which the camera adjusts for the light color (color temperature) of the illumination source (e.g., bluish light with a metal halide lamp). Unlike the human eye, a video camera cannot compensate for variations in the color of light. Before white balancing is performed, all components of the optical system (endoscopic adaptor, endoscope, light-transmitting cable, and light source) must be connected to the camera. The operator then points the endoscope at a white object (e.g., a piece of gauze or a clean white laboratory coat) and depresses the white-balance button on the camera control unit. Once the camera is white balanced, all colors should be accurately represented. With *automatic exposure control,* a patented feature of some cameras, the correct shutter speed for the CCD is automatically selected to provide the best exposure, regardless of scene illumination.

The monitor completes the basic video chain. The image presented on the video monitor is a representation of all previous transformations from the light source, light-transmitting cable, endoscope, camera head, and CCU. Video signals are sent to a monitor in three common formats: composite (or Bnc), Y/C (or S-video), and RGB. The signal formats differ in the way portions of the video signal are transmitted to the monitor. The video signal is comprised of chrominance (color), luminance (bright-

ness), and sync (i.e., synchronization of the signal information on the monitor).

Composite video combines the elements of luminance, chrominance, and sync into one signal. The combined signal reduces the amount of bandwidth available to each individual element. The monitor also has to separate the three elements, with the decoding process often producing artifacts. As a result a sort of herringbone fuzziness occurs at the boundaries between different colors. Composite video offers the least detail at the lowest cost and is the signal format used in most consumer television and VCR systems.

The Y/C or S-video format separates the brightness and color information into two distinct signals. This standard is capable of higher resolution than composite video because of the wide bandwidth available on each channel. With brightness and color already on separate bandwidths, signals do not have to be divided at the monitor; thus artifacts are avoided, and color is better than with the composite standard. In addition, the synchronizing signals are encoded with the luminance signal, providing greater bandwidth for chroma. The S-video format is highly recommended to derive full benefit from high-quality single-chip cameras. This video format is characteristic of super VHS and high-band 8-mm systems.

The RGB standard separates the sync, luminance, and chrominance information into four channels: red, green, blue, and sync. The outcome is true color and high resolution. The RGB format is strongly recommended for use with three-chip cameras. The different types of cables are shown in Figure 1-12.

Monitors vary greatly in size and resolution. Size is a matter of preference, but 13- to 20-inch monitors are most commonly used. To provide the optimal image, the

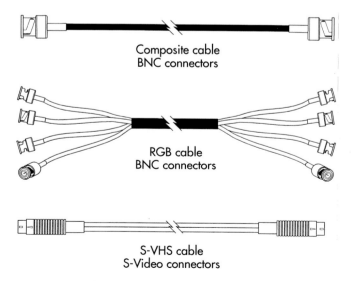

**Figure 1-12** Video connecting cables through which video signals are transmitted to a monitor. (Courtesy Karl Storz Veterinary Endoscopy–America, Inc., Goleta, Calif.)

monitor must match or surpass the horizontal resolution of the video camera. By today's standards the minimum monitor resolution should be 500 lines for single-chip cameras and 600 lines for three-chip cameras. The monitor should also have Y/C or S-video and RGB inputs to maximize the advantages of these video signal formats.

If the desired results are not being achieved from an endoscope system, the operator should start at the beginning of the imaging chain (the light source) and check every device along the way. Over time, bulbs and fiberoptic bundles lose their intensity and need to be replaced. Because endoscopes are somewhat fragile, they can be damaged if they are not handled with care. Video cameras sometimes malfunction, and video monitors often need to be recalibrated. *Always* keep in mind the optical and electronic chain that has been put together, and remember that every piece affects the quality of the image achieved.

A variety of video accessories can be incorporated into the imaging chain. VCRs, video printers, slide makers, digital enhancers, and image-capture systems can be used in conjunction with the basic video system described in this chapter. Perhaps the most useful and affordable accessory is the video printer (Figure 1-13). This machine allows the endoscopist to make a print directly from the video signal, which may contain one or several endoscopic images seen during a procedure. After the initial purchase of the printer, each print costs approximately $1. Many veterinary endoscopists consider the video printer a cost-effective means for creating accurate medical records, educating clients, and communicating with colleagues. Another option is to record live video with a VCR. It is important to choose a recorder or printer with high resolution that is easy to operate. Standard VHS VCRs record only about 240 lines of horizontal resolution. To derive full benefit from a high-resolution camera, a higher quality super-VHS (S-VHS) recorder should be used. Because this piece of equipment is placed in the imaging chain before the monitor, it affects the view displayed on the screen. The resolution of

the VCR or printer needs to be as close as possible to that of the video camera.

Image-capture devices are essentially computers that record and store still images from a live video source. This digitally stored information can then be used to produce reports in a variety of formats (e.g., prints, slides, transparencies). The images are sent by modem to a service for printing. Dictation capabilities make this system ideal for medical records or presentations.

## CLEANING, DISINFECTION, AND STERILIZATION

No general discussion of endoscope care and cleaning can replace the prudent use of the manufacturer's recommendations for each instrument. However, the general guidelines given in this section apply in most situations.

Immediately after a procedure is performed, organic material should be mechanically removed from all surfaces of the endoscope and other instruments. The equipment should then be rinsed thoroughly. The biopsy channel of a flexible scope should be flushed repeatedly with a mild cleaning solution and rinsed until clean distilled or deionized water runs clear for several seconds. Cleaning brushes should also be passed through all channels several times to remove adherent debris before it has an opportunity to dry. The cleaning brush should be passed all the way through a channel until the head of the brush exits the other end before it is pulled back through the entry site. A repeated back-and-forth scrubbing motion within the channel may cause damage.

For each piece of equipment the operator should refer to the manufacturer's instructions for disassembly that may be required for thorough mechanical cleaning of all parts that might have been exposed to organic matter. A soft brush or sponge should be used to clean all surfaces meticulously. Although most modern endoscopes and video camera heads are completely soakable, the manufacturer's instructions should be consulted before a piece of equipment is immersed in fluids. For the initial phase of cleaning, a commercially available enzymatic cleaning solution designed for endoscopes and accessories is highly recommended (e.g., Enzol, Endozime, Metrizyme).

After initial cleaning, all instruments should be thoroughly dried before sterilization, reassembly, or storage. A soft cloth may be used to dry external surfaces. Accessory channels and other unexposed areas where moisture has entered should also be dried with alcohol flushes (70% ethanol) and/or a high-pressure air gun. All lens surfaces and LG faces should be wiped with alcohol to remove residual film that may compromise light transmission. When feasible, flexible endoscopes should be stored in a *hanging position* rather than in storage cases. Storage in a hanging position allows for drainage and

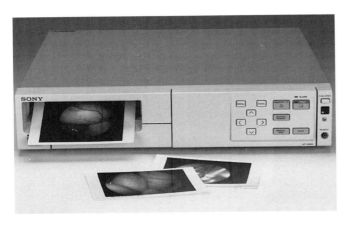

**Figure 1-13** Video printer. (Courtesy Karl Storz Veterinary Endoscopy–America, Inc., Goleta, Calif.)

**Box 1-1   Common User-Related Causes of Fiberscope Damage**

1. Bitten-insertion tube resulting from failure to use a mouthpiece
2. Damage to the channel caused by forced passage of kinked accessories
3. Sticky or inoperable biopsy forceps and other accessories caused by delayed or improper cleaning
4. Kinked biopsy forceps or brushes caused by failure to grasp the accessory close to the channel valve and advance using short, repeated strokes
5. Progressive damage leading to a major repair as a result of postponed repair of minor problems such as loose screws
6. Rough handling such as sharply bending the insertion tube or light-guide cord, closing the instrument in the hinge of the carrying case, or dropping the fiberscope
7. Damage caused by excessive heat during ethylene oxide gas sterilization and aeration
8. Use of inappropriate cleaning agents or disinfectants; use of acceptable agents with improper dilution and contact time
9. Sticky air/water and suction valves caused by improper cleaning and lubrication
10. Obstruction or sticking of small parts of the instrument caused by failure to clean the instrument immediately after the procedure

From Barlow DE: Fiberoptic instrument technology. In Tams TR, editor: *Small animal endoscopy,* St Louis, 1990, Mosby.

airing of residual moisture and also minimizes the stress placed on fiberoptic bundles.

High-level disinfection or sterilization of most endoscopes may be accomplished using ETO sterilization or cold sterilization in a glutaraldehyde solution. (A 2%, 14-day, low surfactant solution such as Cidex, Metricide, or Procide is recommended.) Endoscopes, video camera heads, and LG cables are generally *not* autoclavable, although most associated hand instruments may be autoclaved. The specific manufacturer's instructions should be consulted before an instrument is soaked or gas sterilized because various attachments must be in place to prevent moisture or pressure damage to most flexible endoscopes. Immersible fiberscopes are generally equipped with a pressure tester, or manometer, which is used to detect small leaks before they cause major damage. A leakage test should be performed before an instrument is soaked in a disinfecting solution (see previous discussion of importance of routine leakage testing). After glutaraldehyde soaking or ETO sterilization, endoscopes and instruments must be thoroughly rinsed or aerated, respectively, because residues may be harmful to patients and operators.

Proper care and handling of endoscopes and associated instruments definitely increase the life span of this equipment. User-related damage is commonly caused by inappropriate cleaning practices. (Box 1-1). By thoroughly training selected staff in endoscope care as described by the manufacturer, a veterinary practice should benefit from the routine use of a quality endoscope for many years, with only minimal repairs required.

A troubleshooting guide that reviews various problems and solutions pertaining to flexible endoscopes appears in Table 1-3.

**Table 1-3   Troubleshooting Guide for Flexible Endoscopes**

| Symptom | Possible problem | Remedy |
|---|---|---|
| Image is not clear | Dirty objective lens | Feed water to remove stool, mucus, and other debris from objective lens. |
| | Dirty eyepiece, camera, or adaptor | Clean using cotton swab moistened with alcohol. |
| | Lens not adjusted to operator's eyesight | Rotate diopter adjustment ring until fiber pattern is clear. |
| | Internal fluid damage | Moisture within instrument will permanently cloud lenses in distal end or eyepiece (repair by manufacturer). |
| Image is too dark or too bright | Dirty light guide | Clean light-guide connector and distal tip using gauze moistened with alcohol. |
| | Improper light-source settings | Adjust brightness control knob; check filter. |
| | Old or improperly installed lamp | Properly install lamp; replace old lamp. |

**Table 1-3**     Troubleshooting Guide for Flexible Endoscopes—cont'd

| Symptom | Possible problem | Remedy |
|---|---|---|
| Air or water feeding is absent or insufficient | Air/water nozzle clogged | Soak distal end in warm soapy water; feed water or enzymatic soap solution through air/water channels. |
| | Air/water nozzle missing or deformed | Send instrument for repair. |
| | Air/water valve dirty | Remove valve; clean and lubricate with silicone oil. |
| | Air pump not operating | Turn on switch on light source. |
| | Water bottle cap loose | Tighten cap. |
| No water is feeding | Water bottle either empty or too full | Fill two-thirds full. |
| Air/water valve is sticky | Dirty valve | Remove valve; clean and lubricate with silicone oil. |
| Constant air is feeding | Dirty air/water valve | Remove valve; clean and replace. |
| Suction is absent or insufficient | Suction channel obstructed | Remove suction valve and pass cleaning brush through suction channels in both insertion tube and universal cord. |
| | Dirty suction valve | Remove valve; clean and lubricate with silicone oil. |
| | Leaky or improperly attached biopsy valve | Check and replace with new valve if necessary. |
| | Suction pump problems | Check suction tube connections, pump collection jar cap, float valve and settings. |
| Suction valve is sticky | Dirty valve | Remove valve; clean and lubricate with silicone oil |
| Resistance is present when rotating angulation control knobs | Angulation locks engaged | Place locks in "free" position. |
| Tip deflection is not normal | Amount of tip deflection less than specifications | Send instrument for repair. |
| Accessory does not pass through channel smoothly | Bent or kinked forceps shaft | Discard and replace with new forceps: when inserting accessory, use repeated short strokes, grasping accessory close to biopsy valve. |
| Forceps do not operate smoothly | Bent or kinked forceps shaft | Discard and replace with new forceps. |
| | Dirty forceps cups | Soak in hot soapy water and brush to remove debris; routine use of an ultrasonic cleaner to aid in cleaning small cup hinges is recommended if problem persists; lubricate forceps with silicone oil or surgical instrument milk. |
| Camera cannot attach to fiberscope | Improperly positioned auto focus pin on fiberscope eyepiece | Refer to instruction manual. |
| Camera fails to activate light source | Dirty or bent electrical contacts in adaptor, eyepiece, or light-guide connector | Clean all contacts using cotton swab moistened with alcohol. |
| Exposure is incorrect | Dirty contacts | Clean all contacts using cotton swab moistened with alcohol. |
| | Improper exposure index setting | Refer to instruction manual for proper light-source settings. |
| Image is blurred | Dirty lenses | Clean objective lens, eyepiece lens, and adaptor lenses using cotton swab moistened with alcohol |
| | Water drops on objective lens | Feed air to remove water drops. |
| Color is incorrect | Improper film | Use daylight-balanced film with xenon light sources; use tungsten-balanced film with halogen light sources. |

From Barlow DE: Fiberoptic instrument technology. In Tams TR, editor: *Small animal endoscopy,* St Louis, 1990, Mosby.

## REFERENCES

Barlow DE: Fiberoptic instrument technology. In Tams TR, editor: *Small animal endoscopy,* St Louis, 1990, Mosby.

Coller JA, Murray JJ: Equipment. In Ballantyne, Leahy, Modlin, editors: *Laparoscopic surgery,* Philadelphia, 1994, WB Saunders.

Hulka JF, Reich H: *Textbook of laparoscopy,* ed 2, Philadelphia, 1994, WB Saunders.

Lamar AM: Standard fiberoptic equipment and its care. In Traub-Dargatz JL, Brown CM, editors: *Equine endoscopy,* St Louis, 1990, Mosby.

McCarthy TC, McDermaid SL: Cystoscopy, *Vet Clin North Am* 20:5, 1990.

# Chapter 2

# Endoscopic Documentation

**Hans Joachim Lunemann**

Before photographs or video recordings could be produced, the only way physicians and anatomists could record their findings was by drawing what they saw. Even the first endoscope (Figure 2-1), constructed by Bozzini in the early 1800s, was used in this way. Using the endoscope, the physician looked into the relevant body cavity with one eye but kept the other eye on the drawing pad in order to sketch the endoscopic picture. As can be imagined, this was a very tedious and time-consuming undertaking.

In 1894 Nitze constructed his photocystoscope, a urologic endoscope with a photographic device. This endoscope provided the first pictures from within a human organ, in this case the urinary bladder. However, Nitze's endoscope, like all subsequent ones until 1960, used a lightbulb in the tip of the instrument. If the scope knocked against a hard object (e.g., a bladder stone or bone), the tiny bulb could shatter. Consequently, glass splinters regularly landed in organs being examined. In 1960, "cold light" was used for the first time in endoscopy (Figure 2-2). This meant that light could be generated outside the body and transported to the endoscope via a fiberoptic cable. In following years, 16-mm film technology was introduced into endoscopy, followed by 35-mm camera photography, and finally video documentation.

## ENDOSCOPIC PHOTOGRAPHIC DOCUMENTATION

Today, endoscopic photographic documentation is a well-established component of research and teaching in veterinary medicine. Anatomy textbooks feature endoscopic pictures, lecturers frequently present endoscopic slides, and advanced training for veterinary internists and surgeons is enhanced by endoscopic photographic documentation. However, a sound command of endoscopic techniques is a prerequisite. If, for example, the veterinarian estimates that 20 minutes is required for an endoscopic examination without documentation, that time needs to be increased by at least one third when the procedure is to be documented with high-quality photographs. Effective sedation or general anesthesia of the animal to be examined is obligatory. An assistant who has been trained in photographic techniques is very important because a "third hand" is often required during endoscopy.

A number of pictures should be obtained. A short series of photographs allows the best one (or ones) to be selected. No two pictures are exactly the same, and the endoscopist has too many distractions during a procedure to be able to make a definite decision as to the best photograph on the spur of the moment. Also, when the developed film returns from the laboratory, not every

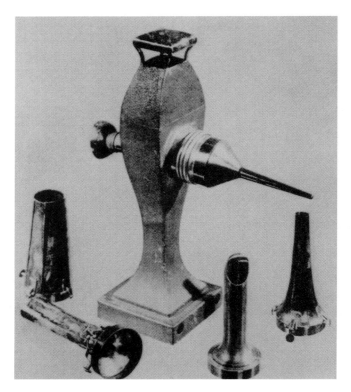

**Figure 2-1** The first rigid endoscope *(lichtleiter)*, built by Bozzini in the early 1800s. The light source was a candle. This instrument was used for the first inspections of human body cavities. (Courtesy Karl Storz GmbH & Co., Tuttlingen, Germany)

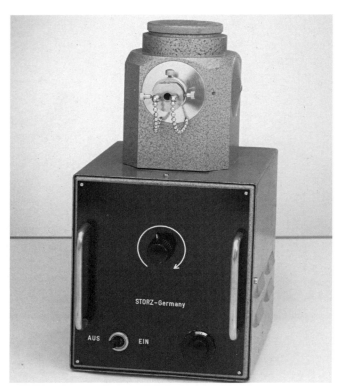

**Figure 2-2** The first "cold" light source, built in 1960. This revolutionary invention was the first extracorporeal examination light. Until 1960, all endoscopes used small bulbs in the distal tip. When these bulbs touched hard objects (e.g., bone), they often broke, leaving pieces of glass in the examined structure. (Courtesy Karl Storz GmbH & Co., Tuttlingen, Germany)

picture is satisfactory. In fact, a good endoscopic view may turn out blurry on the resulting photograph.

## EQUIPMENT SET

The following equipment is recommended for endoscopic photographic documentation:

- Light source with flash generator
- Camera
- Synchronizing cable
- Special lens with through the lens (TTL) metering

A light source with a built-in flash generator (Figure 2-3) is essential for producing the highest quality photographs and slides. No permanent light is bright enough to permit a short exposure time. If a permanent light were used, the camera in automatic mode would select an exposure time in excess of 1/8 second, resulting inevitably in a blurred picture. Only a flash with a maximum firing time of approximately 1/100 second can freeze the content of the endoscopic picture.

High-quality endoscopic photography requires a single-reflex camera that fulfills two requirements. First, the camera must have an interchangeable lens design so that

a special lens with TTL metering can be used. Second, the camera housing must have a removable viewing screen. The viewfinder usually has a matte screen that reduces the amount of light transmitted to the eye and therefore permits focusing. However, the endoscope causes the picture in the eyepiece to be much darker, in part because of the cross section of the scope. Therefore the effect that is desirable in normal photography would be a hindrance in endoscopic photodocumentation. For this reason a transparent screen must be used. The viewing screen of most 35-mm cameras can be modified in this way.

A synchronizing cable serves as the control connection between the light source and camera housing. Its purpose is to ensure that the camera shutter opens at exactly the moment when the required picture demands a fully open picture window.

A special lens with built-in TTL metering is an important component of the photographic documentation system. Although many systems claim to use a TTL method, they have some major differences. TTL means metering the light quantity *through the lens*. A TTL-measuring device in the *lens* is always preferable to a

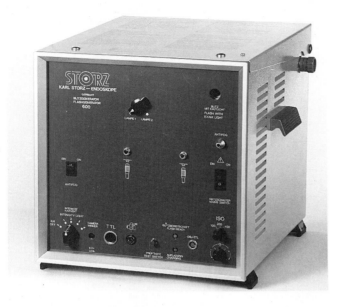

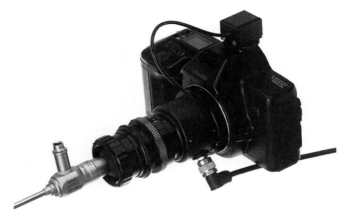

**Figure 2-4** Photographic camera with TTL lens and quick adapter for endoscope attachment. The TTL automatic exposure system in the lens connects directly to the light source via a synchronizing cable. (Courtesy Karl Storz GmbH & Co., Tuttlingen, Germany)

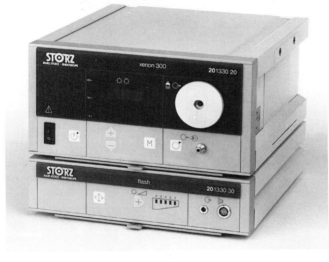

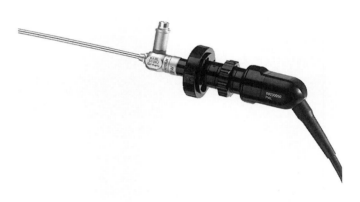

**Figure 2-5** Video camera head attached to a 4-mm rigid endoscope. (Courtesy Karl Storz GmbH & Co., Tuttlingen, Germany)

**Figure 2-3 A,** Combined light source/flash generator. The examination light is a 250-W halogen bulb. The flash unit contains a high-intensity xenon bulb that varies in intensity, depending on the demand registered by the TTL (through the lens) metering system. **B,** A 300-W xenon light source (top) connected to a flash module (bottom) for photographic documentation. This combination offers a higher-power examination light that is ideal for video documentation as well as still photography. (Courtesy Karl Storz GmbH & Co., Tuttlingen, Germany)

## ENDOSCOPIC VIDEO DOCUMENTATION

Endoscopic video documentation has completely replaced the documentation of moving pictures with a 16-mm film camera. Video documentation was initially performed with valvetype cameras, which were larger and heavier than the single-chip and three-chip cameras in present use. The head of a chip camera weighs approximately 160 g.

With video documentation, the results can be seen immediately, with no wait for exposed film to be developed. Perhaps an even more significant advantage is the relative ease of video documentation (Figure 2-5).

Further development of the picture chip for endoscopic color television cameras has resulted in a resolution of

TTL device located in the camera housing, because the TTL lens can be adapted to a variety of camera bodies from different manufacturers.

Finally, the endoscope's eyepiece must fit securely into the quick-release adapter of the lens (Figure 2-4). The quality of the endoscopic pictures depends on a proper connection at this point.

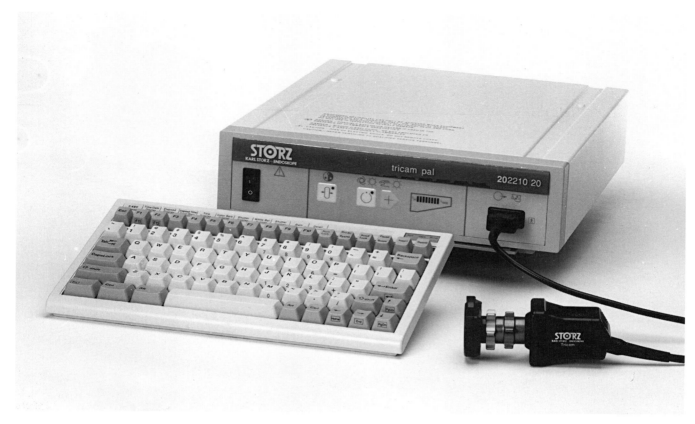

**Figure 2-6** Modern three-chip camera for the highest possible resolution and best color reproduction. An optional keyboard permits the user to add text or numeric identifiers to video or photographic records. (Courtesy Karl Storz GmbH & Co., Tuttlingen, Germany)

approximately 400,000 pixels on a chip surface area of 1/2 inch (approximately 4 × 6 mm). Even higher quality can be achieved with a three-chip camera that has a red, green, blue (RGB) color format (Figure 2-6). However, this camera type has a higher light requirement because light sensitivity is slightly reduced. In terms of weight the three-chip camera can certainly compete with the single-chip camera. A modern unit should be capable of generating a super-VHS (S-VHS) signal. This signal quality optimizes further processing of the picture.

Endoscopic video documentation has become an indispensable tool that is used daily in hospitals, medical colleges, and operating theaters. The full benefit of the latest diagnostic examination methods is only obtained in conjunction with color television technology, which facilitates treatment and makes procedures easier to demonstrate.

## EQUIPMENT SET

The equipment recommended for endoscopic video documentation consists of the following:

- Camera control unit (CCU)
- Camera head
- Endoscope adapter (lens)
- Video recorder
- Monitor
- Color printer
- High-power light source (Figure 2-7)

The camera consists of the CCU, camera head, and endoscope adapter. The video signal is first fed to the monitor to permit endoscopic orientation in the animal's body. A high-quality CCU has a second S-VHS output so that a video recorder can be connected without any signal loss. Three appropriate systems are available:

1. *S-VHS:* This system offers excellent picture quality for endoscopy, and its price-performance ratio is good. However, further processing (editing) of the videotapes obtained with this system cannot always be described as professional. Thus if the videotape of a procedure is to be shown at numerous conferences or in many lectures, a different video system is recommended.

2. *U-matic (SP, high):* At the time of this writing, U-matic is the only world standard in video recording. With this system, further processing (editing) is of a professional standard. However, the U-matic system is much more expensive than the S-VHS system.

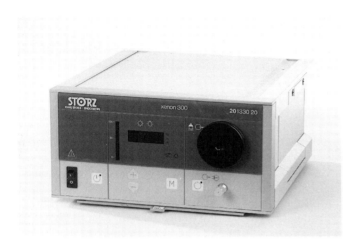

**Figure 2-7** A xenon light source, recommended for video documentation. Performing endoscopy with video always requires a higher light intensity than direct viewing through the endoscope eyepiece. (Courtesy Karl Storz GmbH & Co., Tuttlingen, Germany)

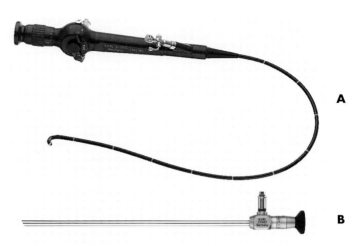

**Figure 2-8 A,** This 5-mm fiberscope is commonly used for bronchoscopy and rhinoscopy. A fiberoptic image is composed of thousands of tiny dots, each representing a single optical fiber that transmits a uniform color and brightness. **B,** This rod lens telescope is 10 mm in diameter and has a 30-degree viewing angle, which is commonly used in laparoscopy. The image seen through a telescope is created by a series of lenses and is therefore comparable to a normal photograph. (Courtesy Karl Storz GmbH & Co., Tuttlingen, Germany)

3. *Betacam:* At present the price of this top-quality broadcast recording system does not permit its widespread use in veterinary medicine.

Video documentation requires a monitor with high resolution. Televisions are limited in their suitability, even if they have video input sockets, because TV monitors cannot display the high picture quality generated by the cameras used in endoscopy. Here too, compatibility with a S-VHS system is critical. The distance between surgeon (endoscopist) and monitor is also important. If the distance is small because space is limited, the monitor's screen diagonal should not be too large (i.e., less than 36 cm). Larger monitors (screen diagonal greater than 36 cm) are only appropriate where plenty of space is available.

Another useful accessory is the color printer (see Figure 1-13). With the S-VHS system, a good, immediately available print of the video picture can be produced. Naturally the quality of this print does not compare with that of a photograph, but the print is certainly suitable adjunctive documentation in a patient's record. The print is also valuable for demonstrating endoscopic findings to clients, colleagues, or referring veterinarians.

Although halogen light sources may be adequate for performing endoscopic procedures with video, the highest quality videotapes and prints are produced using a xenon light source of at least 150 W. If the light quantity is insufficient, the picture on the monitor not only becomes too dark but the colors also change. Viewing an endoscopic image on a monitor with the use of a color

TV camera cannot be compared with direct viewing through the eyepiece of an endoscope.

## DIFFERENCES BETWEEN FLEXIBLE AND RIGID ENDOSCOPY SYSTEMS

The image produced by a flexible fiberscope has an unmistakable faceted appearance. It is made up of many individual parts. A fiberscope transports the image by means of optical glass fibers, each of which transmits a tiny part of the image. For the correct image to be transmitted, the optical fibers must be arranged in the same way at both ends of the endoscope, (i.e., distal lens and eyepiece). However, this means that the image produced by a fiberscope always appears as a faceted picture. In contrast, the picture produced by a rigid endoscope is comparable to a normal photograph, with no facets to disturb the overall impression. However, the rigid endoscope always requires a straight access path to the organ being examined. Various viewing angles (e.g., 30, 45, 90 degrees) allow organs and body cavities to be thoroughly examined (Figure 2-8).

The veterinarian and/or the indication, determines whether a flexible or rigid endoscope is used. As a general rule, flexible endoscopes require greater lighting power than rigid scopes. The thinner the endoscope, the more important lighting power becomes for good image quality. (Diameter is directly proportional to the number of optical fibers.)

## TROUBLESHOOTING IN ENDOSCOPIC DOCUMENTATION

Most endoscopists have, at least once, received a developed roll of film from the laboratory only to find that it contains nothing or at least not the expected result. This mishap is often attributed to incorrect use of the equipment. How does this happen? To answer this question, the examination instruments, such as the endoscope, light cables, and light source, in addition to the photographic and video documentation equipment discussed previously in this chapter, must be considered. Above all, this chapter is intended to illustrate the interrelationships between the examination equipment and documentation instruments.

The endoscope is a precision-made optical instrument. When examining an animal, the endoscopist should never use force because this nearly always results in damage to the endoscope, not to mention possible injury to the animal. Once an endoscope is damaged, documentation (or *satisfactory* documentation) is no longer possible. Bending, and/or twisting should never be used to insert a rigid endoscope into an animal's body. Instead, a flexible scope should be employed to access difficult-to-reach areas.

The endoscope's light entrance and exit faces must be kept clean (Figure 2-9). The glass surfaces should be dry at all times, because moisture may cause dirt to stick to the surface, thereby reducing light transmission. If the examined area is insufficiently illuminated, slides are dark because of underexposure or the image on the video monitor is dark and hence indistinct. Consequently, dirt on the glass surfaces should be wiped off immediately with a soft damp cloth. If dirt becomes firmly attached to the light entrance and exit faces, it should not be removed with hard instruments or abrasives. Once the glass surface has been scratched, it has to be repaired by the manufacturer. Instead, the endoscope should be placed in a storage container filled with lukewarm water. The bottom of the container should be lined with cotton or a surgical pad to prevent the front lens from being damaged by contact with the bottom of the container. Experience has shown that the best cleaning liquid is water with a little mild detergent (i.e., a dilute solution of neutral, nonabrasive dishwashing liquid).

Next, the glass surfaces need to be wiped dry. Even the slightest residual moisture on the endoscope's light-entrance surface can evaporate into a fine mist under thermal influence, causing a reduction in light quantity.

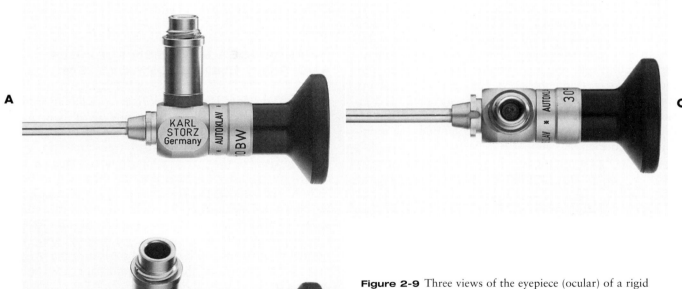

**Figure 2-9** Three views of the eyepiece (ocular) of a rigid endoscope. The light-guide post has two removable, threaded adapters to permit attachment of light-transmitting cables by different manufacturers. The outer adapter should be removed regularly so that the glass surface of the light inlet may be thoroughly cleaned and dried. (Courtesy Karl Storz GmbH & Co., Tuttlingen, Germany)

Detergents used for cleaning surgical instruments may be too caustic or abrasive for use with endoscopy equipment. Therefore information from an instrument's manufacturer should be consulted before the equipment is cleaned. The light guide cable and light source are equally important for successful photographic or video documentation of an endoscopic procedure. The same rules on cleanliness and dryness apply to light cables and endoscopes.

Each time fiberoptic light cables are used, individual fibers break. This is normal and cannot be avoided. Because of broken fibers the image becomes progressively darker. This is a very gradual but continuous process. Because of recent technologic advances, newer model light-transmitting cables and fiberscopes are much more resistant to damage than earlier models were. However, excessive bending may damage a light-guide cable irreparably.

Light sources used in endoscopic documentation are divided into two groups. For photographic use, a light source with an integrated flash generator is recommended. For video use, a high-power light source (preferably xenon) is recommended. However, no lamp burns forever, and no electrical circuit functions indefinitely.

The service life of all light sources varies according to the type of use, frequency of switching on and off, and place of use. If the developed film is too dark but all equipment is in good condition and the light cable appears new, the problem may be decreasing brightness of the flash bulb. In this situation the bulb should be replaced, and pictures obtained with the old and new bulbs should be compared.

Decreasing brightness of the high-power light source used for video documentation is somewhat easier to recognize because the endoscopic examination is seen directly on the monitor. Nevertheless, changing the bulb is the only solution to the problem.

## DIGITAL CAPTURE AND STORAGE OF ENDOSCOPIC VIDEO IMAGES

Personal computer (PC) support adds a completely new dimension to the documentation of endoscopic findings. The S-VHS signal from the CCU can be transmitted directly into a PC. To be able to process this signal, the PC must be equipped with a digitizer that converts the analog signal from the video camera into a digital signal. Unfortunately, direct image capture by a PC requires the presence of a computer in the operation or examination area.

A more practical method of achieving the same result employs a digital still recorder such as the DKR-700 (Figure 2-10). This system, designed primarily for

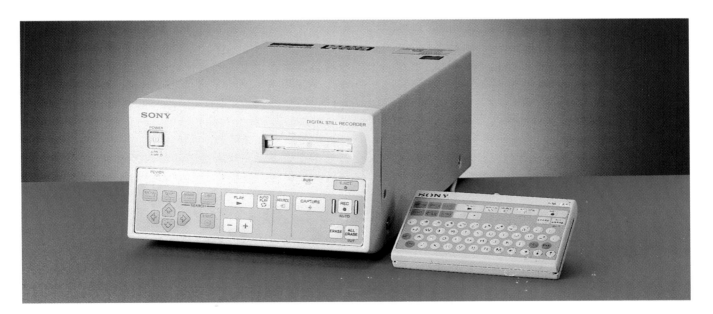

**Figure 2-10** The Sony DKR 700 is a digital still recorder for endoscopic images. Image storage, processing, and editing may be accomplished by downloading files to a personal computer (PC) or a Macintosh computer. Images may then be converted into slides, prints, or other media. Although this system can produce publication-quality pictures, the resolution does not quite match that of traditional photography. (Courtesy Karl Storz GmbH & Co., Tuttlingen, Germany)

the human medical field, is particularly suitable for endoscopic image storage and retrieval. Still images are conveniently stored on a 140 MB MD DATA disk that can hold and play back up to 1000 still images. These images can be retrieved either directly by the DKR-700 for review on a standard analog monitor or by a PC for viewing on a computer display. A well-equipped photo laboratory can then produce slides, color prints, or even customized reports from this stored digital information. It is only a matter of time until digitally produced slides and/or color pictures will achieve the same quality as traditional photographic documentation. PC storage of video sequences or relatively long recordings is not yet possible because storage media with sufficient capacity are not available.

## SUMMARY

Photographic and video documentation have become indispensable in veterinary endoscopy and provide significant support in many important areas:

- Basic and advanced training for veterinarians
- Research and teaching in veterinary medicine
- Diagnosis and treatment
- Development of new examination techniques.

To facilitate advances in endoscopic examination and documentation, veterinarians need to communicate closely with equipment manufacturers. Only then can these manufacturers understand the requirements of veterinary medicine and put them into practice. At the same time, veterinarians need to focus on understanding the latest technologies.

Good documentation often requires expert support from assistants trained in equipment use. The veterinarian should be free to concentrate on the endoscopic examination and management of the patient.

# Chapter 3

# Gastrointestinal Endoscopy: Instrumentation, Handling Technique, and Maintenance

**Todd R. Tams**

Upper gastrointestinal endoscopy is one of the best and yet most fundamental methods of examining the gastrointestinal tract. It is a well-established procedure in veterinary medicine. The opportunity to examine directly and obtain tissue samples from the esophagus, stomach, and intestinal tract has greatly altered the clinical approach to diagnosis and made significantly more accurate the treatment of disorders of the digestive system. Despite the tremendous diagnostic advantages that endoscopy offers, it is still best used by the clinician as an adjunctive procedure in the evaluation of gastrointestinal disease. A thorough history, physical examination, and selected laboratory and radiographic examinations as appropriate for each individual case are still important for thorough patient evaluation. When used judiciously, endoscopy offers a valuable alternative to exploratory surgery for direct examination of tissues, procurement of biopsy samples, retrieval of foreign bodies, and placement of gastric feeding tubes.

Endoscopic equipment is no longer considered a luxury that only large referral centers or veterinarians practicing in affluent areas can justify purchasing. A variety of quality instruments, both new and used, are available. This chapter is concerned with steps to be considered in the purchase of an endoscope, the technical points of maneuvering an endoscope, and proper maintenance to promote maximum lifespan of the equipment. A thorough understanding of the strengths and limitations of endoscopic equipment and its care is essential.

Subsequent chapters on the digestive system deal individually with the technical points of examining the esophagus, stomach, duodenum, ileum, and colon. The beginner learning to perform gastrointestinal endoscopy naturally gives more thought to trying to move the instrument from one point to another than to careful gross examination and diagnosis of the areas being traversed. As the endoscopist becomes more skilled, an almost effortless maneuvering of the endoscope becomes second nature and the greater part of the time used to perform an examination is taken up with careful observation and synthesis of findings in relation to the clinical problem and prior experience. As the reader will find on review of the subsequent digestive system chapters, a *combination* of impressions from observation and microscopic review of biopsy samples is often needed for definitive diagnosis. Because many disorders affect the upper and lower gastrointestinal tract, a variety of appearances may be seen with an endoscope. The gastrointestinal chapters carefully review the technical points of maneuvering the endoscope through these areas and provide an atlas of the things to be "seen" by the endoscopist. Indeed, upper gastrointestinal endoscopy and colonoscopy are a primary means of physical diagnosis for the gastroenterologist.

## THE DECISION TO PURCHASE AN ENDOSCOPE

For the veterinarian, the selection of equipment to be used for performing endoscopy often depends on its versatility of application, durability, and expense. Many practices, recognizing the full range of capabilities of endoscopy, have been able to justify financially the purchase of high-quality endoscope equipment. A single scope can be used for a variety of gastrointestinal and respiratory procedures. In addition, the availability of an endoscope often allows earlier access to examination of the gastrointestinal tract than if surgery is the only other alternative. Clients almost always opt to have a less invasive procedure performed if the capabilities are present, and they often consent to this type of procedure much sooner than they would to surgery. Therefore when consideration is given to purchase of an endoscope, the most important factors to be reviewed should be the probable frequency of usage and versatility of the endoscope rather than the purchase price. Other important considerations are the quality of the optical system and ease of operating the endoscope. Significant differences exist! Too frequently veterinarians rank a lower purchase price as one of the most important factors. This can be a significant mistake because even the most skilled endoscopist may find performing a complete examination and making the correct diagnosis difficult while using an endoscope of poor quality. High-quality endoscopy equipment will pay for itself in most practices in 1 to 3 years. With proper care an endoscope should last many more years.

Once the decision is made to purchase an endoscope, whether new or used, every effort should be made to become proficient in its use. This is best accomplished by the veterinarian's attending one or several formal wet lab courses and then practicing the basic skills of maneuvering an endoscope and procuring biopsy samples. If proper skills of maneuvering and observation are not developed, even the most sophisticated endoscopes are of little value. Frustration resulting from unfamiliarity with proper instrument handling and unavailability of necessary ancillary equipment too often leads to disuse.

## SELECTION OF ENDOSCOPIC INSTRUMENTS

Many types of endoscopes are available. A standard upper gastrointestinal endoscope suitable for esophagogastroduodenoscopy (EGD) in dogs and cats should be a minimum of 100 cm long (working length) and have four-way distal tip deflection with at least 180-degrees upward deflection, water flushing, air insufflation and suction capabilities, independently locking deflection controls, an accessory (working) channel with a diameter of 2 mm or greater, and forward-viewing optics. Most newer endoscopes now feature an upper deflection capability of 210 degrees, and the latest model endoscopes made specifically for use in animals have insertion tube lengths of 140 to 150 cm. Newer instruments that are fluid tight and immersible are easier to clean. Other desirable but not essential characteristics are found.

Veterinarians are cautioned against purchasing endoscopes with two-way, rather than four-way, distal tip deflection capability for use in examining the gastrointestinal tract. Many of these endoscopes are also relatively short (50 to 80 cm) and were originally manufactured as bronchoscopes. Although often considerably less expensive (especially when sold as used equipment), these endoscopes are not versatile enough to facilitate a smooth and thorough examination of the stomach, antral canal, and duodenum. A complete examination can be performed in some cases, but maneuvering through the antral canal, pylorus, and duodenum is more difficult with a two-way than with a four-way endoscope. Also, the shorter length precludes duodenal examination in many dogs. This is an important consideration because an effort should be made to examine the duodenum in all cases in which vomiting, diarrhea, or weight loss is part of the clinical presentation. The ability to routinely perform a thorough examination of the stomach and descending duodenum in a majority of patients who undergo endoscopy is well worth the added expense of a more versatile endoscope.

Careful thought also must be given to the insertion tube *diameter* of the endoscope. Until recently, most endoscopes used in veterinary practice were designed for use in humans and often classified as adult or pediatric. Insertion tube diameters of endoscopes manufactured for examination of the human upper gastrointestinal tract range from 7.8 (pediatric size) to 12.8 mm. Fiberscopes manufactured for veterinary use are available in an insertion tube diameter size as small as 8 mm. Most veterinary endoscopes are in the range of 8 to 8.5 mm. The inner working channel diameter of the human and veterinary endoscopes varies based on insertion tube diameter and ranges from 2 to 2.8 mm.

Veterinarians purchasing their first endoscope should consider a single high-quality endoscope that may be used for a variety of procedures (e.g., EGD, colonoscopy, bronchoscopy, reproductive endoscopy) in cats and small and large dogs. A human pediatric or veterinary endoscope with four-way deflection capability meets these criteria well (Figure 3-1). The insertion tube diameter should range from 7.9 (preferred) to 9 mm. The major

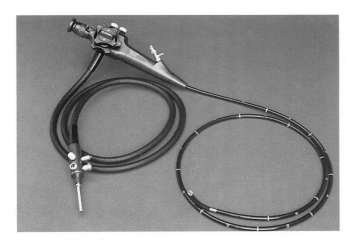

**Figure 3-1** Storz veterinary small animal endoscope. The specifications include 8.5-mm insertion tube diameter, 100-degrees forward-viewing field of view, 140-cm working length, 2.5 mm biopsy channel, and four-way tip deflection. The range of tip bending is 210 degrees up, 90 degrees down, 100 degrees right, and 100 degrees left.

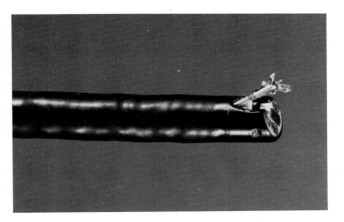

**Figure 3-2** Distal end of an Olympus GIF Type XK10 oblique viewing panendoscope. The specifications include 100-degrees forward viewing and 45-degrees oblique viewing, 11.2-mm distal end diameter, and 103.5-cm working length. A bayonet-type biopsy instrument is in view; its angle is controlled by a forceps raiser knob.

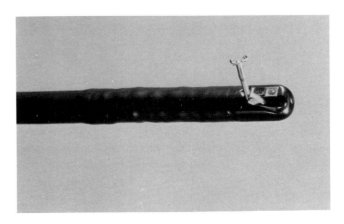

**Figure 3-3** Distal end of an Olympus GIF Type 10 side-viewing endoscope. Specifications include 85-degrees side viewing and 12.5-mm distal end diameter.

limitation of a larger insertion tube (greater than 9 mm) is that passing it through the pyloric canal to the duodenum in cats and small dogs is more difficult. An ability to routinely traverse the pyloric canal to enter the duodenum even in animals as small as 3 to 4 pounds can be achieved with the smaller-diameter endoscopes (7.8 to 8.5 mm) once the endoscopist acquires adequate maneuvering skills. The larger endoscopes can be used effectively in many animals, but a complete examination in very small patients is inherently more difficult. This becomes an important consideration for any urban practice in which many feline and small canine patients are seen.

What is sacrificed when a pediatric or small animal veterinary endoscope rather than a larger-diameter endoscope is purchased? Pediatric endoscopes have working channels of 2 to 2.5 mm, whereas the larger units often have working channels with diameters as large as 2.8 mm. The wider working channel (greater than 2 mm) allows for simultaneous use of suction while a biopsy forceps or other instrument is present in the channel. Simultaneous suction with a smaller working channel is not as effective; the instrument usually needs to be withdrawn from the channel before suction can be used effectively if a large amount of air or fluid needs to be removed. However, this is not a significant drawback because simultaneous use of instruments and suction is not often required. The smaller working channel does not accommodate certain accessory instruments such as bayonet-type forceps, biopsy instruments, and some tripod-type foreign body graspers. However, other instruments can be effectively used for biopsy and foreign body procedures work, and these limitations are quite minor. No substitute exists for a thorough examination, and the pediatric endoscope offers this capability to the endoscopist

better than any other type of endoscope. With the use of proper instruments for biopsy and foreign body retrieval, in addition to good ancillary instument technique, endoscopes with 2-mm biopsy channels work extremely well.

## THE SIDE-VIEWING ENDOSCOPE

Oblique-viewing (Figure 3-2) and side-viewing (Figure 3-3) endoscopes have been designed for use in human medicine for the technique of endoscopic retrograde cholangiopancreatography (ERCP), more thorough visualization of "blind areas" of the duodenum that cannot always be visualized well with a standard forward-viewing endoscope, and accurate biopsy of lesions that may be difficult to maintain in ideal alignment for biopsy with a forward-viewing endoscope. These potentially blind areas in animals and humans include the medial wall of the descending duodenum and the area of the duodenal bulb just beyond the pylorus. A majority of these areas may be seen with a forward-viewing endoscope, however, with skillful maneuvering. Although recesses beyond the pylorus may be difficult to view, lesions in those areas often produce secondary regional changes that can be detected. These changes, which may include edema, erythema, or deformity of the pylorus, alert the endoscopist to examine the area thoroughly because a surgical exploratory examination may be warranted for definitive diagnosis. Lesions in the blind areas include primarily ulcers and neoplasia and are rare in dogs and cats.

Indications for endoscopic cannulation of the biliary and pancreatic ducts are extremely limited in veterinary medicine because cholelithiasis, one of the major indications for ERCP in people, is uncommon. In addition, endoscopes designed for ERCP in people can often only be used in medium to large dogs because of the diameter of these instruments (greater than 10.5 mm). Despite the advantage of more thorough circumferential examination of the duodenal bulb and descending duodenum that side-viewing endoscopes offer, their acquisition for use in animal patients is not practical.

## ANCILLARY EQUIPMENT

A variety of ancillary instruments are available for use in EGD procedures, including biopsy coagulation electrodes. Minimal equipment should include biopsy forceps (alligator jaw or bayonet-type preferred) and foreign body grasping forceps. Use of these accessory instruments is described in subsequent chapters.

## PURCHASE OF USED EQUIPMENT

In the selection of an endoscope, it may be more feasible for a veterinary practice to acquire used equipment, which is often available at reduced cost. The buyer should first be satisfied that no excessive wear or damage to any part of the instrument is present. The objective lens (eyepiece) should be looked through for any clouding of the field, which may indicate that water has entered the insertion tube as a result of damage or mishandling. The covering of the insertion tube should be checked for holes, cracks, or roughened areas that might promote leakage. The instrument should be connected to the power supply and the light transmission bundle checked for intensity of light. If broken fiberbundles exist, they will appear through the eyepiece as black dots (Figure 3-4). An excessive number of broken fiberbundles may preclude proper endoscopic visualization and

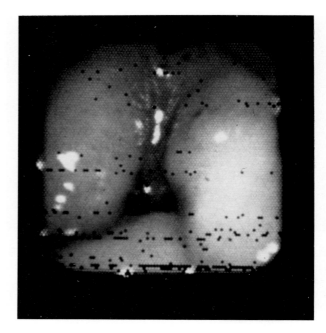

**Figure 3-4** Note the multiple black dots in the field of view. These dots represent broken fiber bundles.

an endoscope damaged in this way should not be purchased. The eyepiece should be checked for scratches and fluid condensation on the inside of both the eyepiece and the distal-tip viewing window.

The distal tip of the insertion tube should be deflected through its full range of motion using the control knobs to determine whether tip angulation approximates original manufacturer specifications and whether the control knobs work smoothly and effectively. Over the course of many procedures the cables that control tip deflection become stretched, causing the degree of tip angulation to gradually decrease. This may cause difficulty in maneuvering the endoscope through the narrow, sharply curving channels of the pylorus and proximal duodenum. The air/water and suction devices should also be checked.

Because repair work on endoscope equipment can be expensive, used endoscopes should not be purchased with the idea that they can be "fixed up." Money would be better spent on a new high-quality scope, which with proper care, can be fully functional for hundreds or even thousands of procedures. Also, the sophisticated technologic advances available with the new endoscopes make many procedures much easier to perform than with the older endoscopes.

## CARE AND HANDLING

Fiberoptic endoscopes should be cared for meticulously. Routine attention to detail promotes maximal endoscope lifespan and efficiency. Mishandling, overly aggressive or forceful use of the controls, failure to prevent an animal from biting the endoscope, and other errors may lead to expensive repair bills or destruction of an endoscope. Fortunately, as endoscope technology has advanced, instrument durability has improved and margin for error has decreased. Nevertheless, an endoscope should always be handled with the greatest possible care.

Proper care involves checking the basic function of the endoscope before each use, using correct and uniform handling methods during each procedure, and employing correct cleaning and storage methods. The insertion tube of a fiberoptic instrument should not be allowed to swing freely when the endoscope is transported because fiberbundles may be damaged. Great care should be taken to ensure that the distal tip is not allowed to strike a hard surface, as can occur if the insertion tube is carelessly allowed to swing into a wall or sink. One blow can result in serious damage. The distal deflecting portion of the insertion tube should never be directly manipulated by the fingers; the control knobs should be used to check range of motion of the deflecting tip. Excessive force on the directional controls should always be avoided. This is especially important to remember in procedures with difficult-to-traverse areas, because the natural tendency is to aggressively force the controls to quickly change the direction of the tip, which enhances the endoscope's movement. Although technologic advances in production of fiberoptic endoscopes have improved durability considerably, all these precautions are still necessary. Demonstrating flexibility to a colleague or client by wrapping the insertion tube in tight circles or into a knot is not recommended. A linear motion is used to connect and disconnect the endoscope from the light source. Twisting or rocking motions during disconnection may cause malalignment of the connecting pins or result in even more serious damage.

An endoscope should be checked before each use to ensure that it works. For verifying that the air/water and suction valves are functional and that the air/water nozzle at the distal tip is not plugged, the best method is to place the distal tip in a bowl of water and check each function independently. The distal tip deflection controls are checked to ensure that they are functional and the objective lens looked through for any clouding of the field or any abnormal accumulation of moisture. This "spot check" takes less than a minute and is especially important when more than one clinician is using the endoscope.

Any ancillary instruments or supplies that might be needed during a procedure should be ready before the procedure is started. If they are not, the procedure may have to be interrupted to search for a necessary piece of equipment. If working with minimal technical assistance, the endoscopist may even have to remove the endoscope from the patient and leave to find needed equipment.

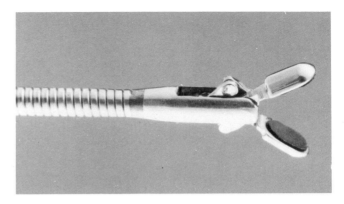

**Figure 3-5** Biopsy forceps cups and adjacent hinge. The cups sometimes lock in an open or closed configuration after drying.

Biopsy forceps and cytology brushes should be readily available. Because biopsy forceps cups tend to lock in the position in which they dry, any tension must be relieved before the instrument can be used. A locked forceps can break if it is opened or closed too forcefully. If the forceps cups are locked in a closed position, they can be soaked in warm water or mineral oil for several seconds, then gently separated using a small-gauge needle or gentle fingernail pressure. Once the forceps cups are freed, the finger control at the top of the instrument is used to open and close the forceps cups several times to ensure that they are moving freely. If the cups are locked in an open position, they are soaked for several seconds in warm water; gentle digital pressure is then applied to the cups to initiate closure and finger control is used as previously indicated to ensure that the cups are moving freely. Dipping the forceps cups and the hinge adjacent to the cups (Figure 3-5) in mineral oil before storage or leaving a small sponge soaked with mineral oil between the cups during storage may help prevent their locking.

A sheathed cytology brush may sometimes be needed to obtain specimens, such as brushings from a gastric or duodenal mass or intestinal mucus to examine for parasites. (See Chapter 10 for further information on use of cytology brushes in GI endoscopy.) Commercially available disposable cytology brushes (e.g., Microvasive, Milford, Mass.) are relatively inexpensive (Figure 3-6). A new brush should be used for each procedure. Because these brushes are difficult to clean adequately, cells from one sample may be transferred to the cytologic sample of another patient if a brush is used on more than one patient. Polyethylene tubing is sometimes used to perform a duodenal wash through the endoscope to examine for evidence of giardiasis or to collect intestinal fluid for identification and quantification of bacteria.

One of the most important pieces of ancillary equipment for any upper gastrointestinal study in small animals is an oral speculum (Figure 3-7). Upper gastrointestinal procedures are performed with the animal under

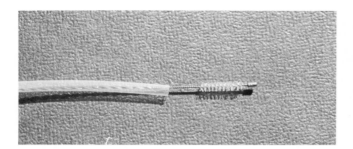

**Figure 3-6** Sheathed (guarded) cytology brush for obtaining mucus samples or brushings from masses.

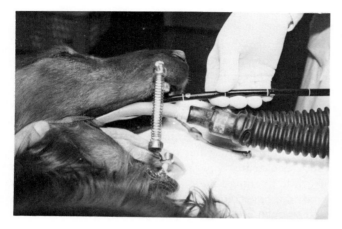

**Figure 3-7** Oral speculum securely in place for an esophagogastroduodenoscopy procedure.

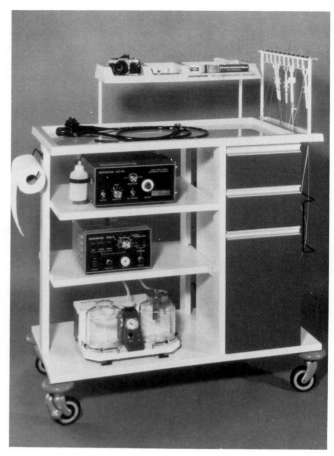

**Figure 3-8** Olympus endoscope cart for convenient transport and storage of an endoscope, light source, electrosurgical unit, suction unit, and ancillary instrumentation.

general anesthesia, and use of an oral speculum is important to guard against an animal biting the insertion tube either when not anesthetized deeply enough or when unexpectedly awaking before the endoscope has been removed. Expensive endoscopes have been ruined by neglecting to prevent this possibility.

If photographs will be taken, the camera should be loaded with film (or the printer if a videoendoscope is being used) and a ledger prepared so that each photograph is recorded. Cleaning solutions should also be ready before the procedure so that the endoscope can be cleaned as soon as each case is completed. Cleaning procedures are discussed in detail at the end of this chapter.

## THE WORK AREA

A limited amount of space is needed to perform endoscopic procedures. It is best to use a sink table with a grate so that any necessary removal of patient secretions or cleaning of equipment can be performed conveniently during a procedure. A single cart with several shelves, such as a unit custom made by the endoscope manufacturing company (Figure 3-8) or a Tuffy Cart (H. Wilson

Co., South Holland, Ill., Figure 3-9), allows for safe storage and easy transport of the light source, suction unit, and all ancillary equipment necessary to perform endoscopy. The cart should be wired with an electrical system so that the light source and suction unit cords can be plugged into the cart. Only a single electrical outlet is then needed for the extension cord from the cart.

A somewhat less convenient alternative is to use either a gurney or adjacent counter space to support the light source and suction unit. A disadvantage is that the light source must be carried manually from its storage area to the procedure area. For lighter portable units this is not a problem, but a large unit can be cumbersome to carry. The greatest advantages of having a cart to permanently house the light source and suction unit are easy mobility, safe storage, and minimal handling of the light source, which minimizes the possibility of damage from its being dropped or knocked from a countertop. A single room for all endoscopy procedures, as exists in some larger institutions, provides for convenient and safe use and storage of the equipment (Figure 3-10). It is best

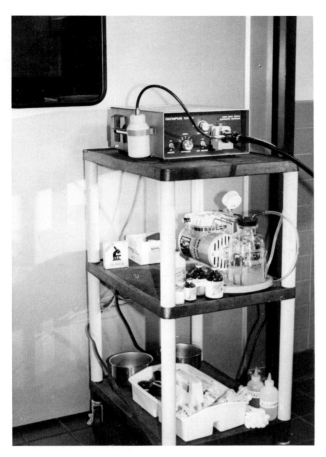

**Figure 3-9** Tuffy Cart with light source, suction unit, preanesthetic agents, emergency drugs, microscope slides, disposable gloves, syringes, and cleaning supplies.

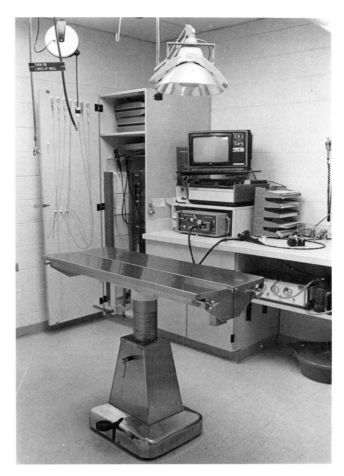

**Figure 3-10** The endoscopy/special procedures room at the Colorado State University Veterinary Teaching Hospital. Note the cabinet for storage of endoscopes and accessory instruments. A videotape deck and television monitor are conveniently located in the work area. (Courtesy David C. Twedt)

that the light source and other ancillary equipment be stored in as safe an area of the hospital as possible (e.g., not on an open countertop) to prevent accidental damage to this fragile and expensive equipment.

## THE ENDOSCOPY ASSISTANT

The number of veterinarians in a private practice or institution who use an endoscope should be restricted to those with the necessary training and expertise to use the equipment safely and effectively and maintain it properly. In some institutions, use of the endoscopy equipment is limited to one or two specialists; in other institutions all clinicians have access to the equipment. Regardless of the situation, a limited number of technicians should also be trained to assist with all aspects of endoscopic procedures, including patient and equipment preparation, patient monitoring during the procedure, and cleanup (Box 3-1).

The endoscopy assistant is responsible for preparing the procedure area before each use. The light source and suction unit should be set up and the anesthesia machine checked carefully to ensure that the equipment is in working order. Biopsy jars, laboratory request forms, preanesthetic agents, an oral speculum, and any needed endoscopy accessory instruments such as biopsy forceps, should be available and ready for use. Because general anesthesia is used for upper gastrointestinal endoscopy, it is strongly advised that intravenous (IV) catheters be placed to facilitate induction of anesthesia and provide ready access to the vascular system in case of any anesthetic complication during the procedure. It is the assistant's job to make sure that the IV catheter is placed before the procedure.

One of the most important roles of the endoscopy assistant is to assist with induction of general anesthesia and monitor the patient's cardiopulmonary status during the procedure. Because the endoscopist is usually

The endoscopy assistant can significantly shorten total procedure time by assisting with sample procurement, handling tissue and cytologic specimens, accurately identifying all samples, and completing the laboratory request forms. Some endoscopists prefer that the assistant operate the biopsy forceps. (Subsequent chapters discuss recommended biopsy and tissue handling procedures in detail.) Specific and simple instructions regarding forceps use, such as "open" and "close," should be given. Because the forceps may break if opened or closed too forcefully, care must be taken to avoid opening them while they are in the working channel of the endoscope. The endoscope may be damaged if this occurs.

Any photographs that are taken should be recorded promptly, including such information as client and patient name, case number, and a brief description of the area or structure photographed. Failure to do this may result in confusion later when the endoscopist tries to identify photographs from cases that can no longer be clearly remembered. A procedure form that can be inserted in the chart provides a convenient means of recording important data, including examination findings, anesthesia parameters, and photographs that were taken.

The endoscopy assistant is responsible for recovering the patient from anesthesia and ensuring that the patient is observed by the assistant or other appropriate support staff until it is fully awake. Complications after gastrointestinal endoscopy are rare but may include retching, vomiting, and abdominal pain.

## HANDLING THE ENDOSCOPE

Proper technique in holding and maneuvering the endoscope is important; improper technique can be a major hindrance to a smooth and thorough endoscopic examination. Every beginning student of endoscopy should concentrate on developing sound technique habits as a foundation for expertise in endoscopy. This section discusses correct methods of holding an endoscope and reviews proper endoscope–body position relationship.

All currently designed endoscopes are made to be held in the left hand. The angulation control knobs are located on the right side of the control housing of the endoscope, precluding use of the right hand to hold the endoscope (see Figure 1-13). The top of the endoscope houses two valves, one for suction and the other for air/water instillation. When the junction of the universal cord and the upper endoscope body is held in the crux of the left hand, the index and middle fingers can each be used to operate one of the valves. The fourth and fifth fingers give stability to this "two-finger" grip (Figure 3-11). For most individuals with long fingers the middle of

engrossed in performing the procedure and not able to monitor the patient closely, the assistant must be able to monitor vital signs and accurately assess any signs of cardiopulmonary problems related to the general anesthesia. The endoscopist should be warned at the earliest sign of any problems.

During gastroscopy, air is usually insufflated into the stomach for dilation purposes to enhance visualization. If too much air is insufflated, especially in cats and small dogs, the stomach can become quite distended, causing significant compromise of respiratory capacity. The endoscopy assistant must watch for this problem and advise the endoscopist to suction air from the stomach if there is evidence that it has become too distended. The problem is usually solved within seconds of suction being applied.

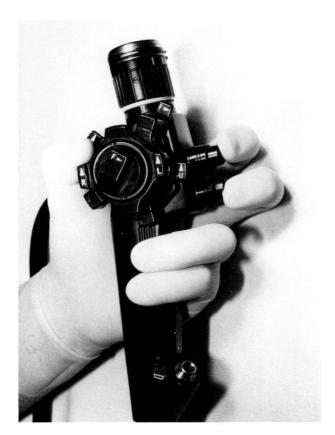

**Figure 3-11** Two-finger method of holding the control section of the endoscope with the fourth and fifth fingers. The left index and middle fingers operate the suction (posterior) and air/water (anterior) valves, respectively. The thumb maneuvers one or both directional control knobs.

the index and middle finger lies across the valves. The fingers are then bent to apply fingertip pressure when use of the valves is indicated. Short fingers in this situation do not cause any disadvantage because in the recommended holding position the fingertips come to lie squarely over the valves. Ease of handling is an extremely important consideration in the purchase of an endoscope. The ergonomic design of the endoscope control area can vary depending on the manufacturer. Some are quite "user friendly"; others are not.

The control knobs can be maneuvered in several ways. Four-direction tip deflection endoscopes have two adjacent control knobs: a larger inner knob to control up/down movement and a smaller outer knob to control side-to-side movement. Most endoscopists are able to use the left thumb comfortably and effectively to maneuver the larger up/down control knob. If the thumb is long enough, it can also be used to deflect the outer knob. Some individuals with long fingers are also able to use the index and middle fingers to manipulate the control knobs by extending them over the valves. One draw-

back is that a firm grip on the control section of the endoscope with the left thumb may be more difficult to maintain.

The right hand is used mostly to advance the insertion tube and apply torque as needed to maneuver the endoscope. The right hand must also be used to assist with movement of the control knobs and operate the control knob locking devices. The goal is to use left hand to operate the valves and control knobs and to use the right hand for assistance as needed. Right-hand assistance is most commonly needed when the endoscope tip is being maneuvered through the antrum, pylorus, and duodenum and during colonoscopy. The right hand is used whenever one of the control knob locking devices is needed. Each knob has one locking device, which will, when activated, hold the endoscope tip in a locked position. This frees the fingers from one or both control knobs, allowing them to perform some other function, such as using an accessory instrument, applying torque to the insertion tube, or obtaining photographs. Using the left thumb solely for support of the endoscope is not recommended because this technique requires the right hand to be used to turn both control knobs. The right hand is then required to perform two major functions: turning the control knobs and advancing and torquing the insertion tube. This prolongs procedure time and makes a smooth, coordinated effort difficult to achieve.

An alternative method of holding the endoscope is the "three-finger" grip, in which the third, fourth, and fifth fingers are used to hold the lower, more narrow area of the control housing (Figure 3-12). This method allows for greater use of the left thumb to work both control knobs, thus minimizing the need to use the right hand for that purpose. The left index finger is used to operate both valves. This method has two disadvantages. First, the last three fingers of the left hand must almost entirely support the endoscope. Second, on newer endoscope models, in which the working channel valve is located close to the insertion tube, the fifth finger (depending on the size of the endoscopist's hand) may lie directly over the valve. This makes the grip more uncomfortable and increases the likelihood that any fluid forced up the insertion tube working channel from the gastrointestinal tract (secondary to a sudden increase in intraabdominal pressure) will spill over onto the hand. On older-model endoscopes the working channel valve is located somewhat closer to the eyepiece, making the three-finger grip more convenient. A major disadvantage of this higher valve location, however, is that it is located uncomfortably close to the endoscopist's face and any reflux of fluid from the working channel could potentially contact the face and hands and also run down over the control housing.

The right hand is usually used to operate the lateral deflection knob (the outer control knob on coaxial

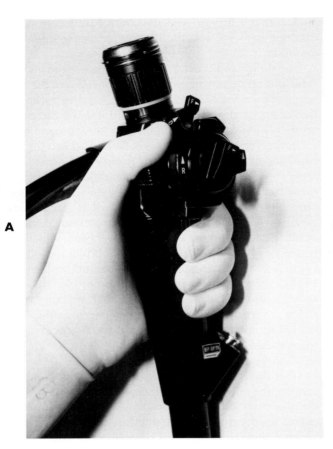
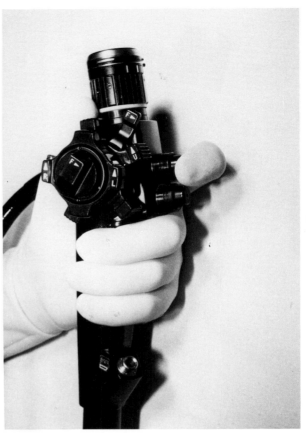

**Figure 3-12** Three-finger method of holding the endoscope with the third, fourth, and fifth fingers. **A,** The left thumb is used to manipulate both control knobs. **B,** The left index finger operates both the suction and air/water valves.

systems) because regardless of the grip used to hold the endoscope, it would be difficult for any but the most dexterous individuals to use the left hand to manipulate the air/water and suction valves and both control knobs during the entire procedure. If proper technique is used to advance the insertion tube, use of the lateral deflection knob is often unnecessary until the antral or pyloric areas of the stomach are reached.

## THE ENDOSCOPE–BODY POSITION RELATIONSHIP

Advancing the endoscope smoothly and efficiently requires that the endoscopist's body position relative to both the patient and the configuration of the control housing and insertion tube be fundamentally correct. It is much easier to advance the endoscope and apply effective torque when the instrument is in a straight configuration. In this position any twisting action applied to the insertion tube as it is advanced will be transmitted along its long axis to the distal tip. Any necessary endoscope tip direction changes can then be made easily by

using the left thumb to maneuver the up/down control. Use of the lateral directional control is not necessary. This technique maximizes use of the right hand for advancing and twisting the insertion tube. Effective use of torque is essential for advancing a two-way tip deflection endoscope through the gastrointestinal tract.

Torque may become significantly less effective for directional control when a loop configuration is allowed to form in the insertion tube, either inside or outside the patient. The loop tends to absorb any twisting force applied proximal to it, therefore the distal tip cannot be controlled as predictably and quickly when proximal torque is applied to the tube. The straighter the instrument, the more precisely it can be controlled.

A mechanically advantageous endoscope–body position relationship clearly enhances maximal endoscope maneuverability and control. Standing too close to the patient, as beginning endoscopists tend to do, promotes loop or coil formation of the proximal insertion tube (Figure 3-13). Maintaining a reasonable distance maximizes the effect of bending the *left* wrist in either direction to enhance a torque effect on the insertion tube. Another position problem typical of be-

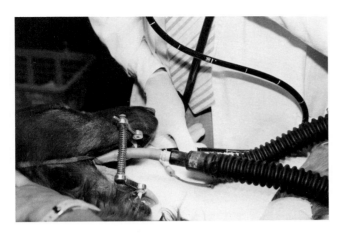

**Figure 3-13** Incorrect endoscope–body postion relationship. A large loop has formed in the insertion tube because the endoscopist is standing too close to the patient. Any attempt to apply torque to the endoscope by rotating the left wrist or by leaning to the left or right will be ineffective. The right hand is shown grasping the insertion tube close to the patient's mouth.

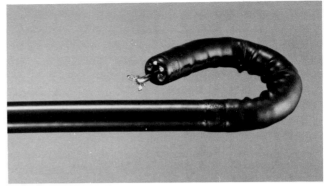

**Figure 3-14** Maximum upward tip bending (210 degrees) of a newer model veterinary gastrointestinal fiberscope.

ginning endoscopists is the tendency to try to advance the endoscope by moving their body toward the patient rather than simply using their right hand to advance the insertion tube.

Among endoscopes, degrees of flexibility (or "stiffness") vary depending on such factors as manufacturer and insertion tip diameter. One advance in technology in newer endoscopes is their increased flexibility, which necessitates that the right hand be positioned on the insertion tube fairly close (approximately 6 to 10 inches) to the patient's mouth for advancing the insertion tube so that the tube does not flex each time an attempt is made to advance it. The beginning endoscopist soon learns that holding the right hand far back on the insertion tube leads to inefficient motion.

The flexibility of the newer small-diameter (less than 9 mm) fiberoptic endoscopes is a disadvantage in some cases in that undesirable coil formation occurs more easily when the insertion tube is in the stomach. This is most commonly a problem in large dogs, in which excess coil formation in the stomach may leave insufficient endoscope length to reach the duodenum. The insertion tube seems to coil more easily in a dilated stomach and other dilated structures such as a megaesophagus and air-dilated colon. Once a loop has formed, it becomes more difficult to advance the tip of the endoscope to the gastric antrum. As the right hand advances the insertion tube farther, the loop formation in the gastric body becomes greater. Also, any torque applied to the insertion tube by the right hand or flexion or rotation of the left arm is absorbed in the coil, causing effective directional control to become minimal or absent. Because the most effective way to control and maneuver an endoscope is to maintain the insertion tube in as straight a line as possible, the correct procedure to remove coil formation is

to retract the insertion tube a sufficient length to straighten the coil. Once the endoscope is repositioned, excess air is suctioned and another advance can be made in a new direction. (Maneuvering techniques for performing a complete examination of the stomach are reviewed in Chapter 5.)

## CONVENTIONAL TERMINOLOGY

Conventional terminology is used to describe directions of endoscopic tip deflection so that written or verbal descriptions of a procedure can be clearly understood. This is especially useful in helping the beginner first learning the art of endoscopy to determine the location of the endoscope tip in relation to various anatomic structures and the movements of the directional controls needed to reach and view important landmarks.

The simple terms *upward, downward, left,* and *right* are used to describe tip deflection. For a starting point of reference, the insertion tube is straight and a standard control housing grip is used with the directional controls to the right. The air/water and suction valves face upward in this configuration. Control knob direction is termed either *clockwise* (forward motion) or *counterclockwise* (backward motion). The distance the knobs can be turned in either direction has a fixed limit. The greatest range of motion of most endoscope tip bending sections is upward. The inner control knob is turned counterclockwise and the corresponding upward deflection bends the tip backward along the insertion tube in the direction of the valves. With the newer endoscopes a deflection angle of 210 degrees can be achieved in this direction (Figure 3-14). For downward direction the inner control knob is turned clockwise and the tip turns away from the valves. The outer control is used for left and right deflection. The endoscope tip can be moved through a circular rotation when both control knobs are used simultaneously. The terms of direction for the endoscope tip do not refer to physical surroundings. Depending on patient position and various axial torque forces applied on the insertion tube during the course of a procedure, the position of the endoscope tip within a patient on upward flexion, for example, may actually not be upward at all. This can be confusing to the beginner, but when the endoscopist develops complete familiarity with the technique required to perform a thorough examination, expertly maneuvering an endoscope becomes almost automatic and the controls can be used with little thought.

For descriptive purposes the endoscopic visual field is divided conventionally (and conveniently) like the face of a clock. Many endoscopes have a small pointed marker clearly visible at the 12 o'clock position of the field. Upward deflection of the endoscope tip causes the visual field to move toward the 12 o'clock position and downward, toward the 6 o'clock position. Clockface terminology is used in this text to describe locations of points of interest on many of the photographs that are presented.

## CLEANING

The endoscope should be cleaned after each examination. Careful, meticulous, and timely cleaning is essential to proper endoscope function and maximum equipment lifespan. If several patients are to be examined, a limited cleaning procedure is usually used between patients, followed by a more thorough protocol after the last patient, before the endoscope is returned to its storage area. Thorough cleaning and disinfection are also necessary after the endoscope is used on a patient that may harbor a transmissible infectious agent or before a bronchoscopy procedure if the same endoscope is used to perform both gastrointestinal and respiratory tract examinations.

The supplies needed for cleaning endoscopes are listed in Box 3-2. Most are kept on the endoscope cart for convenience and efficiency. Two pans of clean water, one containing cleansing solution (e.g., Enzol [enzymatic solution] by Johnson and Johnson, dilute betadine solution, Nolvasan, or dish detergent), are prepared before the start of a procedure and are placed nearby so that the cleaning process can be started as soon as the endoscope is withdrawn from the patient. The cleaning solution (100 to 200 ml) is suctioned through the working channel, and water is then drawn up until the solution exiting the working channel is clear. Transparent suction tubing is used so that the color and contents of the suc-

| **Box 3-2**   Supplies for Cleaning Endoscopes |
| --- |
| Plastic bottles (4)<br>  Soap<br>  Disinfectant solution<br>  70% alcohol<br>  Hydrogen peroxide<br>Bowls (2)<br>  Disinfectant<br>  Clean rinse water<br>Cotton<br>Gauze sponges<br>Cotton-tipped applicators<br>Channel-cleaning adapter<br>Syringe (20 or 35 ml)<br>Cleaning brush for accessory channel and biopsy<br>  forceps<br>Large basin for submersion of endoscope for cold<br>  sterilization<br>Cidex 2% stock solution in basin—change every 14<br>  days |

tioned water can be seen. The working channel should be suctioned clean before any body fluids such as saliva, gastric fluid, and bile are allowed to dry in the working channel. The cleaning brush is then passed through the channel, and water is again suctioned. Finally, air is suctioned to help draw up any residual water droplets.

Next the air/water channel should be cleared. This is done by disconnecting the water bottle and blocking the air/water inlet on the universal cord of the endoscope with a finger while depressing the air/water valve. The light source pump will then blow out the water left in the air/water channel at the completion of each procedure. Air should be pumped through the channel once it is cleared of water.

The endoscope must be kept free of any accumulated organic debris, both in the working channel and on the outer insertion tube. If the endoscope has been cleaned improperly, any subsequent efforts to disinfect or sterilize it will be ineffective. Residual fluid provides an excellent medium for bacterial growth, and debris can shield underlying microorganisms from the action of disinfectants. The routine procedure should be to clean the endoscope thoroughly immediately after use.

The exterior surface is washed with gauze sponges or a brush. Clear or soapy water can be used. After being thoroughly rinsed with water, the insertion tube is wiped down with a gauze sponge soaked in 70% alcohol. Because debris and secretions commonly accumulate in and around the accessory channel valve, this area should be thoroughly cleaned. Alcohol-soaked swabs are used to clean the valve area and the area around the control knobs and suction and air/water valves.

Many newer endoscopes are completely watertight and can be immersed in cleaning or cold sterilization solution. This has been a useful technical advance for human endoscopy units, where disinfecting all equipment after each procedure is routine. Care must be taken in cleaning the control sections of older nonimmersible endoscopes because internal instrumentation can be damaged significantly if water or other fluids enter the control section. *Manufacturer's instructions regarding cleaning and disinfecting procedures should be studied and followed carefully.*

Glutaraldehyde and iodophor solutions are safe for use in cold sterilization of flexible endoscopes. The newer watertight scopes can be fully submerged in these solutions. A glutaraldehyde solution used in many institutions is Cidex. A 2% solution is used and a soak time of 10 to 15 minutes is recommended.

For cold sterilization of a fully immersible endoscope, disinfectant solution (approximately 50 to 70 ml) is flushed through the working channel and then all detachable parts, such as the accessory channel valve, air/water and suction valves, and any attached tubing, are removed before the endoscope is submerged. Cold sterilization solutions are often toxic or irritating to body tissues, so the instrument and all channels should be thoroughly rinsed with clean water and air dried after disinfection. It is important that the endoscope be as dry as possible before storage.

Disinfectant solutions can be used to cold sterilize the insertion tube of nonwatertight endoscopes. After the working channel is thoroughly suctioned and brush cleaned and the outside of the insertion tube of nonwatertight endoscopes is cleaned, as previously described, the working channel is flushed with disinfectant solution. The insertion tube can then be washed with the disinfectant solution or left submerged, as long as great care is taken to ensure that none of the instrumentation above the insertion tube gets wet as well. The insertion tube and accessory channel are then thoroughly flushed with water if a toxic or an irritating solution has been used.

Thorough mechanical cleaning of an endoscope after each upper gastrointestinal procedure is generally sufficient. An endoscope should be thoroughly disinfected before use in the respiratory or reproductive tract and in cases with possible transmission of infectious agents. Automatic washing and disinfecting machines are available from various manufacturers, but such an investment is not practical for most veterinary hospitals. The recommended cleaning procedures are quite adequate for veterinary endoscopy.

Ethylene oxide gas (ETO) sterilization can be used on endoscopic equipment, but an endoscope *cannot* be autoclaved. The fiberscope manufacturer should be consulted for directives on safe sterilization with ETO with regard to the maximum temperature, pressure, and humidity the instrument can withstand during sterilization and aeration cycles.

Ancillary instruments such as biopsy forceps and foreign body graspers can be cleaned with a brush. Ultrasonic cleaners are an excellent means of thoroughly cleaning the difficult-to-reach crevice areas and the delicate hinges of biopsy forceps. Alternatively, these instruments can be soaked in hydrogen peroxide to help remove particulate debris, then gently washed with soapy water. Biopsy forceps and foreign body graspers can be autoclaved if necessary.

## EQUIPMENT STORAGE

Endoscopes can be stored in either a custom padded case, such as the type that the manufacturer delivers the endoscope in, or a hanging position in a cabinet or on a rack (Figures 3-15 and 3-16). The hanging position is strongly recommended for storage. In this position any

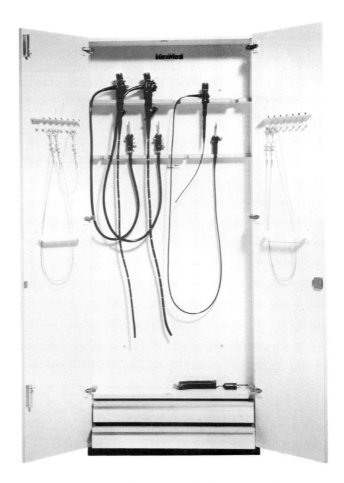

**Figure 3-15** Cabinet for storage of endoscopes and accessory instruments. Two gastrointestinal fiberscopes, a bronchoscope, and biopsy instruments are shown.

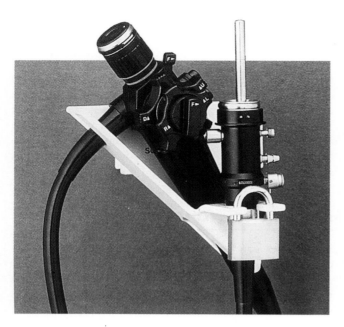

**Figure 3-16** Hanger for storage of endoscopes.

residual droplets of moisture in the insertion tube are more likely to drain. Residual moisture in the working channel can promote growth of bacteria and fungi and can also result in clogging of the tiny air/water channel. When an endoscope is stored in the custom padded case, there is no opportunity for air movement to the channels and residual moisture-related problems are much more likely to develop.

When a cabinet or rack system is available, temporary storage of an endoscope between patient examinations is much more safe and convenient. An endoscope should never be left, even temporarily, on a table or countertop or in any other precarious position from which it could fall or be knocked onto the floor. Great care must be taken if an endoscope is to be stored on an open rack, especially if it is located in a heavily trafficked area of the hospital, because the risk is always present that the instrument might accidentally be bumped and fall from the rack. Serious damage and expensive repair bills can result from such a careless mistake. It is strongly recommended that a storage rack be enclosed in a cabinet that can be locked.

## SUGGESTED ADDITIONAL READINGS

Hagan HW: Clinical observation on sterilizing cystoscopes with glutaraldehyde-phenate, *Urology* 23:224, 1984.

Sivak MV: Technique of upper gastrointestinal endoscopy. In Sivak MV, editor: *Gastroenterologic endoscopy,* Philadelphia, 1987, WB Saunders.

Spada IM, Sivak MV: The gastrointestinal assistant. In Sivak MV, editor: *Gastroenterologic endoscopy,* Philadelphia, 1987, WB Saunders.

# Chapter 4

# Esophagoscopy

Robert G. Sherding,

Susan E. Johnson,

and Todd R. Tams

The term *esophagoscopy* refers to examination of the lumen and mucosal lining of the esophagus with endoscopic equipment. In most cases, esophageal disease is diagnosed by the clinical history combined with contrast radiography of the esophagus, esophagoscopy, or both. Radiography is the most reliable method for documenting megaesophagus. However, esophagoscopy is generally the most precise method for diagnosing disorders that affect the mucosa or cause obstruction of the lumen, including esophagitis, stricture, foreign body, and neoplasia. Esophagoscopy is not only a valuable diagnostic procedure, but it is also a useful therapeutic intervention for removing foreign bodies, performing balloon dilation or bougienage of esophageal strictures, placing indwelling feeding tubes, and providing laser treatment of esophageal neoplasms.

## INDICATIONS

Esophagoscopy is indicated for the evaluation of animals with signs of esophageal disease, including regurgitation, dysphagia, odynophagia, and excessive salivation. This noninvasive modality allows visual examination of the esophageal mucosa and lumen and facilitates the procurement of specimens for biopsy, cytology, and culture. Thus esophagoscopy is most effective for obtaining a definitive diagnosis of conditions involving the mucosa or

abnormalities within the lumen, including esophageal foreign body, esophagitis, esophageal stricture, esophageal neoplasia, diverticulum, vascular ring anomaly, and gastroesophageal intussusception. Compared with contrast radiography, esophagoscopy is less definitive for diagnosing megaesophagus and other motility disorders, diverticulum, hiatal hernia, and compression by periesophageal masses, although it often provides valuable diagnostic information in these situations. Esophagoscopy can also be used as a therapeutic intervention to dilate esophageal strictures, remove esophageal foreign bodies (see Chapter 8), place indwelling gastrostomy (see Chapter 11) or esophagostomy feeding tubes, and ablate neoplastic tissue with lasers.

*Regurgitation* is the passive retrograde expulsion of food or fluid from the esophagus and is influenced by mechanical events within this structure. Regurgitation must be distinguished from *vomiting*, which is a centrally mediated reflex characterized by the forceful ejection of gastroduodenal contents preceded by hypersalivation, retching, and abdominal contractions. The timing of regurgitation in relation to eating is determined by the location of the esophageal abnormality, the presence and degree of obstruction, and the presence of esophageal dilation. Regurgitation immediately after eating is most likely to occur with proximal esophageal lesions or complete esophageal obstruction. However, regurgitation may be unassociated with eating when dilation of the esophagus provides a reservoir for food and fluid. The selective retention of fluids over solid food is more likely to occur with partial obstruction. Regurgitated material is usually composed of undigested food (often tubular) and white to clear frothy liquid (mucus and saliva), but fresh blood may be seen with mucosal lacerations or erosions. Putrefaction of food may occur after prolonged sequestration in a dilated esophagus. In comparison, vomitus usually consists of partially digested food mixed with bile-stained fluid. Both regurgitation and vomiting may occur together in animals with hiatal hernia and gastroesophageal intussusception. Hematemesis is usually a sign of gastric disease but is occasionally seen in animals with esophageal neoplasms that are bleeding extensively.

The age of onset is important because regurgitation related to a vascular ring anomaly or congenital idiopathic megaesophagus usually begins at the time of weaning. The acute onset of regurgitation suggests the presence of an esophageal foreign body or acute esophagitis, whereas a chronic history of regurgitation is more consistent with idiopathic megaesophagus, vascular ring anomaly, or esophageal neoplasia. Intermittent signs are often seen in animals with hiatal hernia and reflux esophagitis. The history may indicate potential exposure to foreign bodies or chemicals, a recent anesthetic procedure that could cause reflux esophagitis and esophageal stricture, or signs of neurologic or neuromuscular dysfunction that could be associated with secondary megaesophagus.

*Dysphagia,* or difficulty in swallowing, is another indication for esophagoscopy. Difficulty in swallowing often suggests the presence of esophageal obstruction, motility disturbance, or pain caused by foreign body, stricture, esophagitis, or another abnormality in the cranial esophagus. Dysphagia is usually associated with repeated or exaggerated attempts to swallow, *odynophagia* (pain on swallowing), and *ptyalism* (excessive salivation). Dysphagia may often be characterized by observing the animal while it is drinking and eating both dry and canned food. Unexplained salivation is also an indication for esophagoscopy. In some cases of esophagitis or neoplasia (especially early in their course), salivation may be the only prominent sign.

Other clinical signs of esophageal disease can also be indications for esophagoscopy. Weight loss occurs secondary to inadequate food intake and is related to the severity of esophageal dysfunction. An animal may have a ravenous appetite when it is otherwise healthy but unable to retain ingested food because of persistent regurgitation. This situation is common in animals with a megaesophagus, esophageal stricture, or vascular ring anomaly. On the other hand, an animal may have anorexia as a result of the pain and difficulty in swallowing that are associated with severe esophagitis,

esophageal foreign body, or neoplasia. Anorexia may also occur in conjunction with cough, dyspnea, and fever in animals that have secondary aspiration pneumonia, esophageal perforation, or bronchoesophageal fistula. Occasionally, laryngeal stridor and change or loss of voice as a result of chronic laryngitis from exposure to gastric acid are the primary presenting signs of severe gastroesophageal reflux.

In dogs and cats, esophageal disorders are less common than disorders of the stomach and intestinal tract, but the clinical signs of these diseases can overlap. As a result, endoscopic examinations limited to the esophagus are not usually appropriate. In most animals with indications for esophagoscopy the entire upper gastrointestinal tract should be examined to obtain the information that is necessary for an accurate diagnosis. Conversely, when the stomach and duodenum are evaluated endoscopically, the esophagus should also be carefully examined (regardless of the presence or absence of clinical signs of esophageal disease) to detect associated or unsuspected abnormalities. This total examination is termed *esophagogastroduodenoscopy (EGD).*

## INSTRUMENTATION

A standard 7.8- to 9-mm flexible endoscope with four-way tip deflection (see Chapter 3) provides the best visualization and manipulative capability for endoscopy of the esophagus, stomach, and duodenum in dogs and cats. However, if the examination is to be limited to the esophagus, a variety of flexible or rigid endoscopes of variable length and diameter can be used. Although esophagoscopy has been performed with rigid scopes for decades, flexible fiberoptic endoscopes and videoendoscopes are now preferred. We highly recommend these newer instruments because of their superior optics, illumination, insufflation, and manipulation capabilities.

Rigid esophagoscopes are available in various lengths and diameters. Even when a flexible endoscope is the primary instrument, one or two multipurpose rigid scopes should be available for use in selected situations, such as esophageal foreign body removal with rigid grasping instruments or flexible endoscope extraction of sharp foreign bodies with the rigid scope used as a protective "overtube" (see Chapter 8). Most rigid endoscopes have a light source, an air-insufflation mechanism, and a blunt-tipped obturator that fits inside the scope to facilitate insertion into the lumen of the esophagus (see Figure 7-2). Pediatric rigid scopes have a diameter of approximately 12 mm, whereas adult rigid scopes are approximately 25 mm in diameter.

The accessory instruments needed for esophagoscopy include a biopsy instrument, foreign body graspers, and either a set of balloon catheters or a supply of bougies for dilation of esophageal strictures. (Instruments for foreign body removal are discussed in Chapter 8.) Although standard alligator-type endoscopic biopsy forceps (especially without a central spike) are adequate for obtaining mucosal and submucosal samples from the stomach, small intestine, and large intestine, they generally cannot procure full-thickness mucosal samples from the esophagus. Forceps with a central spike improve the results of esophageal biopsies. A suction biopsy capsule is usually the most effective instrument for obtaining deeper and larger samples from the esophagus. This instrument is passed alongside the insertion tube of the endoscope and then guided under direct visualization to obtain excellent-quality biopsy samples. Unfortunately, suction biopsy instruments are no longer commercially available but can occasionally be purchased used.

At this time the availability of laser equipment is limited in veterinary medicine. However, in human patients with esophageal cancer, endoscopic laser therapy is often used for the ablation of neoplastic tissue as a palliative measure to relieve obstruction and stop hemorrhage (Figure 4-1).

## PATIENT PREPARATION AND RESTRAINT

General anesthesia is required for any procedure in which an endoscope is to be passed through the mouth. Thus the patient ideally should have no food for a minimum of 12 hours before esophagoscopy is performed. Throughout the procedure the anesthetized patient should be intubated with an endotracheal tube, and a mouth speculum should be in place. The patient is positioned in left lateral recumbency. Routine esophagoscopy requires no other special preparations.

When an esophageal foreign body or stricture is suspected, additional precautions should be taken. Foreign bodies, especially bones and other sharp objects, can cause esophageal perforation. Therefore cervical and thoracic radiographs should be reviewed carefully for signs of perforation such as increased periesophageal mediastinal density, pleural effusion, pneumomediastinum, or pneumothorax. If the esophagus is perforated, esophagoscopy should not be performed, and a chest tube should be placed for drainage and lavage of the thoracic cavity. Esophageal perforation is an indication for surgical exploration rather than endoscopy. If the radiographs reveal no evidence of perforation in the patient with an esophageal foreign body, the esophagoscopic examination can proceed.

Barium contrast radiography should ideally be completed 24 hours before esophagoscopy so that retained contrast medium does not compromise the mucosal examination. Iohexol (Omnipaque), a clear, water-soluble,

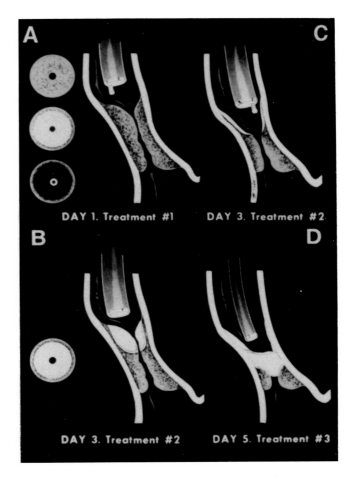

**Figure 4-1** Endoscopic treatment technique using the neodymium:yttrium-aluminum-garnet (Nd:YAG) laser with a quartz waveguide delivery system. **A,** The endoscope is advanced to the superior margin of the tumor, with the waveguide protruding out of the biopsy channel. Treatment (day 1) begins centrally around the residual lumen, proceeding toward but not to the wall. As shown in the cross sections at left, the initial changes are coagulative; with continued thermal damage, vaporization occurs. **B,** On day 3 (48 hours later) the laser-treated tissue is necrotic. **C,** After the necrotic tissue is removed, laser treatment is performed during the same endoscopic session, this time a few centimeters distal to the site treated on day 1. **D,** The same process is repeated on day 5. Treatment progresses until the lumen is opened through the entire length of neoplastic tissue. (From Fleischer D: Lasers in gastroenterology, *Am J Gastroenterol*, 79:406, 1984.)

nonionic iodinated contrast agent, should be used instead of barium when esophagoscopy is likely to be performed within a few hours of contrast radiography. If esophagoscopy has to be done shortly after a barium esophagram, saline lavage may be used to dilute the barium. If barium has pooled because of an esophageal obstruction or motility problem, a suction tube should be used to remove as much of the contrast medium as possible before anesthesia is induced. Alternatively, an animal with a motility disorder may be held upright to facilitate the flow of contrast material into the stomach by gravity. Removing as much barium as possible from the esophagus not only facilitates esophagoscopic evaluation but also minimizes the risk of aspiration during the induction of anesthesia. A flexible endoscope accessory channel should *not* be used to suction a large volume of barium from the esophagus because the barium residue may adhere to the walls and occlude the accessory channel. Furthermore, once the residue dries, it can be difficult to remove.

## ESOPHAGOSCOPY TECHNIQUE

The anesthetized and intubated patient is placed in a left lateral recumbent position with an oral speculum securely in place. The endotracheal tube is particularly important for preventing the aspiration of refluxed or regurgitated material from the oropharynx during the procedure. During rigid endoscopy procedures the endotracheal tube also prevents collapse of the cervical trachea from the pressure of the rigid scope. The insertion tube should be prelubricated with water-soluble lubricant gel to facilitate easy passage. Alternatively, the tube may be lubricated with oral secretions as it is passed into the oral cavity.

With the animal's head and neck extended, the endoscope is directed centrally through the oropharynx and guided dorsal to the endotracheal tube and larynx so that the cranial esophageal sphincter (CES) comes into view. The CES is the entrance to the esophagus and is normally closed, appearing as a star-shaped area of folded mucosa dorsal to the larynx (see Plates 4-1 and 4-20 at the end of this chapter). With insufflation and minimal pressure of the endoscope tip against the CES, the scope is easily advanced through the low-resistance sphincter into the cervical esophagus (see Plates 4-2 and 4-3). Resistance is occasionally felt when the endoscope tip is directed into one of the piriform recesses located on either side of the larynx. This problem is easily corrected by pulling the endoscope back and redirecting it more toward the dorsal midline. If the endoscope tip is passed blindly in large-breed dogs, it may inadvertently be advanced through the laryngeal opening into the proximal trachea. Resistance is felt when the endoscope comes into contact with the endotracheal tube. If this occurs, the endoscope tip should be pulled back to the oropharynx and redirected into the CES.

The cervical esophagus is normally collapsed so that as the endoscope passes through the sphincter, a brief "redout" usually obscures visibility. Thus before the scope is advanced farther, the esophagus should be insufflated with air until the lumen is clearly visualized (see Plates 4-4 and 4-5). Within the esophagus the endoscope should meet little or no resistance as it is advanced. The esophagus is essentially a straight tube except for a slight flexure at the thoracic inlet, where the cervical and thoracic esophagus meet. The operator should advance the scope down the esophagus in a slow continuous motion, using only minor adjustments in tip deflection and torque to maintain a full panoramic view of the lumen and mucosal surfaces. Air should be insufflated intermittently to keep the lumen open. The lumen of the thoracic esophagus generally opens with minimal or no insufflation. Pulsations of the aorta are seen at the level of the base of the heart (see Plates 4-6 through 4-8).

At the gastroesophageal junction the esophagus passes obliquely through the diaphragm to open into the stomach. The gastroesophageal sphincter (GES) is not a true anatomic sphincter but rather a high-pressure zone that keeps the distal esophagus closed between swallows (see Plates 4-9 through 4-13). To move the endoscope into the stomach, the operator deflects the tip of the instrument approximately 30 degrees to the left and simultaneously applies slight upward deflection as the tip is advanced through the slit-like opening of the GES (see Plates 4-14 and 4-15). This can be done easily under direct vision. Minimal or no resistance should be encountered when advancing the endoscope through the GES.

## APPEARANCE OF A NORMAL ESOPHAGUS

The normal esophagus in an animal who has been on a fast is empty or contains a minimal amount of clear fluid or foam. If the esophagus contains ingesta, a large pool of fluid, or bilious fluid, then gastroesophageal reflux, motility dysfunction, or esophageal obstruction should be suspected. In anesthetized animals the normal esophagus becomes flaccid and dilated, which may make the lumen appear very large. Without other supportive clinical findings, this endoscopic appearance should not be overinterpreted as megaesophagus. The cervical esophagus has pliable, longitudinal mucosal folds, more pronounced in dogs than in cats. In a fully inflated cervical esophagus the longitudinal folds disappear; furthermore, as the flaccid esophagus drapes over adjacent structures, the outline of the tracheal rings can be observed against the ventral wall of the esophagus (see Plate 4-5). As the esophagus passes over the base of the heart, the outline of the pulsating aorta against the esophageal wall forms a useful landmark (see Plate 4-7). Because the aorta is pulsatile, its imprint is easily distinguished from the imprints of other extrinsic structures or periesophageal masses.

The feline esophagus is composed of striated muscle in the proximal two thirds and smooth muscle in the distal one third, whereas the canine esophagus is composed almost entirely of striated muscle. Longitudinal folds are found throughout the canine esophagus and in the feline cranial esophagus. In the cat, circumferential mucosal folds in the caudal esophagus form prominent annular ridges (a "herringbone" pattern) that appear endoscopically as a pattern of circular rings (see Plates 4-23 *C, D,* and *E,* and Plate 4-24). This ringlike appearance is not seen in the dog. The normal esophageal mucosa in cats and dogs is smooth, glistening, and pale pink or grayish pink in color. It is noticeably less red than the gastric mucosa. During endoscopy, superficial submucosal vessels are readily visible in the normal feline esophagus (see Plate 4-23) but are not usually seen in the canine esophagus. In heavily pigmented dog breeds such as chow chow and shar-pei, the esophagus may contain variably sized confluent gray or black patches of pigmented mucosa (see Plates 4-17 through 4-19).

When the GES is first visualized, its configuration should be noted. The lumen of the GES usually forms a slitlike opening that is eccentrically located at the confluence of small radial folds configured in a rosette pattern (see Plate 4-9 through 4-13). The GES has many normal appearances. At the gastroesophageal junction the normal pale pink color of esophageal mucosa changes sharply to the vivid pink or red color of normal gastric mucosa. In most dogs and cats, the GES is normally closed at the time of endoscopic examination, even though the tone of the "sphincter" can be decreased by many anesthetic agents. The GES may be gaping open in some normal patients. However, a wide-open GES is unusual and should raise the suspicion of hiatal hernia or gastroesophageal reflux disorder, especially when the open GES is accompanied by esophagitis, pooled fluid in the esophagus, pooled bile in the stomach, or retained ingesta in the stomach of a fasted patient.

## PROCUREMENT OF SPECIMENS

Esophageal biopsy usually is not required for diagnosis of esophageal disease. Primary indications for biopsy of the esophagus include the presence of a mass and suspected esophagitis. It can be difficult to obtain adequate esophageal biopsy specimens (i.e., full mucosal thickness) with standard endoscopic pinch biopsy forceps. Because the esophageal mucosa is often too tough to cut with the forceps, the biopsy cups tend to slide off as they are closed. As mentioned previously, a suction biopsy capsule is probably the best instrument for obtaining esophageal biopsy samples (Figures 4-2 and 4-3). Alternatively, a biopsy forceps (bayonet type) with a central spike within the forceps cup can be used (Figure 4-4). The spike is helpful in fixing the biopsy forceps on the mucosa when the surface is tangential to the trajectory of the forceps as it is advanced toward the lesion.

Standard forceps can often be used to obtain biopsy specimens from proliferative esophageal masses. Preferen-

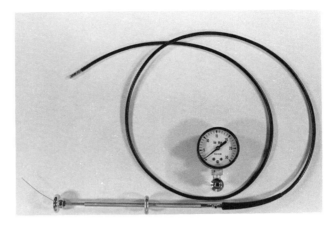

**Figure 4-2** The Multi-Purpose Suction Biopsy Instrument (Quinton Instrument Co.) with vacuum gauge. (Courtesy David C. Twedt.)

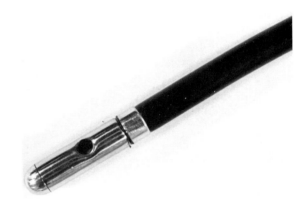

**Figure 4-3** Close-up view of the suction capsule. When negative pressure is applied using a syringe, a section of mucosa is pulled into the aperture. A blade within the capsule, controlled by the handle and pull wire, is used to cut the tissue sample. After the instrument is removed from the patient, the capsule is opened and the biopsy sample is retrieved from the blade apparatus. (Courtesy David C. Twedt.)

tially, the tissue samples should be taken from viable areas of tumors and from border areas between obvious proliferative growth and the area of invasion. Central necrotic, ulcerated areas should be avoided because the diagnostic yield is lower in these areas. With an esophageal mass, 6 to 10 biopsy specimens are usually necessary to obtain adequate tissue for a definitive diagnosis.

Brush cytology specimens are sometimes useful for diagnosing esophageal neoplasia or characterizing unusual forms of esophagitis such as mucosal candidiasis (see Plate 4-48, *B*). A guarded (sheathed) cytology brush prevents contamination and loss of specimen material as the brush is withdrawn through the accessory channel of the endoscope. Brush cytology specimens should be collected first to avoid diluting a cytology specimen with blood from a recent biopsy site.

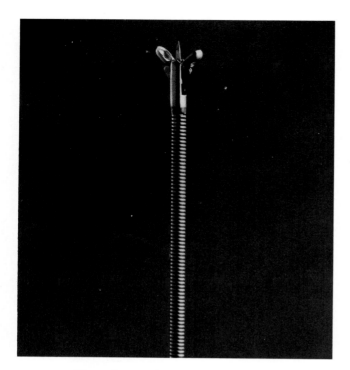

**Figure 4-4** Biopsy forceps that have a central spike within the forceps cups (bayonet type). The spike is helpful in fixing the forceps on the esophageal mucosa.

## TREATMENT OF ESOPHAGEAL STRICTURES

Esophageal strictures result when injury or inflammation extends into the deeper layers of the esophagus and heals by intramural fibrosis. Strictures most commonly occur after injury from an esophageal foreign body or severe gastroesophageal reflux, especially from general anesthesia or hiatal hernia. Other causes include the ingestion of caustic substances (e.g., strong acids or alkalis), persistent vomiting, the vomiting of large hairballs by cats, and thermal injury from the ingestion of microwaved food. The degree of luminal narrowing at the stricture site varies, but the lumen is typically reduced to 2 to 4 mm in diameter. The length of the stricture also varies from a thin band or ridge of fibrotic tissue to a segmental narrowing several centimeters long. Diffuse esophagitis can result in multiple strictures. In one review of six cats and seven dogs, single esophageal strictures were found in 62% of cases and two or three strictures were found in 38% of cases (Harai et al, 1995).

Clinical signs attributable to esophageal obstruction include progressively worsening dysphagia of solid foods, regurgitation immediately after eating, and weight loss despite a ravenous appetite. These clinical signs usually occur 5 to 14 days after esophageal injury and onset of esophagitis or within the same time period after a procedure in an anesthetized patient. Occasionally signs are not evident until 4 to 6 weeks after an injury. With a longstanding stricture, regurgitation may be delayed after eating because the food is "stored" for several hours in a pouch that has developed cranial to the obstruction.

The diagnosis of esophageal stricture can be confirmed by barium contrast radiography or endoscopic examination. Survey radiographs are often normal unless the esophagus contains retained food, fluid, or air proximal to the stricture; however, contrast-enhanced radiography can usually determine the number, location, and length of strictures. It can be difficult to radiographically differentiate a fibrous stricture from intramural thickening caused by severe inflammation or neoplasia. The length of a stricture may also be overestimated radiographically because of associated inflammation and esophageal spasm. With endoscopy, it is possible to evaluate the mucosa visually, estimate the lumen diameter, and assess the pliability of the esophageal wall at the stricture site. Endoscopically an esophageal stricture appears as a white fibrous ring of tissue with adjacent esophagitis (see Plates 4-51 through 4-57). Esophageal neoplasia occasionally causes intramural stricture formation. Stenosis from neoplasia is usually accompanied by a proliferative response or an intramural mass; however, in some cases, the endoscopic appearances of malignant and benign strictures are indistinguishable. If the cause of a stricture is uncertain, biopsy is recommended to determine whether the stricture is benign or malignant. Biopsy samples should be obtained at the stricture site before and after dilation. Brush cytology can provide preliminary information while the biopsy samples are being analyzed.

A benign esophageal stricture may be treated with balloon catheter dilation, bougienage, or surgical procedures such as resection and anastomosis or patch grafting. Conservative management using balloon catheter dilation or bougienage is preferred over surgery. Surgical procedures are successful in fewer than 50% of animals with esophageal strictures. The success rate is between 50% and 75% in animals treated with bougienage and is as high as 85% (Harai et al, 1995) in those treated with endoscopically guided balloon catheter dilation.

Mechanical dilation of the stricture is performed under general anesthesia with endoscopic visualization. Because gastric overdistension can be a significant complication of endoscopy in animals with esophageal stricture, insufflation should be used sparingly. If the stricture precludes passage of the endoscope into the stomach, air introduced during insufflation passes through the stricture and accumulates in the stomach but cannot be suctioned off through the endoscope. Gastric overdistension compromises cardiorespiratory function and increases the complications of anesthesia. The mechanical dilation is repeated every 5 to 7 days as needed to maintain clinical improvement. Sometimes the second dilation procedure is performed 48 to 72 hours after the first. In severe cases, more frequent dilation during the first few weeks increases the chances of a successful outcome. The total number of dilations can range from 3 to 10, depending on the severity of the stricture and the clinical response.

Therapy for esophagitis should be instituted during the series of dilations and for 2 to 3 weeks after the last procedure. The potential for further damage from reflux of gastric acid can be reduced by giving the patient a histamine-2 blocker (i.e., cimetidine, ranitidine, or famotidine in standard dosages), a sucralfate suspension, and metoclopramide or cisapride to promote gastric emptying. A broad-spectrum antibiotic (e.g., ampicillin or amoxicillin) is administered to control mucosal bacterial contamination. Although efficacy is unproved, we typically give corticosteroids to inhibit fibrosis and recurrence of the stricture (e.g., prednisolone, 1 to 2 mg/kg/day for the first 3 weeks and then tapered over the next 2 to 3 weeks). Corticosteroids should not be given to animals with aspiration pneumonia. Animals can usually be fed during the evening of the procedure day once they have completely recovered from anesthesia. However, soft or blenderized food is recommended.

A final esophageal lumen diameter of 10 mm (slightly larger than most endoscopes) usually allows a cat or small dog to be maintained on soft canned food with minimal signs of regurgitation. Medium to large dogs may require an opening 15 to 20 mm in diameter. If balloon dilation is unsuccessful, surgical intervention should be considered, but the prognosis is guarded.

## Bougienage

Bougienage involves the passage of a well-lubricated dilator, such as a bougie, a tapered probe, or the endoscope itself, through the stricture. Excessive force should be avoided because esophageal perforation is a life-threatening complication. The passage of progressively larger bougies results in stretching and dilation of the stricture.

A variety of esophageal dilation devices are available, including mercury-filled bougies and Pilling bougies (Figure 4-5). The diameters of these devices increase in stepwise fashion. Bougies have either rounded tips or tapered ends, and their bases are wider than their tips. The narrow tip is advanced to the stricture site, and the wider area dilates the stricture as the bougie is advanced through it. Other dilators that can be used in selected cases include endotracheal tubes (for cervical esophageal strictures in small patients) and the flexible endoscope itself.

Before each bougienage procedure the stricture site should be carefully assessed by endoscopy. Initial

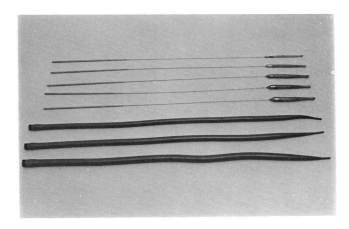

**Figure 4-5** Pilling bougies (upper five instruments) and Maloney mercury-filled bougies (lower three instruments) with tapered ends. Mercury is used in the flexible bougies to achieve the correct balance between flexibility and rigidity. (Courtesy David C. Twedt.)

bougienage should be performed using a dilator one size smaller than the existing lumen diameter at the stricture. The endoscope tip is situated several centimeters proximal to the stricture site so that the dilator can be observed as it is advanced through the stricture. Larger dilators are then used in succession. Excessive force should never be applied because of the risk of causing esophageal perforation, especially at the proximal aspect. The esophageal diameter is enlarged by applying gradually increasing pressure as a tight-fitting dilator is slowly rotated. In most cases a 7.8- to 9-mm endoscope can be readily passed after a stricture has been opened.

The endoscope itself can be used as a dilator under certain circumstances. If the diameter of a stricture is only slightly less than that of the endoscope, a gentle attempt can be made to push the endoscope through to dilate the stricture. The esophageal lumen should be maintained within the center of the field, and excessive force, which could cause either esophageal perforation or damage to the scope, must be avoided. If the endoscope cannot be passed with gentle pressure, another type of dilator should be used.

The key to successful bougienage is to repeat the procedure as often as necessary to improve the lumen diameter to 10 to 15 mm. In some patients, two to three bougienage procedures per week are necessary during the first several weeks of treatment before the desired effect is reached. After a stricture has been forced open, it has a natural tendency to narrow again as collagen forms during healing. The frequency of repetition depends on the patient, severity of the stricture, and resistance that is felt. Each dilation procedure should be initiated with a dilator that is one or two sizes smaller than the largest dilator passed during the previous bougienage. Between 6 and 12 bougienage procedures may be necessary to resolve a stricture problem. In some patients, however, only a few procedures are required.

## Balloon Dilation of Esophageal Strictures

We prefer balloon catheter dilation over bougienage. Balloon dilation of an esophageal stricture can be performed under either endoscopic or fluoroscopic guidance. One advantage of balloon dilation is that it exerts a radial stretch force on the esophageal wall rather than a longitudinal shearing force, as occurs with bougienage (Figure 4-6). Long-term follow-up studies have determined that complete or partial resolution of clinical signs occurs in 85% of dogs and cats with esophageal strictures treated by endoscopic balloon dilation (Harai et al, 1995). In human patients, bougienage and balloon dilation procedures have comparable success rates, but the efficacies of the two procedures have not been compared in dogs and cats.

When inflated, commercially available polyethylene balloon catheters (Rigiflex Balloon Dilator, Microvasive, Watertown, Mass) have an outer balloon diameter of 4 to 20 mm and a length of 4 to 8 cm (Figure 4-7). A balloon catheter with a diameter of 10 mm and a length of 8 cm is adequate for the initial dilation of most esophageal strictures in both dogs and cats. However, if a cat has a stricture that results in a 2-mm lumen diameter or less, a 6- or 8-mm balloon catheter is used initially. For example, in a cat with severe esophageal stricture, 6-, 8-, and 10-mm balloon diameters might be used during the first procedure. Then 8-, 10-, and 12-mm balloon catheters might be used during the next procedure, performed 2 to 3 days later. We strongly advise the use of a conservative approach (i.e., start with a small balloon in dogs and cats with severe strictures), which greatly reduces the chance of esophageal perforation. After the initial procedure a 15-mm balloon catheter may be used in large cats and dogs weighing 5 to 20 kg (11 to 42 lb), and a 20-mm catheter may be used for the final dilations in dogs weighing more than 20 kg.

The catheters are 2.8 mm in diameter when the balloon is deflated. Therefore they can be passed through the lubricated 2.8-mm accessory channel of most larger

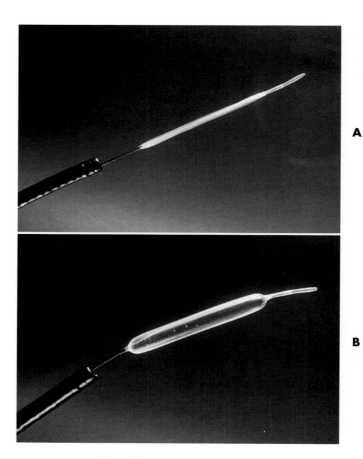

**Figure 4-7** Rigiflex Balloon Dilator catheter (Microvasive) for esophageal stricture dilation. **A,** Appearance of a 10-mm by 8-cm balloon when it is deflated for passage through the 2.8-mm channel of a flexible endoscope and into an esophageal stricture. **B,** Appearance of the balloon when it is inflated with distilled water to 50 psi, used in the endoscopic dilation of an esophageal stricture. The balloon now has a diameter of 10 mm and a length of 8 cm. (From Sherding RG, Johnson SE: *Proceedings of the 17th Annual Waltham/OSU Symposium,* Columbus, Ohio, 1993.)

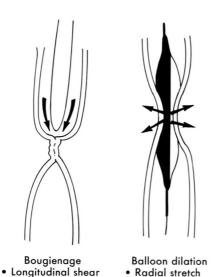

Bougienage
- Longitudinal shear
- Snowplow effect
- Risk of perforation

Balloon dilation
- Radial stretch
- Stationary force

**Figure 4-6** Diagram showing the shearing forces associated with bougienage and the radial forces associated with balloon dilation. (From Dawson SL, Mueller PR, Ferruci JT et al: Severe esophageal strictures: indications for balloon catheter dilation, *Radiology* 153:631, 1984.)

flexible endoscopes, or they can be guided alongside smaller endoscopes with a 2- to 2.5-mm channel. In either case, endoscopic viewing allows the operator to visually guide the balloon into place. Balloon catheters may also be placed under fluoroscopic guidance. Balloon inflation is monitored with a pressure gauge (e.g., Rigiflex Dilation Monitor, Microvasive; Marsh 0 to 200-psi pressure gauge).

With the patient under general anesthesia, the catheter with a deflated balloon is inserted under endoscopic guidance so that the balloon portion is centered across the stricture. A standard disposable syringe is

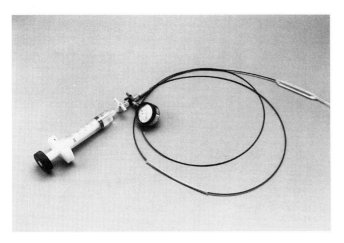

**Figure 4-8** Coiled Rigiflex Balloon Dilator catheter with the balloon inflated and a pressure gauge and LeVeen Inflator (Meditech) attached.

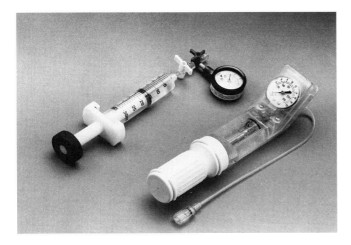

**Figure 4-9** Two types of inflation devices that can be used for endoscopic balloon dilation of esophageal strictures. On the left is a LeVeen Inflator, a screw-press device that compresses the syringe plunger to ensure that adequate dilation pressures are achieved and maintained. A syringe and Marsh pressure gauge for monitoring inflation pressure are attached. On the right is the Indeflator (Advanced Cardiovascular Systems), an inflation device with a built-in pressure gauge.

used to inflate the balloon with sterile or distilled water to the manufacturer-recommended pressure (usually 45 to 50 psi). A pressure monitor is attached between the catheter and syringe to ensure that the pressure in the balloon does not exceed 50 psi, thereby avoiding overinflation and inadvertent balloon rupture (Figure 4-8). The LeVeen Inflator (Microinvasive, Watertown, Mass.) is a screw-press device for compressing the syringe plunger to ensure that adequate dilation pressures are achieved and maintained (Figure 4-9). Alternatively, the Indeflator (Advanced Cardiovascular Systems, Temecula, Calif.) is an inflation device with a built-in pressure gauge (Figure 4-9). If fluoroscopy is available, an iodinated radiographic contrast agent (i.e., diluted Renovist) can be used to inflate the balloon. Fluoroscopic monitoring helps ensure adequate positioning and dilation. The indentation of the balloon at the stricture site produces a "waist" that should disappear as the stricture is fully dilated under maximum pressure (Figure 4-10).

A dilation time of 1 to 2 minutes at maximum inflation pressure of 45 to 50 psi is adequate for treating most strictures. After this time the balloon is deflated, and the catheter is removed to evaluate stricture size and secondary mucosal hemorrhage or tearing (Figure 4-11). If mucosal damage is mild, the procedure can be repeated immediately using the same-size balloon or the next larger size. If multiple strictures are encountered, each one is dilated in a similar manner. This balloon dilation procedure is typically repeated every 5 to 7 days

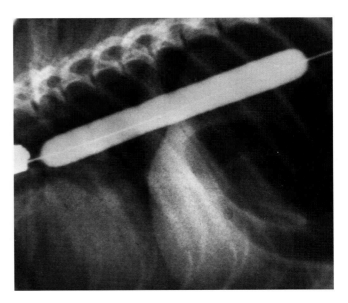

**Figure 4-10** Lateral radiograph of an inflated balloon that has been endoscopically placed in the lumen of an esophageal stricture located just cranial to the gastroesophageal sphincter. The balloon has been inflated with a radioiodide-positive contrast agent (Renovist). Note the slight "waist" in the middle of the balloon at the stricture site.

A          B          C

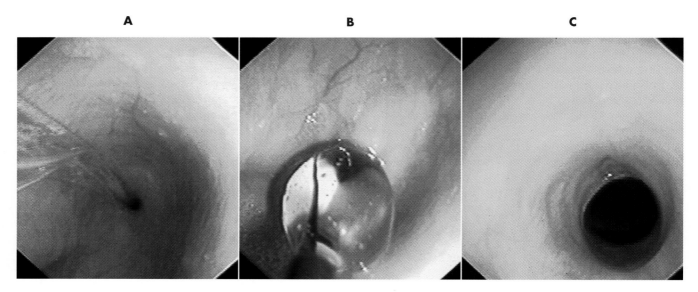

**Figure 4-11** Sequential endoscopic views of a balloon dilation procedure. **A,** The deflated balloon inserted into the stenotic lumen of an esophageal stricture prior to dilation. **B,** The fully inflated balloon catheter within the lumen of the stricture. **C,** The dilated stricture immediately after the balloon has been deflated and removed.

for a total of three to five treatments. However, some may require 10 or more procedures over many months to maintain lumen patency.

Endoscopic examination of the stricture site after each procedure usually reveals a small amount of hemorrhage. Serious hemorrhage or esophageal perforation are occasional complications. In one small series, esophageal perforation occurred in 1 of 50 balloon dilation procedures (Harai et al, 1995.).

## SUGGESTED ADDITIONAL READINGS

Brick SH, Caroline DF, Lev-Toaff AS et al: Esophageal disruption: evaluation with iohexol esophagography, *Radiology* 169:141, 1988.

Callan MB, Washabau RJ, Saunders HM et al: Congenital esophageal hiatal hernia in the Chinese shar-pei dog, *J Vet Intern Med* 7:210, 1993.

Cottrell BD: Post-anaesthetic oesophageal stricture in the cat, *Vet Rec* 118:645, 1986.

Ellison GW, Lewis DD, Phillips L et al: Esophageal hiatal hernia in small animals: literature review and a modified surgical technique, *J Am Anim Hosp Assoc* 23:391, 1987.

Guilford WG: Upper gastrointestinal endoscopy, *Vet Clin North Am Small Anim Pract* 20:1209, 1990.

Guilford WG, Stombeck DR: Diseases of swallowing. In Guilford WG et al, editors: *Strombeck's small animal gastroenterology,* ed 3, Philadelphia, 1996, WB Saunders.

Harai BH, Johnson SE, Sherding RG: Endoscopically guided balloon dilatation of benign esophageal strictures in 6 cats and 7 dogs, *J Vet Intern Med* 9:332, 1995.

Houlton JEF, Herrtage ME, Taylor PM et al: Thoracic oesophageal foreign bodies in the dog: a review of ninety cases, *J Small Anim Pract* 26:521, 1985.

Johnson SJ: Diseases of the esophagus. In Sherding RG, editor: *The cat: diseases and clinical management,* ed 2, New York, 1994, Churchill Livingstone.

Johnson SJ, Sherding RG: Diseases of the esophagus and disorders of swallowing. In Birchard SJ, Sherding RG, editors: *Manual of small animal practice,* Philadelphia, 1994, WB Saunders.

Sullivan M: Upper alimentary tract endoscopy. In Brearley MJ, Cooper JE, Sullivan M, editors: *Color atlas of small animal endoscopy,* St Louis, 1991, Mosby Inc.

Tams TR: Diseases of the esophagus. In Tams TR, editor: *Handbook of small animal gastroenterology.* Philadelphia, 1996, WB Saunders.

Washabau RJ: Swallowing disorders. In Thomas D, Simpson JW, Hall EJ, editors: *BSAVA manual of canine and feline gastroenterology,* Ames, Iowa, 1996, Iowa State University Press.

Zawie DA: Esophageal strictures. In Kirk RW, editor: *Current veterinary therapy X,* Philadelphia, 1989, WB Saunders.

## COLOR PLATES  PAGES 50-96

## COLOR PLATES   PAGES 50-96

## NORMAL CANINE ESOPHAGUS

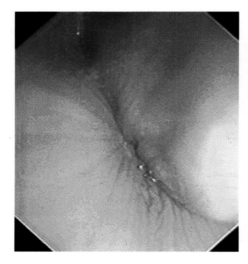

**Plate 4-1** Closed cranial esophageal sphincter as the endoscope is passed dorsal to the larynx.

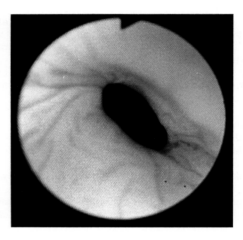

**Plate 4-2** Cranial esophageal sphincter (ovoid area in the center of the field of view) as it becomes dilated during advancement of the endoscope.

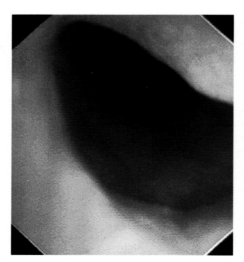

**Plate 4-3** Open cranial esophageal sphincter of the dog shown in Plate 4-1 as the endoscope is advanced through the sphincter into the esophagus.

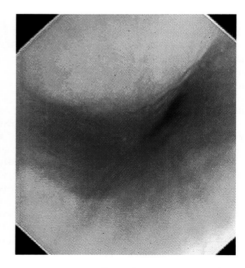

**Plate 4-4** Cervical esophagus in a normal dog. The lumen is partially distended. Before the endoscope is advanced farther, intermittent insufflation of air should continue until the lumen is clearly visualized. Within the esophagus the endoscope should meet little or no resistance.

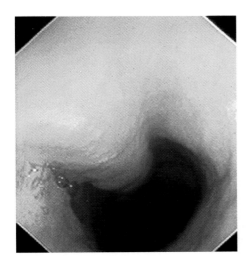

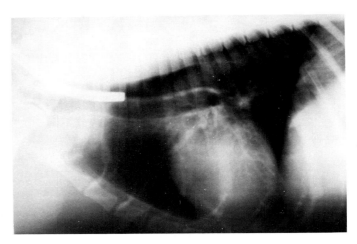

**Plate 4-5** Cervical esophagus of the normal dog in Plate 4-4 after the lumen is fully distended with air. The lumen forms a straight tube with slight flexure at the thoracic inlet. The normal mucosa is smooth, glistening, and pale pink. In the fully inflated cervical esophagus the longitudinal folds disappear, and the outline of the trachea is observed against the ventral wall of the flaccid esophagus (10 to 12 o'clock in the field of view).

**Plate 4-6** Lateral thoracic radiograph showing the position of the endoscope tip when aortic pulsations against the esophageal wall are first observed. The esophagus is dilated as a result of air insufflation through the endoscope.

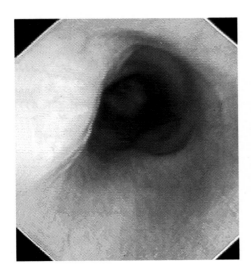

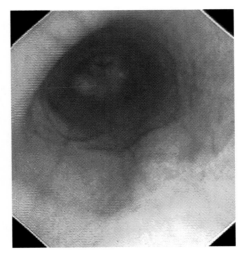

**Plate 4-7** Fully distended mid-thoracic esophagus in a normal dog. The endoscope is approaching the base of the heart (where aortic pulsations are observed) and is in the position shown radiographically in Plate 4-6. The esophagus appears as a pale pink, smooth tube. In the dog, superficial vessels are seen only minimally or not at all. Under anesthesia the normal esophagus becomes flaccid and dilated, which makes the lumen appear very large. This appearance must not be overinterpreted as megaesophagus.

**Plate 4-8** Mid-thoracic esophagus of the normal dog in Plate 4-7. The lumen is empty, and the closed gastroesophageal sphincter is coming into view.

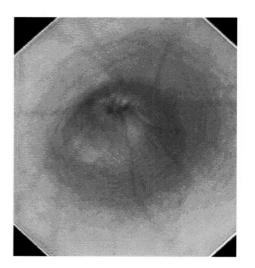

**Plate 4-9** Caudal thoracic esophagus of the normal dog in Plates 4-7 and 4-8. The normal mucosa has slight longitudinal folds and is pale pink in color. The lumen in the fasted animal is empty (as in this patient) or contains a minimal amount of clear fluid or foam. The gastroesophageal sphincter is eccentrically located and closed.

## CANINE GASTROESOPHAGEAL JUNCTION: NORMAL VARIATIONS

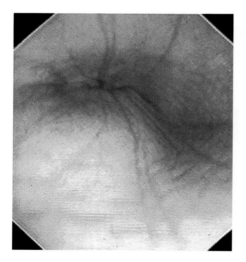

**Plate 4-10** Closer view of the closed gastroesophageal sphincter of the normal dog in Plates 4-7, 4-8, and 4-9. The slit-like lumen of the sphincter is at the confluence of radial mucosal folds. In most normal dogs and cats the gastroesophageal sphincter is closed.

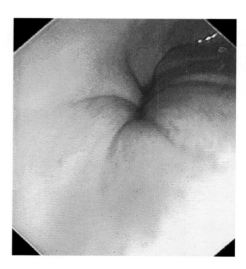

**Plate 4-11** Normal canine gastroesophageal sphincter in the closed position. The radial folds converge to form a rosette-shaped sphincter.

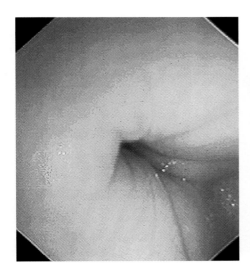

**Plate 4-12** Normal gastroesophageal sphincter, which has been opened slightly with the insufflation of air in preparation for advancement of the endoscope into the stomach.

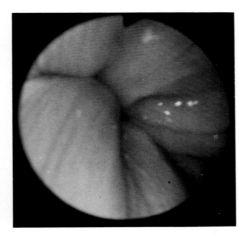

**Plate 4-13** Close-up view of the gastroesophageal sphincter, which appears as a closed rosette in this patient.

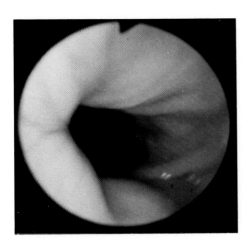

**Plate 4-14** Gastroesophageal junction as the endoscope passes through the lower esophageal sphincter. Left rotation and upward deflection of the tip are required for unobstructed advance to the stomach. (See the text for a description of the technique.) In cats, upward deflection is often sufficient for smooth passage.

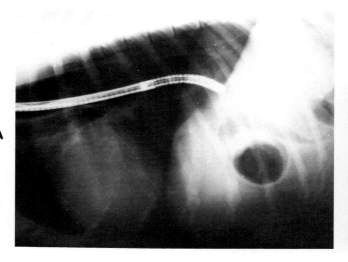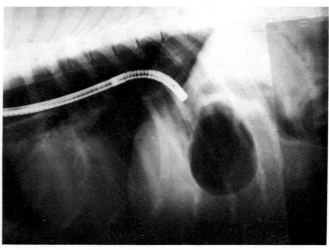

**Plate 4-15 A,** Lateral thoracic radiograph showing the endoscope tip positioned just proximal to the gastroesophageal sphincter. **B,** Radiograph showing the angulation of the endoscope tip that is necessary to advance the scope through the gastroesophageal sphincter and into the proximal stomach.

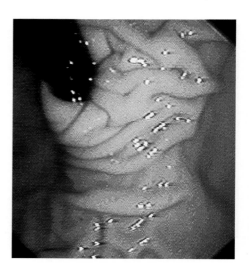

**Plate 4-16** Retroflex view from the stomach of the normal gastroesophageal junction in a dog. The gastroesophageal sphincter and cardia should be evaluated from both the esophageal and gastric retroflex views.

# PIGMENTED ESOPHAGEAL MUCOSA IN DOGS

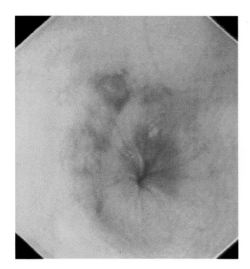

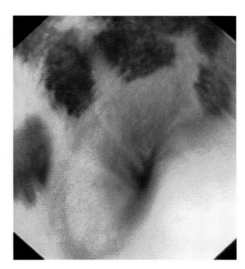

**Plate 4-17** Mildly pigmented mucosa adjacent to the gastroesophageal sphincter in the caudal thoracic esophagus of a normal Chinese shar-pei. In many shar-peis and most chows, mucosal pigmentation is a normal variation. Pigmentation does not affect the stomach or intestines. The transition from the pale pink color of the esophageal mucosa to the dark red of the gastric mucosa is seen at the gastroesophageal sphincter.

**Plate 4-18** Pigmented mucosa of the caudal esophagus adjacent to the gastroesophageal sphincter in a 7-year-old chow. This normal variation is seen in the esophagus of most chows.

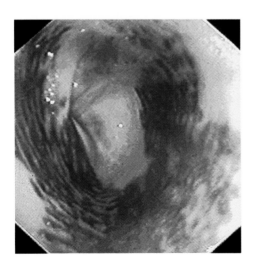

**Plate 4-19** Pigmented caudal esophagus in a 5-month-old female shar-pei with a hiatal hernia and a 1-week history of vomiting. Compare the pigment color with the pale pink color of the distal esophagus and the bright red hemorrhage adjacent to the gastroesophageal sphincter, which is located slightly left of center.

## NORMAL FELINE ESOPHAGUS

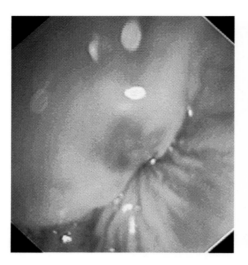

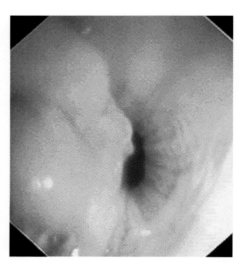

**Plate 4-20** Closed cranial esophageal sphincter in a normal cat as the endoscope is passed dorsal to the larynx.

**Plate 4-21** Partially open cranial esophageal sphincter in a normal cat.

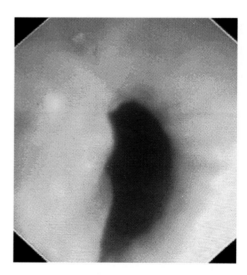

**Plate 4-22** Open cranial esophageal sphincter in a normal cat as the endoscope is advanced into the esophagus.

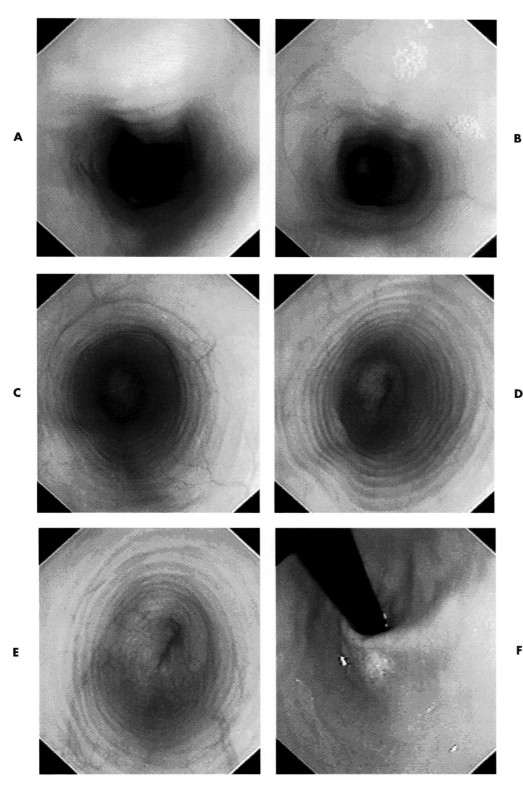

**Plate 4-23** Fully inflated esophagus in a normal cat as the endoscope is advanced from the cervical esophagus to the stomach. **A,** Cervical esophagus. Note the pale pink color of the normal mucosa and the indentation of the tracheal rings against the wall of the esophagus. **B,** Esophagus at the thoracic inlet. Superficial mucosal vessels are normally visible in cats. **C,** Mid-thoracic esophagus. The distinctive circular ring configuration is found in the distal third of the feline esophagus. **D,** Caudal thoracic esophagus with pronounced circular ring (herringbone) pattern. The lumen of the fasted cat is usually empty. **E,** Caudal thoracic esophagus and gastroesophageal sphincter. The gastroesophageal sphincter is completely closed in most cats. **F,** Normal gastroesophageal junction as seen in a retroflex view from the stomach.

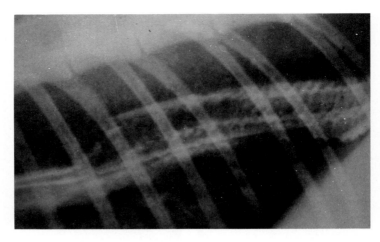

**Plate 4-24** Barium contrast esophagram of a cat. The normal "herringbone" appearance of the caudal thoracic esophagus corresponds to the circular ring pattern seen endoscopically in Plates 4-23, *C, D,* and *E.* (Courtesy Linda J. Konde.)

# MEGAESOPHAGUS

*Megaesophagus* is the term applied to dilation of the esophagus associated with diffuse hypomotility. Regurgitation is the most consistent clinical sign of this abnormality. Megaesophagus can be either congenital or acquired. Most cases are idiopathic. Congenital idiopathic megaesophagus is characterized by severe dilation of the esophagus and the persistent regurgitation of food from the time of weaning. Evidence suggests that this form of megaesophagus is inherited in several canine breeds, as well as in Siamese cats. Acquired adult-onset megaesophagus can be either idiopathic or secondary to various identifiable causes of esophageal hypomotility such as myasthenia gravis, polymyositis, peripheral neuropathies, central nervous system disease, dysautonomia, lead toxicity, hypothyroidism, or hypoadrenocorticism.

Radiography (especially barium contrast esophogography) is generally more reliable than endoscopy for the diagnosis of megaesophagus (Plates 4-25 and 4-26). The normal esophagus is not usually visualized on survey radiographs, but megaesophagus can be identified radiographically when the esophagus becomes distended with gas, fluid, food, or foreign material. Esophageal motility and peristalsis are best evaluated by barium contrast fluoroscopy.

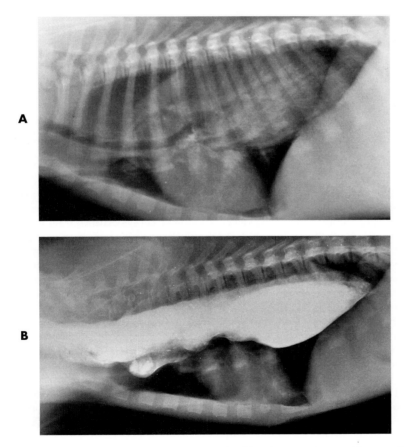

**Plate 4-25** Congenital megaesophagus in a 3-month-old male Great Dane with regurgitation of solid food minutes after eating. Signs began at the time of weaning. **A,** The lateral radiograph shows generalized distension of the esophagus with food and fluid. Note the displacement of the trachea. **B,** Severe megaesophagus and evidence of aspiration pneumonia are seen on the lateral barium esophagram.

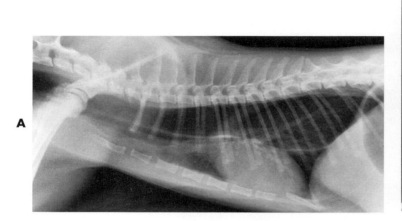
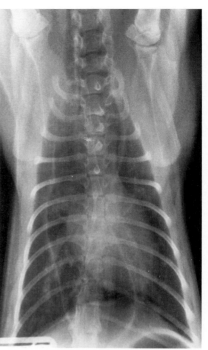

**Plate 4-26** Megaesophagus in a 1-year-old neutered male domestic shorthair cat. The cervical and thoracic esophagus are distended with air. **A,** Lateral radiograph. **B,** Ventrodorsal radiograph.

Endoscopic examination is not necessary for confirming the diagnosis and is rarely beneficial for determining the underlying cause of megaesophagus. The general anesthesia used for esophagoscopy makes the esophagus flaccid and dilated; thus endoscopy is inaccurate for evaluating the caliber of the esophageal lumen and motility. Esophagoscopy may be completely normal in animals with mild hypomotility. Endoscopic findings in severe megaesophagus include a markedly dilated, flaccid esophagus extending from the cranial cervical region to the gastroesophageal sphincter and the pooling of retained fluid, saliva, and fermenting food in the lumen (Plates 4-27, 4-28, and 4-29). If residual contents are discovered in the esophagus of a fasted patient at the start of an examination, a motility disorder should be suspected. Because fluid from the stomach or duodenum may occasionally reflux into the esophagus during gastroduodenoscopy, the esophagus should be examined before gastroscopy or duodenoscopy is performed. Dilation of the entire length of the esophagus distinguishes megaesophagus from vascular ring anomaly, stricture, or other obstructive disorders, in which the dilation occurs proximal to a distinct narrowing of the lumen. The esophageal mucosa in megaesophagus is usually normal in appearance, but secondary esophagitis (mucosal erythema, erosions, and friability) is occasionally observed.

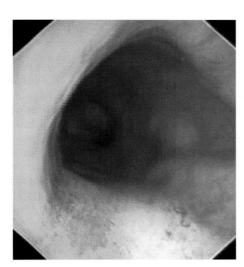

**Plate 4-27** Idiopathic megaesophagus in a 10-year-old spayed female Springer spaniel 10 days after surgery for gastric dilatation-volvulus. The esophagus is markedly dilated and flaccid, and a small pool of foamy fluid is present in the lumen. Because the general anesthesia used for esophagoscopy makes the esophagus flaccid and dilated, endoscopy is less accurate than radiography for evaluating the caliber of the esophageal lumen and motility (see Plates 4-25 and 4-26).

**A**

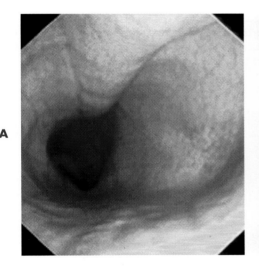

**B**

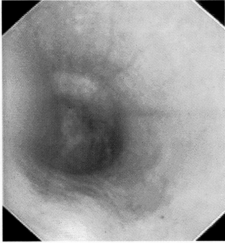

**Plate 4-28** Megaesophagus in a 7-year-old female dog. **A,** Because of marked dilation the esophagus has a cavernous appearance. The flaccid redundant walls of the esophagus are draped against the trachea, producing an outline of that structure. **B,** Fluid is pooled in the caudal esophagus.

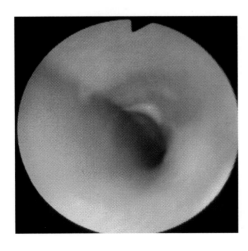

**Plate 4-29** Congenital megaesophagus in a 1-year-old female borzoi. Two other littermates were also affected. Extensive pooling of bile-stained fluid is seen in the dilated esophagus. In some cases of megaesophagus, food residue is also retained.

# DIVERTICULA

Esophageal diverticula are large circumscribed sacculations of the esophageal wall that interfere with the orderly movement of ingesta through the esophagus. These wall sacculations are relatively rare and mostly occur in the cranial mediastinal and epiphrenic regions. Congenital diverticula are caused by abnormalities of embryologic development that result in the herniation of mucosa through a defect in the muscularis. Acquired diverticula can result from external traction and distortion of the esophagus caused by periesophageal adhesions (traction diverticula) or from increased intraluminal pressure and food impaction caused by hypomotility or obstruction (e.g., vascular ring anomaly, foreign body, stricture, tumor) (pulsion diverticula). Small diverticula may be of little clinical significance, but larger ones can become impacted with ingesta, causing postprandial distress, gagging, odynophagia, and regurgitation. Anorexia, lethargy, and fever may also occur.

Diverticula can be diagnosed by radiography or endoscopy (Plates 4-30 through 4-33). Plain radiographs show an air-filled or food-filled mass in the area of the esophagus, and contrast-enhanced radiographs demonstrate filling of the pouch with barium. Esophagoscopy reveals a saclike outpouching from the esophageal lumen with variable degrees of esophagitis in the sac. Food and fluid may have to be removed from the sac before the diverticulum can be adequately visualized. Care must be taken to avoid perforating a diverticulum. Without adequate air distension, the endoscope may enter a blind pouch and be inadvertently forced into the wall. If a diverticulum is small, the only obvious finding may be pooling of fluid. Redundancies in the esophagus that can be mistaken for diverticula are frequently found at the thoracic inlet in normal brachycephalic and Chinese shar-pei dogs. Unlike true diverticula, these false diverticula lack associated impaction or esophagitis, and they decrease or disappear with extension of the neck.

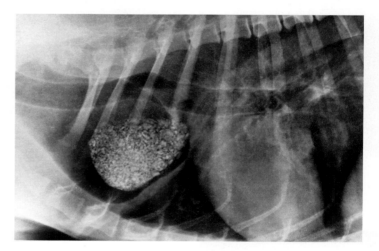

**Plate 4-30** Lateral thoracic radiograph showing a diverticulum of the cranial thoracic esophagus secondary to esophageal stricture in a 5-year-old male German shepherd with a lifelong history of regurgitation. The pouchlike diverticulum is distended with radioopaque bone chips and fluid, and the rest of the esophagus is distended with gas.

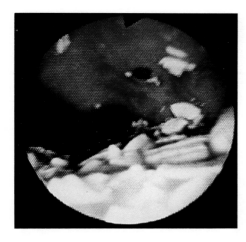

**Plate 4-31** Endoscopic view of the esophageal diverticulum shown in Plate 4-30. Bone chips and fluid are retained in the pouch.

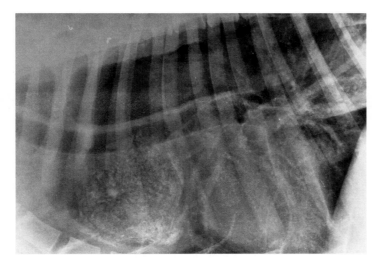

**Plate 4-32** Lateral thoracic radiograph showing a diverticulum of the cranial thoracic esophagus secondary to megaesophagus in a 7-year-old male German shepherd with a 4-month history of intermittent regurgitation and weight loss. The diverticulum is distended with fluid and dense radioopaque fragments (bony remains of a pork roast ingested 10 days previously).

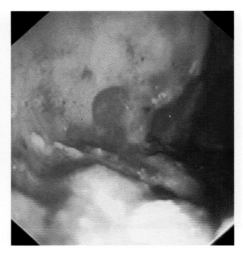

**Plate 4-33** Endoscopic view of the diverticulum and megaesophagus shown in Plate 4-32. **A,** The diverticulum in the cranial thoracic esophagus contains bone fragments and foul-smelling greenish brown fluid. **B,** Prolonged exposure to putrefied food material has caused esophagitis and two well-circumscribed mucosal ulcers in the diverticular pouch.

## VASCULAR RING ANOMALIES

Vascular ring anomalies are congenital malformations of the great vessels and their branches that entrap the intrathoracic esophagus and cause clinical signs of esophageal obstruction. Persistent right aortic arch accounts for 95% of vascular ring malformations and occurs when the functional adult aorta forms from the embryonic right rather than left fourth aortic arch (Plate 4-34). The ligamentum arteriosum continues to develop from the left side and forms a band that crosses over the esophagus to connect the main pulmonary artery and the anomalous aorta. The esophagus is then compressed by the aorta on the right, the ligamentum dorsolaterally on the left, the pulmonary trunk on the left, and the base of the heart ventrally. Dogs and cats with vascular ring anomaly are usually presented because of the regurgitation of undigested solid food beginning at or shortly after weaning. The regurgitation usually occurs immediately after eating. Sometimes, however, it is delayed because ingesta is retained in a large esophageal pouch that develops cranial to the obstruction.

Survey thoracic radiographs usually show an esophagus filled with food and fluid cranial to the heart (Plate 4-35, *A*). On the ventrodorsal view the normal shadow of the aortic arch to the left is absent. A barium esophagram confirms obstruction of the esophagus at the base of the heart (Plate 4-35, *B*). Endoscopy identifies extraluminal compression from the vascular ring anomaly and distinguishes it from other causes of obstruction such as a stricture (Plates 4-36 through 4-40). In animals with persistent right aortic arch, the esophagus becomes entrapped by the base of the heart, the aorta, and the ligamentum. As a result the esophagus becomes circumferentially compressed. Pulsations of the major vessels are seen at the level of the narrowing. An indentation is observed at the level of the base of the heart where the esophagus is externally compressed by the ligamentum, which is an extraluminal band of tissue originating from the right-sided aorta. Entrapment of the esophagus at the level of the heart causes the cranial thoracic esophagus to be dilated and often distended with ingesta and fluid at the time of endoscopy. Putrefaction of food may produce esophagitis cranial to the obstruction. Long-standing obstruction may lead to the formation of a diverticulum pouch in the cranial thoracic esophagus.

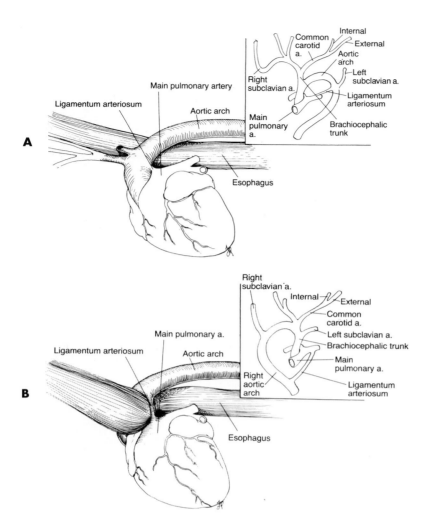

**Plate 4-34** Persistent right aortic arch. **A,** Normal development of the aortic arch viewed from the animal's left side. The inset shows normal embryonic development of the great vessels from a dorsoventral view. **B,** When the embryonic right fourth aortic arch becomes the adult aorta, esophageal constriction occurs. The inset shows a dorsoventral view of the vascular malformation. (From Johnson SE, Sherding RG: Disorders of the esophagus and disorders of swallowing. In Birchard SJ, Sherding RG, editors: *Saunders' manual of small animal Practice*, Philadelphia, 1994, WB Saunders.)

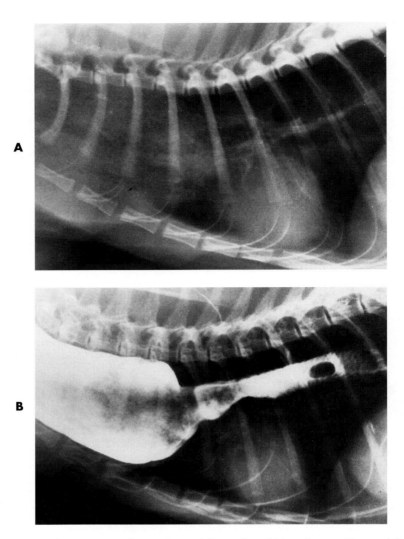

**Plate 4-35** Vascular ring anomaly (persistent right aortic arch) in a 1-year-old spayed female domestic longhair cat with a 2-week history of regurgitation shortly after eating. **A,** The lateral thoracic radiograph shows a mottled cranial mediastinal density from the distension of the esophagus with ingesta and fluid. **B,** The barium contrast esophagram shows marked dilation of the thoracic esophagus cranial to the heart, with a radiolucent bandlike structure (ligamentum arteriosum) superimposed over the esophagus at the base of the heart. (From Johnson SE: Diseases of the esophagus. In Sherding RG, editor: *The cat: diseases and clinical management,* Philadelphia, 1994, WB Saunders.)

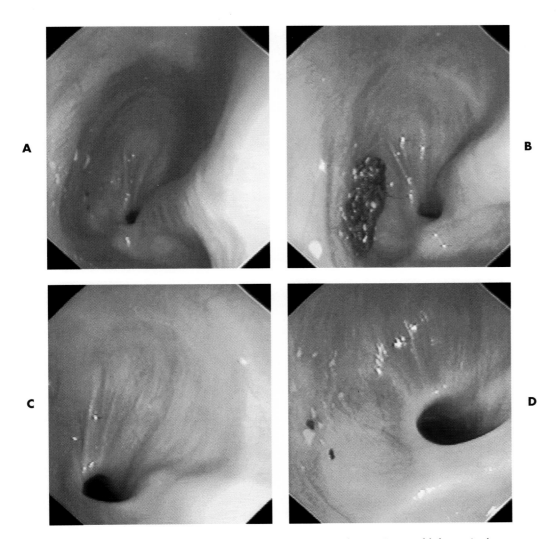

**Plate 4-36** Vascular ring anomaly (persistent right aortic arch) in a 2-year-old domestic short-hair cat that had postprandial regurgitation since it was found as a young kitten. **A,** The esophagus is distended proximal to the constricted lumen of the esophagus where it is compressed by the ligamentum of the vascular ring. The indentation of the trachea in the ventral wall of the esophagus is seen at the right. **B,** A hairball is seen next to the narrowed lumen where the esophagus is constricted by the vascular ring. **C,** Closer view of the narrowed lumen. **D,** Close-up view of the narrowed lumen where the esophagus passes through the vascular ring. The indentation of the ligamentum arteriosum is seen at the left margin of the lumen, which is the dorsal wall of the esophagus.

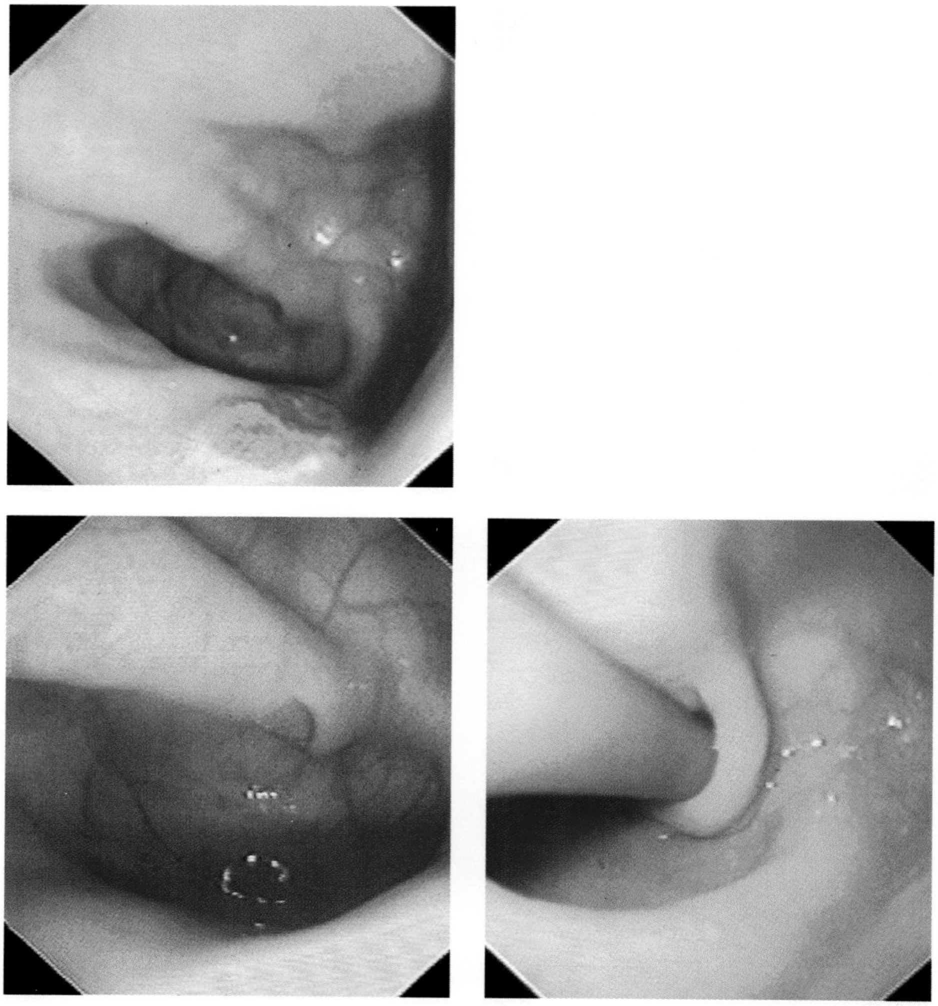

**Plate 4-37** Vascular ring anomaly (persistent right aortic arch) in a 3-month-old female Labrador retriever with regurgitation since 5 weeks of age and a history of one episode of aspiration pneumonia. **A,** Extreme dilation of the cranial thoracic esophagus has occurred proximal to the constriction of the lumen by the vascular ring anomaly. **B,** The lumen is slitlike in the area where the esophagus is constricted by the ligamentum arteriosum as it crosses over the esophagus to the persistent right aortic arch. The indentation of the trachea is seen in the flaccid ventral esophageal wall (top of the photograph). **C,** A feeding tube is passed into the esophageal lumen where it is constricted by the vascular ring anomaly.

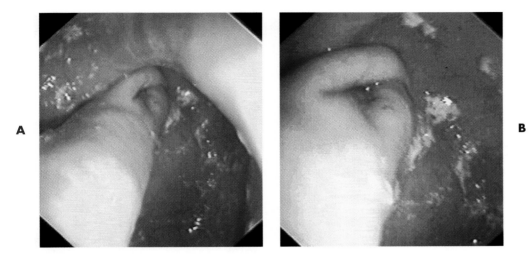

**Plate 4-38** Persistent right aortic arch in a 4-month-old male Labrador retriever that has had regurgitation since it began to eat solid food at 4 weeks of age. **A,** The cranial thoracic esophagus is extremely dilated proximal to the constriction of the lumen by the vascular ring anomaly. The indentation of the trachea is seen in the flaccid ventral esophageal wall. **B,** Close-up view of the slit-like lumen where the esophagus is constricted by the ligamentum arteriosum as it crosses over the esophagus to the persistent right aortic arch.

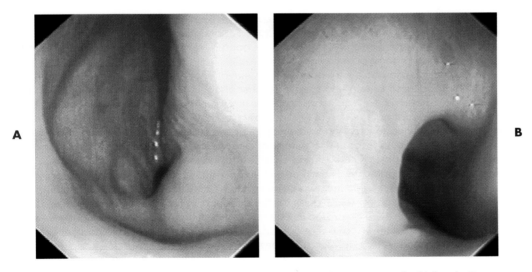

**Plate 4-39** Persistent right aortic arch (vascular ring anomaly) in a 3-month-old female German shepherd with regurgitation. **A,** The lumen is narrow in the area where the esophagus is constricted by the anomaly. **B,** Close-up view of the esophageal lumen where it is constricted by the ligamentum arteriosum.

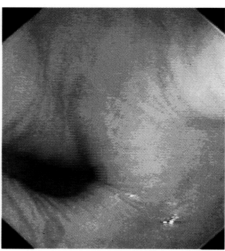

**Plate 4-40** Vascular ring anomaly (persistent right aortic arch) in an 8-year-old Labrador retriever with a lifelong history of intermittent regurgitation and episodes of aspiration pneumonia. Because the opening through the anomalous vascular ring was relatively large, the constriction of the lumen was less severe than in most cases and the condition went undiagnosed for 8 years.

## ESOPHAGITIS

The many possible causes of esophagitis in dogs and cats include the following: injury from esophageal foreign bodies; gastroesophageal reflux secondary to general anesthesia, persistent vomiting of any cause, hiatal hernia, gastric emptying disorders, or indwelling nasogastric tubes; ingestion of caustic irritants; and thermal injury from the ingestion of overheated (microwaved) food. Although the fastidious eating habits of cats makes the ingestion of caustic chemicals unlikely, chemical contaminants on the paws or haircoat may be ingested during grooming behavior.

Esophageal foreign bodies are common causes of esophagitis. Bones are the most frequent foreign bodies to become lodged in the esophagus. Other esophageal foreign bodies include pins, needles, fishhooks, string, toys, and vomited hairballs in cats. Foreign bodies may produce esophagitis when they slide down the esophagus or become lodged in this structure. Most esophageal foreign bodies lodge at the thoracic inlet, the base of the heart, or the hiatus of the diaphragm. The extent of secondary esophageal mucosal injury depends on the type of object, its size and shape, and the length of time it is in contact with the mucosa. Foreign bodies with sharp edges and points, such as bones, may lacerate the mucosa or become embedded in it, whereas tightly wedged objects can cause local-pressure necrosis of the mucosa. Techniques for the endoscopic retrieval of foreign bodies have been well described and are illustrated in Chapter 8. When sharp, pointed, or tightly wedged objects are being extracted from the esophagus, care should be taken to avoid causing further mucosal damage. After a foreign body has been removed, the mucosa should be evaluated endoscopically for secondary esophagitis or perforation.

Gastroesophageal reflux refers to the movement of gastric or duodenal contents into the esophagus unassociated with eructation or vomiting. Reflux is normally restricted by the gastroesophageal sphincter (GES), which in turn is influenced by anatomic, neural, and hormonal factors. Transient reflux events are normal in dogs and cats, but because of efficient esophageal clearance mechanisms these events do not produce esophagitis. Esophageal damage caused by gastroesophageal reflux is primarily attributed to the duration of mucosal contact with refluxed gastric acid, pepsin, bile salts, and trypsin. General anesthesia has been associated with reflux esophagitis and subsequent esophageal stricture in dogs and cats. Contributing factors may include GES relaxation caused by commonly used preanesthetic agents (anticholinergics and tranquilizers), impaired swallowing and secondary peristalsis, increased abdominal pressure during surgical manipulation, and the gravitational effects of a surgery table tilted in a head-down position. Reflux esophagitis may also be associated with impaired GES function caused by a hiatal hernia. A reversible decrease in GES pressure occurs secondary to inflammation in the distal esophagus. Therefore once esophagitis occurs from any cause, including persistent vomiting, it may be perpetuated by gastroesophageal reflux.

The clinical signs of esophagitis are similar to those of other esophageal diseases and include dysphagia, regurgitation, odynophagia, repeated swallowing, and excessive salivation. With mild esophagitis, clinical signs may be subtle or absent. Vomiting and regurgitation may both be observed when esophagitis is associated with a hiatal hernia or is secondary to persistent vomiting. When esophagitis occurs secondary to anesthesia, clinical signs usually are noted within 2 to 4 days of the anesthetic procedure. Nonspecific lethargy and vague discomfort may be seen in the immediate postoperative period, before regurgitation becomes apparent. When esophagitis is severe or is complicated by aspiration pneumonia or esophageal perforation, signs may include anorexia, depression, and fever. Weight loss and dehydration occur when esophagitis is severe enough to interfere with adequate intake of food and water. The ingestion of a caustic chemical should be suspected in any animal with concomitant stomatitis and oral ulcerations.

Esophagitis should be considered whenever signs of esophageal dysfunction are present, but particularly when an animal has a recent history of general anesthesia, foreign body or chemical ingestion, or persistent vomiting. Because reflux esophagitis can be a "silent" disease with minimal clinical signs, it is a difficult disorder to diagnose definitively in dogs and cats. Sometimes radiography may determine the underlying cause (e.g., foreign body, hiatal hernia). Otherwise, survey radiographs in esophagitis are usually unremarkable except for the occasional presence of small amounts of gas in the esophagus. Contrast esophagrams are often normal; however, when esophagitis is severe, the mucosal surface may appear irregular, and secondary hypomotility may cause variable esophageal dilation. When the submucosa and muscles are involved, segmental narrowing of the lumen may occur because of the intramural thickening and focal indistensibility caused by inflammation. This radiographic appearance can be difficult to distinguish from a fibrous stricture. Reflux of contrast media can be demonstrated by fluoroscopy.

Endoscopic examination of the esophageal mucosa is the most sensitive method for diagnosing esophagitis. The endoscopic findings of this inflammatory condition include mucosal erythema, hemorrhage, friability, irregularity, erosions, ulcers, pseudomembranes, indistensibility, and stricture (Plates 4-41 through 4-50). Inflammatory lesions in the caudal thoracic esophagus accompanied by a wide-open GES and the pooling of fluid in the distal esophagus are highly suggestive of reflux esophagitis. Linear erythematous streaks and erosions may be seen on the mucosal folds radiating from the GES. Reflux of gastric contents may be observed during endoscopy. The diagnosis of reflux esophagitis cannot be based solely on the visual examination because in some cases microscopic inflammation occurs before abnormalities can be seen with an endoscope. When reflux esophagitis is suspected, mucosal biopsies should be obtained from an area 2 to 5 cm cranial to the GES. In human medicine, manometry of the GES and continuous monitoring of the distal esophageal pH with a pH probe are used to document gastroesophageal reflux.

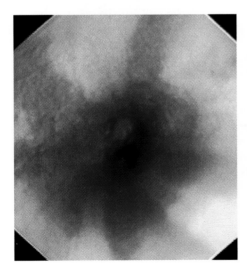

**Plate 4-41** Reflux esophagitis in a dog with chronic vomiting. Erythematous mucosal streaks radiate from the gastroesophageal sphincter into the caudal esophagus.

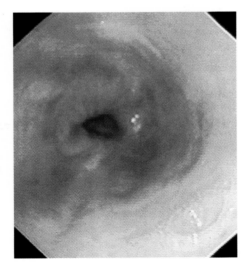

**Plate 4-42** Reflux esophagitis in an 8-year-old male bulldog with chronic intermittent vomiting. Erythema and erosions are present in the caudal thoracic esophagus, and the gastroesophageal sphincter is gaping open.

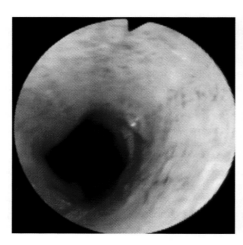

**Plate 4-43** Reflux esophagitis secondary to chronic vomiting and gastric retention disorder in a 9-year-old spayed golden retriever. Widespread focal hemorrhage is seen in the caudal esophagus, and the mucosa is irregular and friable.

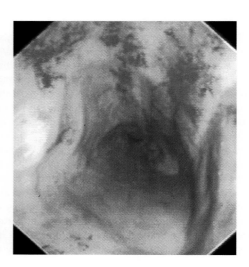

**Plate 4-44** Reflux esophagitis in a 4-month-old male Labrador retriever with vascular ring anomaly (see Plate 4-38). Hemorrhagic mucosal streaks are present just cranial to the gastroesophageal sphincter.

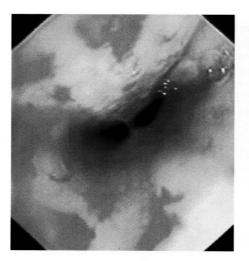

**Plate 4-45** Esophagitis in a 9-year-old female Labrador retriever after the dog underwent an anesthetic procedure (ovariohysterectomy for pyometra). Large, confluent mucosal hemorrhages are seen in the distal esophagus.

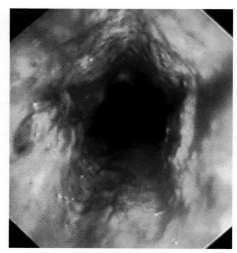

**Plate 4-46** Reflux esophagitis in a 4-year-old castrated male miniature poodle with chronic vomiting and bloating for 3 months, hypergastrinemia (fasting gastrin, 1793 ng/L; normal; 10 to 40 ng/L), and hypertrophic gastropathy. The mucosa is irregular, friable, and hemorrhagic. Esophageal perforation subsequently occurred. Gastrinoma (Zollinger-Ellison syndrome) was suspected but unproved.

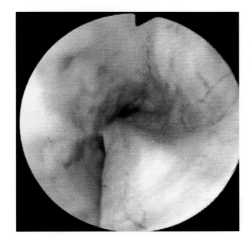

**Plate 4-47** Chemically induced erosive esophagitis with pseudomembrane formation in the cranial esophagus of an 8-month-old male golden retriever that had ingested concentrated chlorine tablets. Note the yellow-gray pseudomembrane separating from the mucosal surface into the lumen. The dog was managed with a gastrostomy tube but was euthanized after it developed aspiration pneumonia.

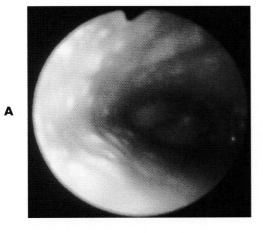

A

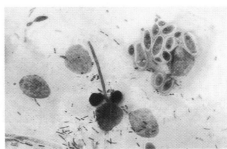

B

**Plate 4-48** Esophageal candidiasis in a 1.5-year-old female English Springer spaniel with megaesophagus. **A,** Endoscopy shows multifocal white mucosal plaques. **B,** Imprint cytology of the lesions reveals abundant yeast (ovoid bodies) and septate nonbranching hyphal forms of *Candida albicans.*

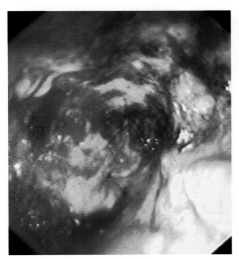

A

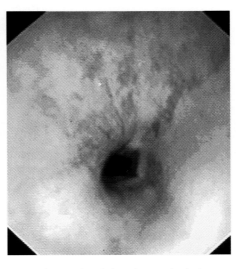

B

**Plate 4-49** Severe esophagitis and mucosal hemorrhage from a hoof-claw foreign body in a 7-year-old spayed female Cairn terrier with with a 5-day history of anorexia, depression, regurgitation, and respiratory distress. The foreign body, which was lodged just cranial to the gastroesophageal sphincter, was pushed into the stomach and removed surgically. **A,** Severe mucosal trauma with hemorrhage and ulceration at the site of the foreign body. The gastroesophageal sphincter is at the bottom center of the photograph. **B,** Progression of esophageal lesion healing after 10 days of treatment with sucralfate suspension, cimetidine, metoclopramide, prednisone, and gastrostomy tube feeding. Some residual superficial mucosal erosions are seen.

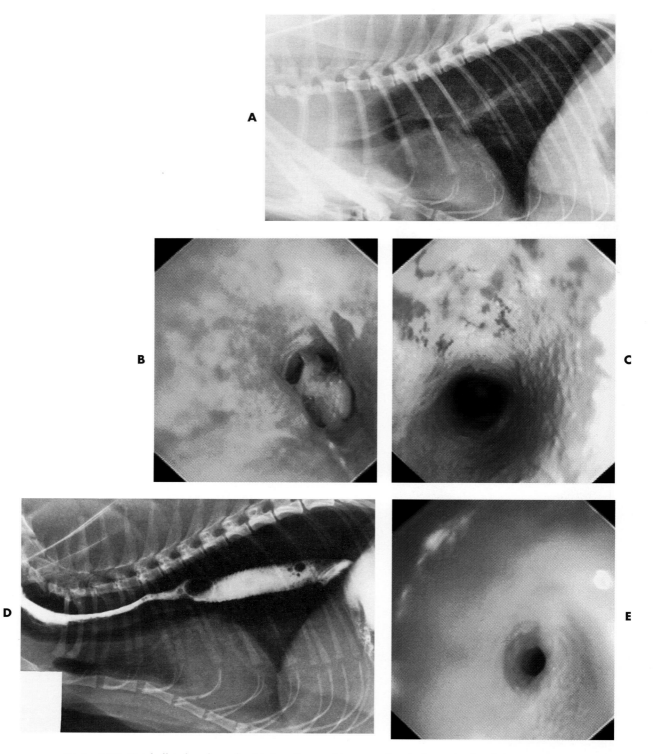

**Plate 4-50** Hairball-induced esophagitis in a 7-year-old castrated male domestic shorthair cat with the acute onset of dysphagia, gagging, and salivation. **A,** The lateral survey radiograph shows a fluid density in the craniodorsal mediastinum in the region of the esophagus. The trachea is displaced ventrally. **B,** Emergency esophagoscopy reveals a large hairball lodged in the esophageal lumen. When vomited from the stomach, large hairballs can become lodged in the esophagus. **C,** Immediately after the endoscopic removal of the hairball, esophagoscopy reveals severe esophagitis with mucosal ulceration and hemorrhage. The effects of pressure from the hairball and prolonged mucosal contact with the acid and pepsin absorbed into the hairball probably contribute to the esophagitis in such cases. **D,** A barium contrast esophagram, obtained because of persistent regurgitation 4 days after extraction of the hairball, shows a narrowed lumen and mucosal irregularity of the cranial thoracic esophagus. (The round filling defects are incidental air bubbles.) Fluoroscopy showed incomplete distension and resistance to the flow of the contrast medium through this region of the esophagus. These findings indicated persistent esophagitis and possibly a developing stricture. **E,** Endoscopy performed 3 weeks later because of continuing regurgitation reveals an esophageal stricture.

# ESOPHAGEAL STRICTURE

The diagnosis of esophageal stricture can be confirmed by barium contrast radiography of the esophagus or by esophagoscopy. Survey radiographs are often normal unless the esophagus is distended with food, fluid, or air proximal to the stricture. However, contrast radiography of the esophagus can determine the number, location, and length of strictures (Plates 4-51 and 4-56).

Endoscopically, an esophageal stricture appears as a focal circumferential narrowing caused by a smooth ridge or ring of fibrous tissue (Plates 4-52 through 4-587). The esophageal lumen at the stricture site is typically 2 to 4 mm in diameter and indistensible. Thus passage of the endoscope is impeded. The adjacent mucosa may be inflamed, hemorrhagic, friable or ulcerated. The esophagus has a variable degree of dilation proximal to the stricture, depending on the duration and extent of obstruction. The deep fibrosis often causes the tubular axis of the esophagus to be angulated rather than straight. Multiple or diffuse stricture formation appears as a series of thin, white, annular or semiannular ridges projecting into the lumen so as to produce a narrow lumen that is poorly distensible and distorted or irregular (nontubular) in shape. In some cases, fibrotic ridges may form a spiral configuration that extends for several centimeters down the esophagus. Occasionally a stricture web may form a membrane that completely occludes the lumen, giving the appearance of a blind pouch (see Plates 4-56 and 4-57). Air must not be overinsufflated into the esophagus during endoscopy of a patient with esophageal stricture. Because the endoscope cannot be readily advanced beyond the stricture, air may accumulate in and overdistend the stomach (especially in cats and small dogs). This could cause complications in an anesthetized patient.

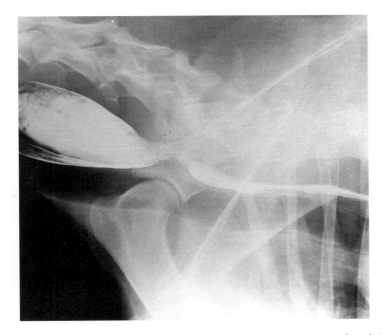

**Plate 4-51** Lateral barium contrast esophagram showing a stricture 1.5 cm in length in the caudal cervical region of a 3-year-old female Doberman pinscher with a 3-week history of regurgitation that began shortly after an anesthetic procedure (ovariohysterectomy). Contrast material is accumulated in the dilated esophagus cranial to the well-delineated narrowing of the lumen caused by the stricture.

Esophagoscopy is useful not only for the diagnosis of esophageal stricture but also for the visual guidance of bougienage or balloon dilation treatment (as described previously in this chapter). Immediately after the stricture has been dilated, the endoscope should be gently manipulated through the strictured area to assess the results of dilation and to evaluate the esophagus distal to the stricture. The esophagus and stomach should be evaluated carefully to determine the severity of esophagitis and to identify underlying causes of stricture formation (e.g., gastroesophageal reflux, hiatal hernia).

In some cases, the mucosa of the strictured area should be biopsied to rule out underlying neoplasia, especially when the stricture is associated with mucosal proliferation or fails to respond to therapy. A benign stricture generally appears as a smooth annular ridge. With neoplasia the surface tends to be ulcerated, lobulated, and friable. In periesophageal compression the mucosa at the site of narrowing appears normal but is indented by an external structure.

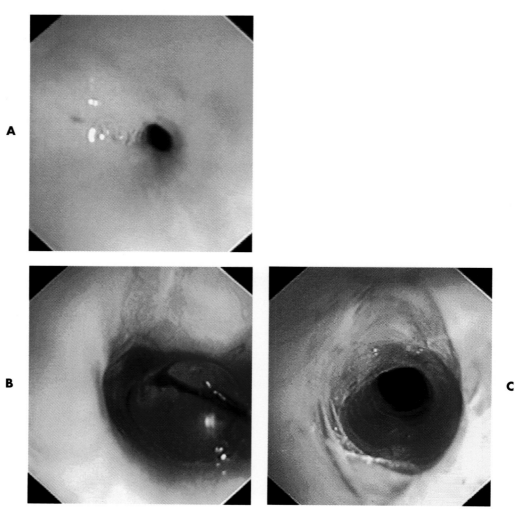

**Plate 4-52** Esophageal stricture in a 3-year-old Siamese cat with a 4-week history of regurgitation that began 1 day after the animal received general anesthesia for routine dental prophylaxis. **A,** The stricture immediately before balloon dilation. **B,** A 10-mm balloon catheter inflated in the lumen of the stricture. **C,** The stricture immediately after balloon dilation. The lumen has been reopened, and remnants of the torn stricture are seen.

A 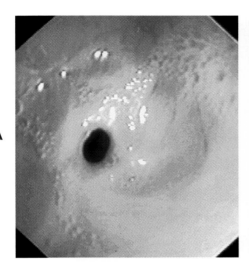 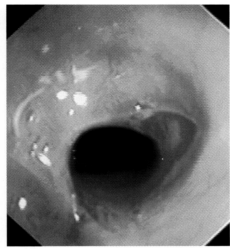 B

**Plate 4-53** Hairball-induced esophageal stricture in an 11-year-old neutered male domestic longhair cat. **A,** The 2-mm stricture before balloon dilation. **B,** Immediately after dilation the stricture site shows evidence of mucosal tearing and mild hemorrhage (typical findings for this procedure).

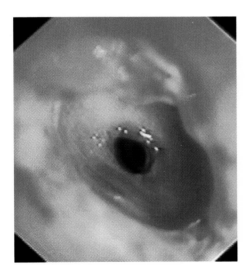 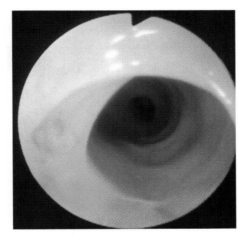

**Plate 4-54** Triple esophageal stricture in a 2-year-old Chinese shar-pei with regurgitation that began 2 weeks after the animal received general anesthesia for the repair of multiple fractures of the pelvis and hind limbs. Through the annular ring of one stricture, a second stricture is seen a short distance down the esophagus.

**Plate 4-55** Esophageal stricture forming thin, spiral-shaped fibrous ridges in the esophagus of a dog.

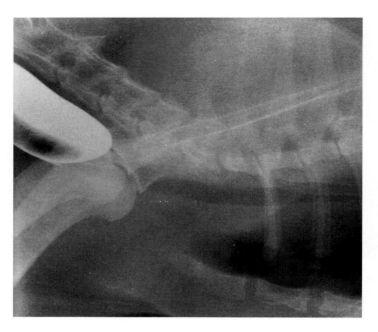

**Plate 4-56** Lateral barium contrast esophagram of an esophageal stricture in a 2-year-old neutered male domestic shorthair cat with a 1-month history of dysphagia and regurgitation. Barium fills a blind pouch in the cervical esophagus proximal to the site of complete obstruction by the stricture. No barium has passed through the stenotic area.

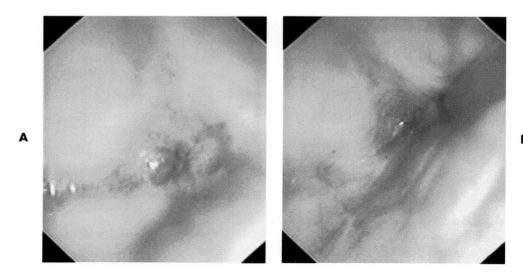

**Plate 4-57** Additional views of the cervical esophageal stricture shown in Plate 4-56. **A,** The stricture has formed a complete occlusive membrane over the lumen (in the center), producing a blind pouch with no identifiable opening. **B,** Probing with the tip of a balloon catheter fails to identify a lumen.

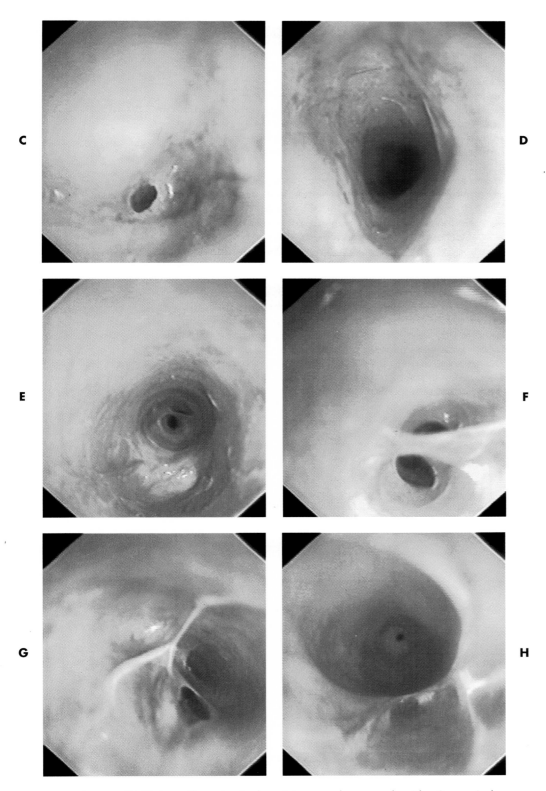

**Plate 4-57—cont'd** C, A small opening in the stricture membrane, made with a 2-mm pinch biopsy forceps, reveals the location of the lumen. D, Stricture site immediately after dilation. E, As the endoscope enters the dilated stricture, a second stricture is seen a few centimeters farther down the esophagus. F, A close-up view of the second stricture shows fibrotic strands that cross the lumen to produce a weblike effect. G and H, The second stricture after balloon dilation.

## ESOPHAGEAL PERFORATION

Esophageal perforation is a rare complication of esophageal foreign bodies, especially objects with irregular or sharp edges such as bones, or chronically lodged foreign bodies that cause deep-pressure necrosis. Iatrogenic esophageal perforation may occur during endoscopic foreign body extraction or stricture dilation (Plate 4-58). Iatrogenic perforation may also occur as a sequela of esophageal surgery or laser treatment. Penetrating injuries of the cervical esophagus can be caused by bite wounds or gunshot injuries. Perforation of the intrathoracic esophagus may have more serious consequences than perforation of the cervical esophagus.

Clinical signs of perforation include anorexia, depression, odynophagia, fever, and pain. Cough and dyspnea occur with perforation of the thoracic esophagus. With cervical perforation, cervical swelling, cellulitis, and draining fistula may occur. A left-shifted neutrophilic leukocytosis is usually present. With perforation of the esophagus, thoracic radiographs may reveal mediastinitis, pneumomediastinum, pneumothorax, soft-tissue emphysema, and pleural effusion. For contrast esophogography in a potential perforation case, a water-soluble nonionic iodinated contrast agent such as iohexol (Omnipaque) is less irritating to periesophageal tissues than barium and is also more readily reabsorbed.

Because of the potential for tension pneumothorax and leakage of contaminated fluids into the thorax, endoscopy should not be performed in patients with perforation of the thoracic esophagus. A deep laceration or tear in the esophagus, discovered during esophagoscopy, can become a full-thickness perforation. Bloody fluid that bubbles from a defect in the thoracic esophagus in synchrony with respirations is indicative of acute perforation. If perforation occurs during endoscopic manipulation of a foreign body or stricture, life-threatening tension pneumothorax may occur that is accentuated by insufflation. This situation requires immediate thoracocentesis and chest tube placement.

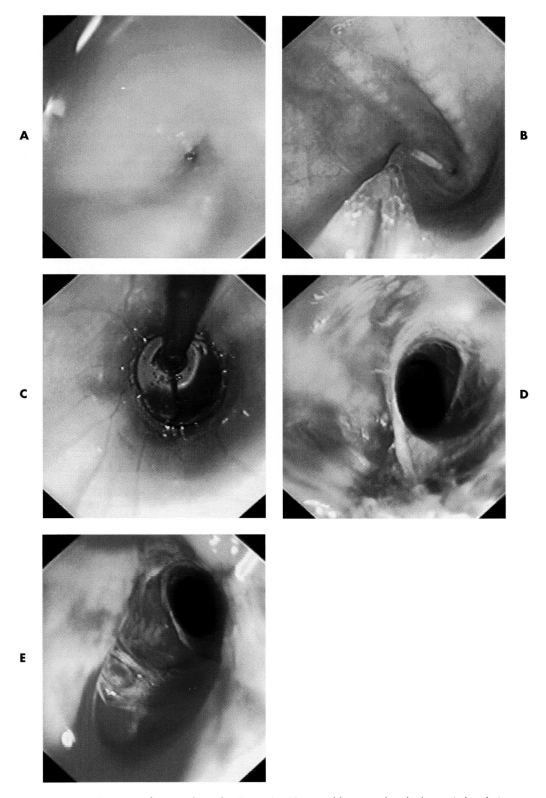

**Plate 4-58** Rupture of an esophageal stricture in a 3-year-old neutered male domestic longhair cat with a 1-month history of regurgitation. **A,** Extremely narrow stricture with a 1-mm lumen, before treatment. **B,** The stricture is so narrow that the endoscopist has difficulty passing the tapered tip of the balloon catheter into it. **C,** A 10-mm balloon catheter inflated within the stricture. **D** and **E,** Examination of the stricture site immediately after deflation and removal of the balloon reveals severe tearing of the mucosa, with mucosal strands, hemorrhage, and perforation. The cat was managed with a gastrostomy tube, but it developed acute septic mediastinitis and was euthanized at the owner's request. This case was the only balloon-induced perforation out of a total of 50 consecutive balloon dilation procedures reported in 13 cases by two of the authors (RGS and SEJ).

## ESOPHAGEAL FISTULA

Esophageal fistulas are congenital or acquired fistulous communications between the esophagus and adjacent structures, such as the tracheobronchial tree, mediastinum, or pleural space. Congenital fistulas resulting from incomplete separation of the embryonic esophagus and the tracheobronchial structures have been reported in the Cairn terrier. Acquired fistulas result from perforations caused mostly by foreign bodies (Plate 4-59). In conjunction with regurgitation the clinical signs are mainly cough and dyspnea from complicating pneumonia, pulmonary abscess, or pleuritis. Chronic perforations that seal off to become blind pouches or fistulas appear endoscopically as dual openings, with one opening being the normal lumen and the other one opening to a blind pouch.

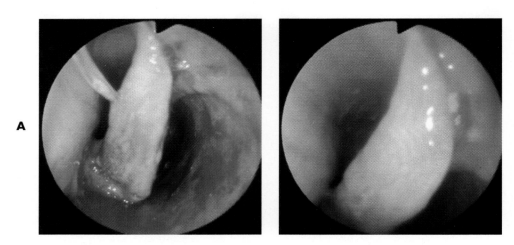

**A**  **B**

**Plate 4-59** Two views of a chronic esophageal fistula in a 2-year-old spayed female Labrador retriever. The fistula developed after the esophagus was perforated by a sharp stick. The fistulous tract extends deep into the cranial mediastinum. **A,** A flap of tissue (free edge of the esophageal wall) is in the center. The lumen of the esophagus passes to the left of the flap, and the fistula is to the right. **B,** Close-up view.

# HIATAL HERNIA

A hiatal hernia is a protrusion of a portion of stomach through the esophageal hiatus of the diaphragm. Hiatal hernia can be congenital or acquired, and in many cases the herniation and clinical signs are intermittent. A sliding hiatal hernia is a protrusion of the abdominal segment of the esophagus and cardia region of the stomach through the esophageal hiatus of the diaphragm into the thorax. A paraesophageal hiatal hernia occurs when a portion of the stomach (usually the fundus) herniates through the hiatus into the caudal mediastinum along the caudal thoracic esophagus. Sliding hiatal hernias are most common, and the majority are diagnosed in young animals.

A congenital hiatal hernia from malformation of the hiatus is most common in the Chinese shar-pei. An acquired hiatal hernia may result from enlargement of the esophageal hiatus and laxity of the surrounding support structures in association with persistently high positive intraabdominal pressure caused by vomiting or persistently high negative intrathoracic pressure caused by chronic airway obstruction. Chronic upper airway obstruction (e.g., laryngeal paralysis, laryngeal collapse, elongated soft palate) has been hypothesized to contribute to the development of hiatal hernia. Presumably, the attempt to overcome high upper airway resistance results in much greater than normal negative intrapleural pressures being generated during breathing, which draws the stomach across the hiatus.

Clinical signs of a hiatal hernia are chronic intermittent vomiting, regurgitation, and excessive salivation. Small hernias may not cause clinical signs, and intermittent stomach herniation may cause signs to be intermittent. Respiratory distress can be a prominent clinical sign in patients with large hiatal hernias. The clinical signs of hiatal hernias are mostly attributable to secondary reflux esophagitis. Displacement of the gastroesophageal junction into the thorax results in a loss of integrity of the gastroesophageal mechanism, thus predisposing to gastroesophageal reflux.

Diseases of the hiatus can usually be diagnosed radiographically, especially when the hernia is persistent (see Plates 4-60, 4-61, and 4-65). Survey thoracic radiographs may demonstrate a soft tissue and gas density mass (the stomach) in the caudal dorsal mediastinum. The normal gastric gas bubble that is usually seen in the cranial abdomen may also be smaller. An esophagram is usually required to confirm the presence of the hernia. The gastroesophageal junction and gastric rugae are visible cranial to the diaphragm, but the linear relationship between the esophagus and stomach is preserved. Gastroesophageal reflux may also be demonstrated (see Plate 4-60). Hiatal hernias that are small and reduce spontaneously are a diagnostic challenge because of their intermittent nature and unknown clinical significance. Fluoroscopy improves the chances of identifying an intermittent hernia and documenting reflux.

Endoscopy is useful for assessing secondary reflux esophagitis and may confirm a hiatal hernia (see Plates 4-61 through 4-65). Pooling of fluid in the esophagus and signs of reflux esophagitis (see previous discussion on esophagitis in this chapter) in the caudal esophagus may be observed secondary to frequent episodes of gastroesophageal reflux or vomiting. The endoscopic diagnosis of the hernia relies heavily on familiarity with normal appearance of the distal esophagus and gastroesophageal junction. A simple hiatal hernia is suggested by enlargement of the esophageal hiatus and cranial displacement of the gastroesophageal sphincter into the thorax. The small, light pink radial folds of the cardia are replaced by the thick, red rugal folds of the stomach that are displaced cranial to the hiatus. A pseudo-pouch effect may result as the endoscope first encounters the cranially displaced gastroesophageal junction. This is followed by dilation of a region of rugal folds representing the intrathoracic portion of the stomach lumen, which is followed by a narrowing of the lumen where the stomach passes through the hiatus of the diaphragm. A retroflex examination of the hiatus as viewed from the intraabdominal region of the stomach may show the rugal folds extending through a wide open hiatus.

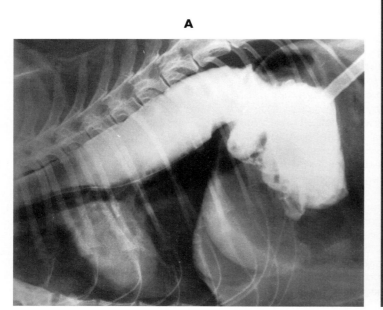

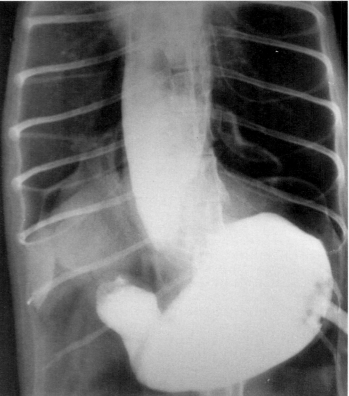

**Plate 4-60** Severe gastroesophageal reflux in a 3.5-year-old neutered male Siamese cat with megaesophagus and hiatal hernia. The clinical signs were chronic intermittent vomiting, chronic respiratory disease, and recent weight loss and dyspnea. Radiographs taken after liquid barium was instilled into the stomach through a gastrostomy tube demonstrate severe gastroesophageal reflux associated with hiatal hernia and megaesophagus. **A,** Lateral radiograph. **B,** Ventrodorsal radiograph.

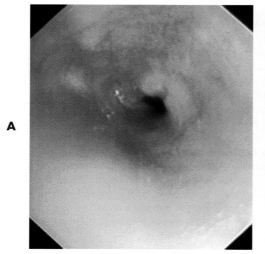

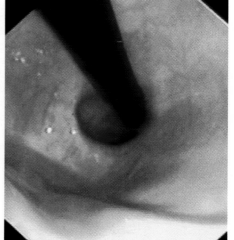

**Plate 4-61** Endoscopic views from the cat with megaesophagus, hiatal hernia, and gastroesophageal reflux (see Plate 4-60). **A,** Fluid is pooled in the caudal thoracic esophagus and the gastroesophageal sphincter is dilated. Reflux episodes occurred repeatedly during the examination. **B,** This retroflex view of the cardia from the stomach lumen shows a widely dilated gastroesophageal junction. The endoscopic findings are suggestive but not conclusive for the diagnosis of hiatal hernia, but barium contrast fluoroscopy was confirmatory.

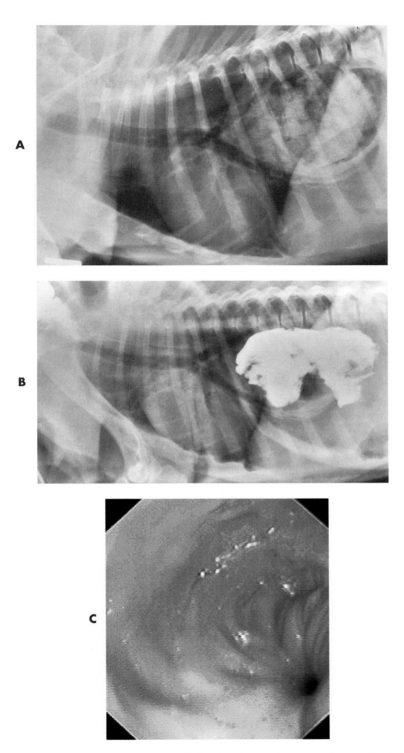

**Plate 4-62** Hiatal hernia in a 5-month-old female Chinese shar-pei with regurgitation. **A,** The lateral thoracic radiograph shows a caudal mediastinal fluid density in the region of the esophagus along with the mottled appearance of ingesta. **B,** A lateral barium contrast esophagram shows cranial displacement of the stomach into the thorax through a hiatal hernia. **C,** This endoscopic view of the gastroesophageal junction shows the hiatal hernia with displacement of the cardia and rugal folds of the stomach through the diaphragm.

**Plate 4-63** Two views of a
hiatal hernia and reflux
esophagitis in a 1-year-old
male bulldog with syncope,
vomiting, and chronic ob-
structive upper airway disease (everted laryngeal saccules). **A,** Gastroesophageal
reflux of food and hemor-
rhagic fluid is filling the
esophagus. The caudal
esophageal mucosa is hemorrhagic from reflux esophagitis. **B,** The gastroesophageal
junction is wide open, allowing direct viewing of the gastric rugae from the esophagus.

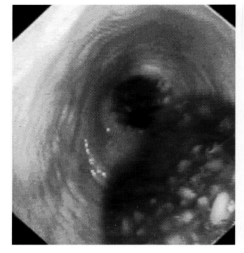
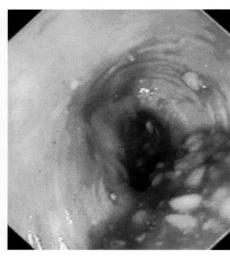

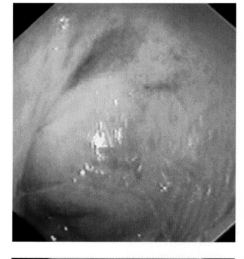

**Plate 4-64** Paraesophageal
hiatal hernia with displacement of the stomach, spleen,
and duodenum into the thorax in a 7-year-old male Chinese shar-pei with a 3-year
history of occasional vomiting (once per month). For 3
days before this examination
the animal vomited fre-
quently. The vomitus con-
sisted of 3-day-old food and
dead rabbit parts. **A,** Refluxed gastric fluid is pooled
in the esophagus. The bulge
of herniated viscera alongside the wall of the esophagus is seen cranial to the gastroesophageal sphincter.
**B,** Refluxed bile and food
are seen in the distal esophagus, but the sliding hernia
has replaced itself. **C,** Erythematous mucosal streaks
in the caudal esophagus indicate reflux esophagitis. Gastroesophageal reflux causes
most of the signs associated
with hiatal hernia.

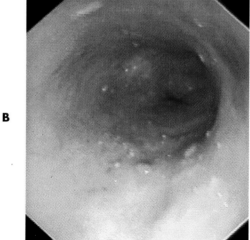
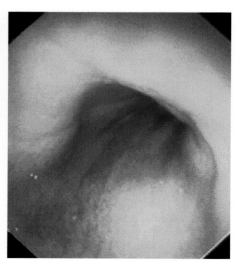

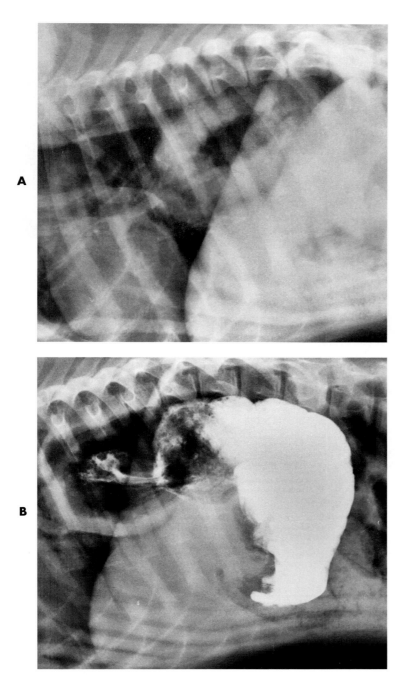

**Plate 4-65** Hiatal hernia and gastroesophageal intussusception in a 6-month-old male Chinese shar-pei with a 1-month history of chronic vomiting, weight loss, lethargy, and retching 15 to 60 minutes after eating. **A,** The lateral thoracic radiograph shows a gas-filled structure in the dorso-caudal mediastinum. **B,** A barium contrast esophagram outlines the esophagus passing around the gas-filled structure with rugae, which is the stomach displaced into the thorax through a right-sided hiatal hernia.                                              *Continued*

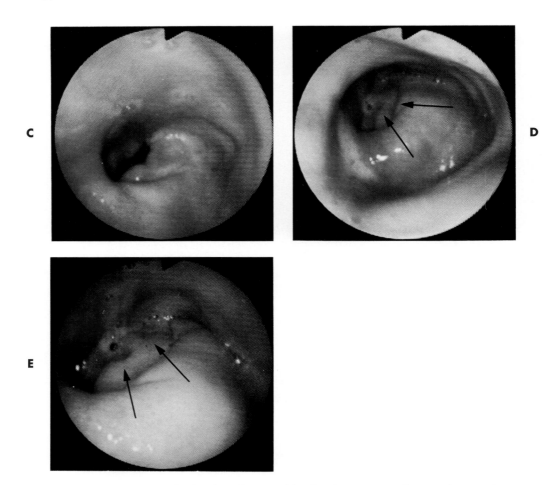

**Plate 4-65—cont'd** C, The distal esophagus is dilated and contains small accumulations of foam. The gastroesophageal junction is slightly dilated. Note the outpouching appearance of esophagus in the lower right aspect of the field of view. This is most likely caused by marked laxity of the diaphragmatic hiatus. **D,** Gastric rugal folds *(arrows)* have filled the lumen at the lower esophageal sphincter. **E,** Close-up view showing the rugal folds *(arrows)* running up into the hernia pouch of the distal esophagus. At times marked gastroesophageal intussusception was observed.

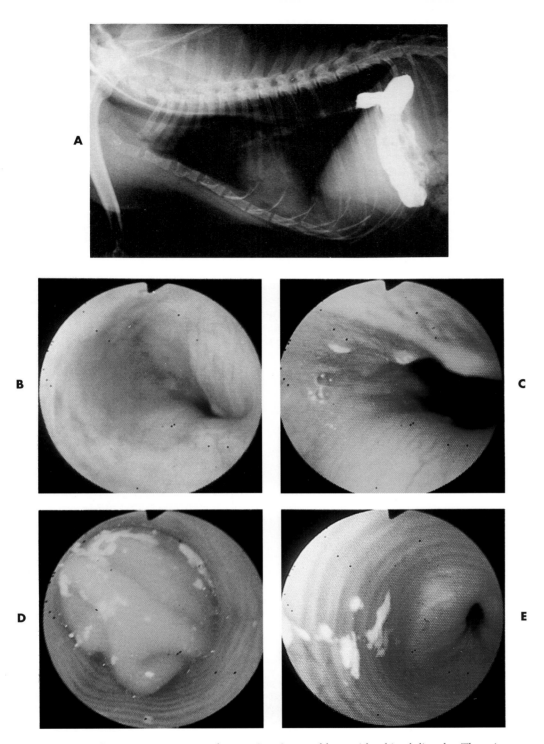

**Plate 4-66 A,** Barium contrast esophagram in a 9-year-old cat with a hiatal disorder. The primary clinical sign was long-term intermittent vomiting 10 to 30 minutes after eating. The vomiting had recently become more frequent. The cat was evaluated with fluoroscopy. The barium bolus was consistently not transported correctly across the distal esophagus and gastroesophageal junction. This lateral radiograph shows an accumulation of barium that crosses the diaphragm in association with the terminal esophagus. The radiographic diagnosis was paraesophageal hernia or gastroesophageal intussusception. **B,** The endoscopic examination revealed mild erythema and outpouching of the distal esophagus to the left of the lower esophageal sphincter. **C,** This close-up view of distal esophagus shows the lower esophageal sphincter to be moderately dilated. **D,** During gastroscopy the cat began to retch. The endoscope was withdrawn to the esophagus, and the gastric mucosa momentarily prolapsed into the distal esophagus (gastroesophageal intussusception). (Note the gastric fold and the barium adhering to the mucosa.) Although gastric prolapse occurs fairly often during vomiting episodes in cats, its occurrence in this case was considered clinically significant. **E,** The stomach returned to normal position, and residual barium from the retching episode is visualized in the distal esophagus. Dietary manipulation and metoclopramide (used twice daily indefinitely) completely controlled the clinical signs. Gastric and duodenal biopsies were normal.

# GASTROESOPHAGEAL INTUSSUSCEPTION

Gastroesophageal intussusception is an invagination of the stomach into the lumen of the caudal esophagus. Like hiatal hernia, it can be a consequence of laxity of the esophageal hiatus and may occur intermittently. It can also be a complication of esophageal hypomotility or megaesophagus. Gastroesophageal intussusceptions can cause both esophagitis and esophageal obstruction. The severity of the clinical signs depends on the degree of intussusception and whether it is spontaneously reversible. Chronic intermittent gastroesophageal intussusception with a mild degree of invagination can cause mild and intermittent signs, similar to those of hiatal hernia. A large gastroesophageal intussusception with gastric dilation can cause hematemesis, depression, dyspnea, and circulatory collapse. In such cases, death may occur rapidly.

Gastroesophageal intussusception can be diagnosed by radiography or esophagoscopy (Plates 4-65 through 4-70). Endoscopically the invaginated stomach appears as an intraluminal mass covered with rugal folds and filling the lumen of the distal esophagus. If intussusception is encountered, the endoscopist should maximally insufflate the esophagus and occlude it in the cervical region to retain the air. The combination of inflation pressure and advancement of the endoscope tip against the invaginated rugae may reduce a small intussusception and allow entry into the repositioned stomach.

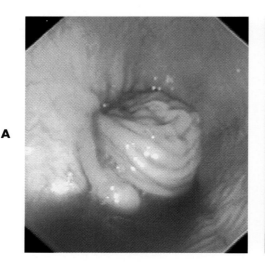 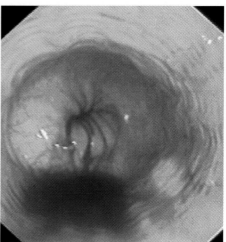

**Plate 4-67 A,** Gastroesophageal intussusception in an adult cheetah with chronic intermittent vomiting. Invagination of the rugal folds through the gastroesophageal sphincter into the caudal thoracic esophagus has occurred, and hemorrhagic fluid is pooled in the esophagus. **B,** Gastroesophageal sphincter moments after the intussusception is reduced by pushing on it with the tip of the endoscope.

A
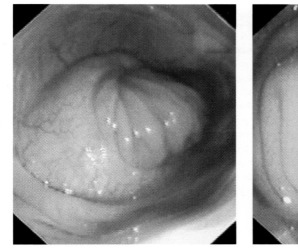

B
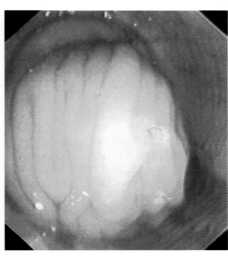

**Plate 4-68** **A,** Gastroesophageal intussusception protruding through the gastroesophageal sphincter in a second adult cheetah with chronic intermittent vomiting. **B,** During the few minutes of observation, the amount of stomach that prolapsed into the esophageal lumen progressively increased until the rugal folds filled the caudal esophageal lumen.

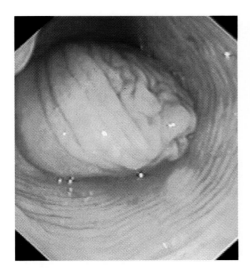

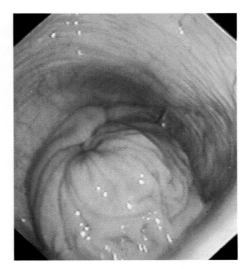

**Plate 4-69** Gastroesophageal intussusception in a third adult cheetah with chronic intermittent vomiting.

**Plate 4-70** Gastroesophageal intussusception in a fourth adult cheetah with chronic intermittent vomiting. Note the lumen in the center of the mass of rugal folds.

## ESOPHAGEAL NEOPLASIA

Primary esophageal neoplasms are rare. Squamous cell carcinoma in old cats is the most common primary esophageal neoplasm. In regions where *Spirocerca lupi* is endemic, fibrosarcomas and osteosarcomas may develop from spirocercal granulomas.

Esophageal neoplasia causes progressive signs of regurgitation, dysphagia, ptyalism, weight loss, and anorexia. Survey radiographs may be normal, or they may reveal a soft-tissue mass in the region of the esophagus. An irregular intraluminal filling defect on a barium esophagram is indicative of esophageal neoplasia (Plates 4-71 and 4-74).

Endoscopy and biopsy are indicated for the definitive diagnosis of esophageal neoplasia (Plates 4-71 through 4-77). With obstruction the esophagus may be dilated with air, fluid, or food proximal to the tumor site. Endoscopically, squamous cell carcinoma usually appears as a proliferative mass with a friable ulcerated surface (Plates 4-71 and 4-72). Lumenal occlusion varies, depending on the size and position of the mass.

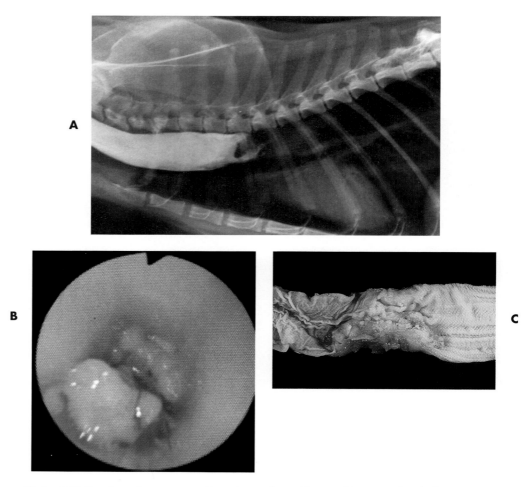

**Plate 4-71** Esophageal squamous cell carcinoma in an 11-year-old castrated male domestic shorthair cat with a 3-week history of progressively worsening regurgitation. **A,** The lateral barium esophagram shows an irregular filling defect causing obstruction of the cranial thoracic esophagus. **B,** Endoscopic view of the irregular proliferative mass in the lumen of the thoracic esophagus. **C,** Necropsy view of the esophagus opened up (cranial end on the left), showing the intramural neoplastic mass. The histopathologic diagnosis was squamous cell carcinoma. (From Johnson SE: Diseases of the esophagus. In Sherding RG, editor: *The cat: diseases and clinical management.* Philadelphia, 1994, WB Saunders.)

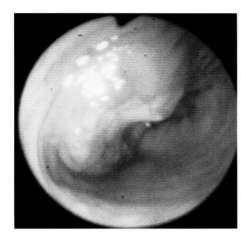

**Plate 4-72** Esophageal squamous cell carcinoma in an 8-year-old female-spayed domestic shorthair cat with chronic progressive regurgitation and weight loss. An ulcerated intramural mass is protruding into the lumen of the caudal thoracic esophagus.

**A**

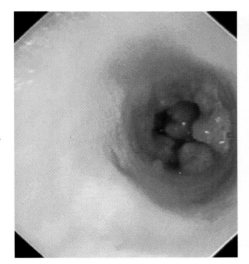

**B**

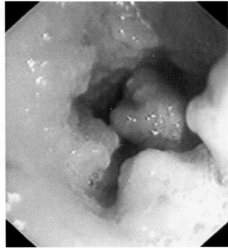

**Plate 4-73** Papillary carcinoma of the terminal esophagus and cardia in the stomach in a 13-year-old pug with intermittent vomiting, anorexia, and dyspnea for 1 week. Thoracic radiography showed pulmonary nodules (metastases) and pleural effusion. Thoracic ultrasonography showed a large hypoechoic mass in the caudal esophagus. **A,** Irregular proliferation at the gastroesophageal junction. **B,** Close-up view showing the irregular proliferations circumferentially at the gastroesophageal sphincter and cardia. This mass is causing extreme disfigurement of the lumen.

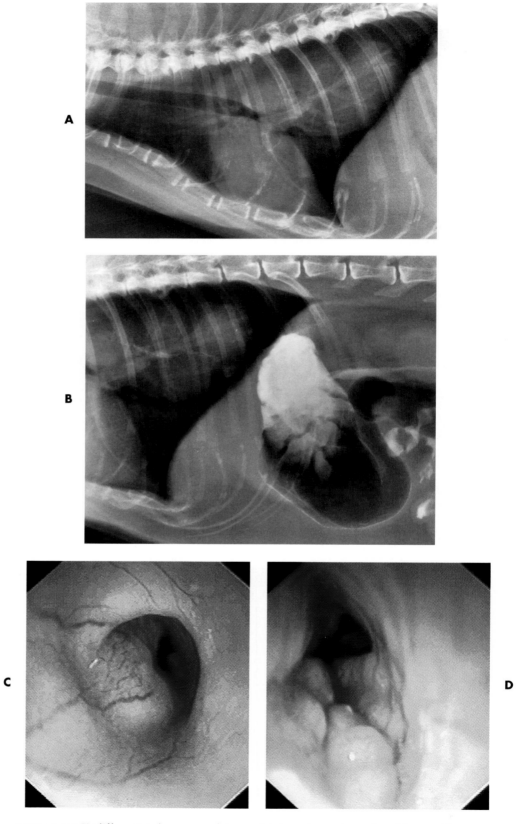

**Plate 4-74** Undifferentiated sarcoma of the caudal thoracic esophagus in a 15-year-old castrated male domestic shorthair cat. **A,** The lateral thoracic radiograph shows a large caudal mediastinal mass in the dorsocaudal thorax. **B,** A lateral barium contrast esophagram shows compression of the lumen, with nearly complete obstruction except for a thin line of barium. **C,** Endoscopic view of the cranial edge of the intramural mass. Normal-appearing mucosa and mucosal vessels are seen on the surface of the bulging tumor mass. **D,** The center of the mass shows irregular, lobulated neoplastic proliferations.

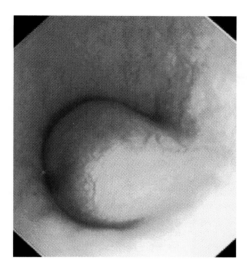

**Plate 4-75** Leiomyoma at the gastroesophageal junction discovered as an incidental finding in a 14-year-old male Cairn terrier with pharyngeal dysphagia. A large protruding mass is seen in the caudal esophagus in front of the gastroesophageal sphincter. Normal-appearing mucosa covers the surface of the mass.

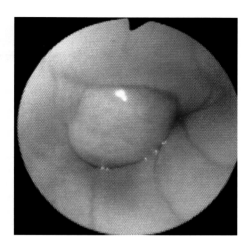

**Plate 4-76** Leiomyoma at the opening of the gastroesophageal sphincter in a 12-year-old male Maltese. As is often the case with leiomyomas, this benign tumor was an incidental finding. Leiomyomas commonly occur in the cardia and therefore are often best seen with retroflex viewing from the stomach lumen.

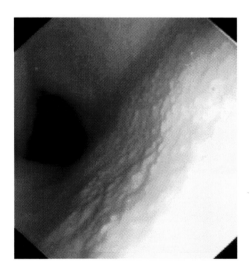

**Plate 4-77** Esophageal lymphoma in an 8-year-old male golden retriever with vomiting, diarrhea, and protein-losing enteropathy (total protein, 4.2 g/dl; albumin, 1.9 g/dl) associated with diffuse lymphoma concurrently in the small intestine. Numerous smooth mucosal nodules from lymphomatous infiltration have produced a diffuse cobblestone pattern in the esophageal mucosa.

# PERIESOPHAGEAL MASSES

Mass lesions arising from periesophageal tissues may cause extraluminal compression of the esophagus or may invade locally into the wall of the esophagus. Mediastinal lymphoma is most common, although any large tumor or abscess arising from cervical or mediastinal structures (e.g., thyroid, thymus, lymph node, lung, heartbase) can cause secondary esophageal compression.

The clinical signs associated with external compression of the esophagus include regurgitation, dysphagia, and hypersalivation. Lymphoma also causes dyspnea (pleural effusion), decreased thoracic compressibility, and Horner's syndrome. Survey thoracic radiography usually identifies the compressive mass. If not, a barium esophagram identifies the location and extent of obstruction (Plate 4-78, *A*). Large mediastinal and pulmonary masses can be examined by fine-needle aspiration cytology. Thoracocentesis and cytology of the pleural fluid may also be diagnostic.

Endoscopy is useful for evaluating the extent of obstruction and determining whether the mass is extramural or intramural (Plate 4-78, *B*). A stenotic region of esophagus with normal-appearing mucosa suggests extraluminal compression by a periesophageal mass rather than stricture or primary esophageal neoplasia.

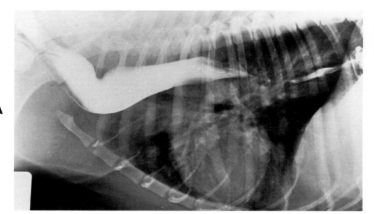
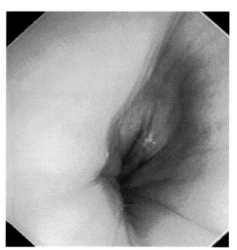

**Plate 4-78** Periesophageal mass (poorly differentiated sarcoma) in a 3-year-old male shar-pei with a 3-week history of weight loss and a 1-week history of coughing, gagging, vomiting, and anorexia. **A,** The lateral barium contrast esophagram shows the esophagus to be distended with barium. The esophagus narrows abruptly just caudal to the heart because of compression by an intramural or extramural mass. Indistinct pulmonary nodules (metastases) are also noted. **B,** This endoscopic view of the thoracic esophagus at the base of the heart shows compression of the lumen suggestive of a periesophageal mass. The mucosa appears normal, and no evidence of intraluminal strictures or masses is seen. Necropsy revealed a poorly differentiated sarcoma surrounding the esophagus and aorta just caudal to the base of the heart.

# Chapter 5

# Gastroscopy

**Todd R. Tams**

Gastroscopy mainly identifies abnormalities of the gastric mucosa, but it may also reveal distortion of the stomach's normal anatomic relationships by displacement or extrinsic compression as a result of a mass or enlargement of an adjacent organ. Gastroscopy has become the most valuable diagnostic method available for evaluating primary gastric disorders because it permits unparalleled observation of the gastric mucosa. This modality significantly increases diagnostic yield in comparison with contrast radiographic studies, which are somewhat less sensitive in the evaluation of mucosal disorders. Endoscopy-guided biopsy provides rapid and reliable assessment of many disorders. Endoscopic examination of the stomach has improved early diagnostic capability significantly and has highlighted the fact that gastric mucosal disorders occur fairly often.

## INDICATIONS

Indications for gastroscopy include clinical signs referable to gastric diseases, including nausea, salivation, vomiting, hematemesis, melena, unexplained abnormal breath changes, and anorexia. The most common disorders diagnosed include chronic gastritis (with or without overgrowth of *Helicobacter* organisms), superficial gastric erosions, gastric foreign bodies, and gastric motility disorders. Ulcers and neoplasia can be readily diagnosed but are somewhat less commonly found. The antral-pyloric canal can be examined, and significant narrowing

of the pylorus or the presence of prominent folds of tissue in the antrum may suggest the possibility of hypertrophic gastropathy.

Vomiting is one of the most common reasons animals are presented to veterinarians for examination. In many cases a history of dietary indiscretion (e.g., overeating, acute dietary change) or foreign body ingestion can be elicited. Gastroscopy is not commonly performed in acutely vomiting patients unless a gastric foreign body or gastric ulceration is suspected. This examination is much more commonly done in animals with a history of acute vomiting that has continued for a period of time without relief (i.e., greater than 3 to 4 days), chronic intermittent vomiting (i.e., recurrent for more than 2 to 3 weeks), and vomiting that includes blood. (Gastroscopy should be considered any time hematemesis is observed.) The most common causes of hematemesis in dogs and cats are chronic gastritis and acute gastric mucosal erosions from factors such as drugs (especially nonsteroidal antiinflammatory medications) and hypotension with subsequent decreased gastric mucosal blood flow. Gastric ulcers and neoplasia are somewhat less common causes of hematemesis. Occasionally the only clinical manifestations of chronic gastritis are inappetence and salivation.

An initial diagnostic plan for an animal with a chronic vomiting disorder should include a complete history, physical examination, complete blood count, biochemical profile (including thyroid evaluation for vomiting cats), urinalysis, fecal examination for parasites, evaluation for heartworm disease in cats (starting with a heartworm antibody test), and survey abdominal radiographs. Once metabolic disorders are ruled out (e.g., renal failure, diabetes mellitus, and liver disease), the decision to perform a barium contrast study, gastroscopy, or both is made. Considering the insensitivity of barium contrast studies for diagnosing mucosal disorders, the thoroughness of a complete gastric endoscopic examination, and the cost-containment factor that concerns many pet owners, the decision to choose gastroscopy over radiography is usually a sound one. To the increasing number of small animal practitioners who are performing endoscopy, the conclusion that endoscopy is clearly superior should come as no surprise. If radiographs identify a lesion or foreign body, gastroscopy or surgery is still necessary for definitive diagnosis and treatment. Furthermore a normal gastric contrast radiographic examination does not rule out the presence of a gastric disorder.

In patients with chronic upper gastrointestinal disorders, gastroscopy should be performed in conjunction with esophagoscopy and duodenoscopy. Important diagnostic clues may be evident in any or all of these areas during the course of an examination. Follow-up gastroscopy is a valuable aid for monitoring therapeutic response in patients with chronic gastritis or ulcers. Follow-up biopsies are especially important in animals with chronic, severe histiocytic and granulomatous gastritis, chronic fibrosing gastritis, and gastric lymphosarcoma. Important information that is useful in treatment protocol decisions can often be obtained. (Case examples highlighting this point can be found in the atlas at the end of this chapter.)

Finally, esophagogastroduodenoscopy (EGD) is a most useful aid when clients have limited financial means but earnestly wish more than palliative treatment for their pet's discomfort. If inexpensive routine tests have proved unrewarding in diagnosing a disorder characterized by gastrointestinal signs, money may be better spent on early endoscopic examination.

## INSTRUMENTATION

For small animal patients a complete evaluation of the stomach is best accomplished using a flexible endoscope with a diameter of 9 mm or less and four-way tip deflection capability (see Chapter 3). In cats and in dogs weighing less than 5 kg (11 lb) an endoscope insertion-tube diameter of 8.5 mm or less is highly preferred. Use of a smaller endoscope makes it much more likely that the pyloric canal and proximal duodenum can be traversed and examined in these small patients than when a larger diameter scope is used, especially if the operator has limited experience. The degree of endoscope flexibility is also an important factor in small animals because maneuvering through

tight angles around the incisura angularis (angulus fold) and pyloric canal can be very difficult.

## PATIENT PREPARATION

The main requirement for a successful gastroscopy is that the patient's stomach be empty. No food should be given for 12 to 18 hours before the examination, and water should be withheld for 4 or more hours.

Under certain circumstances, fasting alone is insufficient to ensure an empty stomach. If gastric emptying is significantly impaired because of abnormal gastric motility (e.g., idiopathic gastric hypomotility or severe chronic gastritis) or obstruction (e.g., hypertrophic gastropathy, or antral or pyloric neoplasia), significant amounts of ingesta, debris, or retained gastric or duodenal fluid may compromise the examination. In these situations, biopsies may still be obtained if areas of mucosa can be visualized, but because lesions can be easily missed, the examination may need to be repeated later. Finding retained ingesta in a properly fasted animal can be an important diagnostic clue. For example, the presence of retained ingesta may strongly suggest that the patient has a gastric motility disorder.

When clots or pooled blood is present, the endoscopist may find it difficult to determine the source of bleeding. Free fluid can be suctioned through the accessory channel, but copious lavage through a large-bore tube may be necessary to dislodge clots before the endoscope is reintroduced.

Gastroscopy is generally not performed within 12 to 24 hours of a barium contrast examination unless a gastric foreign body has been identified. This usually allows sufficient time for complete clearing of the barium and subsequent thorough mucosal evaluation. The accessory channel of an endoscope should *not* be used to suction barium because residue may become adhered to the channel wall.

## RESTRAINT

As with any endoscopic procedure of the upper gastrointestinal tract, general anesthesia is required for gastroscopy. Atropine and other anticholinergic agents are not used unless they are required to increase heart rate. These drugs alter gastric motility patterns, which may cause increased gastric flaccidity and dilation. In addition, pyloric tone may increase, making it difficult to advance an endoscope through the pylorus. Atropine can also decrease lower esophageal sphincter tone. In most animals, however, the lower esophageal sphincter is closed on initial examination regardless of whether atropine was administered before the procedure. Finally, opioid drugs should not be used because they may increase pyloric tone.

The patient should always be placed in *left* lateral recumbency for gastroscopy. With the animal in this position the antrum and pylorus are away from the tabletop. This significantly improves the endoscopist's ability to completely examine and more readily traverse these structures with the scope. When an animal is in *right* lateral recumbency, it is much more difficult to clearly identify and pass the endoscope around the incisura angularis and through the antrum to the pylorus.

## PROCEDURE

All areas of the stomach should be examined completely in every patient that undergoes gastroscopy. Therefore the beginning endoscopist must learn to identify landmarks properly (Figure 5-1). Only after the endoscopist has become familiar with luminal gastric anatomy do maneuvering the endoscope to obtain a retroflexed view of the cardia, advancing the scope around the incisura angularis to reach the antrum, and traversing the pyloric canal become consistent and effortless procedures.

## GASTROESOPHAGEAL JUNCTION

Because the esophagus is essentially in a posterior plane compared with the stomach, the endoscope tip needs to be deflected in the distal esophagus before it can be successfully advanced to the stomach. As the endoscope is advanced to the distal esophagus, the position and configuration of the gastroesophageal junction are noted (see Chapter 4). The endoscope tip should be centered at the gastroesophageal orifice. As the scope is advanced, the tip is deflected to the left approximately 30 degrees

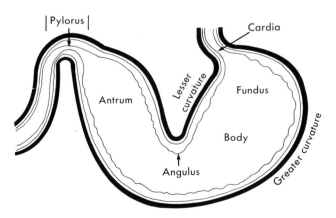

**Figure 5-1** Five basic regions of the stomach. The most important landmarks for endoscopy are the cardia, angulus, and pylorus.

with simultaneous slight upward deflection as the gastroesophageal junction is passed. In most patients this is easily accomplished by rotating the outer control knob counterclockwise for left deflection and the inner control knob counterclockwise for upward deflection. In some patients, minimal or no upward deflection is needed. When the endoscope tip is properly directed, no resistance should be encountered as the scope is advanced to the stomach. If the tip is advanced too far before deflection is begun, the endoscope is usually directed into the esophageal wall bordering against the posterior aspect of the lesser curvature of the stomach. If this occurs, the endoscope tip should be retracted and repositioned. Variable degrees of air insufflation of the distal esophagus may be necessary to aid visualization and positioning.

## PROXIMAL STOMACH AND GASTRIC BODY

The endoscope tip should be positioned just through the gastroesophageal junction so that the endoscopist can become spatially oriented and obtain an overview of the gastric lumen. As the tip enters the stomach, the rugal folds, generally on the greater curvature of the body, are seen. Often the stomach walls are partially or completely collapsed, especially in medium- to large-sized dogs or if only a small volume of air was insufflated during esophagoscopy. In this situation the view of the stomach is quite limited, and it is necessary to pause and insufflate air.

The ideal degree of gastric distension is a matter of judgment. Generally the distension should be at least to the point that the rugal folds begin to separate. This allows for spatial orientation and the identification of most gross abnormalities, such as an ulcer, a mass, or a foreign body. In cats and small dogs the degree of insufflation can be achieved within seconds; in giant breeds, constant insufflation may be necessary for 30 to 120 seconds before adequate distension is achieved. Later in the procedure it may be necessary to distend the stomach to a greater degree so that the entire gastric mucosal surface can be carefully examined.

During insufflation the endoscopist must be careful not to overdistend the stomach because this may result in significant cardiopulmonary compromise. When the stomach is overdistended, the rugal folds become almost completely flattened or undetectable, superficial blood vessels can sometimes be observed, and the mucosa may appear blanched. The respiratory rate may increase significantly. The endoscopy assistant should be aware of changes in the character of the patient's respirations and any increase in anterior abdominal distension. As soon as possible a sufficient volume of air should be suctioned off to moderately deflate the stomach. During most gastric examinations, both *air insufflation* and *suction* are commonly used to maintain a proper and safe balance of distension.

Several observations should be made during the initial examination of the stomach. These include the presence of fluid or ingesta, the ease with which the gastric walls distend when air is insufflated, and the gross appearance of the rugal folds and mucosa.

In most properly fasted patients the stomach is completely empty. Occasionally a small pool of fluid is present in the fundus or at the proximal aspect of the greater curvature. This is not considered abnormal. However, the presence of larger volumes of fluid, especially green or yellow bilious fluid, may be abnormal. This finding suggests the possibility of reflux of intestinal fluid to the stomach, which may occur in animals that have undergone enemas or that have a duodenogastric reflux disorder, an intestinal obstruction, or a primary gastric motility disorder. Bile is irritating to the gastric mucosa. Thus if significant bilious fluid is retained, the gastric mucosa may appear reddened. Mucosal erythema should be noted, but the patient should not be assumed to have gastritis. The diagnosis of gastritis requires histologic evidence.

If only a small amount of fluid is present, aspiration of the fluid is probably unnecessary. If, however, a pool of fluid obscures the rugal folds, aspiration should be done. The endoscope tip should be positioned as parallel to the gastric wall as possible, and alternating suction *and* air insufflation should be used. When suction is applied with the endoscope tip perpendicular to the mucosa, the tendency is to draw a portion of the mucosa into the accessory channel. This delays aspiration and may cause superficial mucosal lesions. Great care should be taken when attempting to suction fluid that is present in conjunction with particulate matter such as food or foreign body debris. The accessory channel can become obstructed if debris is suctioned along with fluid. In one instance a fragment from a small pebble obstructed the accessory channel of one of my endoscopes, and it could not be dislodged. Replacement of the accessory channel was required.

As the scope is gradually advanced through the proximal stomach, the endoscopist can thoroughly evaluate the gastric body by using the control knobs to deflect the endoscope tip or by rotating the insertion tube with the right hand. With the patient in left lateral recumbency and the endoscope held in a conventional manner (i.e., buttons up), the endoscopic view is predictable. The smooth lesser curvature is on the endoscopist's right, and the rugal folds of the greater curvature are seen below and to the left (Figure 5-2). Required directional changes can usually be made with the left thumb on the inner

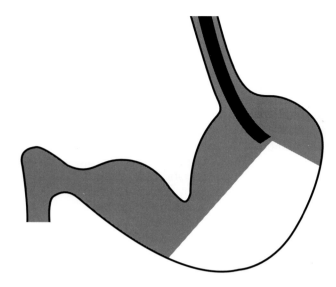

**Figure 5-2** Areas of the stomach not in view (shaded) as a standard forward-viewing endoscope is advanced into the proximal stomach. A retroversion maneuver is required to completely view the cardia and fundus.

control knob and the right hand controlling rotation (torque) of the insertion tube. In most cases, only minor directional changes are needed to provide a panoramic view. The endoscope is advanced along the greater curvature until the angulus is identified. The angulus appears as a large fold that extends from the lesser curvature. The angulus is an important landmark that separates the body of the stomach from the antrum. Once the angulus is identified, the lesser curvature can be easily differentiated from the greater curvature of the stomach. With the patient in left lateral recumbency, the antrum is directed up or away from the tabletop. As viewed from the gastric body, the angulus and entrance to the antrum usually appear as a circular or crescent-shaped orifice that is smaller than the distended body of the stomach (see Plates 5-5, 5-23, and 5-24). The endoscopist must be able to maneuver around the angulus to advance the endoscope to the antrum, pylorus, and duodenum. This is one of the more difficult gastroscopic techniques to master.

Once the angulus and antrum are reached, the endoscopist has the option of advancing directly through the pyloric canal to the duodenum or completing the gastric examination. The cardia and fundus have not yet been completely evaluated. Depending on the particular endoscope's angle of illumination, a portion of the proximal stomach cannot be seen as the scope enters the stomach (see Figure 5-2). For the cardia and fundus to be visualized the endoscope must be retroflexed (J maneuver) so that it is possible to see the portion of the scope entering through the cardia, as well as the surrounding

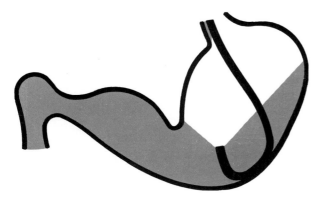

**Figure 5-3** Retroversion maneuver (J maneuver). The endoscope tip has been deflected fully in the upward direction.

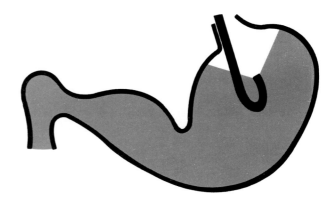

**Figure 5-4** To provide a close-up view of the fundus and gastroesophageal junction, the insertion tube has been rotated 180 degrees to the left and retracted toward the esophagus.

area (Figure 5-3). The retroversion maneuver should either be done at this point or after duodenoscopy. It can be advantageous to proceed directly from the angulus to the pylorus and duodenum. The physiologic function of the pylorus is to close in response to gastric distension. When gastric distension has been kept to a minimum and the antrum is not actively contracting, the pylorus is in a relatively lax state and the endoscope can pass through it with only minimal resistance. However, if a large volume of air has been insufflated and the endoscope has been significantly manipulated in the stomach, the pylorus may be tight and difficult to traverse. In my experience this is a greater problem in large-breed dogs. Also, as the endoscopist becomes more experienced, it becomes easier to maneuver through difficult areas. I usually prefer to perform at least a cursory examination of the *entire* stomach before proceeding to the duodenum. In most cases I perform a final, more thorough gastric examination and procure biopsy specimens after duodenoscopy.

## RETROVERSION (J MANEUVER)

The importance of the retroversion maneuver is that it provides an en face view of the angulus and the cardia and fundus. On forward view only a tangential view of the angulus is obtained, and the cardia and part of the fundus are not seen at all. Failure to thoroughly examine the proximal stomach may cause the endoscopist to miss lesions (e.g., erosion, ulceration, or neoplasia) or a foreign body wedged in the cardia or fundus.

To provide an en face view of the angulus, the endoscopist must initiate the retroversion maneuver at a point proximal to or opposite the angulus (see Plates 5-6, 5-7, and 5-8). The scope is advanced along the greater curvature to the level of the distal body. The inner con-

trol knob is turned counterclockwise with the left thumb, and as the endoscope is gradually advanced, the angulus can be seen en face. Variations of normal appearance may be present (see plates at end of chapter). The endoscope tip is then deflected upward as far as possible (full counterclockwise rotation of the inner control knob) as the scope is advanced a little farther. This maneuver generally requires at least 180 degrees of tip deflection. Many newer endoscopes are capable of 210 degrees of upward tip deflection. This deflection provides a retroflexed view of the endoscope as it enters the stomach through the cardia (see Figure 5-3 and Plate 5-6, *D*). Pulling the endoscope back once this view is attained draws the endoscope tip closer to the cardia (see Figure 5-4 and Plate 5-8). A circumferential examination of the proximal stomach is completed by rotating the insertion tube or by turning the outer control knob in each direction for lateral deflection. Air insufflation is usually necessary to keep the proximal stomach dilated. During most of the examination the right hand is kept on the insertion tube to keep the tube in place with respect to forward and backward motion.

In cats the retroversion maneuver is started when the endoscope tip is in the mid-body area (see Plate 5-25). The tip is deflected upward as the endoscope is advanced. Because the working area is smaller than in most dogs, an en face view of the angulus is not achieved as often in cats.

Retroversion should be reversed gradually so that the mucosa can be further inspected. This can be accomplished by moving the deflection controls to a neutral position while the instrument tip is still in the proximal stomach. Alternatively the tip can be advanced to the proximal antrum while it is still in the retroflexed configuration. This provides an additional view of the proximal stomach and lesser curvature. When the angulus comes into view, the deflection knobs are returned to a neutral position. The antrum and pylorus should then be in view.

## PARADOXIC MOTION

Once the endoscopist has mastered a few basic techniques, the body and antrum can be quickly traversed in most cats and small- to medium-sized dogs. However, in some medium- to large-sized dogs, advancing the endoscope to the antral canal and pylorus can be quite difficult. Many beginning endoscopists often feel "lost" as they try to maneuver a scope in the stomach of a large dog. The most bothersome occurrence is the formation of a loop in the insertion tube as it passes along the greater curvature. As the tip of the endoscope is advanced toward the antrum and pylorus, the insertion tube invariably comes to lie along the greater curvature. The stomach can stretch considerably to accomodate intralumenal forces, and much of the forward force generated by the advancement of the scope is absorbed by the greater curvature so that the curvature is pushed caudally in the abdomen. A loop may form against the greater curvature (Figure 5-5). Endoscopically it may appear that as the insertion tube is advanced farther, the instrument tip is not moving in response or is actually moving away from the pylorus; this is termed *paradoxic motion.* Loop formation can occur readily, especially with newer, more flexible endoscopes and longer narrow-diameter instruments, as well as when the stomach contains a large volume of air. To reach the pylorus the endoscopist should continue to advance the endoscope until the greater curvature loop is fully formed and the tip begins to move forward again (see Figure 5-5, *B*). Further upward deflection of the tip using the left thumb on the inner control knob may be necessary.

Occasionally, if the gastric wall is considerably stretched, getting the endoscope into position to advance from the gastric body to the antrum may seem quite difficult. This is especially true if a narrow-diameter (9 mm or less), very flexible endoscope is being used. Rather than advancing into the antrum, the tip of the scope "swings by" the angulus and curves back into the gastric body as the endoscopist pushes it forward, despite efforts to control tip direction with the control knobs (Figure 5-6); this is called *inadvertent retroversion.* In this situation the insertion tube usually "hugs" a considerable length of the wall of the greater curvature (see Figure 5-6, *B*). The shape of the wall curvature may then be more in control of the direction of advance than is the endoscopist, who is only able to direct the short distal tip with the control knobs. This problem is best solved by withdrawing the endoscope tip to an area proximal to but still in view (forward view) of the angulus and antral canal, suctioning much of the lumenal air, and then read-

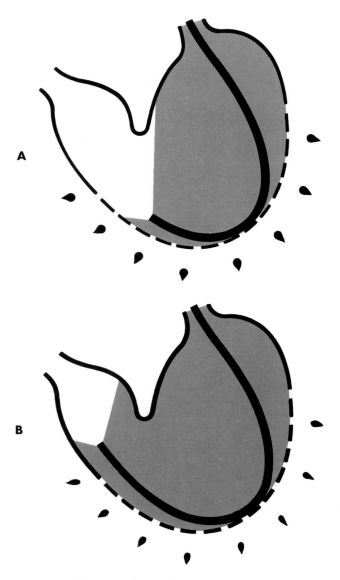

**Figure 5-5 A,** Effect of forward force by the endoscope as it pushes against the flexible greater curvature wall. The endoscope tip may not move forward in response to advancement of the insertion tube because the wall stretch accommodates some of its length. **B,** The point of paradoxic motion has been passed, and the endoscope tip is being advanced to the pylorus.

vancing the scope as close to the lesser curvature and angulus as possible. It is often useful to rotate the patient from left lateral to dorsal recumbency to change the configuration of the stomach and the approach angle to the antrum.

Use of *both* tip directional changes using the control knobs and simultaneous torque on the insertion tube with the right hand provides the best means for advancing the endoscope to the antral canal. This does not have to be done as one continuous motion. In some cases, it is best to advance the scope gradually,

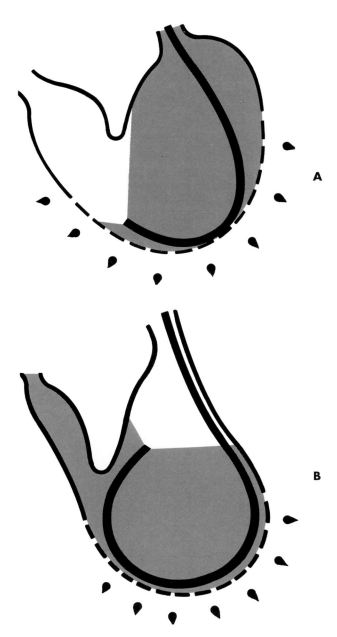

**Box 5-1** Maneuvering Tips for Overcoming Inadvertent Retroversion in the Stomach

- If loop formation continues to occur, retract the endoscope to the lower gastric body.
- Suction air from the stomach if it is too distended.
- Use both tip directional changes (by manipulating the control knobs) and rotation (torque) of the insertion tube to provide optimal maneuverability when advancing the endoscope.
- If advancing the endoscope into the antral canal remains difficult, rotate the patient from left lateral to dorsal recumbency to alter the approach angle to the antrum.

trol knobs and torque are important maneuvering components in this situation. For torque the right hand grasps the insertion tube close to the patient's mouth and applies a twisting motion.

It may still take several attempts before the antrum and pylorus are successfully reached. The beginning endoscopist needs to maintain patience while working through these "problem cases." With experience the maneuvers become routine. Important maneuvering steps are summarized in Box 5-1.

## ANTRUM

The antrum differs from the body of the stomach in that it has no rugal folds. Furthermore, peristaltic contractions are sometimes observed in the antrum, but not in the gastric body. To advance the scope from the distal body to the antrum, upward deflection (counterclockwise rotation of the inner deflection knob) is applied as the instrument tip is passed along the distal greater curvature. This usually reveals a view of the angulus. From this position the endoscopist can appreciate the appearance of two separate "tunnels," one on each side of the angulus (see Plate 5-6, *A*). The upper area is the gastric body—the first area viewed is the lesser curvature as it extends beyond the angulus—the more dependent tunnel is the antrum. From this location the retroversion maneuver can be performed, or the endoscope can be advanced to the antrum. As previously discussed, the endoscopist may elect to complete a thorough examination of the cardia and fundus at this time or may proceed directly to the duodenum with the intention of examining the proximal stomach later.

In *cats* the antrum can be easily entered in one of two ways. It is often helpful to rotate the insertion tube to the right when the endoscope tip is in the distal body. Once

**Figure 5-6 A,** Effect of forward force by the endoscope as it pushes against the greater curvature wall (same as Figure 5-5, *A*). The endoscope tip may not move forward in response to advancement of the insertion tube because the wall stretch accommodates some of its length. **B,** Excessive wall stretch causes inadvertent retroversion as the endoscope is advanced. In this situation the endoscope should be repositioned to a forward view of the angulus, and air should be suctioned before another attempt is made to advance the scope toward the antrum.

then stop to reorient the tip, then advance again, etc. (The same maneuvering technique is used to traverse the pylorus in difficult cases.) Once the endoscopist becomes more adept at the maneuver, the advance can be made more quickly. The *key point* is that both conthe insertion tube is rotated, it is advanced and the tip is simultaneously deflected upward (i.e., the inner control knob is turned counterclockwise). This reveals a view of both the antrum and pylorus. In some cats the crescent-shaped angulus is not located in the typical upward position (i.e., away from the tabletop). If the angulus is in a deviated position, the tip of the endoscope should be advanced to a position just beyond the angulus, and the control knobs should be used as indicated by the direction of the antral canal to point the tip in the proper direction. The insertion tube should be advanced *simultaneously* as the tip direction is adjusted. Applying rotation to the insertion tube is often quite effective in achieving necessary directional changes in cats.

Antral peristaltic waves may be observed when the endoscope is in the mid-gastric to distal gastric body. These are seen as round, symmetrical rings that form in the proximal antrum and sweep toward the pylorus as a rolling wave (see Plate 5-9). The contractions are generally not observed in cats unless metoclopramide or cisapride has been administered. When present, they usually occur at a frequency of three to four contractions per minute. Occasionally the endoscopist may find it difficult to keep the endoscope tip in proper position in the distal antrum to facilitate smooth passage through the pylorus when antral contractions are occurring. The pylorus is often persistently closed during periods of antral contractions.

Usually the antrum has no folds. Refluxed duodenal bile may be present, and in some cases active reflux can be observed during the procedure. The antrum should be evaluated carefully for the presence of mucosal hypertrophy or folds that may result from chronic inflammatory diseases or chronic gastric hypertrophy, polyps, ulcerations, and masses. When present, gastric neoplasia commonly involves the antrum and lesser curvature of the body. In dogs, adenocarcinoma is the most common malignant tumor of the stomach. Lymphosarcoma is the most common gastric malignancy in cats. (Various antral lesions are shown at the end of this chapter.)

## PYLORUS

In most animals the pylorus can be easily identified as the endoscope is advanced through the antrum. Variable degrees of dilation of the pyloric canal may be observed. In some cases the pylorus is persistently closed, and occasionally the exact location of the pyloric opening may be quite difficult to identify because of an overlapping fold of the pyloric ring or because the opening is obscured by fluid.

The cardinal rule in successfully advancing the endoscope through the pylorus is to keep the pylorus in the center of the endoscopic field. Because the pyloric position commonly changes slightly every time the patient breathes, small adjustments of the up/down deflection knob and minor changes in insertion tube rotation are required as the endoscope tip is gradually advanced toward the pylorus. These adjustments are made using the left thumb to turn the inner control knob and the right hand to rotate the insertion tube. In some large-breed dogs only a little of the insertion tube length is outside the dog's mouth at this point. It must be remembered that when the pyloric area is being examined, slow, gradual forces applied to the endoscope tip are generally more productive than rapid, "spastic" tip directional changes.

In many canine patients the endoscope tip can be passed through the pyloric ring without difficulty. This is especially true when the pyloric canal is open to any degree. In some cases the endoscope can be advanced from the mouth to the duodenum in as little as 30 seconds. Usually what has happened is that the endoscope is advanced through the stomach at a uniform rate to the angulus, and as the antrum is viewed, the pylorus can be clearly identified and is open. Because minimal air insufflation and manipulation of the stomach have occurred, the pylorus remains open and can be readily traversed. In this situation, it may be best to perform duodenoscopy and biopsies and to examine the stomach later. This approach is more common when an animal is suspected of having a primary small intestinal disorder rather than a gastric disorder.

In some cases the pylorus may be closed and offer significant resistance when the endoscopist tries to advance the scope into the duodenum. This may represent normal pyloric closure, or it may be an indication of disease, such as pyloric mucosal hypertrophy, an extrinsic mass, or another disorder. Based on experience, the endoscopist must judge how hard to push the tip of the scope against the pyloric ring. If considerable resistance is encountered and the endoscope tip can be only slightly advanced into the pylorus, it may not be possible to enter the duodenum. In my experience with dogs closure of the pylorus strongly suggests a diagnosis of pyloric mucosal hypertrophy. In Siamese, Burmese, and Tonkinese cats the pyloric canal tends to be quite narrow, but in most cases the duodenum can still be entered. Once adequate experience and manual dexterity are developed, the endoscopist can usually recognize a situation in which it is highly unlikely that the pylorus can be traversed. It is significantly more difficult to advance an endoscope greater than 9 mm in diameter through the pylorus of some cats. It is best not to apply excessive force in attempting to enter the duodenum.

The most important rule in negotiating a "spastic" or persistently closed pylorus is to keep the pyloric ring in the center of the endoscopic field as the endoscope tip is advanced. The pattern of motion of the pylorus as the animal breathes should be carefully noted. It may be beneficial to leave the endoscope tip stationary in the distal antrum for a minute or two while the pylorus is studied.

Then as the endoscope tip is *gradually* advanced, it should be kept in line with the most common location of the pylorus. Gentle but constant forward pressure should be maintained. In small patients the pressure is applied with the right hand as it advances the insertion tube.

When the proximal end of the insertion tube has already been advanced through the mouth in large dogs, the endoscopist places both hands on the endoscope control housing and applies pressure by leaning in toward the patient. At this point the endoscopist is in kneeling, crouching, or bent-over position. Occasionally the entire control housing is in the dog's mouth before the endoscope tip reaches the duodenum. Several maneuvers can provide sufficient insertion tube length for examination of the proximal duodenum when a 100-cm-long endoscope is being used. The newer, longer veterinary pediatric endoscopes have insertion tube lengths ranging from 125 to 150 cm. These insertion tubes provide extra length for advancing the scope to the duodenum in large dogs (see Chapter 6). When both hands are on the control housing, the right hand is used to make necessary directional changes by adjusting the control knobs.

A distinct sensation is often felt as the pylorus relaxes and allows the endoscope to enter the duodenum. Recognizing this sensation is important because the endoscopic view is obscured by a reddish hue as the tip advances through a compacted area. Because of the sharp angle between the pylorus and duodenum, it is necessary to make a directional change as soon as the pylorus is passed, so that the endoscope tip falls into the duodenal canal. If the directional change is not made, the endoscope tip can become wedged against the wall of the proximal duodenum (Figure 5-7). Turning both control knobs clockwise to deflect the endoscope tip in a downward and right direction facilitates advancement to the proximal duodenum. Once there, a view of the duodenal canal is obtained by turning the inner control knob counterclockwise. (This technique is described in detail in Chapter 6.)

Occasionally the opening of the pyloric canal is difficult to identify, usually because pooled fluid, a fold, or a mucosal rosette formation is obscuring the opening of the canal, or the pyloric canal is at an obtuse angle in relation to the antrum. In the latter instance a forward edge of the canal may be detectable, but it is quite difficult to turn the endoscope tip sharply enough to enter the canal (see Plate 5-20). In these occasional instances it is sometimes beneficial to rotate the patient from left lateral to dorsal recumbency. The change in position may alter the antral-pyloric configuration enough that the canal can be identified and then traversed. Once the endoscope is advanced to the duodenum, the patient is returned to lateral recumbency. (Various pyloric configurations are shown at the end of this chapter.)

Even when all proper steps are taken, advancing the endoscope through the pylorus can still be difficult in

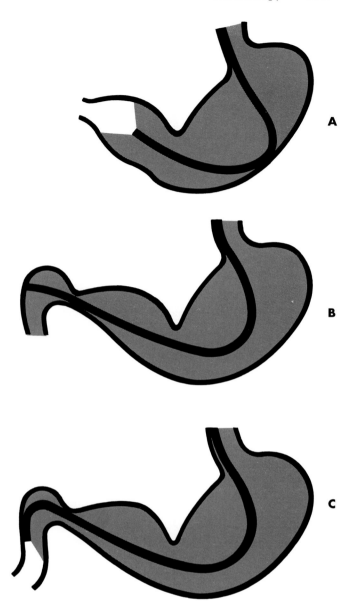

**Figure 5-7** Advance of the endoscope through the pylorus. In **B**, the endoscope tip is wedged against the wall of the most proximal aspect of the duodenum. A directional change is required to obtain a view of the duodenal lumen.

some patients. The most commonly encountered problem is deflection of the endoscope tip away from the pyloric canal as a result of excessive force against a tightly closed pylorus. The endoscopist feels considerable resistance as the scope is moved into the pyloric orifice; then as the tip is deflected away from the orifice, the scope suddenly advances easily. The shaft of the insertion tube can usually be seen as the endoscope becomes retroflexed (Figure 5-8). During subsequent attempts, every effort should be made to align the endoscope tip properly with the pyloric canal. If the stomach is overinflated, air should be suctioned. Occasionally it may help to lock the lateral deflection knob (outer knob) in place,

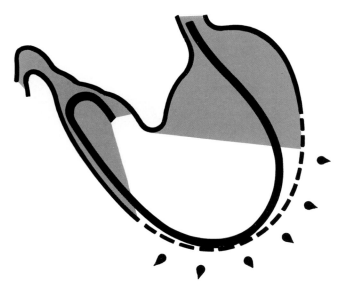

**Figure 5-8** Retroversion at the antral-pyloric junction. This occurs when the endoscope tip is not the correct angle to enter the pylorus.

but I usually prefer to maintain control of the endoscope tip by leaving the knobs free to move. This is especially important as the pyloric sphincter is passed.

An additional step that can be tried is to pass the biopsy instrument blindly through the pylorus and then use it as a "guide wire" over which the endoscope can be passed to the duodenum (see Plate 5-22). However, in some cases, it is difficult to pass the biopsy instrument through the tight angle between the pylorus and duodenum and far enough into the proximal duodenum to make this maneuver effective. In addition, when this maneuver is used, the endoscopist must be careful not to cause undue damage to the duodenal mucosa as the scope is advanced over the "guide wire." Sometimes as the endoscope is advanced over the biopsy instrument, the force generated by the scope pushes the tip of the biopsy instrument more deeply into the duodenal mucosa. Then the instrument "troughs" along the duodenum as it is advanced farther. In this situation, once the scope begins to pass through the pylorus the best way to prevent damage is to *retract* the biopsy instrument simultaneously and gradually as the scope is advanced. By the time the endoscope is in the duodenal canal, the biopsy instrument should be fully retracted inside the tip of the scope.

Traversing a narrow pylorus can be difficult and frustrating. In this situation the endoscopist should maintain patience and maneuver the endoscope methodically rather than abruptly and forcefully.

Some endoscopists occasionally use pharmacologic intervention to decrease pyloric tone and thereby facilitate passage of the endoscope through the pylorus. Glucagon can be administered intravenously (0.05 mg/kg [0.023 mg/lb] to a maximum of 1 mg) to suppress gastrointestinal motility and relax the pylorus. The promotility drug

metoclopramide is not beneficial for this. However, pharmacologic intervention is not needed for most diagnostic gastroscopy and duodenoscopy procedures. Once sufficient expertise is gained and a proper-diameter endoscope is used, the endoscopist can routinely advance an endoscope through the pylorus of most cats and dogs.

## FELINE GASTROSCOPY: SPECIAL CONSIDERATIONS

In cats, several special factors must be considered when maneuvering the endoscope through the pylorus. Because considerable force may be generated against the opening of the canal or at the angle of the pyloroduodenal junction as the endoscope is being advanced through a relatively narrow area, it is often necessary for the endoscopy assistant to hold the patient's body stationary to prevent it from being pushed along the table by the endoscope. Placing a hand behind the patient's head is usually sufficient. In addition, the endoscope can sometimes be advanced even if the tip cannot be lined up directly with the pylorus. In these instances, as the endoscope tip contacts a peripyloric wall, it often deflects into and through the canal in response to stretching of the orifice area by the advance of the insertion tube. The amount of force that should be applied is a matter of judgment and experience. Although a 9-mm-diameter endoscope can be passed through the pylorus of most cats, it is often easier to advance smaller scopes (e.g., 7.8 to 8.5 mm in diameter). These smaller endoscopes can more routinely be advanced to the duodenum in cats weighing less than 2.25 kg (5 lb). The endoscope configuration as the scope is advanced toward the antrum and pylorus of a cat is demonstrated in Figure 5-9.

Great care must be exercised in monitoring cardiopulmonary status during passage of the endoscope through the pylorus, especially in small cats and in any cat in which the pylorus seems narrow and particularly difficult to traverse. The pylorus of the cat is unique in that it is narrow and has a high constant resistance. In response to stretching and displacement of the gastric body and the pylorus, transient bradycardia secondary to vagal stimulation may occur. Significant respiratory depression also occurs occasionally. More commonly, the respiratory rate increases when moderate force is required to advance the endoscope through the pylorus. If cardiopulmonary status is significantly compromised, the endoscope should be withdrawn to the proximal stomach or esophagus and the stomach should be completely deflated. Once the patient is stabilized, the procedure can be resumed. It is rarely necessary for an endoscopist who is proficient in gastroscopy and duodenoscopy in cats to cancel a procedure because of transient complications. The cardinal rule is to recognize complications at their outset and to work as efficiently as possible to minimize procedure time in patients with a greater-than-normal anesthetic risk.

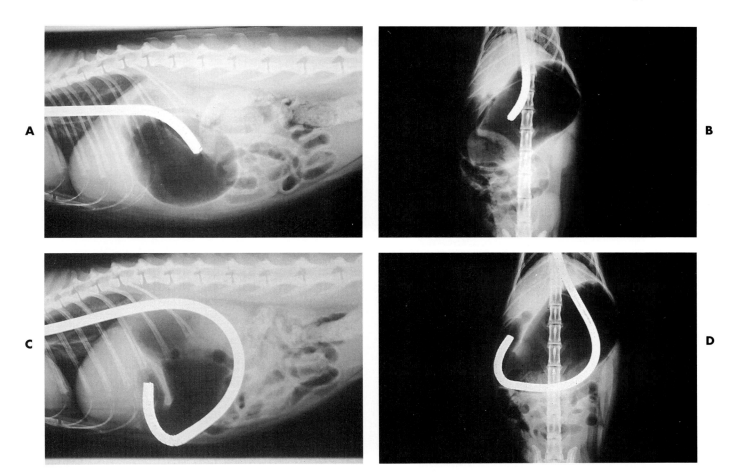

**Figure 5-9** Endoscope position and configuration during routine gastroscopy in a cat. (See also Plates 5-23 and 5-24 [gastric body] and Plates 5-29 and 5-30 [antrum and pylorus]. Lateral (**A**) and ventrodorsal (**B**) radiographs with the endoscope tip situated in the mid-gastric body. The stomach has been insufflated with air through the endoscope. This degree of distension allows for very thorough assessment of the gastric mucosa. Lateral (**C**) and ventrodorsal (**D**) radiographs with the endoscope tip positioned in the antral pylorus. In both views the incisura angulus fold can be seen as a distinct band of tissue (just to the right of the endoscope tip). Note the length of endo-scope that is in contact with the greater curvature of the stomach. In this position any advance of the endoscope tip is a result of force generated by the endoscopist pushing the insertion tube against the greater curvature. As the insertion tube slides along the greater curvature, the tip of the endoscope is advanced closer to the pyloric orifice and then into the duodenum. In the lateral view two distinct gas bubbles are seen in the descending duodenum (center of the field of view).

## GASTRIC BIOPSY TECHNIQUES

Gastroscopy is usually used to obtain biopsy samples. Samples should be obtained regardless of whether gross abnormalities are present. The purpose of endoscopic biopsy is to confirm the nature of a lesion and to exclude other diseases that have a similar endoscopic appearance. Many patients with a histologic diagnosis of mild to mod-erate gastritis have no gross gastric mucosal lesions, whereas patients with gastric motility disorders may have mucosal erythema but no histologic abnormalities. Gastric biopsy with endoscopic forceps is a *very safe* procedure.

Biopsy forceps with serrated edges or bayonet-type in-struments usually obtain good-quality mucosal biopsy samples. Commonly the submucosa is also sampled. Sample size is often smaller when straight-edge forceps are used. An adequate number of biopsy specimens must be taken to establish whether the stomach is normal. The best area to obtain biopsy samples is the *rugal folds* of the gastric body. These elevated areas are easy to grasp with the forceps, and adequate size samples for histo-logic evaluation are routinely obtained (Figure 5-10).

The entire biopsy procedure can be performed by the endoscopist. Alternatively an assistant can manip-ulate the biopsy instrument for the endoscopist. Gas-tric biopsy samples are usually obtained after duo-denoscopy has been completed. Once the entire stomach has been thoroughly examined, biopsy sites

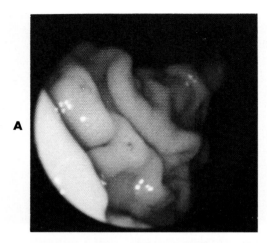

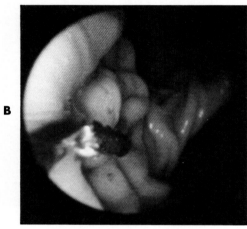

**Figure 5-10 A,** If the stomach is grossly normal, prominent rugal folds are the best area to obtain samples. If the rugal folds are flat, air should be suctioned so that the folds become more prominent and therefore easier to grasp. **B,** Advance of biopsy forceps onto a rugal fold.

are selected. If the stomach is grossly normal, four to eight samples are obtained from various areas of the gastric body. The antrum is not routinely sampled unless gross lesions are seen. Because the antrum generally has no folds, it is difficult to obtain adequate-size samples from this area. The stomach should *not* be overinflated during the biopsy procedure. If the rugal folds are markedly decreased in size or are completely flattened as a result of overinflation, the biopsy samples obtained are likely to be quite small and thus are more likely to be lost during processing. Meaningful histologic evaluation is also more difficult when small tissue samples are examined. The most common errors made in obtaining gastric biopsy samples are summarized in Box 5-2.

The biopsy forceps are extended beyond the endoscope tip and advanced to the area to be sampled (Figure 5-11). The endoscopist maintains control of endo-

**Box 5-2   Most Common Errors in Attempting to Obtain Gastric Biopsy Samples**

| ERROR | REASON |
|---|---|
| Overdistending the stomach with air | Rugal folds are too flat, which makes it more difficult to obtain adequate tissue purchase. |
| Attempting to obtain routine samples from the antrum rather than the gastric body | Normally the antrum has no folds; it is difficult to obtain adequate tissue purchase unless a raised fold or lesion is present. |
| Using straight-edge biopsy forceps rather than serrated-edge or bayonet-type biopsy forceps | Samples, although adequate in some cases, are often smaller when straight-edge forceps are used. |

scope tip direction using the left thumb on the inner control knob or on both controls if the thumb is long enough. When the biopsy instrument is close to the sampling site, it is opened and advanced firmly into the tissue. The stomach wall is usually pushed away to some degree as the instrument is advanced against the tissue. Once resistance to movement is met, the forceps are closed firmly. If an assistant is manipulating the forceps, the endoscopist should use simple, agreed-upon directions such as "open" and "close." As the forceps are withdrawn in the closed position, the mucosa that has been grasped is drawn up to the objective lens. A tissue sample is then torn off as the forceps are withdrawn into the accessory channel (see Figure 5-11). The endoscopist learns by experience the correct degree of force to apply on the biopsy instrument to remove a quality tissue sample. It is best not to tease a sample free gently or to tear a sample abruptly or forcefully away once mucosal contact is made with the accessory channel. These actions often result in a distorted or damaged sample. Rather, the biopsy forceps should be pulled to the endoscope tip, and then a firm steady tug should be applied to tear a tissue sample free. Once the sample is freed, the narrow area of gastric wall that was drawn up quickly returns to its normal position. The biopsy instrument is removed from the endoscope as the scope remains in position in the stomach. Biopsy-related mucosal hemorrhage is usually minimal (Figure 5-12). When gastritis or some other disorder causing mucosal damage (e.g., bile retention) is present, biopsy sample size and mucosal hemorrhage are often a little greater than normal.

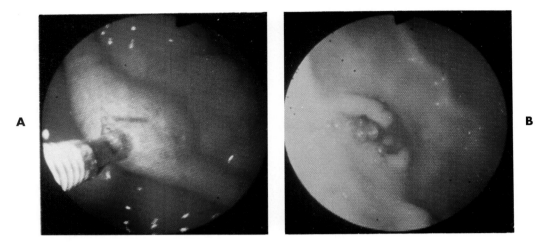

**Figure 5-11** Gastric biopsy technique. **A,** A rugal fold has been grasped and is being drawn up toward the objective lens. **B,** The sampled area quickly returns to its normal position as soon as the biopsy sample is torn free. Note hemorrhage at the biopsy site (center of field).

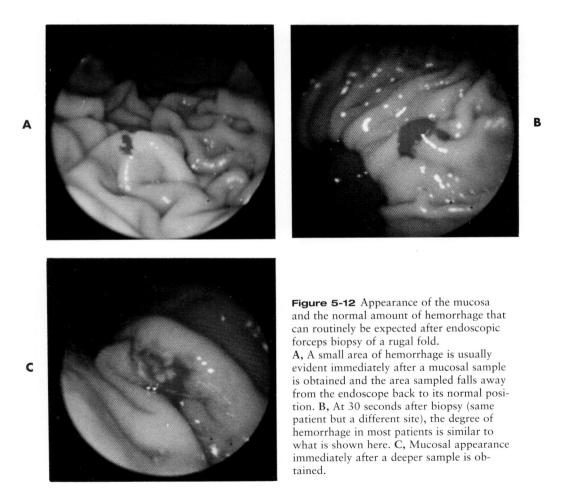

**Figure 5-12** Appearance of the mucosa and the normal amount of hemorrhage that can routinely be expected after endoscopic forceps biopsy of a rugal fold.
**A,** A small area of hemorrhage is usually evident immediately after a mucosal sample is obtained and the area sampled falls away from the endoscope back to its normal position. **B,** At 30 seconds after biopsy (same patient but a different site), the degree of hemorrhage in most patients is similar to what is shown here. **C,** Mucosal appearance immediately after a deeper sample is obtained.

It is usually preferable to advance the forceps directly into the mucosal folds at a 45- to 90-degree angle rather than to make a parallel approach in which the forceps tend to slide along the mucosal wall rather than make a firm tissue purchase. This may not be possible in some small patients with a narrow lumen. Because of this lumen it may be difficult to turn the endoscope tip to a precise degree so that the biopsy forceps can be directed into a small lesion (Figure 5-13). In this situation, serrated-edge or bayonet-type biopsy forceps are often quite effective for obtaining an adequate sample. Removing air from the lumen to create more of a fold effect may also be helpful. If a specific lesion is to be sampled, the endoscope should be maneuvered into position before a biopsy attempt is made. Samples can be obtained from the prominent angulus if difficulty is encountered in sampling other areas.

Biopsy samples of *erosive* or *ulcerative lesions* should be obtained at the *upper wall* where the lesion merges with normal-appearing mucosa. Caution must be exercised when maneuvering around the pit of an ulcer because of concern about causing perforation. Biopsy samples of superficial erosions can be obtained without concern.

*Masses* should be sampled as *deeply* as possible. Lymphosarcoma and benign gastric polyps can be readily diagnosed on biopsy, but adenocarcinoma and other neoplastic masses often must be sampled deeply to obtain diagnostic tissue. Superficial biopsy attempts may only retrieve fibrous or granulomatous tissue. Because it is not possible to obtain deep biopsy samples from a firm mass with standard endoscopy forceps on any one attempt, the endoscopist should sample the same site sev-

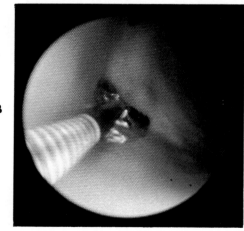

**Figure 5-13** Biopsy of a focal gastric erosion in a cat. **A,** Forward view of the distal gastric body with two small erosive lesions. The angulus is at the upper right. **B,** The endoscope tip could not be positioned at a 45- to 90-degree angle to the lesions. Obtaining biopsy samples from this type of lesion can be difficult because the forceps tend to slide along the mucosa when the endoscope is parallel to the wall. In this case, serrated-edge forceps were used to obtain biopsies.

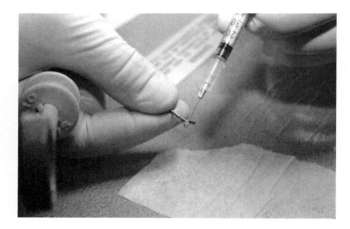

**Figure 5-14** The biopsy sample is gently removed with a small-gauge needle.

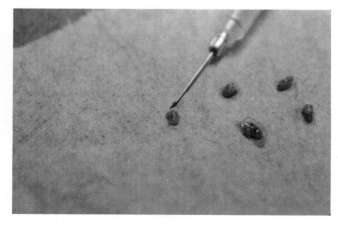

**Figure 5-15** Size of a typical gastric biopsy sample obtained with endoscopic forceps.

eral times, each time advancing the forceps a little deeper. Closure of the forceps should not be too abrupt or forceful. Brusque closure may cause the forceps cups to shear off a firm lesion without obtaining a specimen. On closing the forceps, an experienced endoscopist or biopsy assistant can usually appreciate that a lesion is unusually firm or hard. This tactile perception is often associated with malignancy. Usually, 10 to 20 biopsy samples are obtained when neoplasia is considered a likely diagnostic possibility so that the pathologist has adequate tissue to examine. A skilled endoscopist can accurately identify the site that is most likely to yield a positive biopsy.

Biopsy samples can be handled and prepared for shipment to the laboratory in several ways. (See Chapter 10 for a detailed discussion of sample handling.) I prefer to lift samples out of the forceps cups with a 22- to 25-gauge needle and gently place them on formalin- or saline-moistened lens paper (Figure 5-14). A typical biopsy sample size is shown in Figure 5-15. After all samples from a particular organ area are obtained, the thoroughly moistened paper is folded in several different directions to form a packet that is then submerged in a jar of 10% formalin solution (Figure 5-16). Filter paper, small cassettes, or small sections of cucumber can also be used for affixing samples (see Chapter 10). The samples should not be allowed to dry on the paper material because they may then adhere tightly to the paper and subsequently be damaged when they are removed at the histopathology laboratory. I do not attempt to orient the specimen in any way because attempts to rearrange the specimen may damage the tissue. The number of tissue samples obtained from each organ area should be indicated on the histopathology request form so that the histopathology technician knows how many "nippet" samples have been submitted. Biopsy samples obtained from each area (e.g., stomach, duodenum, ileum, colon)

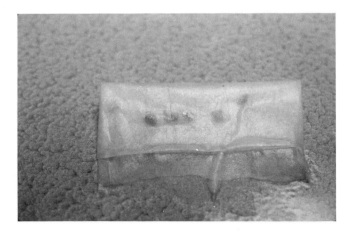

**Figure 5-16** Biopsy samples gently wrapped in moistened lens paper before submersion in formalin.

are placed in separate containers. If dissimilar lesions in the stomach or other area are sampled, a separate biopsy jar should be used for each lesion (e.g., one container for gastric body samples and a separate container for antral samples if specimens are procured from the antrum).

## CYTOLOGY

It is sometimes useful to obtain cells from the surface of a lesion for cytologic study. This can be done with a sheathed cytology brush or by making impression smears from a biopsy sample. A tentative diagnosis of gastric lymphosarcoma can often be made based on cytology. A new cytology brush should be used for each procedure and then discarded because this instrument is difficult to clean adequately. If a cytology brush is reused, malignant cells from one patient may be transferred to the cytologic sample of another animal. (See Chapter 10 for a more detailed description of the clinical utility of cytology in endoscopic procedures.)

## COMPLICATIONS OF GASTROSCOPY

Complications related to gastroscopy are uncommon. In cats and small dogs, retching occasionally occurs as a result of endoscope manipulation in the pyloric area. In this situation, air should be suctioned from the stomach, and the endoscope should be withdrawn to the distal esophagus. In some cases, forceful retching results in transient prolapse of a portion of the stomach into the esophagus (see Plate 4-66). An attempt should be made to suction any fluid that is forced into the esophagus. Once the retching subsides, the examination can be resumed.

Gastric perforation by an endoscope can occur but is extremely uncommon. To my knowledge, most reported cases of gastric perforation have occurred at the hands of experienced operators and have been directly related to excessive force applied during attempts to advance the scope through a region that was narrow and difficult to pass (especially the pyloric canal of a small cat). Significantly compromised gastric tissue can increase the risk of perforation. Experienced endoscopists have learned the range of force that can safely be applied in tight areas. When this degree of pressure is exceeded, perforation occasionally occurs. The keys to avoiding perforation are to always proceed with caution in difficult areas, use maneuvering skills to keep the tip of the endoscope as close to the lumen of narrow areas as possible, and if resistance is too great (e.g., a narrow pyloric canal in a small cat), know when to back off (see Plate 5-34). Occasionally, even a very talented and experienced endoscopist encounters a pyloric canal that cannot be safely traversed. Good technique and the use of proper instrument size can minimize the occurrence of complications.

Cardiac and pulmonary complications can result from anesthesia-related problems or prolonged overdistension of the stomach with air. Gaseous distension of the stomach can cause hypotension and bradycardia, which result from interference with venous return to the right heart, vasovagal stimulation, and compromise of respiratory muscles. Careful monitoring during the procedure and avoiding excessive gastric distension can prevent the majority of complications.

Perforation related to examination of an ulcer pit, an endoscopic biopsy, or the maneuvering of a sharp-edged gastric foreign body can occur but is extremely rare in small animals. The integrity of the gastric wall would have to be severely compromised for a routine biopsy technique to cause perforation. Great care should always be exercised when obtaining biopsies from deep ulcers.

## SUGGESTED ADDITIONAL READINGS

Cotton PB, Williams CB: Upper gastrointestinal endoscopy. In *Practical gastrointestinal endoscopy,* Oxford, England, 1982, Blackwell Scientific Publications.

Fox JG: *Helicobacter*-associated gastric disease in ferrets, dogs, and cats. In Bonagura JD, editor: *Current veterinary therapy XII,* Philadelphia, 1995, WB Saunders.

Graham DY: Peptic diseases of the stomach and duodenum. In Sivak MV, editor: *Gastroenterologic endoscopy,* Philadelphia, 1987, WB Saunders.

Guilford WG, Strombeck DR: Chronic gastric diseases. In Guilford WG et al, editors: *Strombeck's small animal gastroenterology,* ed 3, Philadelphia, 1996, WB Saunders.

Jenkins CC, Bassett JR: *Helicobacter* infection, *Compend Contin Ed Pract Vet* 19(3):267, 1997.

Johnson GF: Gastroscopy. In Anderson NV, editor: *Veterinary gastroenterology,* Philadelphia, 1980, Lea & Febiger.

Magne ML, Twedt DC: Diseases of the stomach. In Tams TR, editor: *Handbook of small animal gastroenterology,* Philadelphia, 1996, WB Saunders.

Serna JH et al: Invasive *Helicobacter*-like organisms in feline gastric mucosa, *Helicobacter* 2 (1):40, 1997.

Sivak MV: Technique of upper gastrointestinal endoscopy. In Sivak MV, editor: *Gastroenterologic endoscopy,* Philadelphia, 1987, WB Saunders.

Twedt DC: Diseases of the stomach. In Sherding RG, editor: *The cat: diseases and clinical management,* New York, 1994, Churchill Livingstone.

## COLOR PLATES   PAGES 114-172

## COLOR PLATES   PAGES 114-172

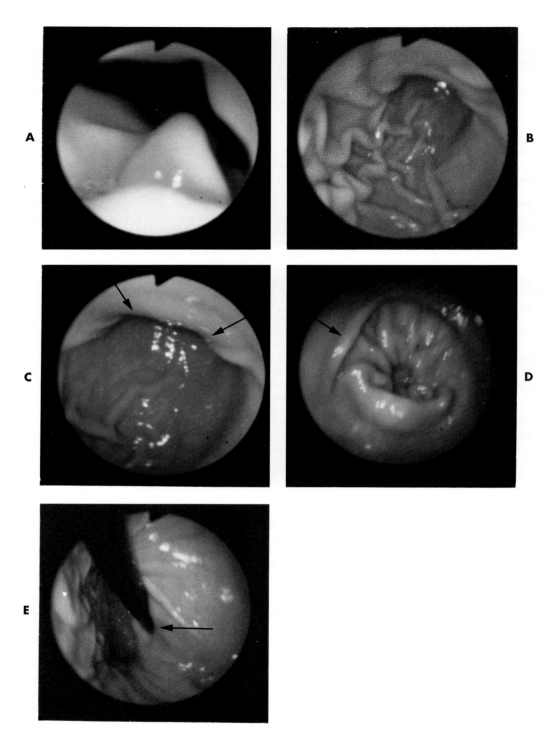

**Plate 5-1 A,** The first view of the stomach as the endoscope is advanced through the gastro-esophageal junction. The stomach walls often are collapsed as shown here, and the way forward may not be readily apparent. **B,** Moderate inflation quickly makes orientation easier. Rugal folds are in the forefront, and the angulus appears as a short curved fold in the upper right aspect of the field from the 12 to 2 o'clock position. **C,** Advancing the endoscope tip and deflecting the tip slightly to the right (outer control knob clockwise) bring the angulus into central view *(arrows)*. The stomach has been further distended with air. **D,** The endoscope tip is stationary in the same location as in C. An antral wave has changed the configuration of the angulus (long narrow fold in left aspect of the field at *arrow)*, distal body, and proximal antrum. **E,** Retroversion (J maneuver) provides a view of the cardia and fundus. The gastroesophageal junction is in the center of the field *(arrow)*, and the endoscope insertion tube is seen extending to the 11 o'clock position.

## RUGAL APPEARANCES

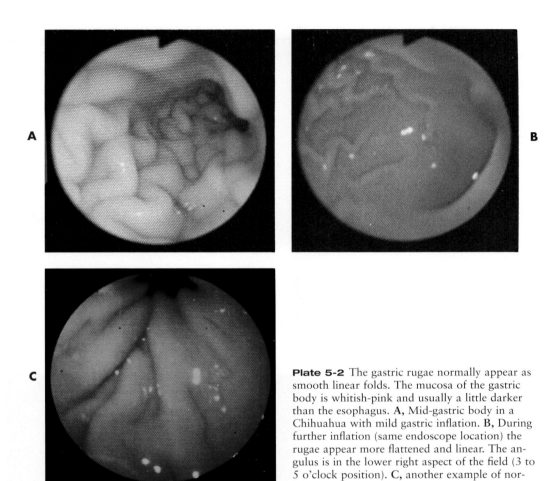

**Plate 5-2** The gastric rugae normally appear as smooth linear folds. The mucosa of the gastric body is whitish-pink and usually a little darker than the esophagus. **A,** Mid-gastric body in a Chihuahua with mild gastric inflation. **B,** During further inflation (same endoscope location) the rugae appear more flattened and linear. The angulus is in the lower right aspect of the field (3 to 5 o'clock position). **C,** another example of normal color and appearance of the rugal folds.

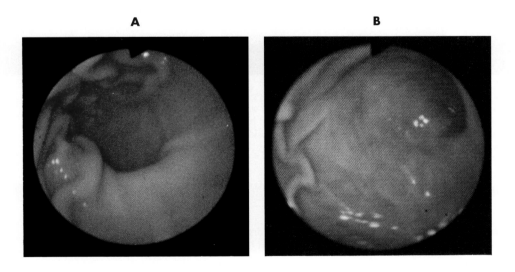

**Plate 5-3 A,** The rugae covering the greater curvature and posterior wall are more prominent than those of the lesser curvature (right and lower aspect of field of view). The angulus is just below center in the field of view. **B,** Occasionally, patchy color changes of the mucosa may be observed (here pink- and cream-colored changes). These changes, which are not considered abnormal, may occur in response to alterations in mucosal blood flow as a result of the effects of anesthesia or insufflation.

## RESIDUAL GASTRIC JUICE

It is not always possible to obtain good views when entering the stomach. Refluxed bile-stained duodenal fluid or residual gastric juice may obscure visualization of gastric mucosa. Small amounts of fluid are not considered abnormal. Fluid may be present in the stomach in animals that have undergone enemas or that have a gastric motility disorder.

**Plate 5-4 A,** Frothy saliva and bile-stained fluid in a schipperke that had received several enemas. No clinical signs suggested a gastric motility disorder. **B,** Froth and bile-stained fluid. Residual fluid can usually be easily aspirated, but the excessive use of suction may traumatize the mucosa, causing suction artifacts.

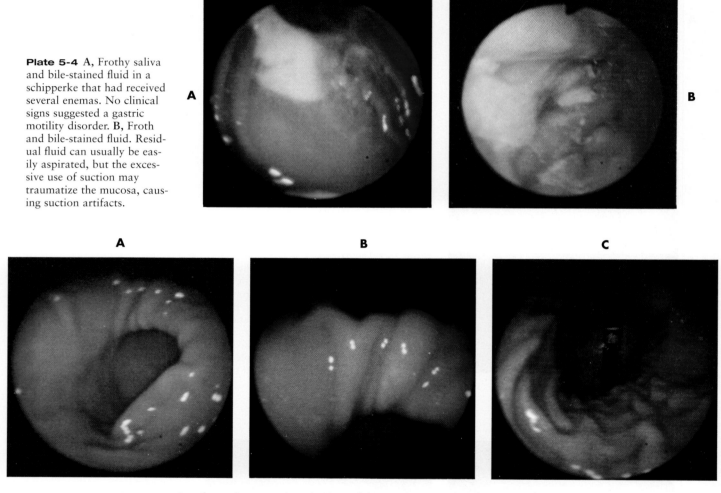

**Plate 5-5** Angulus and retroversion. **A,** View of the angulus (upper and right aspect of field) from the mid-gastric body. **B,** En face view of the angulus at the start of the retroversion maneuver. The antral canal is at the bottom of the field, and the gastric body is at the top. **C,** Increasing insufflation and further withdrawal of the endoscope in the J position provide a view of the gastric body, fundus, and cardia. The endoscope is seen in the central background.

## ANGULUS AND RETROVERSION (J-MANEUVER)

The angulus appears as a fold that extends from the lesser curvature. In medium to large size dogs the angulus may not be seen until the endoscope is advanced to the lower gastric body. In small dogs it can sometimes be identified after insufflating a small amount of air in the proximal stomach. The angulus may appear as either a sharp or flattened fold.

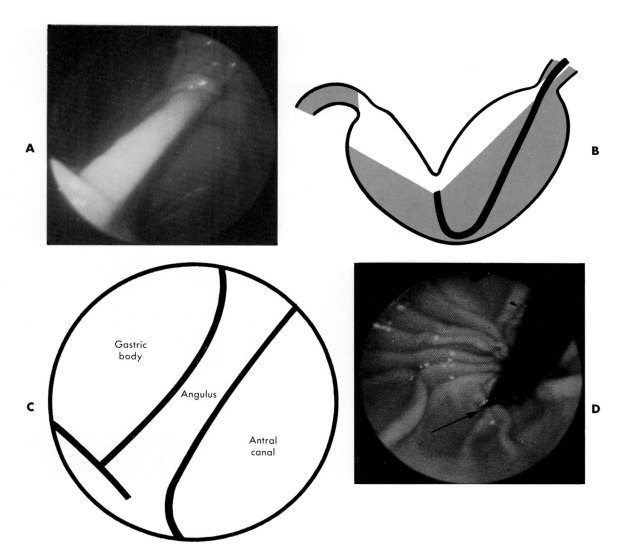

**Plate 5-6 A,** In this patient the angulus appears as a sharp fold in the center of the field. The endoscope tip has been retroflexed (same position as in Plate 5-5, *B*). The antral canal is at the right aspect of the field. The gastric body is to the left. **B** and **C,** Schematics depicting the endoscope position and the view seen in Plate 5-6, *A.* **D,** Completion of the J maneuver. After the angulus is viewed, the insertion tube is retracted while the endoscope tip is still flexed. The shaft of the insertion tube is observed in the right aspect of the field. The gastroesophageal junction *(arrow)* and surrounding folds appear normal.

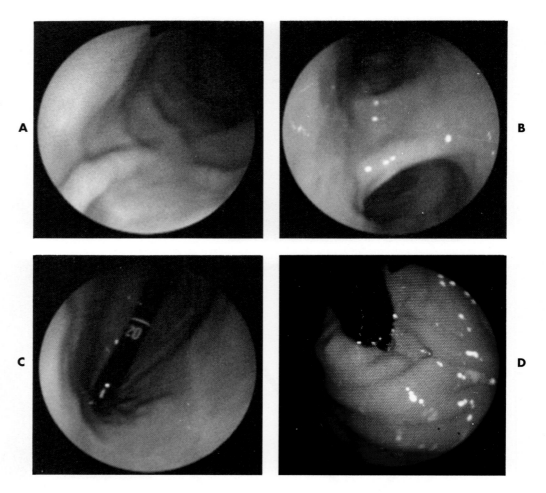

**Plate 5-7** Retroversion maneuver technique. **A,** Midgastric body with moderate insufflation. Tip deflection is initiated in the distal body to provide an en face view of the angulus. **B,** This flatter-appearing angulus is a normal variant. Deflection of the tip or rotation of the endoscope provides a more thorough view of the antrum (4 to 6 o'clock position) and pylorus. **C,** For a view of the cardia and gastroesophageal junction the insertion tube is retracted while the endoscope tip is still flexed. Panoramic views to thoroughly examine the fundus and cardia in large dogs are best attained by rotating the endoscope shaft with the right hand or by deflecting the control knobs to rotate the endoscope tip through various angles. **D,** Close-up view of the gastroesophageal junction from below, in retroversion.

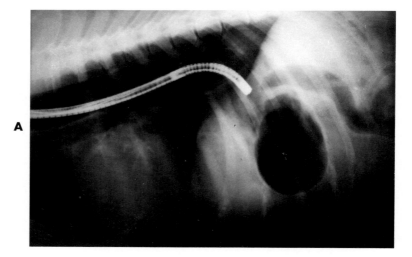

**Plate 5-8** Endoscope positions in the stomach of a 35-kg (77-lb) dog through a retroversion maneuver. **A,** The endoscope tip is angled to enter the proximal stomach from the esophagus.

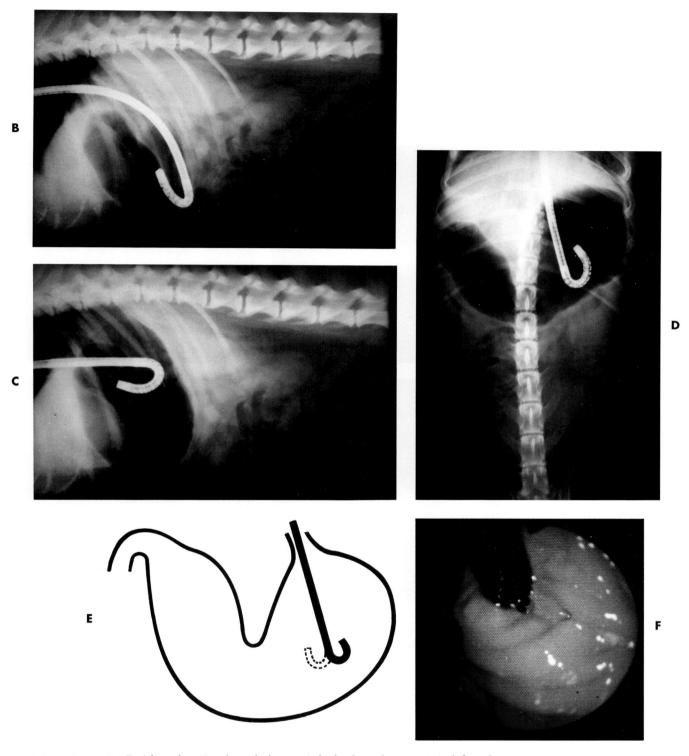

**Plate 5-8—cont'd** B, After advancing through the gastric body, the endoscope tip is deflected to a maximal degree in the area of the distal body and proximal antrum to provide an en face view of the angulus (the fold beyond the endoscope tip in this radiograph). The position corresponds to Plates 5-5, *B*, 5-6, *A*, and 5-7, *B*. This radiograph shows an air-filled antrum anterior to the endoscope. Lateral (C) and ventrodorsal (D) projections made after the insertion tube is retracted in the flexed position to provide a close-up view of the fundus, cardia, and gastroesophageal junction from below. In **D** the endoscope tip has been rotated through 180 degrees by applying torque to the insertion tube to provide a more complete view of the fundus. **E,** Endoscope position before *(dashes)* and after *(solid)* rotation of the entire insertion tube described in **D.** The degree of tip deflection can also be adjusted to provide a thorough view of the fundus. **F,** Endoscopic view of the gastroesophageal junction from below after nearly maximal withdrawal of the endoscope in the flexed position.

## ANTRAL CONTRACTIONS

Antral contractions are occasionally observed during gastroscopy. The contractions travel along the antrum in circumferential symmetrical fashion and sweep toward the pylorus as a rolling wave.

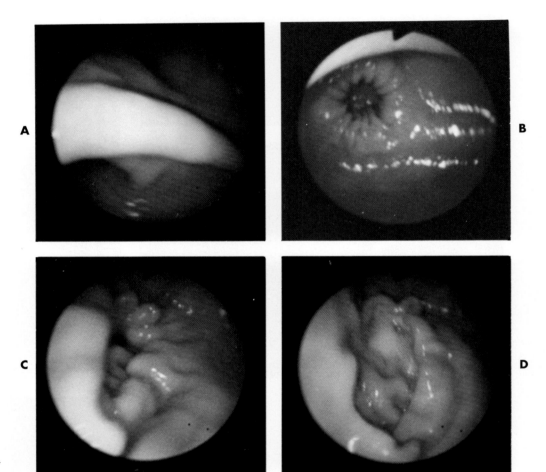

**Plate 5-9 A,** The endoscope tip is in the distal gastric body. The angulus is in the center of the field, and the antral canal is at the 7 o'clock position. **B,** As the wave begins, the angulus is seen at the uppermost aspect of the field. **C,** The pylorus is at the center of the field. **D,** The pylorus is obscured by white foam. The endoscope tip has not moved during this sequence.

## ANTRUM AND PYLORUS: NORMAL APPEARANCES

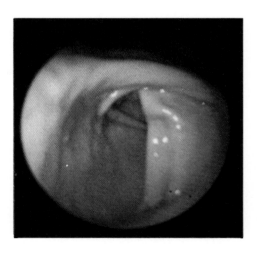

**Plate 5-10** Proximal antral canal in a greyhound as viewed from the distal body. The fold at the upper aspect of the field is the angulus. The pyloric orifice is not in view.

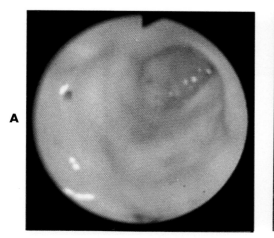

**A**

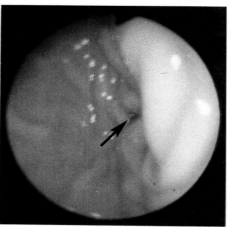

**B**

**Plate 5-11 A,** Antral canal in a Chihuahua. The pylorus is at the 2 o'clock aspect of the field and is closed. Two focal erosions are visualized (6 and 9 o'clock positions). Normally no folds are present in the proximal and mid antrum. **B,** The endoscope has been advanced toward the closed pylorus, which is visualized as a small darkened area just to the right of the center of the field *(arrow)*. In this situation, changes in tip deflection are necessary to properly align the endoscope with the pylorus.

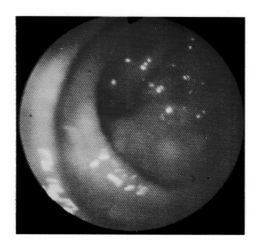

**Plate 5-12** Occasionally, small circular rings or a single flap surrounds the pylorus. This is a normal variant, as shown here in a Doberman.

**A**

**B**

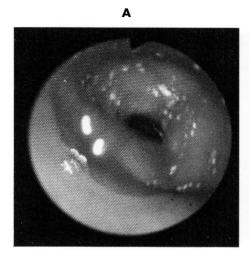

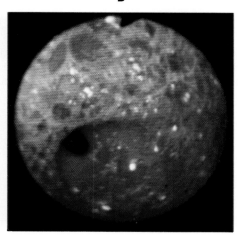

**Plate 5-13 A,** The pyloric orifice in a German shepherd was readily traversed with a 9-mm endoscope. Note the alignment of the pylorus in the center of the field. **B,** It is not unusual to see yellow bile-stained froth being blown into the antrum through the pylorus. Water flushing followed by suction usually restores clear vision and a readily identifiable path.

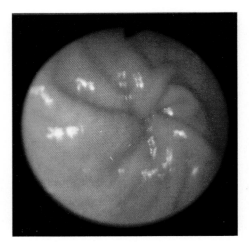

**Plate 5-14** Closed pylorus with rosette formation in a German shepherd. With minimal
gastric insufflation before antral examination,
careful alignment, and smooth control of tip
deflection, the pylorus was not difficult to traverse.

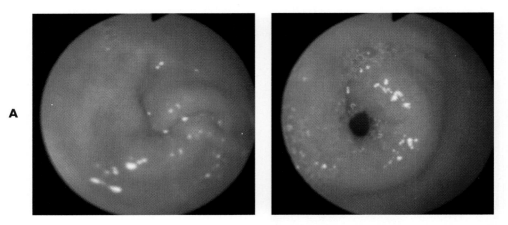

A

B

**Plate 5-15** Normal pylorus in a mixed-breed dog. **A,** The orifice is in the center of the field of
view. The pylorus remained closed on approach but was readily traversed with steady pressure.
A closed pyloric orifice is best traversed using slow steady motion and keeping the orifice as close
to the center of the field as possible. **B,** Appearance of the pylorus after the endoscope has been
retracted to the stomach following duodenoscopy. The orifice is slightly open.

## PYLORUS: DIFFICULT CASES

In some dogs the duodenum can be easily entered within 15 to 30 seconds of beginning the
endoscopic procedure at the esophagus. In others, however, great skill and patience are
required to advance an endoscope to the duodenum. The following cases illustrate some
of the difficulties that may be encountered.

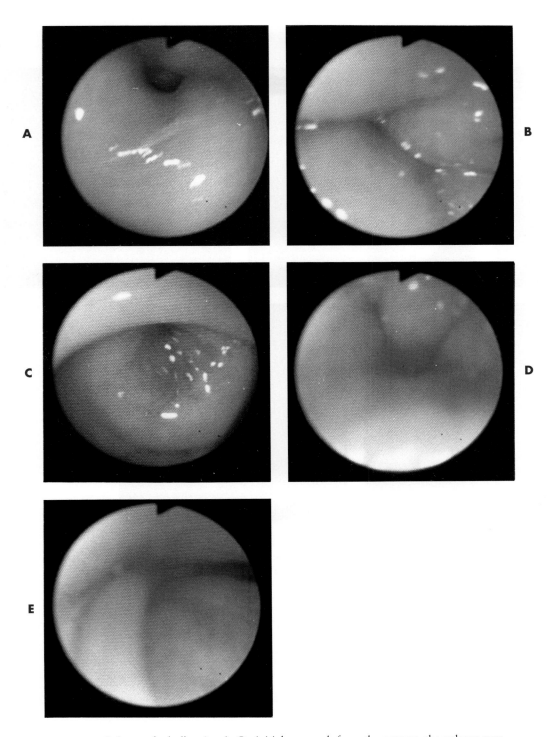

**Plate 5-16** Pylorus of a bullterrier. **A,** On initial approach from the antrum, the pylorus was slightly open. **B,** The orifice closed on initial contact, however, and the endoscope tip was deflected away to the distal body when an attempt was made to advance the scope. **C,** The pylorus configuration changed slightly. Note the flap above the pylorus, the appearance of a thickened rim around the orifice, and the mild mucosal erythema caused by endoscope trauma. The pyloric orifice is the slightly darkened area just beneath the upper flap. The endoscope tip was gradually advanced (fourth attempt), and the tip direction was adjusted based on changes in pyloric position. An adept operator can do this by using the fingers of the left hand to deflect *both* control knobs while advancing and withdrawing the insertion tube with the right hand. The insertion tube is grasped fairly close to the patient's mouth. The beginning endoscopist may find it easier to have an assistant control the advance of the scope, while the endoscopist uses the right hand to make control knob adjustments. **D,** Once the pyloric canal was entered, the walls pressed tightly around the endoscope. **E,** End of the pyloric canal just anterior to the duodenum. The linear off-white object in the left aspect of the field is a roundworm. Visualization routinely remains obscured through the pylorus until the duodenal canal is reached and insufflated.

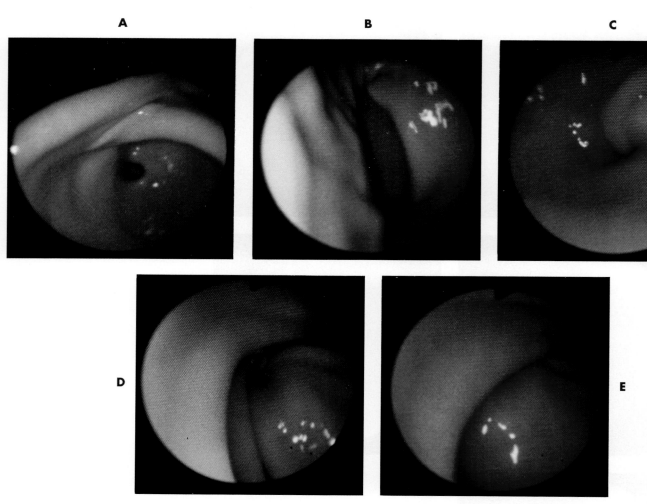

**Plate 5-17** Gastroscopy of a greyhound in which the entire working length of the endoscope (110 cm) was taken up by the time the endoscope tip reached the antrum. The endoscope had formed a large loop along the greater curvature. **A,** Angulus, antrum, and pylorus (slightly open). The endoscope could be advanced no farther using the current position and approach. In this situation the endoscope should be withdrawn to the proximal stomach. Then the stomach should be moderately deflated to shorten the distance to the antrum. **B,** The endoscope was then readvanced as directly to the antrum as possible. The angulus is the crescent-shaped fold in the right aspect of the field. Minimizing inflation often helps slightly decrease the length of insertion tube used during the advance along the greater curvature. **C,** The first several attempts to traverse the then tightly closed pylorus were unsuccessful. The endoscope control housing was nearly in the dog's mouth at this point. **D,** The configuration around the pylorus changed slightly during the course of the procedure. This is not uncommon when more than several attempts are made to traverse the pylorus. **E,** The dog was moved from left lateral to dorsal recumbency. This maneuver occasionally provides improved visualization or a better approach angle and consequently may facilitate entry to the pyloric canal. In this case the pyloric orifice has become obscured but is in the center of the field immediately below the flap. Because rotation was not particularly beneficial, the dog was returned to left lateral recumbency, and the endoscope was finally advanced successfully to the duodenum. The endoscopist negotiated the final short distance through the pylorus by placing both hands on the control housing (the right hand controlled tip deflection) and slowly leaning in, while in a kneeling position, to provide forward movement.

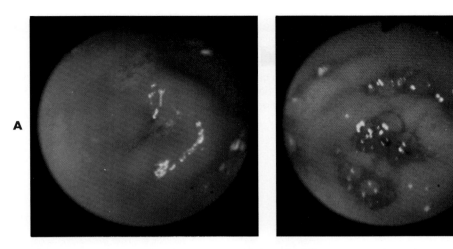

**Plate 5-18 A,** Tightly closed pylorus in a greyhound (different patient from Plate 5-17). The orifice is obscured by a small amount of white foam. The pylorus is properly aligned with the endoscope tip (i.e., in the center of the field). **B,** A small amount of hemorrhage has occurred because of trauma from several attempts to pass the 7.9-mm-diameter endoscope through the pylorus. The endoscope was passed after 4 minutes of maneuvering. The minor mucosal hemorrhage here is inconsequential.

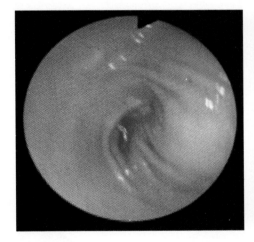

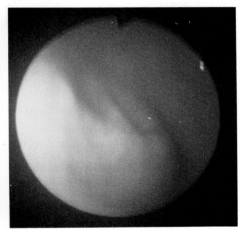

**Plate 5-19** In some dogs it is at first difficult to identify the exact location of the pyloric orifice. In this standard poodle the pylorus is closed and the orifice is located at the upper confluence of the vertical folds (immediately above the small pool of hemorrhage). The endoscope was successfully passed to the duodenum. *If the pyloric orifice cannot be identified after examination of the distal antrum and folds, the dog should be rotated to dorsal recumbency.*

**Plate 5-20** In this dog the edges of the pyloric orifice are flat, and the pyloric canal is at a sharp angle to the left. It would be extremely difficult to gain proper alignment of the endoscope with the pylorus in this configuration. Rotating the dog to dorsal recumbency allowed for better alignment, and the pylorus was successfully traversed.

# PYLORUS: OBSTRUCTED VIEW

Food or other material (e.g., hair, foreign body) in the antrum at the time of gastroscopy may obscure the pylorus. The endoscope tip can be deflected in various directions to move soft material away, and water flushing may help displace cloudy liquid. Suction should be used cautiously to avoid blocking the accessory channel particulate matter.

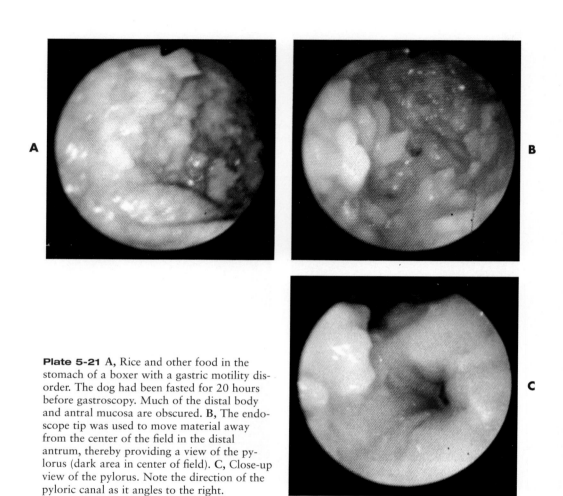

**Plate 5-21 A,** Rice and other food in the stomach of a boxer with a gastric motility disorder. The dog had been fasted for 20 hours before gastroscopy. Much of the distal body and antral mucosa are obscured. **B,** The endoscope tip was used to move material away from the center of the field in the distal antrum, thereby providing a view of the pylorus (dark area in center of field). **C,** Close-up view of the pylorus. Note the direction of the pyloric canal as it angles to the right.

A                                    B                                    C

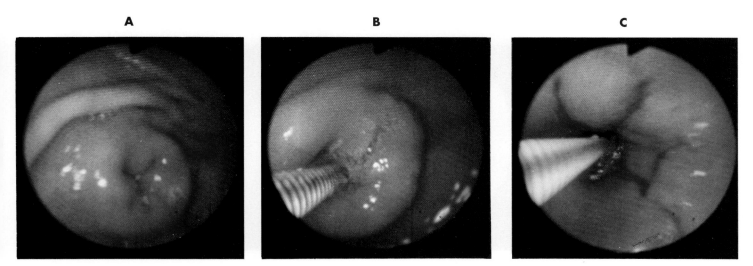

**Plate 5-22** If the pylorus proves particularly difficult to traverse, the biopsy forceps can sometimes be used as a guide wire over which the endoscope can be advanced to the duodenum. With the endoscope situated in the distal antrum, the closed forceps are advanced through the pylorus and down the descending duodenal canal. Because of a sharp angle at the pylorus, duodenal bulb, and descending duodenum, the forceps cannot be advanced far enough in some dogs for this maneuver to be successful. Excessive force should not be applied to the duodenal bulb. **A,** This closed pylorus in a collie was particularly difficult to enter. **B,** The biopsy forceps has been advanced through the pylorus and into the descending duodenum. **C,** View of the descending duodenum. The streaks of hemorrhage resulted from duodenal mucosal trauma that occurred during attempts to pass the biopsy forceps.

## NORMAL APPEARNACES: FELINE STOMACH

The normal feline stomach is pale pink and has smooth rugal folds that are more prominent along the greater curvature, as well as a readily identifiable angulus and flat antral walls. Small folds are present in the distal antrum around the pylorus in some cats. Although the stomach is completely empty in almost all cats that have been properly fasted, it is not unusual to find small amounts of hair material present. Occasionally a small pool of residual gastric fluid or streaks of bile-tinged fluid are present, and this is not considered abnormal. Only minimal intermittent air insufflation is generally necessary to maintain gastric dilation sufficient for thorough examination in cats.

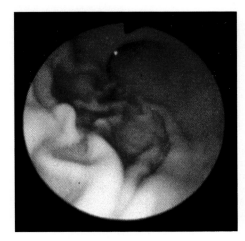

**Plate 5-23** Gastric body as viewed from the proximal stomach in a cat. A small amount of air was insufflated to separate the gastric walls. Note the crescent-shaped angulus at the upper aspect of the endoscopic field of view.

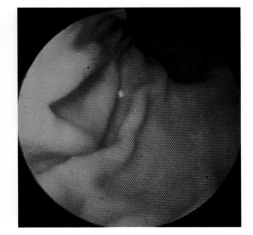

**Plate 5-24** Mid-gastric and distal gastric body. The angulus in this cat extends toward the middle of the field from the 2 o'clock position. The antrum can be reached by rotating the insertion tube to the right while deflecting the endoscope tip upward (turning the inner control knob counterclockwise) and simultaneously advancing the insertion tube.

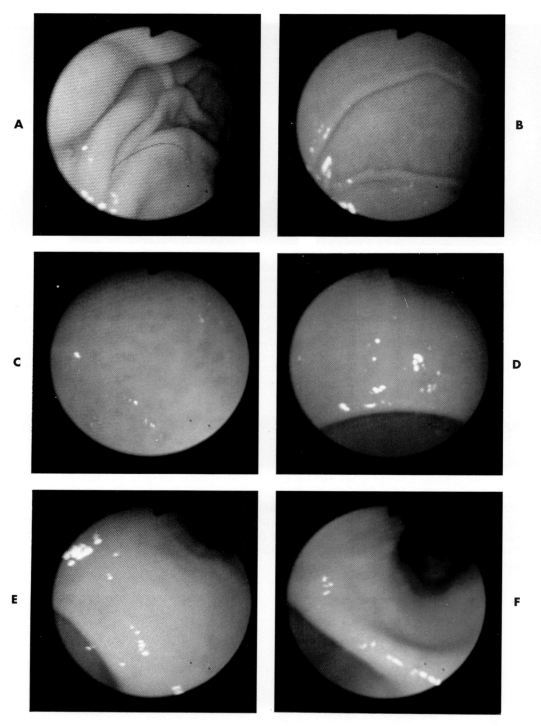

**Plate 5-25** Gastric examination in an 8-year-old male Burmese cat with hyperthyroidism and primary clinical signs of vomiting and diarrhea. The gastric examination and biopsies were normal, but enterocolitis was identified on duodenal and colonic biopsies.
**A,** Greater curvature with mild gastric distension. A single hair is present in the foreground. This view was obtained by deflecting the endoscope tip to the left (turning the outer control knob counterclockwise) in the distal esophagus as the endoscope was directed through the gastroesophageal junction. Invariably the greater curvature is the first area of the stomach that is visualized. **B,** View of the same site as in Plate 5-24, *A,* after air has been insufflated to moderately distend the stomach. This allows for more thorough mucosal examination. **C,** Small pocklike lesions in the fundus are a normal variant occasionally found in cats. This view can be obtained by pulling the endoscope back and deflecting the tip downward (turning the inner control knob clockwise) or by deflecting the tip downward immediately after entering the stomach. **D, E,** and **F,** En face view of the angulus in the sequence of its examination. **D,** Retroversion was begun in the distal body and proximal antrum. The antrum is in the lower aspect of the endoscopic field of view (5 to 7 o'-clock position). **E,** The insertion tube was then advanced farther with the endoscope tip in the flexed configuration. The wall of the lesser curvature fills most of the field. A small area of the antrum is seen at the 6 to 8 o'clock position. The shaft of the insertion tube can be faintly seen as it enters the stomach (1 o'clock position). **F,** With advancement of the insertion tube, which is in part wedged against the greater curvature, the angulus could be visualized at a different angle. The proximal stomach is in the upper right aspect of the field, and the antrum is in the lower left.

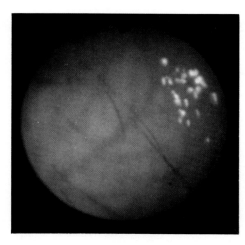

**Plate 5-26** Proximal stomach at maximal distension. Note the mucosal blood vessels and hair strands. This degree of gastric distension is not necessary for a thorough examination. If this much distension occurs, air should be suctioned before significant cardiopulmonary compromise occurs.

A

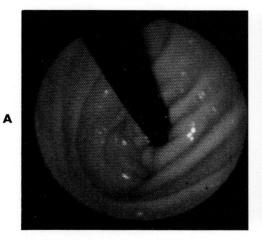

B

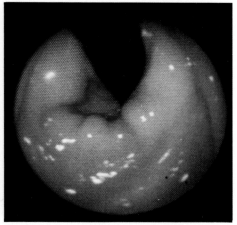

**Plate 5-27** Gastroesophageal junction as viewed from below (retroversion). **A,** Normal fundus. The endoscope is seen coming through the junction. **B,** The endoscope has been withdrawn with the tip in the flexed position to provide a close-up view of the cardia and gastroesophageal junction.

# FELINE ANTRUM AND PYLORUS: NORMAL APPEARANCES

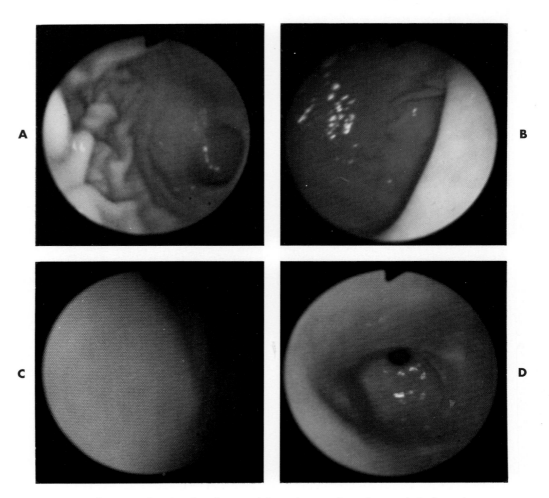

**Plate 5-28** Sequence showing the advance of the endoscope from the gastric body to the py-lorus. **A,** View from the mid-gastric body with moderate distension. The greater curvature rugal folds are in the left aspect of the field of view, and the angulus fold is at the 3 o'clock position. **B,** The endoscope has been advanced to the distal body. The angulus fills the right aspect of the field. Immediately after the endoscope tip passes the angulus, the insertion tube is rotated to the right (using the right hand) and the endoscope tip is deflected upward. Gradual forward motion is continued throughout this maneuver. **C,** Close-up view of the proximal antral mucosa as the endoscope is passed through the tight angle between the gastric body and the antrum. **D,** Mid-antrum with the pylorus in the center of the field. Note the flat antral walls. In cats the pylorus is commonly open to the degree shown here.

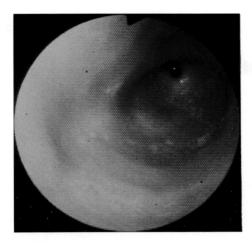

**Plate 5-29** Proximal antral canal. Note the flat walls. It is not unusual to observe small amounts of refluxed duodenal fluid or active reflux occurring during examination of the antrum and pylorus. Note the slightly open pylorus at the 2 o'clock position.

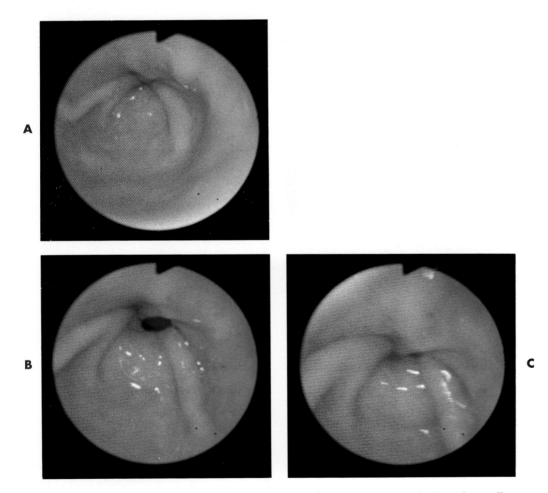

**Plate 5-30** Sequence of antrum and pylorus photographs in a Siamese cat. **A,** Note the small folds around the pylorus. **B,** The pylorus has opened slightly. As this structure is gradually approached, it should be kept in the center of the field. **C,** The pylorus has closed as the endoscope is advanced to the orifice. The endoscope tip is properly aligned. With minimal force the 7.9-mm endoscope was advanced through the pylorus. (Time sequence: of A through C—10 seconds.)

# ENTERING THE PYLORUS

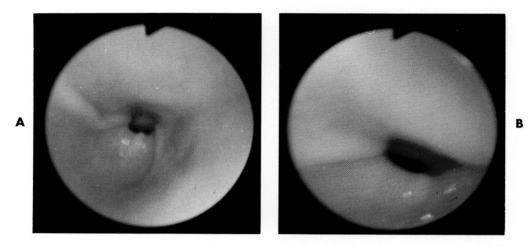

**Plate 5-31 A,** View of the distal antrum as a slightly open pylorus is approached. **B,** The pylorus has remained open. Note the curving wall within the pyloric canal (just beyond pyloric orifice). To advance the endoscope through the pylorus to the duodenum, the endoscopist should deflect the tip of the scope downward and to the left (turning both control knobs clockwise) once the canal has been entered.

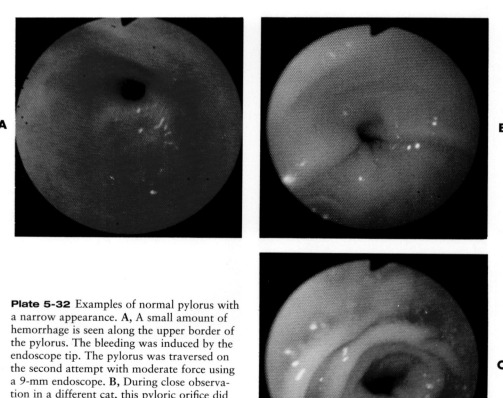

**Plate 5-32** Examples of normal pylorus with a narrow appearance. **A,** A small amount of hemorrhage is seen along the upper border of the pylorus. The bleeding was induced by the endoscope tip. The pylorus was traversed on the second attempt with moderate force using a 9-mm endoscope. **B,** During close observation in a different cat, this pyloric orifice did not dilate to any significant degree. However a 7.9-mm endoscope was advanced without significant difficulty. **C,** The same pylorus immediately after duodenoscopy was completed and the endoscope was withdrawn back through the pyloric orifice.

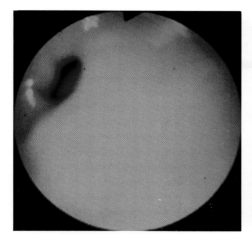

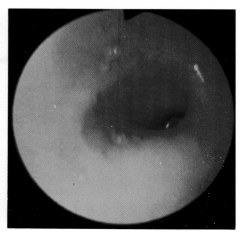

**Plate 5-33** In some cats it is difficult to align the pylorus in the center of the endoscopic field. In this view, the endoscope tip is almost touching the antral wall adjacent to the pyloric orifice. The pylorus was entered by sliding the endoscope tip along the wall and applying steady forward pressure until the scope slipped into the orifice.

**Plate 5-34** Narrow pyloric canal in a Siamese cat that could not be traversed with a 7.9-mm endoscope. Although the orifice could be entered, the pyloric canal was quite narrow and did not stretch sufficiently. The pylorus of Siamese cats commonly seems to be more narrow than that of other cats. After making several attempts, the experienced endoscopist is able to recognize that the pylorus cannot be successfully traversed. When this point is reached, no further efforts should be made.

## CHRONIC GASTRITIS: VARIOUS APPEARANCES (CANINE)

Various endoscopic appearances can be seen in patients with gastritis, ranging from normal in some patients with mild gastritis to marked mucosal irregularity and friability in patients with severe gastritis. Since gastritis is a diagnosis that can be established and characterized based on biopsy, tissue should be routinely obtained during gastroscopy for histologic evaluation. *A diagnosis of gastritis cannot be excluded based on normal gastric mucosal appearance.*

**A**
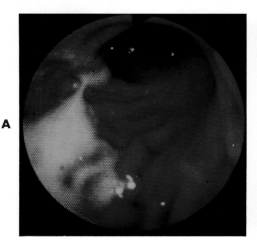

**B**
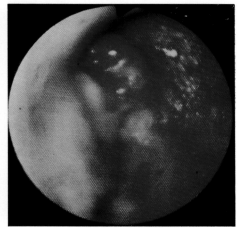

**Plate 5-35** Moderate lymphocytic, plasmacytic gastritis with mild fibrosis in a 6-year-old Irish setter with chronic intermittent vomiting. The vomiting had recently increased in frequency. **A,** Note the generalized mucosal erythema. The rugal folds of the greater curvature are in the foreground, along with foam and several streaks of bile-tinged fluid. The angulus is at the uppermost aspect of the field of view (at the pointer), and the proximal antral canal is just below it. **B,** Erythema of the distal antrum and pyloric orifice. The pylorus is to the left of the pointer at the 11 o'clock position.

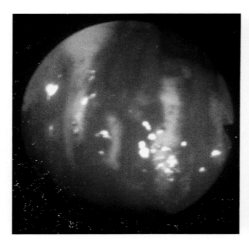

**Plate 5-36** Severe erythema, mucosal hemorrhage, and bile-stained foam along the mucosa in a 3-year-old Great Dane with severe acute gastritis. This is an en face view of a wide angulus. The gastric body is to the left.

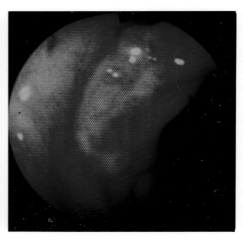

**Plate 5-37** Thickened gastric folds and a superficial "blister" (upper middle in the field of view) in a 5-year-old German shepherd dog with eosinophilic gastritis. The antral canal is to the right (3 o'clock position).

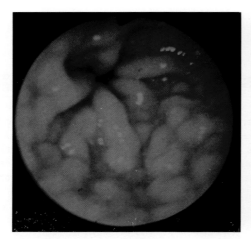

**Plate 5-38** Thickened raised areas of mucosa in the antrum of a mixed-breed dog with chronic intermittent vomiting. Note the pylorus at the convergence of folds at the 11 o'clock position. The histologic diagnosis was moderate fibrosing lymphocytic, plasmacytic gastritis. Gastric lymphosarcoma was a leading differential.

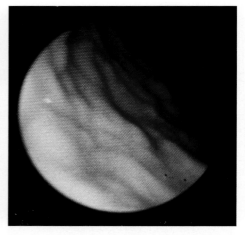

**Plate 5-39** Irregularity of the rugal folds in a basset hound with intermittent vomiting and salivation. The histologic diagnosis was mild to moderate lymphocytic, plasmacytic gastritis with fibrosis. No erosive changes or erythema is seen.

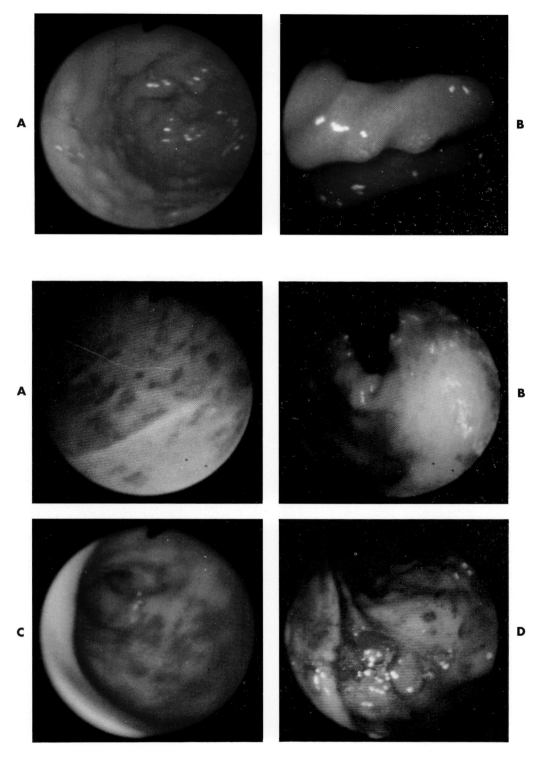

**Plate 5-40 A,** Multiple follicular, raised areas in the antrum of a 10-month-old standard poodle with chronic vomiting of 6-months duration. The pylorus is closed (to the right of midline at the 2 to 3 o'clock position). **B,** En face view of the angulus, showing two follicular lesions on the lower border. Bile-tinged fluid is seen on the surface. The histologic diagnosis was mild to moderate lymphocytic, plasmacytic, eosinophilic gastritis.

**Plate 5-41** Chronic gastritis in a 13-year-old schnauzer with recent onset of persistent vomiting. **A,** Multifocal superficial erosive lesions in the distended gastric body. **B,** Mucosa of the fundus and cardia as viewed on retroversion maneuver. Foam and erosions are seen. **C,** Mucosal erythema of the antral canal. The pylorus is at the upper left (11 o'clock position). **D,** Greater than normal hemorrhage that occurred after a single mucosal biopsy (foreground). This is a retroversion view with the angulus at the bottom right, (5 o'clock position), the lesser curvature in the right foreground, and the greater curvature rugal folds in the left foreground. The insertion tube is barely visible at the top, just to the right of midline. The histologic diagnosis was multifocal erosive gastritis with fibrosis.

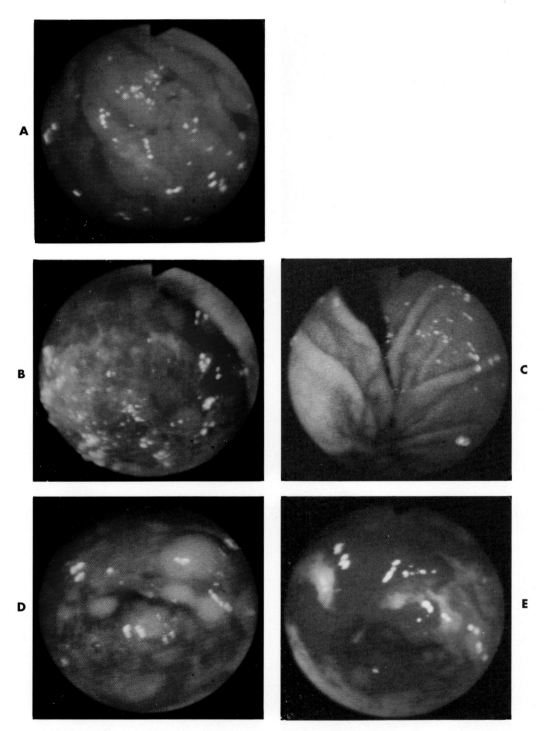

**Plate 5-42 A,** Close-up view of the rugal folds of the distal greater curvature (moderate gastric distension). The folds appeared edematous and bled easily on contact (note the focal areas of hemorrhage). **B,** Distal greater curvature just beyond the view shown in **A.** The angulus extends from the 12 to 4 o'clock positions at the edge of the field. Note the severe erythema and the friability of the mucosa. **C,** Proximal stomach (mild distension) as viewed on retroversion maneuver. The insertion tube shaft is at the 11 o'clock position. The proximal one-half of the stomach was grossly normal. **D,** Distal antrum and pylorus (narrow horizontal opening in center of field) as seen before biopsy. Note the vesicle-like changes around the pyloric orifice. **E,** After two biopsy samples were obtained, marked hemorrhage occurred around the pylorus. Normally it is quite difficult to obtain adequate-size tissue samples from the antrum and pylorus. Furthermore, minimal to no hemorrhage usually occurs. The cause of the pyogranulomatous gastritis was undetermined.

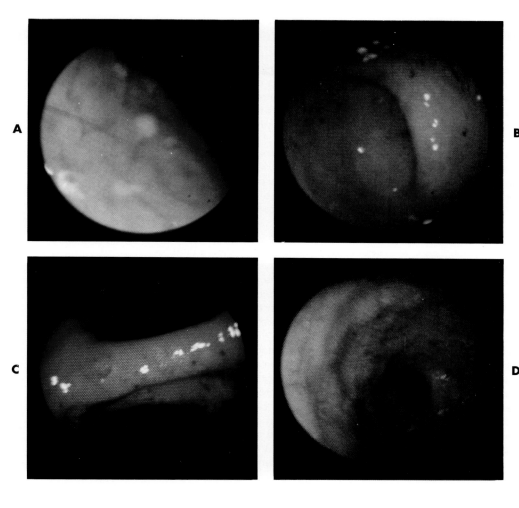

**Plate 5-43** Follow-up gastroscopy conducted 6 weeks after the initial diagnosis in the patient depicted in Plates 5-41 and 5-42. The animal's clinical condition had improved, and no vomiting had occurred for 4 weeks. Treatment included prednisone, metronidazole, famotidine (2 weeks), and sucralfate (4 weeks). **A,** Distal gastric body mucosa (compare with Plate 5-41, *A*). The mucosa has a reticular pattern. **B,** Distal gastric body with the angulus just to the right of midline (from the 11 to 5 o'clock positions). The dark spots in the upper right, middle right and far left are focal areas of hemorrhage ("coffee-ground" color). This is nearly the same endoscope position as in Plate 5-41, *B*. **C,** En face view of the angulus showing the pinpoint areas of hemorrhage. The mucosa was significantly less friable at follow-up. **D,** Antrum and pylorus. A small amount of fluid residue is present in the antral canal. Note the dramatic improvement compared with Plate 5-42, *D* and *E*.

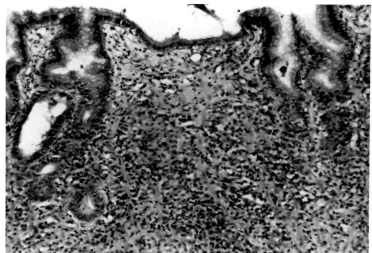

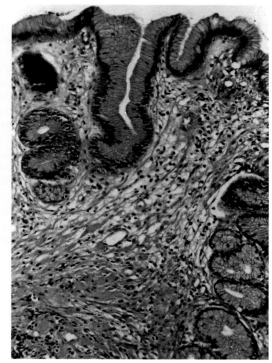

**Plate 5-44** Comparison photomicrographs. **A,** The photomicrograph of a biopsy sample obtained at initial endoscopic examination shows a massive infiltration of neutrophils, histiocytes, and lymphocytes × 200). Surface erosion and necrosis are also seen. The diagnosis was severe, erosive, ulcerative necrotizing and pyogranulomatous gastritis. **B,** Photomicrograph obtained at 6-weeks follow-up shows dramatic resolution of the erosive and inflammatory lesions (×200). Mild fibrosis, probably a sequela to the previous necrotizing process, is the only significant lesion. (Courtesy Stephen J. Engler.)

# Helicobacter-Associated Gastritis

The gastric spiral bacteria *Helicobacter pylori* is now well recognized as a significant cause of various forms of upper gastrointestinal problems in humans, including chronic gastritis with varying degrees of inflammation (nonerosive nonspecific gastritis is the most common type seen), nonulcer dyspepsia, and gastric and duodenal ulcers. Furthermore, epidemiologic evidence supports an association between *H. pylori* infection and gastric cancer in humans.

*Helicobacter* organisms have long been known to be present in the stomachs of animals, and it is speculated that these organisms are normal inhabitants. However, in some animals, it is likely that *Helicobacter* infection can cause chronic gastritis and in rare cases gastric ulceration. *Helicobacter felis* and *Helicobacter heilmanii* appear to be the most common species affecting dogs and cats. In ferrets, *Helicobacter mustelae* is known to cause significant gastrointestinal disease (both ulceration and neoplasia).

Endoscopic examination and biopsy have become very important to the diagnosis of *H. pylori*-associated disease in humans. Endoscopy is also important in the ongoing investigation of *Helicobacter*-associated problems in animals as researchers and clinicians work to determine more specifically the true role of these bacteria in animal diseases.

Tests for *Helicobacter* infection include histopathologic examination, rapid urease testing (frequently done in conjunction with gastric biopsy), polymerase chain reaction testing, culture, immunoglobulin G antibody titers, and the urea broth test. A fecal test is expected to be available soon.

Endoscopy plays an important role in the diagnosis of *Helicobacter*-associated disease in animals. Clinical signs of *Helicobacter* gastritis may include chronic vomiting (food, bile, and sometimes mucus), intermittent inapettence, unthriftiness, weight loss, breath changes, belching, and abdominal discomfort. However, a variety of gastrointestinal disorders can cause these clinical signs. Endoscopy is highly useful for more clearly defining a specific problem or problems based on the findings of gross examination and the identification of histopathologic abnormalities. *Helicobacter*-associated disease is considered a possibility when the histologic examination shows evidence of gastric inflammation in conjunction with the presence of a significant number of *Helicobacter* organisms. Variable degrees of inflammation may occur.

Biopsies should be obtained from various regions of the stomach, including the fundic area, gastric body, and antrum (mid-region and close to the pyloric orifice). As was described in the text section of this chapter, it can be difficult to procure adequate-sized tissue samples from the antral region because the mucosa is denser in this area. I usually do not obtain antral samples from animals that have no upper gastrointestinal signs. (Gastric body samples are always obtained during upper endoscopy.) However, I always try to procure tissue samples from both the gastric body and antrum in animals with any type of upper gastrointestinal symptoms. I place the antral samples in a separate jar or cassette from the samples obtained from the gastric body and fundus, primarily so that the pathologist can clearly differentiate what is in each region of the stomach. Good biopsy technique is essential to helping the pathologist determine whether significant inflammation is present and to identify *Helicobacter* organisms. In the future, veterinarians may be able to use noninvasive tests such as antibody titers or antigen tests to make a presumptive diagnosis of *Helicobacter*-associated disease. At present, however, correlation of biopsy findings with other tests is very important. Endoscopy and urease testing of tissue samples may be done concurrently.

Endoscopic findings in the stomach of dogs and cats range from a normal gastric appearance to variable degrees of inflammation (e.g., erythema, superficial patchy erosions). The appearance may be the same as the examples of chronic gastritis shown in this atlas section, but in my experience, gross changes are more commonly minimal in animals thought to have significant *Helicobacter* gastritis.

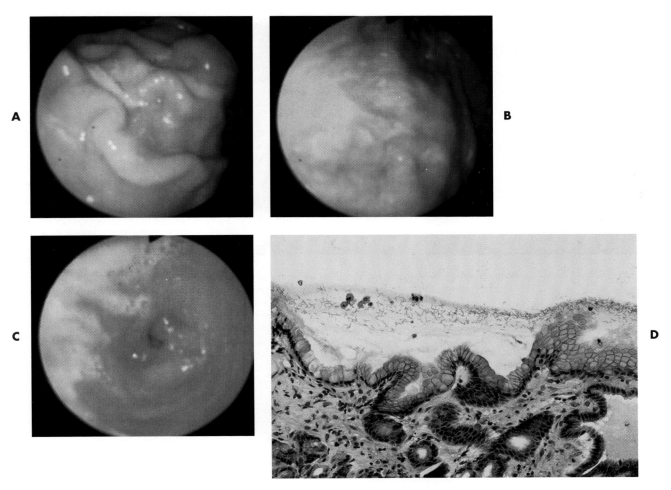

**Plate 5-45** Mild, multifocal subacute hyperplastic gastritis with *Helicobacter* organisms in a 2-year-old cocker spaniel with chronic intermittent vomiting. The animal responded well to amoxicillin, omeprazole, and metoclopramide. **A,** Normal appearance of the rugal folds in the gastric body (foreground) and erythema of a rugal fold (top right) **B,** Patchy erythema with bilious fluid retention in the upper gastric body. **C,** Mild patchy erythema in the antrum and peripyloric region. **D,** Chronic gastritis. Examination of multiple sections revealed patchy foci of fibrosis with infiltrates of lymphocytes, plasma cells, and neutrophils. This photomicrograph shows numerous *Helicobacter* organisms in the overlying surface mucus layer (×20).

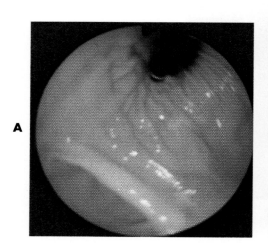
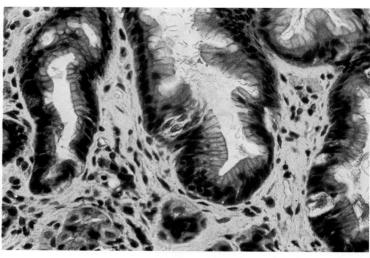

A

B

**Plate 5-46** *Helicobacter* overgrowth in a 7-year-old dachshund with a 2-month history of intermittent vomiting after eating. **A,** Lesser curvature (retroversion) with the angulus fold in the lower field (6 to 8 o'clock positions). The endoscope can be seen in the 12 to 1 o'clock area. No significant gross abnormalities of the gastric mucosa were seen. **B,** Photomicrograph showing substantial *Helicobacter* overgrowth in the gastric pits with minimal attendant inflammation (×40). The gastric pits are mildly dilated. Because inflammation is minimal, it is unlikely that *Helicobacter* was a significant cause of this dog's problem.

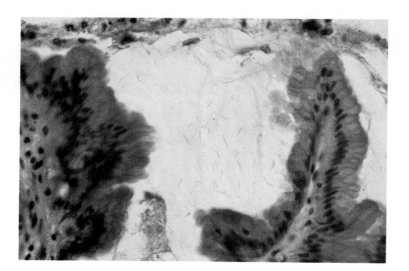

**Plate 5-47** Photomicrograph from an 11-year-old chow with a 3-week history of intermittent vomiting and 10 days of anorexia. A gastric ulcer was found in the lesser curvature of the stomach (endoscopic photo not available) with marked thickening around the upper rim. Multiple biopsies were obtained and a suspected diagnosis of gastric carcinoma was confirmed. This photomicrograph shows large numbers of *Helicobacter* organisms in the gastric pits. The pits are widened. Many organisms were also present in the surface mucus. The accumulations of *Helicobacter* organisms were most prominent in regions of the stomach away from and not around the ulcer and carcinoma tissue. Mild diffuse subacute gastritis and mild lymphocytic, plasmacytic, eosinophilic duodenitis were also present.

# GASTRITIS: VARIOUS APPEARANCES (FELINE)

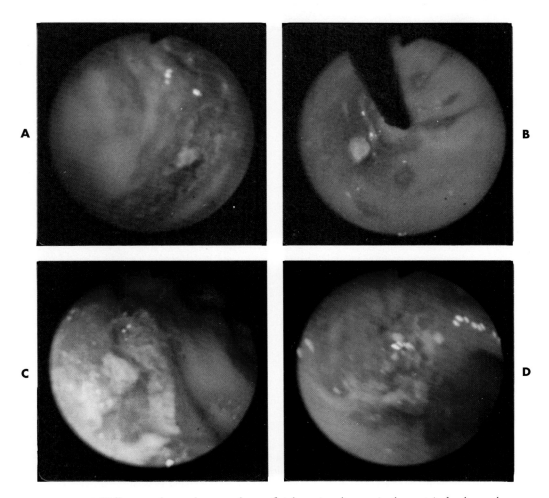

**Plate 5-48** Diffuse patchy erythema and superficial erosive changes in the gastric fundus and body of a 1-year-old cat that was presented for evaluation of acute vomiting. Gastroscopy was performed 18 hours after hospital admission, primarily because of marked depression and hematemesis. **A,** Moderate distension of gastric body at the greater curvature. Note the diffuse erythema. An area of normal mucosa is at the left aspect of the field of view. **B,** Retroversion view of the cardia and gastroesophageal junction from below, revealing focal erosive and ulcerative lesions. The white object to the left of the endoscope is a fragment from a sucralfate tablet. **C,** Gastric mucosa of the proximal gastric body. The erosive lesions have been covered by the gastric protectant agent sucralfate. Biopsies of the lesions revealed severe pseudomembranous and erosive gastritis. **D,** Distal gastric body. A small section of the angulus is observed at the 3 o'clock position, and the antrum extends to the right. The erosive lesions extended only slightly into the antrum. The cause of this cat's acute gastritis was not proved, but the owner thought the animal had ingested parts of fresh flowers recently brought into the house. Treatment consisted of sucralfate, cimetidine, and chlorpromazine (first 2 days only). The follow-up examination is shown in Plate 5-49.

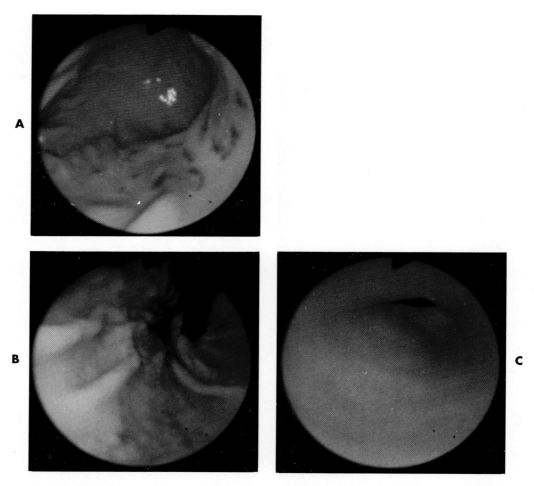

**Plate 5-49** Follow-up gastroscopy on day 5 in the cat shown in Plate 5-48. **A,** Distal gastric body and angulus (upper right aspect of the field at the 1 to 3 o'clock position). The remaining erosive changes are much more focal than on initial examination (compare with Plate 5-44, *C* and *D*.). Follow-up biopsies were markedly improved. **B,** Retroversion view of the proximal stomach **C,** The antrum and pylorus were normal. The lesions were confined to the gastric body and fundus.

**Plate 5-50** Multiple raised follicular lesions in the gastric body of a cat with a 3-month history of intermittent vomiting and peripheral eosinophilia (a white blood cell count of 24,000/mm³ with 4500 eosinophils). The histologic diagnosis was eosinophilic gastritis. Although some cats with *Helicobacter* gastritis have follicular changes in the stomach, this particular animal showed no significant evidence of *Helicobacter* overgrowth. Only transient improvement occurred with dietary therapy conducted prior to biopsy. However, the animal responded well to corticosteroid therapy.

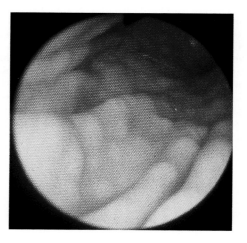

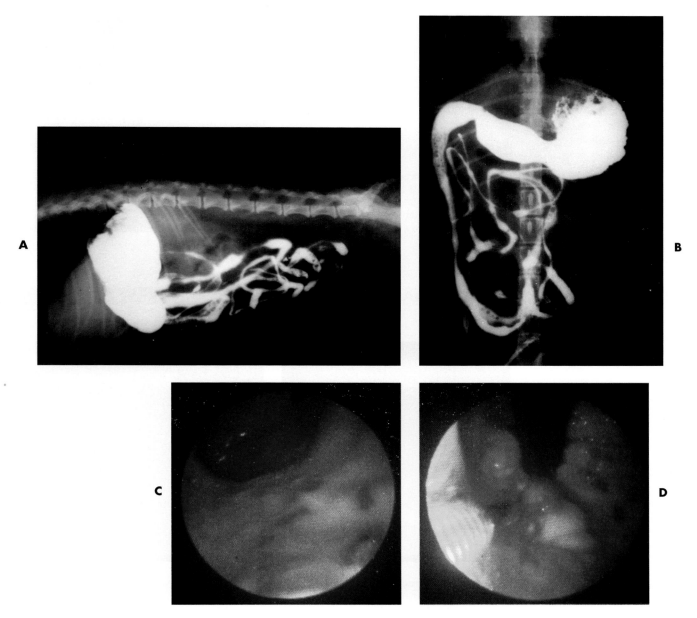

**Plate 5-51** Moderate to severe lymphocytic, plasmacytic gastritis in a 16-year-old cat with chronic intermittent vomiting (2 years) that had recently increased in frequency. Several episodes of hematemesis occurred during the 2 days before contrast radiography. **A** and **B,** Lateral and ventrodorsal radiographs obtained 5 minutes after the administration of barium. A filling defect is seen in the cardia area. **C,** Endoscopic examination revealed focal erosions of the gastric body mucosa. **D,** Proliferative and erosive mucosal lesions are present around the gastroesophageal junction. The biopsy forceps are seen below the endoscope shaft. The lesions visualized in the cardia and fundus caused the filling defects identified on the contrast radiographs. Although the proliferative lesions were grossly suggestive of neoplasia, no neoplastic cells were found on microscopic examination. Multiple biopsies were obtained in an effort to rule out neoplasia. Biopsies revealed moderate to severe lymphocytic, plasmacytic gastritis. The animal responded well to corticosteroids.

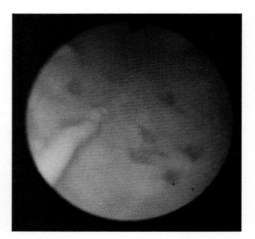

**Plate 5-52** Superficial pock-like lesions in the distal gastric body of a cat with intermittent vomiting. The histologic diagnosis was mild focal fibrosis of the lamina propria. These lesions may have been chronic.

## CHRONIC FELINE HISTIOCYTIC GASTRITIS

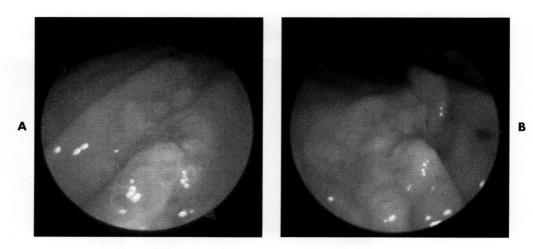

**Plate 5-53** A 12-year-old, 9-kg (20-lb) cat with a history of chronic vomiting, most recently on a daily basis. **A,** Gastric body with normal rugal fold on the left and an irregular adjacent fold with an erosive lesion. **B,** Area of the greater curvature with marked disruption of the continuity of the rugal folds and thickening and irregularity of the folds in view.

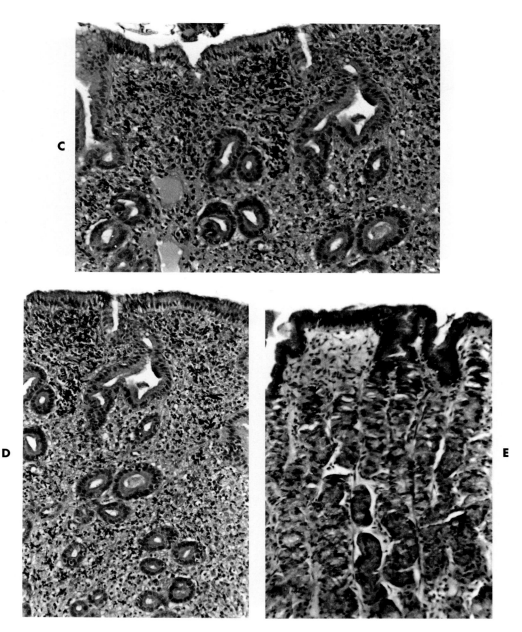

**Plate 5-53—cont'd** C and D, Photomicrographs showing distorted mucosal architecture with marked widening of the rugae and marked infiltration by sheets of large histiocytes. (Note the dense superficial infiltration.) **E,** Normal feline stomach for comparison. All biopsy samples were obtained with endoscopic forceps. (Courtesy Stephen J. Engler)

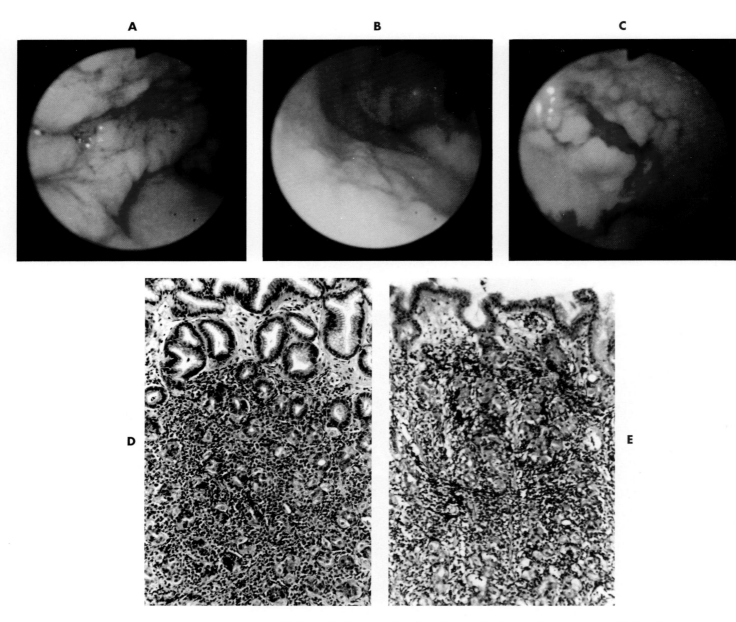

**Plate 5-54** Endoscopic photographs taken six months after moderate to severe histiocytic gastritis was diagnosed in a 4-year-old Siamese cat with chronic vomiting and weight loss. The animal was treated aggressively with corticosteroids. **A,** Irregularity and distortion of the greater curvature rugal folds. Note hemorrhage at bottom of photo. **B,** Retroversion view with moderate gastric distension. Note the follicular changes in the mucosa along the greater curvature. The endoscope is visualized at the edge of the field at the 2 o'clock position. **C,** Greater-than-normal degree of hemorrhage after a single mucosal biopsy. **D,** For comparison, this photomicrograph of a gastric biopsy sample taken at the time of original diagnosis shows focally severe infiltrations of macrophages and smaller numbers of lymphocytes and plasma cells (severe focal granulomatous gastritis). **E,** At 6-month follow-up, histologic changes were considered to be slightly worse, with focally severe infiltrations of small lymphocytes and histiocytic cells. Azathioprine was added to the therapeutic regimen, and the animal showed mild clinical improvement. NOTE: Histiocytic gastritis is a rare but serious disorder in cats. Aggressive treatment is required, and surveillance of lesions via periodic endoscopic examination (every 3 to 6 months) is recommended. (Courtesy Stephen J Engler.)

# EROSIONS AND HEMORRHAGES

Erosions and hemorrhages may be found anywhere in the stomach and may be single or multiple. An *erosion* is a shallow defect in the mucosa that does not extend through the muscularis mucosa into the submucosa. Typically an erosion is flat or minimally depressed and is focal. The base may be reddish, yellowish, or black. Many beginning endoscopists tend to incorrectly identify erosions as ulcers.

The term *hemorrhage* refers to the endoscopic appearance of discrete petecchiae or bright-red confluent streaks that are not associated with any visible breaks in the mucosa. The intactness of the mucosa can be ascertained from the appearance of mucosal highlights. The hemorrhages are usually described as subepithelial.

Biopsies from grossly hemorrhagic areas or from erosions commonly reveal no histologic abnormalities. Occasionally partial- or full-thickness necrosis with minimal inflammation is identified. It is rarely necessary to obtain more than one or two biopsies from erosions or areas of hemorrhage. In many cases it is doubtful that erosions cause symptoms. They are usually associated with another disorder, which is responsible for the patient's discomfort. When identified endoscopically, hemorrhages and erosions should not automatically be incriminated as the cause of clinical signs.

*Clinical settings* for nonspecific erosions or hemorrhages include stress lesions, critical illness, localized gastric trauma (e.g., retching or vomiting, foreign body), ingestion of corrosives, radiation, drugs (especially nonsteroidal antiinflammatory drugs [NSAIDs]), a discrete ischemic insult, and idiopathic chronic erosions.

A 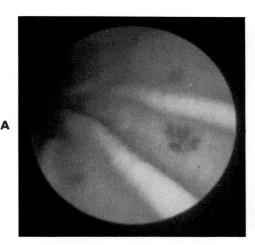 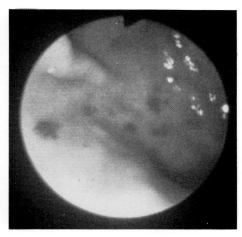 B

**Plate 5-55** Focal streaks of subepithelial hemorrhages in a cat with chronic diarrhea. A Mid-gastric body. **B,** Gastric body. Biopsies were unremarkable, and the history did not suggest a gastric disorder.

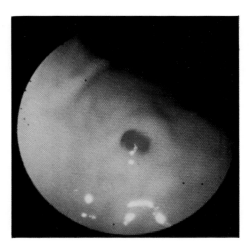

**Plate 5-56** Isolated erosion in the stomach of a cat with mild lymphocytic, plasmacytic gastritis.

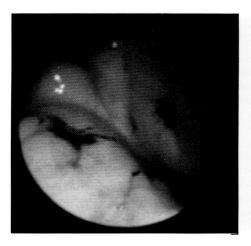

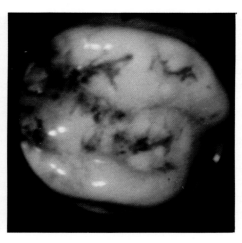

**Plate 5-57** Focal erosions in the distal gastric body of an 8-year-old Labrador retriever with intermittent nausea. No histologic abnormalities were found.

**Plate 5-58** Superficial gastric erosions with hemorrhage along the greater curvature of the stomach in a 3-year-old boxer with intermittent vomiting, chronic diarrhea, anorexia, and weight loss. Gastric biopsies showed histologic evidence of mild erosive subacute gastritis. Histiocytic ulcerative colitis was also identified.

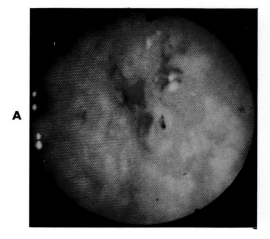

A

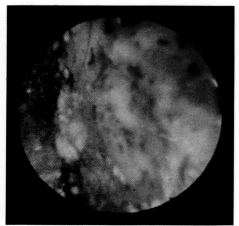

B

**Plate 5-59** Erosions in the distal antrum of two dogs that were receiving both prednisone and flunixin meglumine in an experimental study. **A,** Day 4 of combination drug administration. **B,** Multiple erosions at day 2 in a dog receiving prednisone at 1.1 mg/kg (0.5 mg/lb) once daily and flunixin meglumine at 1.1 mg/kg (0.5 mg/lb) bid. It is recommended that NSAIDs not be used in combination or in conjunction with corticosteroids because of the risk of gastric ulceration. (Courtesy Steven W. Dow.)

# GASTRIC ULCERS

Breach of the muscularis mucosa distinguishes an *ulcer* from an erosion. The pathogenesis of ulcer disease is not yet completely understood. Ulcers have a variety of causes, including drugs, foreign bodies, disorders that cause higher than normal release of gastric acid, *Helicobacter* infection,* and others. Ulcers probably begin as erosions, which then increase in depth of damage. Fortunately, erosions rarely become ulcers in animals. The incidence of gastric ulcers in dogs and cats is quite low. In dogs, ulcers most commonly occur in conjunction with the use of NSAIDs or in the presence of hepatic disease or mastocytosis. Ulcers associated with the use of NSAIDs most often occur in the antral-pyloric area. To avoid missing a lesion such as an ulcer, the endoscopist must carefully examine the *entire* stomach.

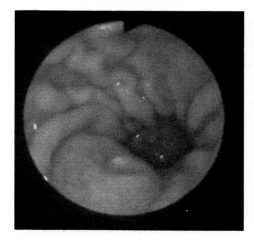 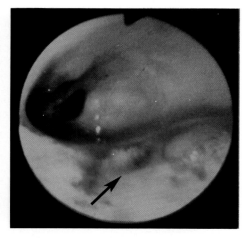

**Plate 5-60** Large ulcer with a shallow crater in the gastric body of a cat (6 o'clock position). Note the normal appearance of the surrounding mucosa. (From Twedt DC and Tams TR: Diseases of the stomach. In Sherding RG, editor: *The cat: diseases and clinical management,* New York, 1989, Churchill Livingstone.)

**Plate 5-61** Shallow ulcer in the proximal antrum of a cat *(arrow)*. A small amount of hemorrhage is associated with the ulcer. An open pylorus is seen at the far end of the field.

*Helicobacter* infection rarely causes ulcers in animals but is a more common factor in the development of ulcers in humans.

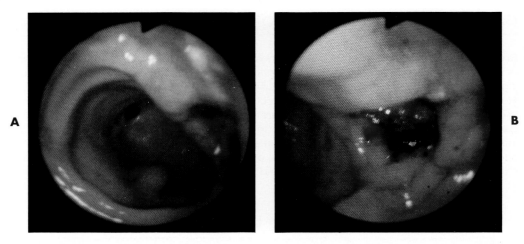

**Plate 5-62** Large antral ulcer in a 14-year-old cocker spaniel. Methylprednisolone acetate had been administered for severe degenerative joint disease, and the dog's owner instituted ibuprofen without notifying the clinician. **A,** Antral canal from the distal gastric body. A large ulcer is seen in the right aspect of the field of view (3 to 4 o'clock position), and the pylorus is in the center of the field. The tissue projection on the antral wall at the 6 o'clock position is a polyp (an incidental finding and insignificant lesion). **B,** Close-up view of the gastric ulcer. Much of the ulcer pit is filled with hemorrhage. The antral canal is to the left. On initial approach this ulcer was poorly visualized because it was covered by thick foam, mucus, and bile. Once the fluid and mucus were suctioned away, the ulcer was clearly seen.

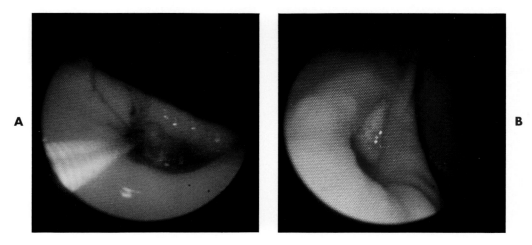

**Plate 5-63** Large angulus ulcer in a 12-year-old chow with severe degenerative joint disease. Aspirin and corticosteroids were administered simultaneously. **A,** Ulcer in the angulus. Biopsy samples were obtained from the upper wall (shown here) and the rim. No evidence of neoplasia was found. Treatment included famotidine and sucralfate. **B,** Early signs of healing at 14-day follow-up. Large ulcers may take 8 to 16 weeks to heal.

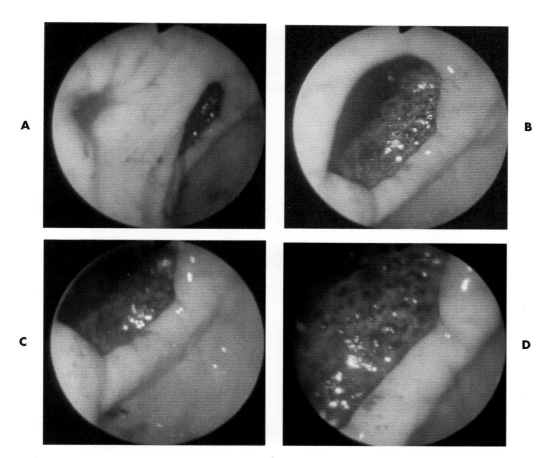

**Plate 5-64** Perforated gastric ulcer in an 8-year-old chow that had received naproxen (an NSAID) once daily for 7 days. On the sixth day, vomiting and inappetence were first noted by the owner. Naproxen was discontinued after the seventh day, but the clinical signs persisted. Famotidine and misoprostol were started 3 days later. The vomiting soon subsided, but inappetence persisted. Nine days after naproxen was discontinued, the dog was presented for endoscopy. The dog was bright and alert. The complete blood count and biochemical profile were completely normal except for mild leukocytosis. The packed cell volume was 48%. **A,** View toward the antrum from the lower gastric body. Two ulcers are seen: a smaller lesion at the 9 o'clock position and a much larger ulcer to the right of center (mid-antrum). **B,** On advancement into the antrum the endoscope revealed a very deep ulcer with a thick rim (entire upper left quadrant). The pyloric orifice is at the lower left (7 o'clock position). **C,** Straight-forward view into the ulcer. The whitish meshlike tissue seen through the ulcer crater is omentum. **D,** Close-up view of the ulcer crater with an omental seal.                    *Continued*

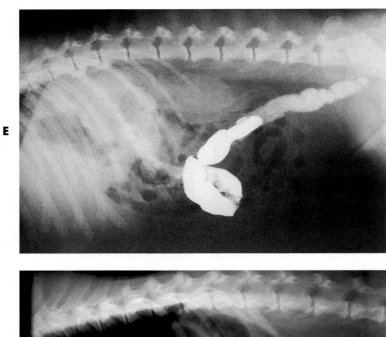

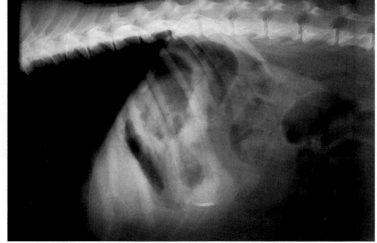

**Plate 5-64—cont'd** E, To determine whether the omental seal was incomplete and whether surgery needed to be performed immediately rather than on the following day (the endoscopy was being conducted late in the day), survey abdominal radiographs were obtained to look for evidence of free air in the abdominal cavity (air was insufflated to the stomach as for routine gastroscopy). The radiograph shows no evidence of free air in the abdominal cavity. Barium was present in the colon from a contrast series started by another veterinarian a few days before. Barium transit was thought to be delayed by anticholinergic therapy that had been started several days earlier in an effort to control vomiting. (Anticholinergic treatment is not advisable.) F, For comparison, a survey abdominal radiograph from a *different patient* with a perforated gastric ulcer shows free air in the abdominal cavity between the liver and stomach. *Note:* The chow underwent surgery the following day, and the ulcer was found to have a firmly adhered, complete omental seal. A partial antrectomy was done, and the histologic diagnosis was focal chronic ulcerative gastritis. (Ulcer tissue should always be biopsied to rule out neoplasia.) An incidental finding at surgery was a mass in the left medial lobe of the liver. The lobe was resected, and the mass was determined to be a hepatocellular carcinoma. The dog was fed via jejunostomy tube for 12 days and had an uneventful recovery. The chow lived for 3 years after surgery with no evidence of tumor recurrence.

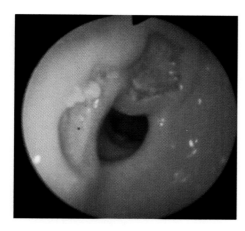

**Plate 5-65** Two peripyloric ulcers in a 14-year-old dog that was receiving NSAID therapy for severe osteoarthritis. The pyloric orifice (center) is open, and ulcers are seen to the left and above (with hemorrhage) the pylorus. In animals that are sensitive to NSAIDs the prostaglandin drug misoprostol has proved very effective in preventing gastrointestinal ulceration.

# ABNORMAL GASTRIC MOTILITY

Gastric motility disorders are usually diagnosed based on the history, clinical signs, and radiographic findings (e.g., prolonged retention of liquid barium, radiopaque markers [BIPS], or a barium meal or decreased antral contractions observed at fluoroscopy). When used alone, endoscopy is of limited value in assessing disorders of gastric motility. However, important clues can sometimes be recognized during gastroscopy. This is important because some animals with a gastric motility disorder do not have diagnostic contrast radiographic studies (i.e., a normal liquid barium series does not rule out a gastric motility disorder). Endoscopic examination is also important in patients with clinical signs of a motility disorder because mucosal biopsies should be evaluated whenever possible for evidence of gastritis or fibrosis. These disorders can alter gastric motility. Findings that should alert the endoscopist to the possibility of a motility disorder include retention of food or fluid admixed with bile in a properly fasted patient and generalized erythema with or without presence of streaks of bile-stained fluid.

Fluid may be present in the stomach as a result of reflux from the colon after high enemas. Also, any time a large pool of fluid is found in the stomach, the possibility of fluid retention as a result of a small intestinal obstruction (e.g., foreign body, stricture, or mass) must be considered. In this situation fluid is usually pooled in the duodenum as well. As much fluid as possible should be suctioned from the stomach so that the mucosa can be thoroughly evaluated.

Gastric mucosal erythema commonly occurs in animals with gastric retention of bile-stained fluid. Erythema may be secondary to superficial mucosal damage from bile. Biopsies are routinely unremarkable in idiopathic gastric motility disorders.

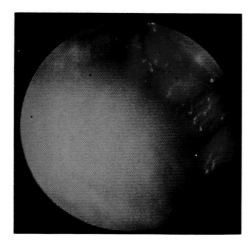

**Plate 5-66** Gastric fluid and bile retention in a 7-year-old Pekingese with an idiopathic gastric motility disorder. Note the mucosal erythema. Mucosal biopsies were normal. Clinical signs included intermittent vomiting, frequent nausea and loud gastric gurgling sounds, periodic inappetence, and occasional bloating episodes

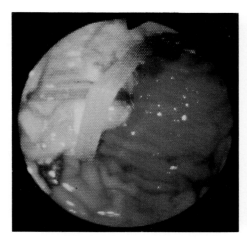

**Plate 5-67** Grass blades and food in the gastric body of a 3-year-old Doberman with lymphangiectasia. The dog was quite weak and had a total protein concentration of 2.3 g/dl. The dog had not eaten or been outdoors in 3 days. Gastric mucosal biopsies were normal.

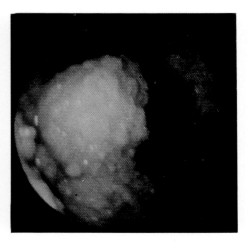

**Plate 5-68** Large amount of retained food (canned) in a 6-year-old cocker spaniel with a disorder characterized by the vomiting of undigested or partially digested food 18 to 24 hours after eating. At the time of endoscopy the dog had not eaten in 30 hours. The endoscope was maneuvered beyond the food, and the pylorus was traversed without difficulty. A thyroid-stimulating hormone test was consistent with hypothyroidism. Gastric and duodenal biopsies were normal. The animal responded well to thyroid supplementation and metoclopramide.

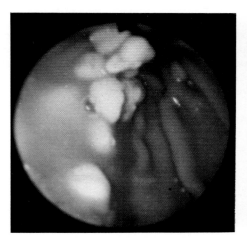

**Plate 5-69** Food and fluid retention in the gastric body of a 10-year-old miniature poodle. The surrounding mucosa appears normal.

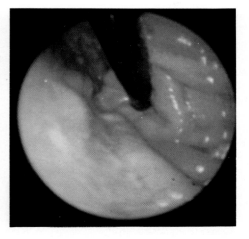

**Plate 5-70** Retroversion view of the proximal stomach of a 1-year-old Kuvasz with a 6-month history of intermittent vomiting. Note the presence of bile-stained fluid. No metabolic abnormalities were found, and gastric and duodenal biopsies were normal. An idiopathic gastric motility disorder was diagnosed, and the animal responded well to metoclopramide.

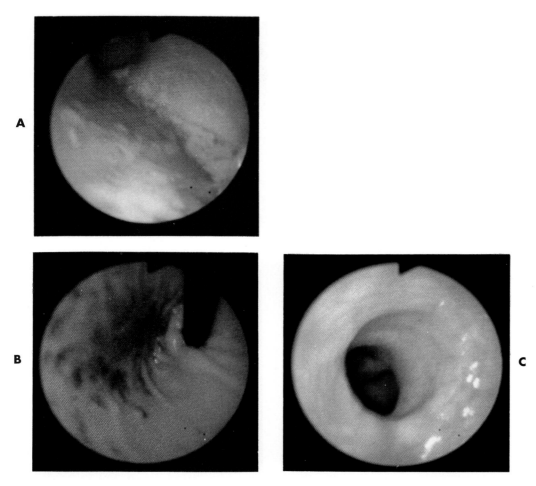

**Plate 5-71 A,** Gastric fluid retention in a 2-year-old Balinese with anorexia (5 days) and vomiting. Several of the vomiting episodes were projectile in nature. **B,** Retroversion view of the fundus and gastroesophageal junction. Most of the gastric fluid was suctioned so that a thorough examination could be completed. No evidence of a foreign body was found. **C,** The pylorus was unusually dilated in this cat. The duodenal wall can be seen at the far end of the canal. Duodenal biopsies revealed chronic active enteritis. Esophagitis was most likely secondary to vomiting. A barium series done after endoscopy to rule out a lower small bowel obstruction was normal. The increased gastric fluid was most likely secondary to marked duodenal-gastric reflux and abnormal gastric motility. Treatment included metoclopramide and prednisone.

## ABNORMAL APPEARANCES OF THE ANTRUM

Pronounced folds are occasionally identified in the antrum. This is a rare finding in cats. Pronounced folds may be secondary to chronic mucosal hypertrophy or chronic inflammatory disease, or they may be a healing sequela to an ulcer, neoplasia, or chronic hypergastrinemia. In some cases the pronounced folds may not be clinically significant, but their appearance should always be noted in the endoscopy report. Examples of antral neoplasia appear in a later section in this atlas.

**Plate 5-72** Pronounced antral folds in a 16-year-old dog with chronic diarrhea and a ravenous appetite. The animal had no clinical signs that were specific for gastric disease. Biopsies showed antral fibrosis, which was probably the sequela of a previous inflammatory disorder. **A,** Endoscopic view from the proximal end of the insufflated antrum. **B,** Distal antrum with smooth folds. The pylorus is just below the pointer at the 12 o'clock position.

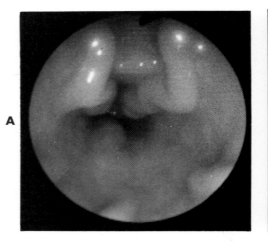

A

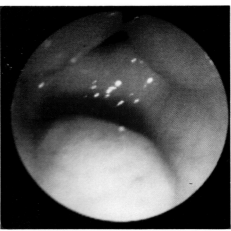

B

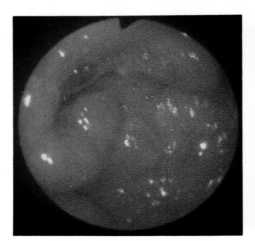

**Plate 5-73** Pronounced folds in the distal antrum of a 10-year-old beagle with intermittent vomiting. This dog had mild hypertrophic gastropathy. The pyloric orifice is obscured by foam to the left of center (directly below the pointer)

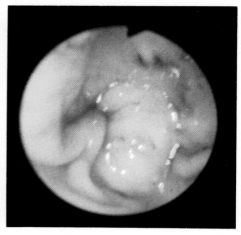

**Plate 5-74** Pronounced folds around the pylorus of a 14-year-old cat with intestinal and hepatic lymphoma. The closed pylorus is to the left of center at the 9 o'clock position. Biopsy samples obtained from the thickened tissue around the pylorus showed no histologic evidence of neoplasia. (This was confirmed at necropsy.) The diagnosis was proliferative gastropathy with mild inflammation.

**Plate 5-75** Hypertrophic gastritis in a 10-year-old poodle with a 3-month history of intermittent vomiting. Survey abdominal radiographs showed marked gastric distension with fluid and gas, and a barium series revealed marked delay in the emptying of barium from the stomach. At endoscopic examination the pyloric orifice was extremely narrow *(arrow),* and it did not open to any degree during the examination. The tissue around the pylorus tended to bulge up (as shown here) any time gastric contractions occurred. A y-u pyloroplasty was performed, and hypertrophic gastritis was diagnosed based on the results of full-thickness biopsy. (Courtesy Susan E. Johnson)

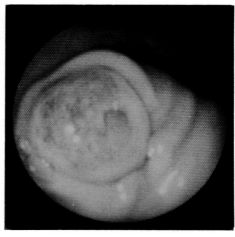

# GASTRIC POLYPS

Gastric polyps usually are not clinically significant, and they are often discovered incidentally on gastrointestinal radiographs or at endoscopy or surgery. Rarely, there may be bleeding from an eroded surface or transient obstruction of the pylorus by an antral polyp protruding into the pyloric canal. Bloating, nausea, and vomiting may occur during periods of obstruction. Gastric polyps are only rarely found in dogs and cats. Endoscopically they appear as sessile or pedunculated protuberances that do not disappear with maximal insufflation. Polyps are most commonly found in the antrum and pyloric areas. These growths are usually benign. Biopsies should be obtained to confirm the histologic nature of a polyp. If clinically significant, the polyp should be removed with a polypectomy snare loop and cautery or by surgical excision.

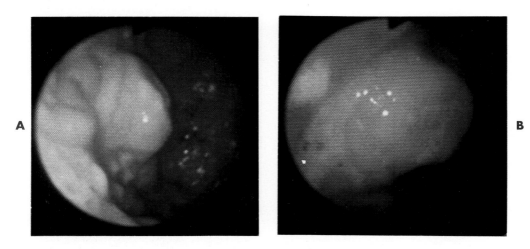

A                                                                              B

**Plate 5-76** Large, benign polyp in the mid-gastric body of a 12-year-old chow. This is an unusual location. The polyp was not clinically significant. **A,** Forward view from the proximal gastric body. **B,** Close-up view of the polyp.

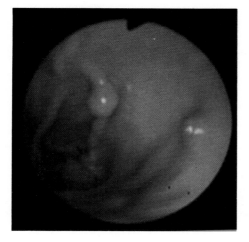

**Plate 5-77** Two small antral polyps, an incidental finding in a 16-year-old dog.

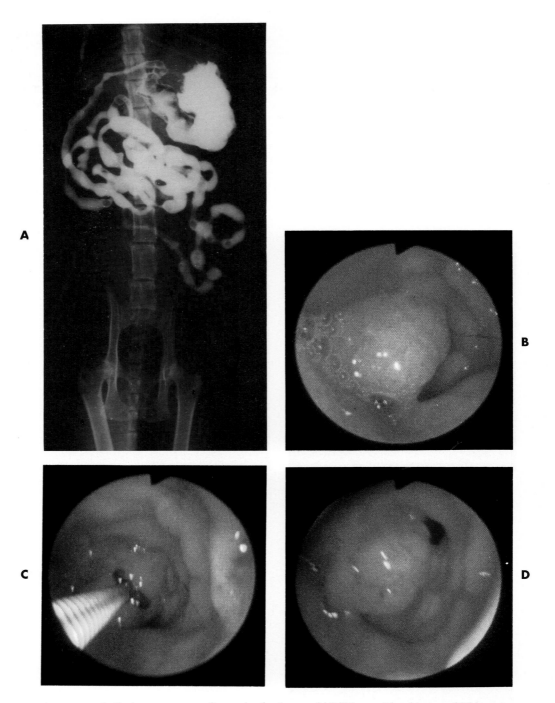

**Plate 5-78 A,** Barium contrast radiograph of a 6-year-old DSH cat with a history of lifelong intermittent vomiting. For some time before this presentation the cat had been vomiting daily, with some episodes being projectile in nature. The pyloric antrum has a filling defect (a consistent finding throughout the series). **B,** A large polyp with irregular surface was identified in the distal antrum. In this view the polyp occludes the pyloric orifice. The antral mucosa also displayed erythema and irregularity. **C,** Biopsy forceps were used to move the polyp to the side, providing a partial view of the pyloric orifice. The polyp was freely movable on a stalk. **D,** Polyp biopsy procedure. The polyp had a soft surface. Note the irregularity of the antral walls. The histologic diagnosis was benign inflammatory polyp. Chronic gastritis and moderate lymphocytic enteritis were also present.

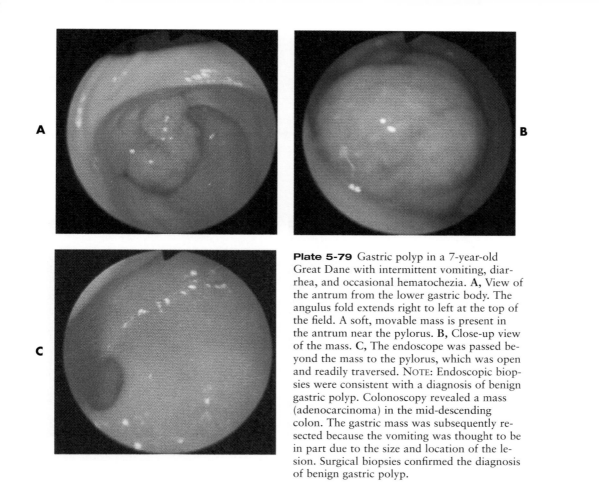

**Plate 5-79** Gastric polyp in a 7-year-old Great Dane with intermittent vomiting, diarrhea, and occasional hematochezia. **A,** View of the antrum from the lower gastric body. The angulus fold extends right to left at the top of the field. A soft, movable mass is present in the antrum near the pylorus. **B,** Close-up view of the mass. **C,** The endoscope was passed beyond the mass to the pylorus, which was open and readily traversed. NOTE: Endoscopic biopsies were consistent with a diagnosis of benign gastric polyp. Colonoscopy revealed a mass (adenocarcinoma) in the mid-descending colon. The gastric mass was subsequently resected because the vomiting was thought to be in part due to the size and location of the lesion. Surgical biopsies confirmed the diagnosis of benign gastric polyp.

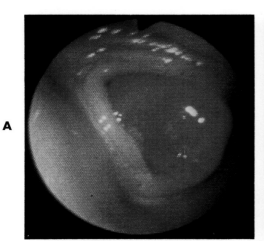

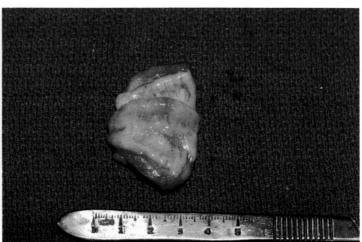

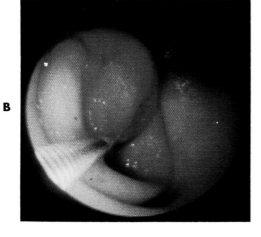

**Plate 5-80** Pyloric polyp in a 7-year-old pug with frequent vomiting. Some episodes were projectile in nature. **A,** The polyp caused distortion of the pyloric orifice and occlusion of the pyloric canal. In this photograph the pyloric orifice appears as an inverted V with the polyp protruding through it. **B,** The biopsy forceps have been passed through the pyloric canal. Note that the polyp has compromised the lumen. This is an unusual location for a polyp. **C,** Surgically excised tissue from the pylorus.

# GASTRIC NEOPLASIA

Adenocarcinoma is the most common malignant tumor in the stomach of the dog, and lymphosarcoma is the most common malignant tumor in the cat. Cancerous lesions may appear as raised plaques, as polypoid lesions projecting from the lumen, or as a firm, diffusely infiltrating mass invading the stomach wall.

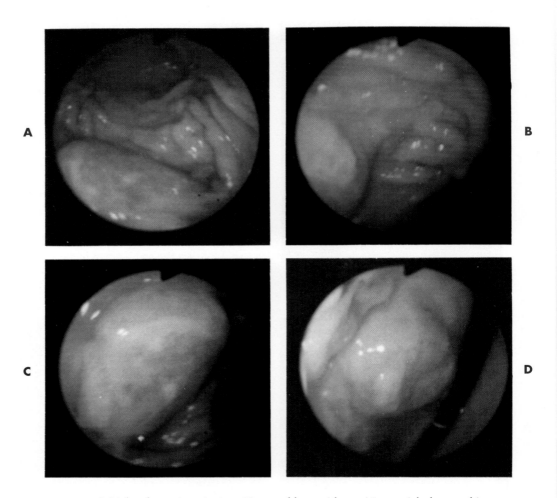

**Plate 5-81** Initial endoscopic series in a 10-year-old cat with vomiting, weight loss, and inappetence. **A,** Immediate view upon entering the stomach. A small amount of air has been insufflated. A large mass is seen at the lower aspect of the field of view. The angulus is at the 12 to 1 o'clock position. **B,** The edge of the mass is at the 7 to 8 o'clock position. Note the irregularity and thickening of the rugal folds around the mass in both views. **C,** Close-up view of the large mass in the proximal stomach. **D,** View of the mass and surrounding irregular folds after the retroversion maneuver. The cat lived for 8 years after the diagnosis was made.

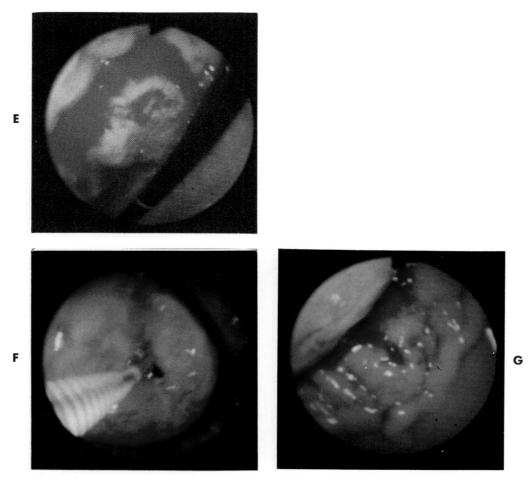

**Plate 5-81—cont'd**   E, A significant amount of bleeding occurred after a single biopsy sample was obtained from the center of the mass. F and G, Samples were obtained from the mass and surrounding tissue. The mass was sampled several times in the same location in an effort to obtain tissue as deeply as possible. G, The mass is in the upper left aspect, and hemorrhage from a mucosal-fold biopsy site is seen in the center of the field.

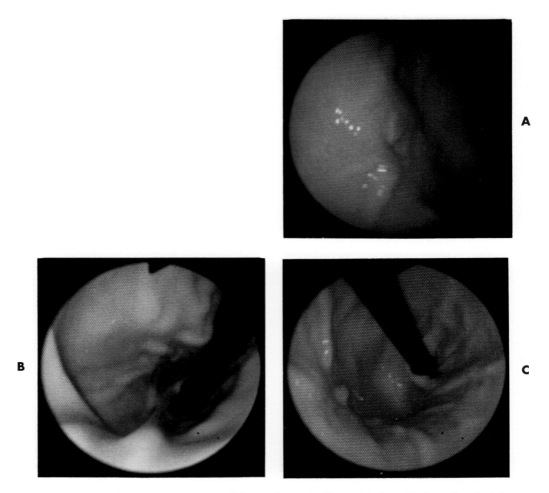

**Plate 5-82** Endoscopic examination of the cat shown in Plate 5-81, done 19 days after the initial examination. Treatment involved only chemotherapy (prednisone, cyclophosphamide, and vincristine). **A,** Forward view of the proximal stomach at slightly more than moderate distension. The mass, which had decreased dramatically in size, is in the center of the field. (Compare with Plate 5-81, *C.*) **B,** Retroversion view. The site of the mass is barely detectable (focal reddened area to left of center). (Compare with Plate 5-81, *D.*) **C,** Retroversion view at a different angle. The mass can be seen at the 7 o'clock position.

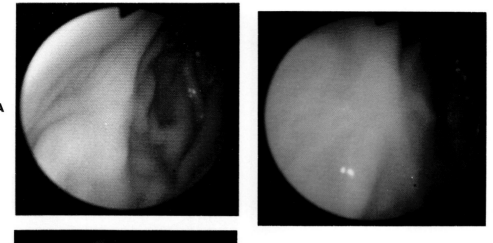

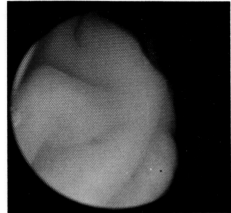

**Plate 5-83** Endoscopic photographs of the cat discussed in Plates 5-81 and 5-82, obtained 19 weeks after the initial examination. The animal was doing extremely well on chemotherapy. No evidence of a gastric mass is seen, and the mucosa at the original site of the lesion appears whiter than the surrounding mucosa. **A,** Forward view of the proximal stomach in mild distension. Note that the rugal folds no longer appear thickened or irregular. **B,** Same site as in **A** but with moderate distension. **C,** Close-up view of the gastric mucosa. Note the smooth mucosal surface.

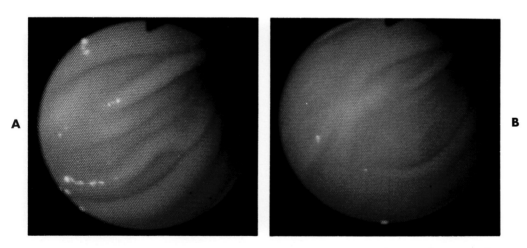

**Plate 5-84** Endoscopic photographs of the cat in Plates 5-81, 5-82, and 5-83, taken 9 months after the animal was first examined. **A,** Forward view of the proximal stomach in mild distension. **B,** Forward view of the stomach in moderate distension. The stomach is grossly normal except for the small, whitened area where the mass was previously located. (Compare with Plates 5-81, *C*, 5-82, *A*, and 5-83, *A*.) Biopsy samples showed no evidence of lymphosarcoma. The cat was still receiving chemotherapy and was clinically normal. Chemotherapy was discontinued at 12 months; at 18-months, no evidence of tumor recurrence was found. NOTE: The cat lived 8 years after the diagnosis was made. Chemotherapy never had to be resumed. This case highlights the importance of using endoscopy relatively early in animals with unexplained chronic vomiting. This cat's history was easily consistent with a diagnosis of inflammatory bowel disease or chronic gastritis. Yet endoscopy revealed lymphosarcoma. Early initiation of the most indicated therapy resulted in an excellent outcome.

**Plate 5-85** Lymphosar-
coma involving the gastric
body and fundus in a 12-
year-old Siamese cat. A readily palpable mass was found
in the anterior abdomen
(stomach). Lymphosarcoma
was also identified in the
colon. **A,** Forward view in
the gastric body. The stomach has not been insufflated.
Note the dramatic distortion
of the normal rugal fold
structure and the ulcerative
change at the 5 o'clock position. **B,** Retroversion view
showing the multiple mass
effect in the proximal stomach and fundus. **C,** Forward
view in the gastric body.
Note the irregular rugal fold
adjacent to the mass. The
animal responded fairly well
to chemotherapy for 6
weeks, but then clinical signs
worsened and the cat was
euthanized. **D,** Distal gastric
body. A short edge of the angulus is seen at the far lower
right (5 o'clock position).
The proliferative effect from
the lymphosarcoma stopped
abruptly in the lower body.
The antrum was completely
normal.

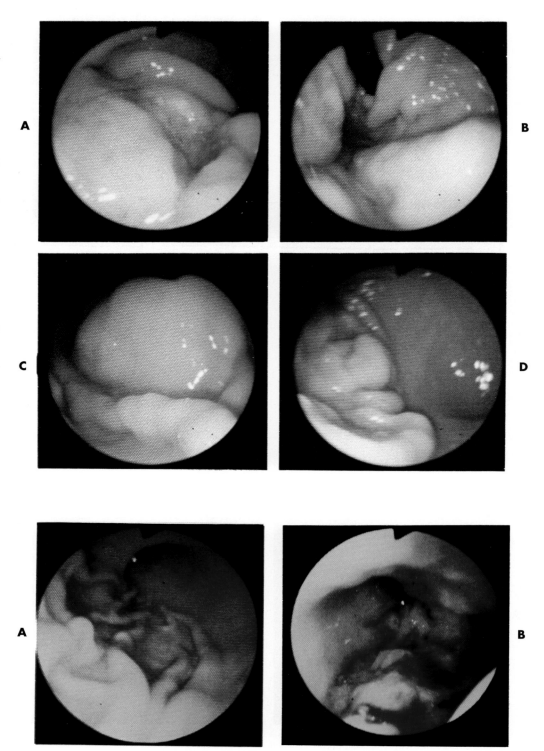

**Plate 5-86** Antral lymphosarcoma in a 14-year-old cat with a short history of inappetence and
occasional hematemesis. **A,** The gastric body was completely normal. **B,** The antrum was infiltrated with proliferative tissue. The pylorus is directly below the pointer. Failure to examine the
antrum would have resulted in a missed diagnosis. The histologic diagnoses were normal gastric
body, antral lymphosarcoma, and moderate lymphocytic, plasmacytic enteritis. The cat did well
on chemotherapy for 5 months, but then bilateral renomegaly developed quite rapidly. The cat
was subsequently euthanized because of anorexia and vomiting. The blood urea nitrogen and
creatinine levels were normal. Histologic examination of tissues obtained at necropsy identified
lymphoma in both kidneys and the antrum.

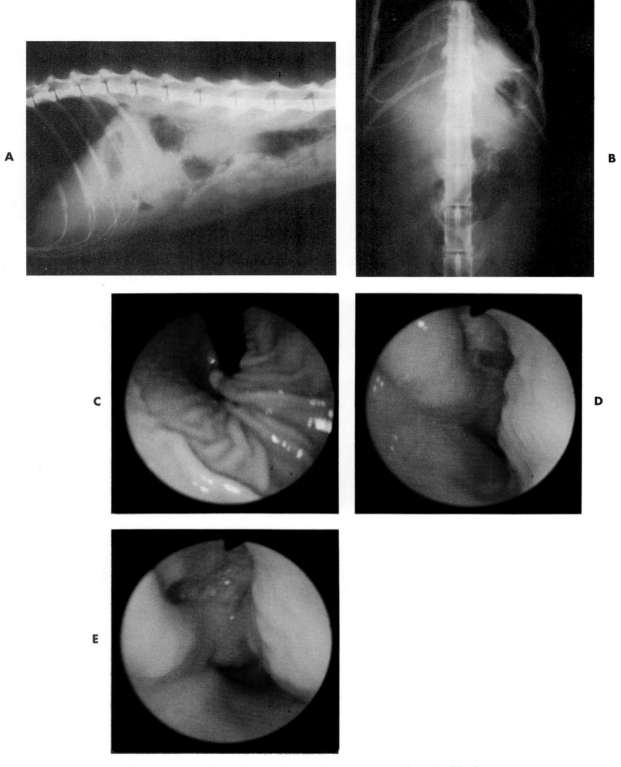

**Plate 5-87** Gastric lymphosarcoma in an 8-year-old cat with inappetence. The animal had tested positive for the feline leukemia virus. A physical examination revealed a palpable abdominal mass. **A** and **B,** Lateral and ventrodorsal radiographs showed a soft tissue mass involving the stomach. Gastroscopic examination showed a single mass along the distal lesser curvature and several prominent linear masses in the antrum. **C,** Retroversion view showing the normal fundus and gastroesophageal junction. **D** and **E,** Mass effect in the antral canal has caused marked occlusion. At the top of the field of view, note the cavernous area with debris. The pylorus is not in view. The endoscope was advanced to the pylorus through the tunnel seen at the bottom of the photographs.

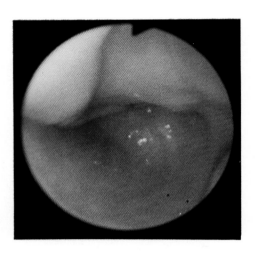

**Plate 5-88** Examination of the cat shown in Plate 5-87, performed 5 weeks after presentation. Chemotherapy dramatically decreased the size of the antral masses. The endoscope is in the same position as in Plate 5-87, *D* and *E.* The pylorus is closed, but its orifice is seen in the center of the field. One of the antral masses, although somewhat smaller, is still evident in the left aspect of the field. The debris-filled cavern is no longer present.

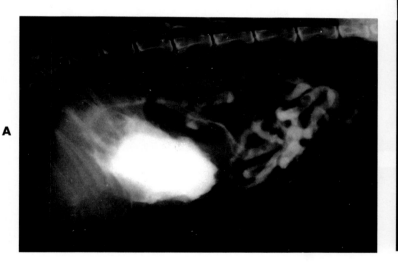

A

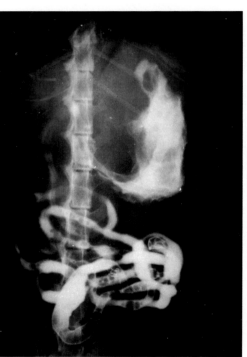

B

**Plate 5-89** Gastric adenocarcinoma in a 14-year-old Siamese cat with a 2-week history of anorexia but only occasional vomiting. **A** and **B,** Barium contrast radiographs showed incomplete gastric filling and mucosal irregularity.

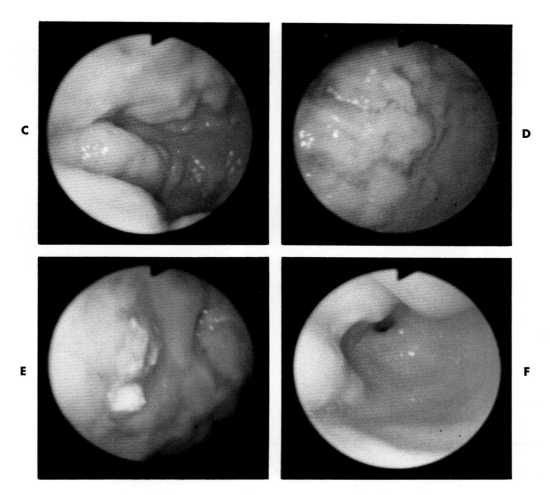

**Plate 5-89—cont'd**   C, Immediate view when the endoscope entered the stomach. Note the
thickened, irregular rugal folds. The walls of the stomach were poorly distensible in response to
air insufflation. **D,** Mucosal irregularity and focal hemorrhages along the distal greater curvature.
**E,** White plaque material (left of center) adhering to the mucosa of the greater curvature.
**F,** Prominent folds in the antral canal. The pylorus is to the left of center at the 11 o'clock position. Multiple biopsy samples were obtained from the gastric-body lesions. The tissue felt unusually hard when the biopsy forceps were closed. This tactile perception is often associated with
malignancy.

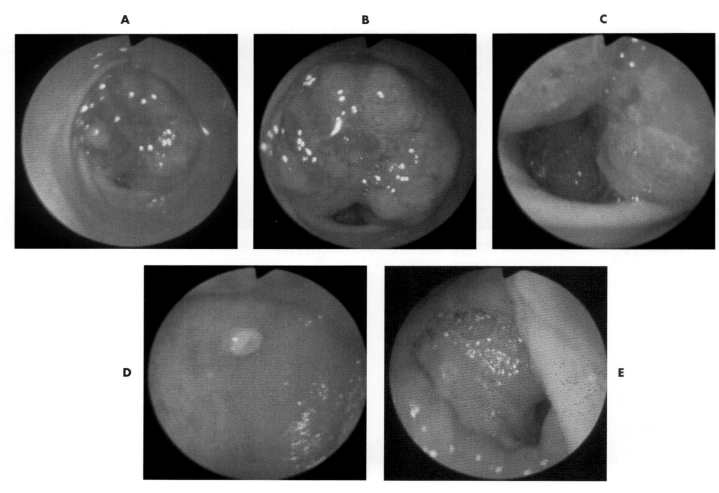

**Plate 5-90** Gastric adenocarcinoma in a 9-year-old male Bouvier with a 5-month history of intermittent vomiting (one or two episodes per week and no worrisome associated signs). The complete blood cell count, biochemical profile, serum thyroxine concentration, urinalysis, fecal examination for parasites, and survey radiographs of the thorax and abdomen were unremarkable. The dog was referred for endoscopy because the owner was anxious to determine why the animal was vomiting. **A,** View from the proximal antrum. The antral walls are smooth and normal. However, a proliferative mass was found in the pylorus. **B,** Close-up view of the pyloric mass, which is occluding most of the pyloric orifice. **C,** View of the pyloric canal near the pyloroduodenal junction after the endoscope was advanced into the pyloric canal, beneath the mass. The mass extended into the proximal duodenum. The histologic diagnosis was adenocarcinoma. **D,** Grossly normal duodenum in the area of the major duodenal papilla (upper center). This very important finding indicates that resection would not need to extend very far down the descending duodenum. The duct area appeared unaffected. NOTE: A 30-cm section of antrum, pylorus, and duodenum was resected during a 4-hour surgical procedure. No evidence of metastasis was found, and the adenocarcinoma did not involve the deep layers of the pylorus. The dog's recovery was uneventful. Long-term metoclopramide therapy was prescribed to help decrease duodenogastric reflux because the animal no longer had a pylorus. The dog lived 3 years after surgery, with no evidence of tumor recurrence. **E,** Endoscopic view of the antral-duodenal junction (site of the anastomosis) 8 months after the dog was first examined. The anastomosis site between the proximal gastric antrum and the duodenum is in the field of view. (Note the ridged area extending from the 5 o'clock to 12 o'clock position). Biopsies obtained from the area were normal (as they were at 12 and 24 months after surgery). (From Tams TR: Gastrointestinal symptoms. In Tams TR, editor: *Handbook of small animal gastroenterology,* Philadelphia, 1996, WB Saunders.)

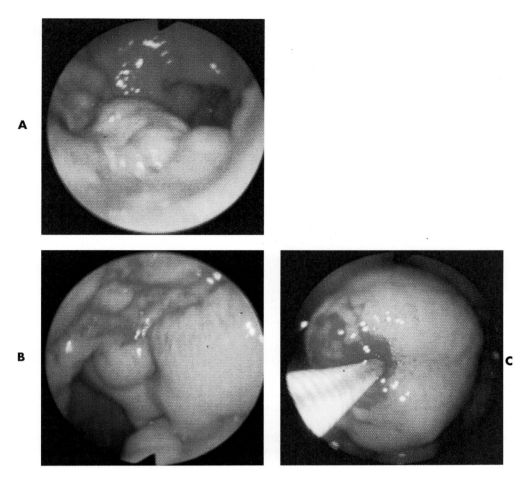

**Plate 5-91** Gastric adenocarcinoma. **A,** Marked proliferative changes in the lower gastric body; with complete loss of the normal rugal fold architecture. **B,** Lower gastric body with an area of superficial ulceration seen in the lower field. **C,** Close-up view of a mass in the mid-gastric body. The mass was rigid and had a very dense wall (suggestive of neoplasia). Masses such as this one should be biopsied as deeply as possible. If only superficial tissue is obtained, the endoscopist may fail to retrieve neoplastic cells. The first four attempts to biopsy the mass yielded very small tissue samples, but on the fifth attempt the biopsy instrument advanced inside the mass. A number of large tissue samples were obtained, and the diagnosis of adenocarcinoma was confirmed. Biopsies were also obtained from the ulcerated area shown in **B.**

## MISCELLANEOUS FINDINGS

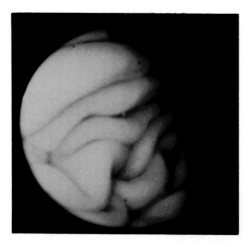

**Plate 5-92** Secondary changes (thickening) of the rugal folds in a 12-year-old mixed-breed dog with Zollinger-Ellison syndrome. In this syndrome, gastrin is released into the circulation by a gastrinoma (a tumor usually located in the pancreas). The release of gastrin leads to expansion of the parietal cell mass with an enhanced capacity to secrete gastric acid. The rugal folds thicken because of the trophic effect of gastrin. This dog also had hyperemia of the distal esophagus. Between 90% and 95% of humans with Zollinger-Ellison syndrome have upper gastrointestinal ulceration at some time during the course of their disease. No ulceration was identified in this dog. Vomiting was completely controlled by cimetidine. A gastrinoma was found in the pancreas at surgery. (Courtesy Robert G. Sherding.)

## HAIRBALLS IN CATS

It is not unusual to encounter small accumulations of hair during gastroscopy in cats. In many cases a hairball is an incidental finding and is not diagnostic of a specific disorder. Occasionally a large tubular hairball in the antrum causes outflow obstruction. Hairballs can usually be easily removed using a foreign body grasper. Gastric and duodenal biopsies should still be obtained if clinical signs include vomiting, inappetence, or weight loss. Vomiting in cats is less likely to be caused by hairballs than by inflammatory disorders, which may disrupt normal motility patterns.

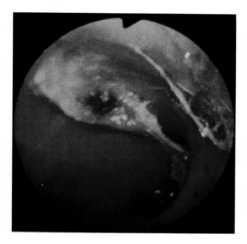

**Plate 5-93** Small accumulation of hair in the distal gastric body and proximal antrum of a cat with chronic intermittent vomiting. The angulus is at the lower right aspect of the field. Gastric biopsies were normal, and duodenal biopsies revealed inflammatory bowel disease. The hair was thought to be an incidental finding.

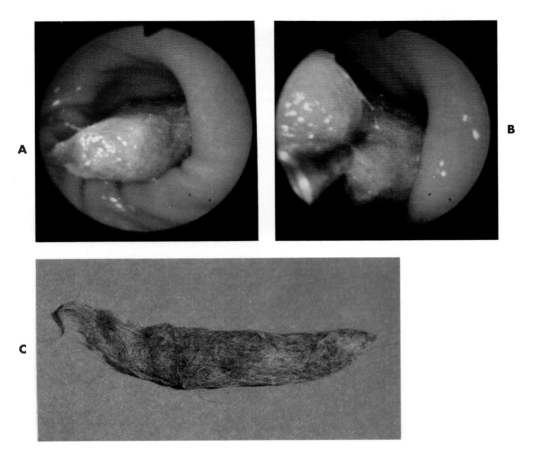

**Plate 5-94 A,** A large tubular hairball extends slightly into the distal gastric body from the antrum. The angulus is in the right aspect of the field. **B,** The hairball has been grasped with a two-prong foreign body grasper and is being pulled into the gastric body. **C,** The retrieved hairball. NOTE: These photographs are of the cat with gastric lymphosarcoma that was discussed in Plates 5-81 through 5-84. The owner reported recurrence of intermittent vomiting 19 weeks after the animal began receiving chemotherapy. Based on gastroscopy and the cessation of vomiting after the hairball removal, the vomiting was caused by the hairball and *not* loss of remission from lymphosarcoma.

# PHYSALOPTERA

*Physaloptera* species are small, stout nematode parasites occasionally found in the stomach and anterior small intestine of dogs and cats. Adult worms are creamy white, sometimes tightly coiled, and ½ to 1½ inches long and about 1/12 inch wide. Chronic intermittent vomiting is the most common clinical sign of Physaloptera infection. Anorexia and melanous stools may be observed. Treatment involves manual removal of the parasite followed by a 3-day course of fenbendazole or a single dose of pyrantel.

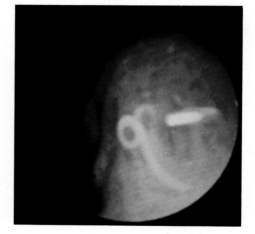

**Plate 5-95** *Physaloptera* parasite on the gastric mucosa of a dog (center of field). The white image at the right (3 o'clock position) is due to light reflection. (Courtesy Michael S. Leib.)

# Chapter 6

# Endoscopic Examination of the Small Intestine

**Todd R. Tams**

Endoscopy of the small intestine *(enteroscopy)* is an extremely valuable and minimally invasive means of examining the small bowel and procuring biopsy samples in animals. The value of small bowel biopsy in the diagnosis of diseases that affect the small intestine is well recognized. After appropriate insufflation the small intestinal lumen is usually well visualized during enteroscopy. The descending duodenum can be examined in all animals in which the endoscope can be advanced through the pylorus, and the jejunum can often be reached in cats and small dogs. Furthermore, in most dogs weighing more than 5 kg (11 lb) a pediatric endoscope can be used to perform retrograde ileoscopy after complete colonoscopy, which makes, it possible to evaluate segments of both the upper and lower small intestine. The newer pediatric veterinary endoscopes with insertion tube lengths of 140 to 150 cm can be advanced at least along the entire descending duodenum in even large- to giant-breed dogs.

Enteroscopy primarily identifies abnormalities of the intestinal mucosa, but it may also reveal distortion of the normal anatomic relationships by displacement or extrinsic compression as the result of a mass or enlargement of an adjacent organ. Enteroscopy with biopsy is excellent for detecting diffuse mucosal small bowel disease. It has become an extremely valuable means of diagnosing inflammatory bowel disease, a common cause of vomiting and diarrhea in dogs and cats. In fact, the frequency of inflammatory bowel disease came to be recognized as animals with various patterns of gastrointestinal symptoms began to be evaluated more thoroughly by endoscopic examination and biopsy. Before endoscopy became available, intestinal biopsies could only be obtained during surgery or by passing a suction capsule biopsy instrument through the pylorus under fluoroscopic control. (The latter procedure can be difficult and is not commonly used.) Endoscopic examination with biopsy of the small intestine significantly increases the yield of diagnostic information in comparison with radiographic contrast studies, which are often less sensitive when a mucosal disorder is involved. The main disadvantage of endoscopy compared with contrast radiography is that the entire length of the intestinal lumen cannot be examined with an endoscope. Ultrasound scanning, an excellent modality for evaluating the small intestines, is commonly used in conjunction with enteroscopy to provide a very thorough evaluation of the intestinal tract. The combination of ultrasonography and endoscopy is far superior to contrast radiography.

When esophagoscopy or gastroscopy is performed, the endoscopist should make every effort to examine the duodenum. *Complete* esophagogastroduodenoscopy (EGD) should be routine practice any time an examination is undertaken to evaluate a specific area of the upper gastrointestinal tract. With experience the endoscopist can conduct this thorough examination in a relatively short period. Lesions are far less likely to be missed when a complete examination is performed.

## INDICATIONS

Indications for enteroscopy include the clinical signs associated with small-bowel diseases, such as vomiting, diarrhea, hematemesis, melena, change in appetite (a ravenous or decreased appetite or complete anorexia), and weight loss. When clinical signs are acute, symptomatic treatment is provided, and a number of baseline diagnostic tests are performed. These tests may include survey abdominal radiograph complete blood count, biochemical profile, urinalysis, and fecal studies (to evaluate for parasitic, viral, and bacterial disorders). When a patient is presented for the evaluation of predominantly acute clinical signs, enteroscopy is generally undertaken only when a foreign body, ulcer, or tumor is suspected. Enteroscopy is most commonly recommended when clinical signs are chronic or acute signs fail to resolve in a reasonable period. If vomiting is the predominant clinical sign, enteroscopy is mainly limited to the upper small intestine. However, particularly in cats, vomiting with or without diarrhea may occur secondary to a lesion in the lower small bowel, ileocecal area, or proximal colon. Therefore, in some vomiting cats both upper and lower gastrointestinal endoscopy may be necessary to establish a definitive diagnosis. In animals with vomiting the endoscopic examination must not be limited to the esophagus and stomach because vomiting is a common clinical sign of inflammatory bowel disease. If only gastric biopsies are obtained, the diagnosis may be missed.

When chronic small bowel diarrhea or weight loss occurs, especially in conjunction with panhypoproteinemia, the endoscopist should try to perform ileoscopy or at least attempt to obtain ileum biopsies blindly by advancing biopsy forceps through the ileocolic valve. In the clinical setting the upper small intestine is *routinely* examined because it is easier to enter and significantly less patient preparation is necessary. The patient must be prepared for complete colonoscopy before any thought can be given to reaching the ileum with an endoscope. When chronic nonspecific diarrhea is the dominant clinical sign, biopsies ideally should be obtained from the duodenum, jejunum (if it can be reached with the endoscope or biopsy forceps), ileum, and colon. This approach often provides representative tissue for making an accurate diagnosis.

Intestinal involvement is diffuse in the majority of dogs and cats with inflammatory bowel disease. In such cases it is usually sufficient to obtain biopsy samples from the duodenum if the endoscope is not long enough to be advanced to the jejunum. However, in disorders with patchy intestinal involvement, such as regional enteritis and intestinal lymphoma, the diagnosis can be missed if only duodenal biopsies are obtained. Regional enteritis is an *uncommon* disorder in which inflammatory changes are more focal, and obtaining a biopsy sample of the proximal small intestine is helpful only if an involved area is sampled. When inflammatory bowel disease is suspected, an attempt should be made to obtain biopsies from the ileum if colonoscopy is performed in conjunction with EGD. In this way the histologic characteristics of the small intestine can be more thoroughly evaluated. In my experience, if inflammatory changes are found in the ileum, they are often of the same type but less severe than those found in the duodenum. Occasionally a different cell type predominates, but usually no alteration of the treatment protocol is necessary. Rarely in canine and feline patients, the duodenum is completely normal and significant inflammatory changes are identified in the ileum. I have also observed several cases in which dogs had ileal lymphoma but benign disease or no significant histologic changes in the duodenum. Diarrhea was the predominant sign in these dogs. A definitive diagnosis in these cases was reached by following the policy of performing endoscopy of both the upper and lower gastrointestinal tract in animals with chronic diarrhea, even if no large bowel signs were evident.

At this point it appears that biopsy samples obtained from the upper small intestine are reliably representative of the type of intestinal disorder that is present in a majority of patients with inflammatory bowel disease. The most significant advantage offered by endoscopic examination and biopsy of the small intestine is the opportunity to diagnose inflammatory bowel disease relatively early, as clinical signs become evident, *without* having to procure tissue samples surgically.

Endoscopy offers an alternative approach to obtaining small bowel biopsies in protein-losing enteropathy cases in which there is a concern that full-thickness biopsy sites may heal slowly. This is an especially important consideration in patients with a total protein level less than 3.5 g/dl. Multiple biopsies can be safely obtained using endoscopic biopsy forceps. In addition, compared with surgery, endoscopy requires a significantly shorter hospital stay, which makes it a cost-effective procedure. In dogs, inflammatory bowel disease is by far the most common cause of protein-losing enteropathy and occurs much more often than lymphangiectasia and intestinal lymphoma. Intestinal lymphoma occurs somewhat more commonly in cats than dogs. Lymphangiectasia, a disorder of the intestinal lymphatics that results in malabsorption, has a characteristic mucosal histologic appearance; in some cases, pronounced gross changes can be seen at endoscopic examination (see Plates 6-43 and 6-44). Rarely the diagnosis of lymphangiectasia is missed when only the descending duodenum is examined and sampled.

Duodenal fluid aspirated into tubing passed through the endoscope can be examined for *Giardia* organisms.

Because the combination of zinc sulfate concentration and enzyme-linked immunosorbent assay (ELISA) testing of fecal samples for *Giardia*-specific antigen is quite reliable for detecting *Giardia* species, duodenal aspiration is rarely required to establish the diagnosis of giardiasis. In the upper small intestine of the dog and the lower small intestine of the cat, *Giardia* trophozoites attach to the brush border of the villous epithelium, usually at the basal regions of the villi. Direct smears of the aspirates should be examined within 20 minutes of collection, using light microscopy at magnifications of 100× and 400×.

Occasionally enteroscopy is useful for evaluating patients with obscure gastrointestinal bleeding. In humans, possible causes of intestinal bleeding are identified in 30% to 40% of patients with unexplained hemorrhage who undergo enteroscopy. Retrograde ileoscopy is often done if an examination of the upper small bowel proves unrewarding. Ulceration of the small intestines occurs less commonly in animals than humans. Sources of bleeding in animals may include benign ulceration, various benign mucosal inflammatory disorders, drug-induced hemorrhage (e.g., nonsteroidal antiinflammatory medications), and neoplasia. If routine procedures such as radiography and gastroscopy fail to identify a source of bleeding, enteroscopy should be considered and as much of the small intestine as possible should be examined.

Tumors that involve the small bowel mucosa can be reliably diagnosed by biopsy if a large enough sample of *representative* tissue is obtained. Occasionally it is difficult for a pathologist to differentiate lymphocytic enteritis from lymphosarcoma. In this situation, full-thickness surgical biopsies may be necessary to clarify the diagnosis. Benign lymphocytic enteritis (inflammatory bowel disease characterized by a pure infiltrate of lymphocytes) is a well-recognized disorder in cats but appears to be quite uncommon in dogs. Focal areas of lymphoma in the jejunum or ileum may be easily missed because of insufficient endoscope length. Also, if lymphoma involvement is primarily in the deeper muscle layers of the intestinal wall, mucosal and submucosal biopsy samples obtained with endoscopy forceps may not be deep enough to obtain representative tissue. When lymphoma is present but not definitively diagnosed on the samples submitted for examination, the mucosal tissue that is obtained is rarely normal. Varying degrees of inflammatory changes are usually found. Positive biopsy findings such as this may give the clinician false assurance that a definitive diagnosis has been reached. A poor response to treatment that is initiated based on biopsy results may then be an indication that some other more significant disorder is present. If lymphoma is strongly suspected, more tissue samples should be obtained with biopsy forceps. Alternatively, the patient should undergo exploratory laparotomy for a more detailed gross examination and the procurement of full-thickness biopsies. Surgery is the *recommended* procedure at this juncture because a much more extensive evaluation can be accomplished. It should be noted that in dogs and cats, idiopathic inflammatory bowel disease occurs much more commonly than intestinal lymphoma.

## INSTRUMENTATION

The endoscope specifications for small bowel examinations are the same as those described in Chapters 3 and 5. An endoscope diameter as large as 9.8 mm can be used in most dogs and some cats, but the success rate for advancing through the pylorus to the duodenum is estimated to be only 50% to 60% when this size endoscope is used in cats. (This success rate is higher for very experienced operators.) My personal preference is to use a 7.8- to 7.9 mm endoscope with four-way tip deflection (e.g., an Olympus GIF Type XP20 or XP10, respectively, or a Storz 512 VG [150 cm long, 8.5 mm in diameter]). A 8.5-9-mm diameter endoscope can be used successfully in many feline patients, but the smaller diameter scopes *routinely* allow enteroscopy to be performed in canine and feline patients even as small as 1.4 kg. Four-way rather than two-way tip deflection capability is definitely preferred because it considerably improves maneuverability through the pylorus and intestinal lumen.

## PATIENT PREPARATION

Patient preparation for upper small intestinal examination is the same as for gastroscopy (see Chapter 5). No food should be given for 12 to 18 hours before the examination, and water should be withheld 4 or more hours. If a barium contrast radiographic examination has been done, the small bowel should be relatively empty before an endoscope is introduced. Pools of barium should not be suctioned through the working channel because residue is likely to adhere to the channel walls. Small flecks of barium residue along the mucosal lining do not need to be suctioned, however, and pose no hindrance to completing a thorough examination (see Plate 6-10).

Ileoscopy requires that the patient be prepared for complete colonoscopy. This is discussed in detail in the section on patient preparation for colonoscopy in Chapter 7.

## RESTRAINT

As with any endoscopic procedure of the upper gastrointestinal tract, general anesthesia is required for enteroscopy. The guidelines recommended for gastroscopy should be followed (see Chapter 5). Both duodenoscopy and ileoscopy are performed with the patient positioned in *left* lateral recumbency.

## PROCEDURE

To successfully maneuver an endoscope into the duodenum, the endoscopist must first become proficient at gastroscopy. Techniques for maneuvering the endoscope around the incisura angularis (angulus) of the stomach, evaluating the antrum and pylorus, and advancing the endoscope through the pyloric canal are described in detail in Chapter 5. Techniques for traversing the pylorus are reviewed in this chapter, which also discusses in detail the examination of the duodenum and ileum, as well as techniques for obtaining biopsy samples from the small intestine.

## PYLORUS TO PROXIMAL DUODENUM

As the endoscope is advanced through the gastric antrum toward the pylorus, minor tip adjustments are made so that the pyloric orifice position is maintained in the center of the field of view. Depending on the size of the scope, the endoscopist can often apply minimal forward pressure to advance the tip directly through an open pyloric orifice and into the first segment of the duodenum. If the pyloric orifice is closed or only slightly dilated, varying degrees of resistance can be expected. If the pylorus is closed, several fairly predictable maneuvers can facilitate entrance to and advancement through the pyloric canal. Based on the endoscope that is used, the following recommendations may vary slightly. Often the endoscope tip can be directed into the pyloric canal by applying leftward tip deflection (turn outer control knob in a counterclockwise direction) alone or in some cases along with slight to moderate upward tip deflection (turn inner control knob counterclockwise) while gradually advancing the scope. Once the tip of the endoscope is in the pyloric canal, only a blurred image is seen because the pyloric walls are usually pressed in around the tip of the scope. Turning both control knobs in a clockwise direction as the endoscope is advanced provides a downward and right tip deflection change that facilitates entry into the proximal duodenal segment, a small area immediately beyond the pylorus. Although the first part of the duodenum is not expanded to form a pronounced "duodenal bulb" or "cap" (as occurs in humans), its functional independence is retained. The initial portion of the duodenum continues from the pylorus and passes toward the right body wall before being deflected caudally to become the descending duodenum.

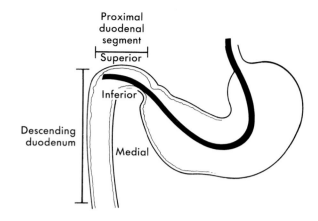

**Figure 6-1** The endoscope has been advanced through the pylorus, but a clear view of the descending duodenal canal cannot be attained until the tip of the scope is directed away from the wall of the proximal duodenal segment.

A convex curve is formed by the junction of the antrum and descending duodenum; and this area, along with the pylorus, provides some resistance to passage of the endoscope. In large dogs it is sometimes possible to clearly visualize the mucosa along this curved area, but in most cases the image remains blurred because the endoscope tip is still tightly confined. Despite the lack of a clear view, the endoscopist is usually aware that the proximal segment of the duodenum has been reached and because a distinct sensation is felt as the pyloric resistance is passed. In addition, the color of the mucosa usually changes from cream (antrum and pylorus) to pinkish red (duodenum). The color change is quite subtle in some cases. In a particularly tight pyloric canal, the color change provides an important landmark that determines the point at which directional changes are made to help guide the endoscope tip to the proximal duodenal segment (both control knobs forward). In cats and most dogs the duodenum still is not viewed clearly at this point because the endoscope is wedged against or is close to the wall of the proximal duodenal segment (Figure 6-1). One final maneuver is performed to direct the tip into the descending duodenal lumen (the second duodenal segment). *Excessive force should never be used in this area.* As the tip lies against the superior wall of the proximal duodenal segment (see Figure 6-1), it is angled acutely up (turn inner control knob counterclockwise) and in some cases also to the left (turn outer control knob counterclockwise). Further gentle advance usually provides a tunnel view of the descending duodenum (Figure 6-2). Air insufflation is usually continued to distend the walls. In some cases, minor forward or backward movements of the entire insertion tube (using the right hand placed close to the patient's mouth) are also necessary to help free the endoscope tip. If a clear view

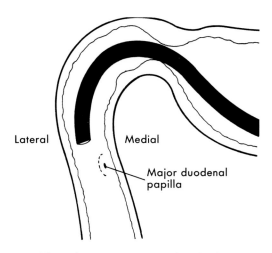

**Figure 6-2** The endoscope is positioned in the descending duodenal canal. Air insufflation is used to distend the walls to provide maximal visualization.

cannot be obtained after these collective maneuvers have been attempted, the endoscope should be retracted a short distance rather than forced forward against resistance. *If in doubt, it is almost always best to retract and insufflate to regain one's bearings.* Once the technique is mastered, an endoscope can usually be advanced from the antrum to the proximal descending duodenum in a matter of seconds. When a patient is small or the pyloric canal and proximal duodenal areas are normally narrow, successful passage to the duodenum can usually be accomplished using the maneuvers described here in sequential order and observing for important color change landmarks. As described in Chapter 5, occasionally (especially in patients with pyloric mucosal hypertrophy) even a pediatric endoscope cannot be advanced through the pylorus. The patient's heart rate and respiratory rate and character should always be monitored carefully during difficult passages in which the pyloroantral and proximal duodenal areas can be stretched considerably or distorted. Although significant cardiopulmonary changes as a result of an increase in vagal tone occur only occasionally, the endoscopy team should remain alert for these changes because they may require pharmacologic intervention. Chapter 5 provides further information on the potential complications of pyloral passage in cats.

## EXAMINATION OF DESCENDING DUODENUM

Once the proximal duodenal segment has been passed, the endoscope can usually be easily advanced along the lumen of the descending duodenum. A stomach curvature loop has usually been formed by the time the endoscope

is advanced to the proximal duodenum. Paradoxically, in some cases the endoscope tip may be best advanced along the descending duodenum by *withdrawing* the endoscope shaft. This maneuver removes the stomach curvature loop and effectively presses the endoscope tip forward along the duodenal canal. In fact, forward movement of the endoscope tip is often accelerated at this point. This maneuver is especially helpful in large dogs in which very little insertion tube length may remain after a stomach curvature loop forms and the endoscope tip has reached the proximal descending duodenum.

Varying degrees of insufflation are usually necessary to maintain a clear view of the lumen of the small intestine as the endoscope is advanced. This is easily accomplished by using the air insufflation button on the control housing. As in gastroscopy, great care must be taken to monitor the degree of gastric distension, especially in cats and small dogs. Air insufflated to the intestine may reflux into the stomach and cause significant *gastric dilation,* which may subsequently cause *respiratory compromise.* Moderate gastric distension usually is not a significant problem, except in some obese patients whose conformation may potentiate respiratory difficulty under general anesthesia. Marked gastric distension should be quickly relieved because it can significantly compromise respiration. To relieve gastric distension, the endoscopist withdraws the tip of the scope to the stomach so that the air can be effectively suctioned. Traversing the pylorus again usually is not difficult after it has already been done one or more times.

The intestine should be carefully examined as the endoscope is advanced and as it is retracted after the furthest point of advance has been reached. It is usually easier to view parts of the proximal duodenal segment during retraction than on entry. The major limiting factor of enteroscopy is that only a limited length of intestine can be visualized using standard endoscopes. A minor limitation is that certain portions of the duodenum, including the area immediately beyond the pylorus and parts of the medial wall of the descending segment, are sometimes difficult to view other than tangentially. A special effort is made to obtain full circumferential views by rotating the endoscope tip in various directions during *retraction.* Under the different conditions of motility and organ shapes determined by distension and endoscope position during retraction, areas previously seen only tangentially may be brought into direct view. This minimizes blind areas that cannot be examined thoroughly on entry. Examination on entry is most important for recognizing general mucosal appearance and obvious lesions. In small patients the endoscope itself sometimes causes minor mucosal trauma, which usually appears as streaks of erythema or mild superficial hemorrhage (see Plates 6-47 and 6-48). Comparison of the examination findings during advance and retraction can confirm whether lesions are iatrogenic or were present before the evaluation was undertaken.

## ASCENDING DUODENUM AND JEJUNUM

In cats and small- to medium-sized dogs a pediatric endoscope can often be advanced to the proximal jejunum (see Plate 6-7). With the tip of the scope situated in the mid-descending duodenum, the endoscopist can see a fold or curve that represents the junction between the descending and ascending duodenum. This curve is situated at a point between the right kidney and the pelvic inlet. After a short medially directed section, the duodenum ascends for a short distance (ascending duodenum or third duodenal segment). The next bend is directed ventrally and represents the continuation of the small intestine as jejunum. Endoscopically this juncture is more difficult to recognize than the junction of the descending and ascending duodenum. Depending on the remaining insertion tube length outside the patient, gradual advance of the endoscope can be continued as long as no significant resistance is met. Minimal manual changes in tip deflection are often required as the scope is advanced through the small intestine because the junctional curves are usually freely movable and accommodating to passage of the scope. However, in some cats and dogs the junction between the descending and ascending duodenum and ascending duodenum and jejunum is not easily traversed, especially if a gastric greater curvature loop remains and the pyloroduodenal junction continues to resist advancement of the insertion tube. In such cases it is not particularly worthwhile to continue efforts to advance the endoscope tip as far as possible. Continued efforts may cause considerable stretch and caudal displacement of the stomach and pyloroduodenal area. If resistance is met, it is usually best to begin retracting the endoscope. At this point in the procedure the mucosa of the proximal bowel is examined in detail and biopsy specimens are obtained.

If for some reason the endoscope tip must be advanced along the small intestine as far as possible and resistance is met before this is accomplished, several maneuvers may help facilitate passage. Gently sliding the insertion tube forward and backward may slightly alter the intestinal loop configuration. Alternatively, an assistant can help "milk" the endoscope through the intestine by palpating and massaging the small intestinal loops transabdominally. This maneuver is most useful in cats and small dogs because it is easy to identify the endoscope on abdominal palpation. Glucagon can be used to reduce duodenal or jejunal motor activity if such motion interferes with visualization or scope advancement. Finally, during laparotomy it is sometimes desirable to examine long sections of mucosa (e.g., areas of focal hemorrhage, neoplasia, or segmented enteritis) in search of lesions. Direct mucosal examination may add considerably to the value of an evaluation limited solely to external bowel manipulation and palpation. In addition to potentially guiding the surgeon to an important lesion for resection or biopsy, intraoperative enteroscopy may identify diffuse lesions throughout the intestine, which may effectively rule out surgical resection as a viable option. Once the endoscope is advanced to the duodenum, the surgeon can manually feed the endoscope along the intestine using a pleating technique. The surgeon then examines the mucosa during both advance and retraction.

## NORMAL APPEARANCE OF UPPER SMALL INTESTINE

The normal duodenal and jejunal mucosa appears reddish pink to yellow-red in dogs and cream to slightly reddish pink in cats. Because of the presence of villi the mucosa has a velvety or shaggy appearance, especially on close visualization. Aggregated lymphatic nodules (Peyer's patches) can routinely be identified in the descending duodenum of dogs (see Plate 6-3). The nodules, some as large as 2 cm by 1.5 cm, are found on the lateral wall. A shallow central crater effect (approximately 2 to 3 mm deep) is associated with these nodules. Although aggregated lymphoid nodules also occur in the cat, they are not readily identified on endoscopic examination.

With newer endoscopes that have wide-angle illumination, one or both duodenal papillae of dogs can often be visualized. The major duodenal papilla is located along the medial wall approximately 5 cm from the pylorus. This papilla represents the common opening for the bile duct and the pancreatic duct (the duct of Wirsung). The appearance of the papilla varies from a flattened white disk to a small thickened projection from the medial wall. Occasionally an active bile discharge can be seen emanating from the papilla. A second papilla, the minor papilla, is located on the upper wall, approximately 2 cm distal to the major papilla. The accessory pancreatic duct (the duct of Santorini) opens onto the minor duodenal papilla. This papilla is generally flattened and appears as a small (1.5 to 2 mm in diameter) white, round to oval disk against the reddish pink of the surrounding mucosa. Cats have only one papilla (the major duodenal papilla) for the pancreatic and biliary ducts. As a result of its location close to the convex curve formed by the antrum, pylorus, and proximal duodenum, this papilla is sometimes difficult to visualize endoscopically. Various normal appearances of the duodenal papillae are shown in Plates 6-19 through 6-24.

# EXAMINATION OF THE TERMINAL ILEUM

As previously described, examination and biopsy of the ileum are most important in animals with chronic diarrhea or weight loss that is clinically consistent with a small intestinal disorder. Although it is not always possible to enter the ileum in dogs, the ileocolic valve can often be identified during complete colonoscopy, and a biopsy instrument can usually be passed blindly into the terminal ileum. With practice, an endoscopist can routinely enter the ileum of dogs weighing over 5 kg (11 lb), especially when a pediatric endoscope is used. It is essential that the ascending colon contain minimal to no residue. It is rarely possible to advance a pediatric endoscope into the ileum of a cat, but blind biopsies can be obtained from cats with sufficiently clean colons in which the ileocolic orifice can be clearly visualized.

For ileoscopy the colon must be thoroughly cleansed. Retained fecal material prevents thorough mucosal evaluation and makes it extremely difficult to see clearly enough to maneuver through the curves of the colon. Therefore when ileoscopy is contemplated, every effort must be made to ensure that the colon is completely evacuated. Procedures for cleansing the colon and examining this organ to the level of the ileocolic junction are described in Chapter 7.

The ileal orifice usually protrudes into the lumen of the terminal ascending colon as a papillary form and as such is easily recognized (Figure 6-3 and Plates 6-25 through 6-28). A close-up view of the orifice reveals either a narrow opening or more commonly a closed opening represented only by a small depression in the center of the raised valve structure. In contrast, the cecocolic junction is often open to some degree and is flattened. In some cases the ileocolic orifice is difficult to identify ei-

ther because it also is both flattened and closed or because it is tucked behind a fold. In the former instance the ileocolic valve may be correctly identified after observing intestinal contents issue from the valve. It may be necessary to suction pooled fluid from the area at various times during the procedure to improve visualization.

Occasionally the ileocolic valve is open and easily traversed. In the majority of cases, however, the valve is closed, and precise tip control is required for entry into the ileum. The raised valve structure may be pliable and is often easily deflected when the endoscope tip touches it. Therefore unless the approach angle is straight, entering the valve channel is difficult. If several attempts to ease the endoscope tip through the valve fail to achieve entry to the ileum, the endoscopist can attempt to guide biopsy forceps through the valve. If the forceps instrument can be advanced at least several centimeters beyond the valve, it can be used as a guide wire over which the endoscope insertion tube is advanced. Once the endoscope enters the ileum, the forceps instrument is retracted so that the scope can be advanced along the lumen. Occasionally, however, this maneuver is not successful. For example, the forceps tip can become wedged into a mucosal wall of the valve or the most terminal section of the ileum when these structures are positioned at an oblique angle relative to the proximal section of the endoscope. If the approach angle is difficult, the patient may be rotated from left lateral to dorsal recumbency. This may shift the position of the ileocecocolic area sufficiently to provide a more favorable angle of approach. Once the endoscope tip is in the ileum, the patient is returned to left lateral recumbency.

Undue force should *never* be used to gain entry to the ileum. Excessive forward pressure on the endoscope shaft may cause considerable stretch and displacement of the colon. For the most effective maneuverability the endoscopist should rely on the tip deflection controls, insertion tube torque, air insufflation, suction, and gradual advance and withdrawal techniques.

With the endoscope tip in the ileum, air is insufflated to improve visualization. The ileal mucosa often has a more mottled or patchy appearance than colonic mucosa. Toward the junction with the large intestine, Peyer's patches tend to be more numerous than in the upper small intestine. On average, a 5- to 10-cm section of terminal ileum is examined; however, the endoscope should be advanced farther if no resistance is encountered. Depending on gross appearance, six to eight biopsy specimens should be obtained before the endoscope is retracted to the ascending colon. These tissue samples are placed in a separate formalin container from the proximal small intestine and colon samples.

Air insufflation of the ascending colon and ileum may cause significant dilation of the upper small bowel and stomach. This dilation is of greatest concern in small patients. Therefore patients should be observed carefully for

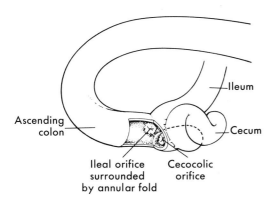

**Figure 6-3** The ileocolic junction and its relation to the cecum in the dog. Note the positions of the ileum, cecum, ascending colon, ileal orifice surrounded by annular fold, and cecocolic orifice. (From Dyce KM et al: *Textbook of veterinary anatomy,* Philadelphia, 1987, WB Saunders.)

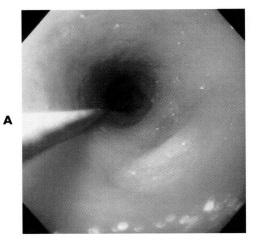

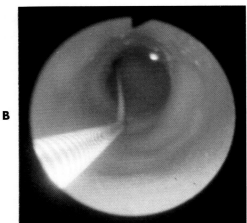

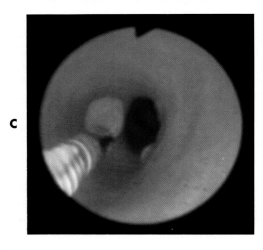

respiratory distress, a potentially serious problem that can result from overdistension of the stomach. Rarely a stomach tube must be passed to relieve the distension. If moderate or marked gastric dilation is present after ileoscopy and colonoscopy are completed, I usually advance the endoscope from the mouth to the stomach to facilitate *complete* evacuation of air from the stomach before the patient is awakened from anesthesia. This makes vomiting much less likely to occur during recovery.

## SMALL INTESTINE BIOPSY TECHNIQUES

Several techniques are useful for obtaining tissue samples from the small intestine. Unlike gastric mucosa, the mucosa of the small intestine is generally not drawn up to the tip of the endoscope before a biopsy sample can

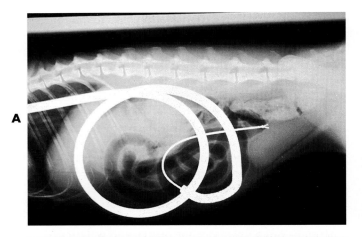

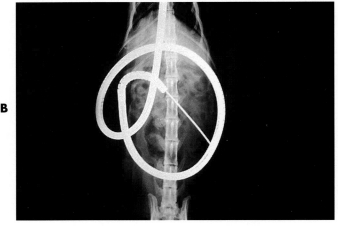

**Figure 6-4 A,** The tip of the biopsy instrument is being advanced along the descending duodenum. The forceps cups remain closed during the advance. Air is insufflated as needed to maintain distension. A Peyer's patch is visualized from the 4 to 6 o'-clock position in the field of view. **B,** The biopsy instrument is advanced as far as possible until resistance is met. Note that the forceps shaft has bowed slightly against the resistance, indicating that it will be difficult to advance the instrument any farther. The forceps instrument is retracted slightly, the cups are opened, and the instrument is readvanced. **C,** The biopsy forceps have been retracted, and the tissue sample is seen within the cups. This sample is larger than normal.

**Figure 6-5** Lateral (**A**) and ventrodorsal (**B**) abdominal radiographs in a cat, showing the configuration of an endoscope (100-cm insertion tube length) with the tip positioned in the proximal jejunum. Endoscopic biopsy forceps have been advanced along the jejunum. Excellent biopsy samples can be obtained by advancing the open forceps cups against resistance. In this case the forceps have been advanced around a curve, well beyond the area the endoscopist can see.

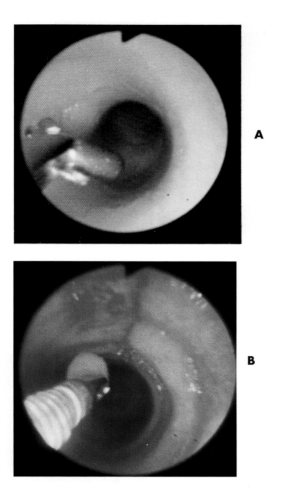

**Figure 6-6 A,** The forceps cups were opened as soon as they were advanced beyond the endoscope tip. The forceps can then be buried in an adjacent section of mucosa or advanced along the small intestinal canal until resistance is met. **B,** A biopsy sample is obtained at the 11 to 12 o'clock position.

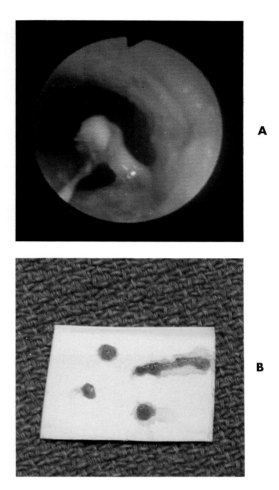

**Figure 6-7 A,** A large linear section of tissue is lifted from the duodenum of a 14-year-old cat with a 10-month history of chronic diarrhea resulting from severe lymphocytic, plasmacytic, fibrosing enteritis. In such cases, bowel perforation from the biopsy technique is not a concern because the samples are long but not deep (no greater depth than deep mucosa). **B,** Three small intestinal mucosal samples of routine size and one long tissue sample (the same tissue segment shown in Figure 6-7, *A*) were obtained from this patient.

be torn free because the intestinal mucosa is somewhat more friable than gastric mucosa. Consequently, samples are lifted off as the forceps cups are snapped shut. Only occasionally, when fairly deep samples are obtained, is the intestinal wall drawn up toward the endoscope tip as the forceps cups are closed and retracted.

I generally use two biopsy techniques when obtaining small intestinal samples. First, after the endoscope is advanced as far as possible, the biopsy instrument is passed through the working channel and along the lumen until resistance is met (see Plate 6-7, *E*). The forceps cups are usually beyond view when this is done (Figure 6-4). Once resistance is met, the forceps are retracted slightly so that the cups can be opened, and the forceps are then firmly readvanced into the mucosal wall. After closure the forceps cups are withdrawn, usually with minimal resistance (Radiographs demonstrating forceps positioning in a cat are shown in Figure 6-5.) Alternatively the forceps cups can be opened as soon as they are passed beyond the en-

doscope tip (Figure 6-6) and then advanced until resistance is met. Further slight advance against resistance may seat the forceps cups more deeply and may help procure a larger tissue sample. The purpose of these blind biopsy techniques is to obtain samples from as far down the small intestine as possible. Even if the jejunum cannot be visualized, it is often possible to obtain biopsy samples from this section of the small bowel. Biopsy samples vary in size. They are often small when the intestinal mucosa is normal. When the intestinal mucosa is compromised by some disorder, sample size is invariably larger. Occasionally a long linear strip (1 inch) of tissue is lifted off when marked inflammatory disease alters the mucosal and submucosal integrity (Figures 6-7 and 6-8). These large samples are most likely to be obtained using the technique described above.

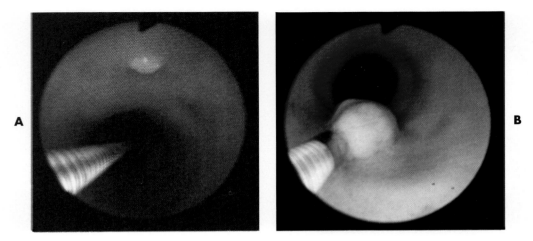

**Figure 6-8 A,** Blind biopsy technique used in a dog to obtain a tissue sample from the jejunum. The mucosa appears grossly normal, and the minor duodenal papilla is visualized at the 12 o'-clock position. **B,** A larger than normal tissue sample was procured using standard alligator-jaw biopsy forceps advanced through a pediatric endoscope with a 2-mm accessory channel. Normally only a small amount of tissue can be seen outside the forceps cups once they have been closed.

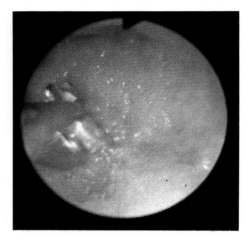

**Figure 6-9** The endoscope tip has been directed toward the bowel wall, and the forceps cups are buried in the mucosa. (The lower shaft of the instrument is seen at the 8 to 9 o'clock position.)

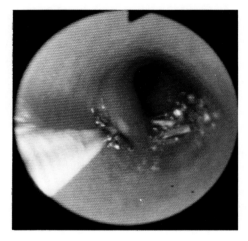

**Figure 6-10** With the endoscope tip positioned straight in the center of the lumen, it is more difficult to seat the forceps cups in a site close to the scope. As shown here, the forceps tend to slide along the wall. At best only a small sample is usually obtained if the endoscopist even manages to seat the forceps in the mucosa. Bayonet forceps help avoid this sliding problem. Whenever possible, the endoscope tip should be directed into the wall (i.e., more perpendicular than parallel) for the procurement of intestinal samples.

As the endoscope is retracted toward the stomach, additional biopsies (usually six to eight per procedure) are obtained from various sites. If an area of mucosa in view is to be sampled, the tip of the endoscope is angled as much as possible toward the wall so that the forceps can be adequately seated (Figure 6-9). Otherwise the forceps cups tend to slide along the wall of the lumen without firm tissue purchase (Figure 6-10). Although bayonet-type forceps with a central needle are useful for preventing the problem of sliding along the lumen, adequate-size tissue samples can be obtained using standard alligator-jaw forceps and good technique.

After biopsy samples are procured from the small intestine, bleeding is usually minimal. In contrast more than a normal amount of bleeding may occur after mucosal samples are obtained from an abnormal bowel. However, not enough blood is lost to cause a significant clinical problem. Figure 6-11 shows the amount of hemorrhage that can be expected after a large biopsy sample is obtained. A corresponding photomicrograph is included.

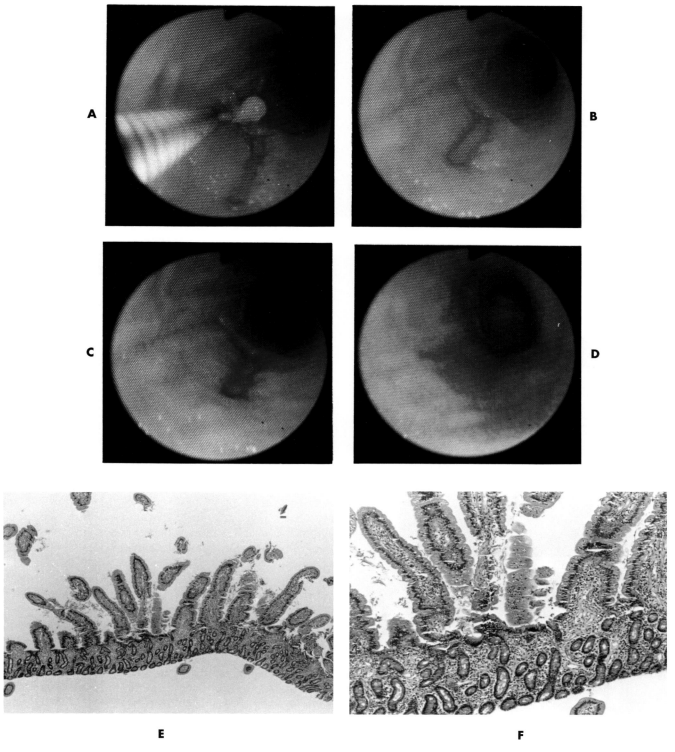

**Figure 6-11** A sizeable tissue sample has been procured (**A**). Once the biopsy instrument was seated in the mucosa in the immediate foreground, it slid distally and lifted off a large sample. Hemorrhage after 3 (**B**), 6 (**C**), and 12 (**D**) seconds. Low-power (**E**) and high-power (**F**) photomicrographs show sample depth to the level of the crypts (deep mucosa). (Photomicrographs courtesy Emily J. Walder.)

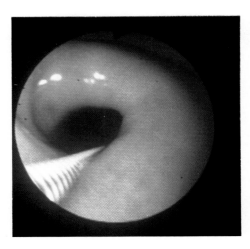

**Figure 6-12** Duodenal blind biopsy technique in a 70-kg (154-lb) Great Dane. A 110-cm endoscope had insufficient length to reach the duodenum. Biopsy forceps were easily passed through the open pylorus, and good-quality tissue samples were obtained blindly from the duodenum.

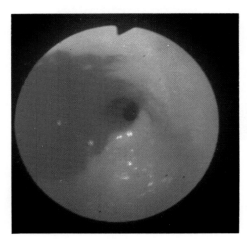

**Figure 6-13** Hemorrhage in a cat resulting from superficial pyloric mucosal trauma caused by forward and backward action of the biopsy forceps during a blind duodenal biopsy procedure. No clinical problems resulted from the superficial trauma.

In the event that an endoscope cannot be advanced through the pylorus to the duodenum, blind biopsies of the descending duodenum can sometimes be obtained. The endoscope tip is positioned in the distal antrum with the pyloric orifice as close to central view as possible, and the biopsy forceps are guided through the pylorus. The forceps slide most easily when the pylorus is open (Figure 6-12). If the pylorus is tightly closed or the pyloric orifice cannot be approached from an appropriate angle, it may be difficult to traverse either the pyloric canal or the proximal duodenal segment to reach the descending duodenum. Adjusting the endoscope tip angle, changing the patient's position to dorsal recumbency, or using a series of gentle forward and backward moves

with the forceps may facilitate passage to the descending duodenum. Occasionally, superficial pyloric mucosal trauma from the biopsy forceps shaft results in hemorrhage (Figure 6-13). If the forceps still cannot be advanced, biopsies can at least be obtained from the short proximal duodenal segment. Fortunately, ulcers in this area are a rare occurrence in dogs and cats, so the risk of perforation through a compromised duodenal wall is extremely small. The only risk associated with blind biopsy of the proximal descending duodenum is the slight possibility of damaging the duodenal papilla. With this in mind the biopsy forceps should be advanced as far along the duodenal lumen as possible. As proper maneuvering skills are gained, the need for blind biopsy of the small intestine is minimized.

## ENTEROSCOPY: THE FUTURE

Future advances in enteroscopy primarily involve the manufacture of longer endoscopes that allow greater lengths of the bowel to be examined. In human enteroscopy, various techniques have been devised to maximize the extent of insertion. Techniques used in the past include ropeaway-type enteroscopy and sonde-type enteroscopy.

In the ropeaway method the patient swallows one end of a considerable length of a string and waits several days for the string to pass from the rectum. At the time of the procedure the string, exiting from mouth and anus, is used as a guide over which the endoscope is passed. General anesthesia is required to relieve pain because as the string is stretched taut, the intestines begin to plicate. The advantage of this procedure is that as long as sufficient endoscope length is available, the entire length of the small intestine can be examined. However, as a result of patient discomfort, the length of time necessary for string passage, and the development of better tolerated techniques, the ropeaway method has largely been abandoned in human medicine.

Another technique involves the use of a long endoscope (e.g., the Olympus SIF-10L with a working length of 217.5 cm and an insertion tube diameter of 11.3 mm) and a stiffening tube that is placed over the endoscope to prevent excessive loop formation in the stomach and resultant loss of usable endoscope length. During the course of the procedure the stiffening tube is often advanced sequentially as far as the duodenojejunal junction to prevent duodenal loop formation. This maximizes the extent of the examination.

One of the newest instruments available for use in humans is a long, small-caliber, sonde-type transnasal endoscope. This instrument allows most of the small bowel to be examined during a relatively short (6 to 8 hours) ambulatory procedure. For sonde-type enteroscopy a long scope is propelled by peristalsis throughout the intestine. Two channels are present: one for air insufflation of the intestinal lumen and the other for inflation of a balloon at the instrument's tip. The inflated balloon provides a bolus upon which peristalsis acts to pull the instrument through the small intestine.

Multiple prototype sonde enteroscopes have been developed by the Olympus Corporation. The SSIF-VII prototype has a 90-degree field of vision and a 5-mm tip diameter. In humans the scope is passed transnasally and is well tolerated. Because these enteroscopes do not have tip deflection capability, procedure time can be prolonged (14.7 hours on average) with passive passage through the pylorus. However, when the transnasal enteroscope is guided "piggyback" through the pylorus and descending duodenum using a conventional endoscope, the procedure time is decreased to 6 to 7 hours. During sonde-type enteroscopy, the mucosa is inspected in detail during withdrawal of the instrument.

Although it may be some time before specialized enteroscopes are used routinely in small animals, the advantages of this type of instrumentation should be recognized. With complete enteroscopy it is possible to identify obscure sites of intestinal hemorrhage, focal neoplastic lesions, and the patchy involvement of benign inflammatory disease. In many patients enteroscopy may obviate the need for diagnostic exploratory laparotomy.

## SUGGESTED ADDITIONAL READINGS

Barkin JS et al: Enteroscopy and small bowel biopsy— an improved technique for the diagnosis of small bowel disease, *Gastrointest Endosc* 31:215, 1985.

Dyce KM, Sack WO, Wensing CJG, editors: *Textbook of veterinary anatomy: the digestive apparatus,* Philadelphia, 1987, WB Saunders.

Johnson GF: Duodenoscopy. In Anderson NV, editor: *Veterinary gastroenterology,* Philadelphia, 1980, Lea and Febiger.

Lewis BS, Waye JD: Small bowel enteroscopy in 1988: pros and cons, *Am J Gastroenterol* 83:799, 1988.

Pitts RP, Twedt DC, Mallie KA: Comparison of duodenal aspiration with fecal flotation for diagnosis of giardiasis in dogs, *J Am Vet Assoc* 182:1210, 1983.

Shimizu S, Tada M, Kowai K: Development of a new insertion technique in push-type enteroscopy, *Am J Gastroenterol* 82:844, 1987.

Sivak MV: Technique of upper gastrointestinal endoscopy. In Sivak MV, editor: *Gastroenterologic endoscopy,* Philadelphia, 1987, WB Saunders.

## COLOR PLATES   PAGES 187-215

## NORMAL CANINE DUODENUM: VARIOUS APPEARANCES

The color of normal canine duodenal mucosa varies from pinkish white to light red. The mucosa often appears slightly irregular or velvety because of its digitate villi. Air insufflation is usually necessary to maintain a clear view of the small intestine.

**A** 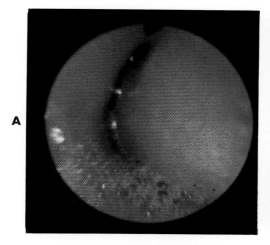   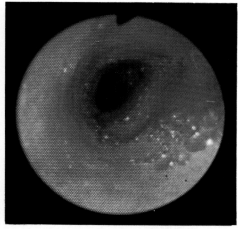 **B**

**Plate 6-1** Proximal descending duodenum before (**A**) and after (**B**) air insufflation, with the endoscope tip in same position. After adequate distension a full circumferential view of the small intestinal lumen can be attained.

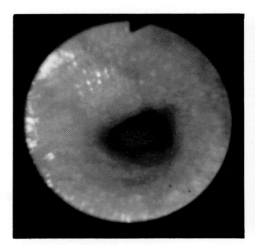   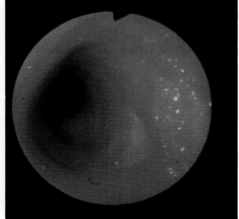

**Plate 6-2** Close-up of duodenal mucosa. Its "shaggy" appearance is due to the presence of villi. When fully distended, the intestinal walls often appear smoother.

**Plate 6-3** The duodenal mucosa in an Irish setter appears more erythematous than normal. Biopsies were normal. Note the Peyer's patches, which appear as circumscribed, slightly depressed, cream-colored aggregates in the right aspect of the field of view.

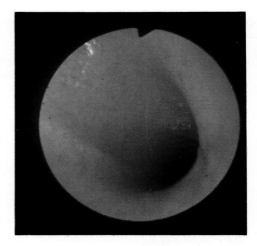

**Plate 6-4** Normal duodenum. Note a slight color variation compared to other examples of a normal duodenum.

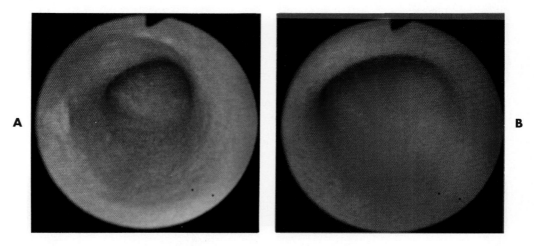

A                                                                 B

**Plate 6-5 A,** Distal descending duodenum. **B,** Close-up of the function (at fold) between the descending and ascending duodenum. Small patches of bile are present along the walls of the duodenum (a normal finding). The endoscope is advanced to the ascending duodenum using gentle forward pressure. Minor manual changes in tip deflection may be necessary to facilitate the advance. The junctional curves of the small intestine are usually freely movable and accommodating to the passage of an endoscope, especially a highly flexible pediatric model.

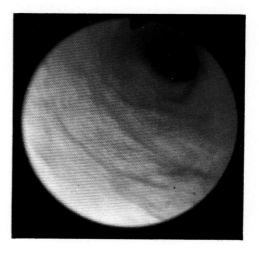

**Plate 6-6** Normal jejunum. The mucosal appearance is identical to that of duodenum.

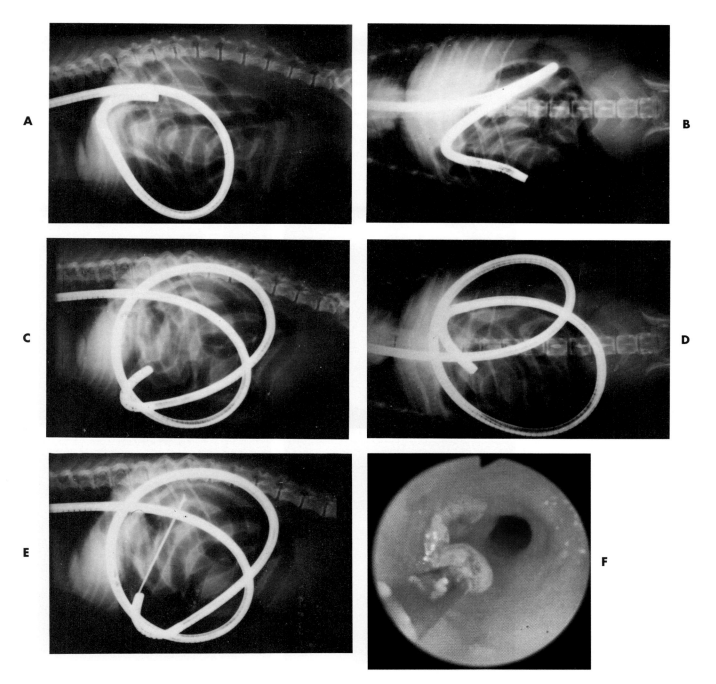

**Plate 6-7** Radiographs showing endoscope positions in the small intestine of an 8-kg (17.6-lb) dog during routine upper enteroscopy using a pediatric endoscope with a 7.9-mm diameter and a 100-cm working length. **A** and **B,** Lateral and ventrodorsal projections with the endoscope tip positioned in the proximal descending duodenum. Note the large stomach-curvature loop. The stomach has been displaced caudally by the endoscope as it advanced along the greater curvature. The formation of this loop decreases the usable endoscope length for small bowel examination. Note the curve at the distal end of the endoscope as the insertion tube passes through the antrum and pylorus to the descending duodenum. **C** and **D,** Lateral and ventrodorsal projections showing the endoscope tip positioned in the proximal jejunum. The curve at the distal end of the endoscope is located at the junction between the ascending duodenum and proximal jejunum. **E,** The biopsy forceps have been advanced along the jejunum to the point of resistance. **F,** A long tissue sample obtained from the jejunum at the point of resistance. The mucosa appears grossly normal, but histologic examination revealed moderate lymphocytic, plasmacytic enteritis. Using this technique of advancing biopsy forceps as far as possible beyond the scope, the endoscopist can obtain biopsy samples from the jejunum in cats and small dogs and from at least the ascending duodenum in larger dogs, even if the endoscope is not long enough to reach beyond the distal descending or ascending duodenum.

## DUODENAL CONTRACTIONS

Active duodenal contractions are occasionally observed during enteroscopy. These appear as contractile rings and usually do not hinder advancement of the endoscope. Duodenal contractions are part of normal small intestinal motility activity. If the contractions partially compromise the view on entry, the full circumference of the lumen should be carefully evaluated while maintaining air insufflation as the endoscope is retracted toward the stomach at the conclusion of the small bowel examination.

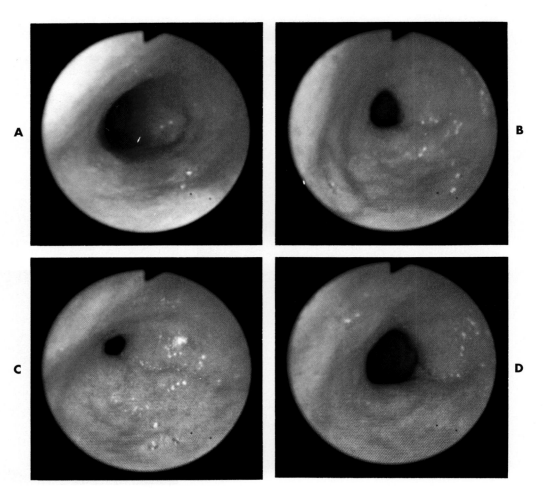

**Plate 6-8** Duodenal contraction sequence (total time; several seconds). **A,** Normal duodenal lumen. **B,** The lumen diameter begins to narrow as a contractile ring starts to form. **C,** At maximal contraction the lumen diameter decreases considerably in size. **D,** Contractile ring as it begins to relax.

## DUODENAL FROTH

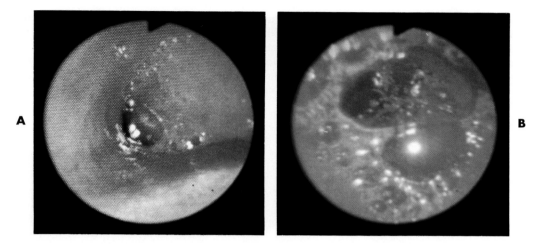

**A**    **B**

**Plate 6-9** Yellow bile-stained froth is commonly seen in the upper duodenum. In rare cases, visualization is significantly impaired when the froth is particularly thick. **A,** Mild accumulation of bile-stained froth. Air insufflation would be sufficient to improve visualization by dispersing the froth and distending the duodenal walls. **B,** Thicker accumulation of froth. Water flushing and suction were effective in removing most of the froth.

## BARIUM RESIDUE

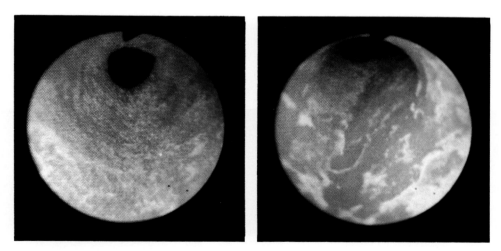

**Plate 6-10** Small bowel mucosa shortly after the completion of a barium series. These photographs were taken approximately 6 hours after a barium series was begun to investigate for the presence of a gastric foreign body in a dog with acute severe vomiting. The barium series was unremarkable, and endoscopy was performed later the same day to expedite a complete work-up. The stomach examination was normal, and the duodenum was subsequently evaluated. Residual barium adhered to the mucosa, but adequate visualization was still possible. Enteroscopy should be postponed if large pools of barium remain in the stomach or intestine because the accessory channel of an endoscope should not be used to suction barium.

# NORMAL FELINE SMALL INTESTINE: VARIOUS APPEARANCES

The small intestinal mucosa of cats is lighter in color (primarily cream to slightly pink) than the intestinal mucosa of dogs. Before insufflation distends the intestinal walls, the mucosa sometimes has a somewhat irregular surface texture that may include small fissures. This appearance can be consistent with either histologically normal small intestinal mucosa or a variety of disorders, including inflammatory bowel disease and lymphosarcoma. This irregular appearance often abates when insufflation distends the intestinal wall. Diagnostic assumptions usually cannot be made based on gross appearance alone. Histologic examination is *essential* for accurate diagnosis.

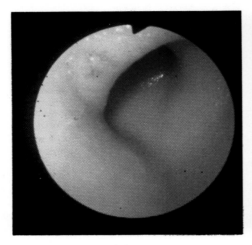

**Plate 6-11** Normal feline duodenum. The fold in the upper aspect of the field is at the junction of the descending and ascending duodenum.

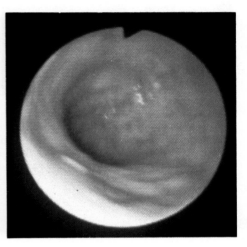

**Plate 6-12** Normal duodenum with a patchy color pattern. The small white flattened area at the 7 o'clock position is the duodenal papilla.

**A**                    **B**                    **C**

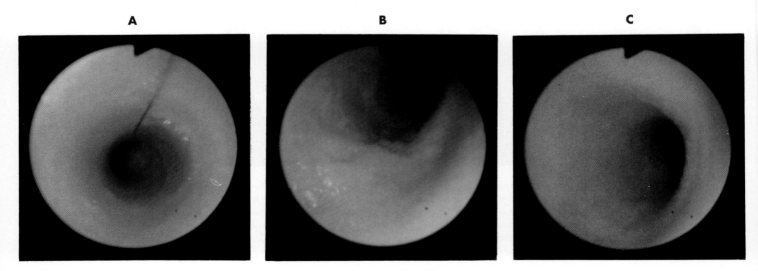

**Plate 6-13** Various appearances of the upper small intestine during routine enteroscopy in a cat. **A,** Proximal descending duodenum containing a small amount of bile-stained (yellow) fluid. A single hair is seen in the upper aspect of the field. **B,** Ascending duodenum. Note mild irregularity of mucosa (a normal finding). **C,** Proximal jejunum. The mucosa appears quite smooth in this patient.

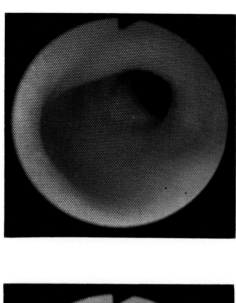
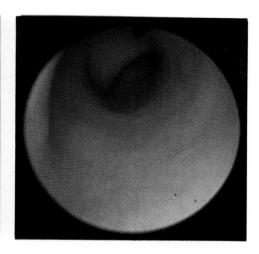

**Plate 6-14** Folds and curves encountered during examination of the upper small intestine in a cat. If necessary, air insufflation can be used to distend the folds.

**A**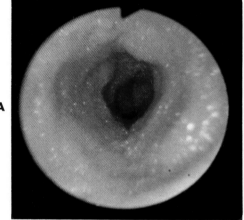
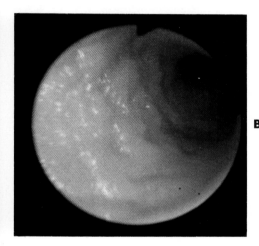 **B**

**Plate 6-15** Mild to moderate mucosal irregularity in a cat with normal duodenal histology. This appearance can also be seen in cats with inflammatory bowel disease (see Plates 6-20 and 6-41, *A*). **A,** Mild insufflation. Note the grainy appearance caused by villi. **B,** Close-up view with the endoscope tip directed more toward the duodenal wall.

**A**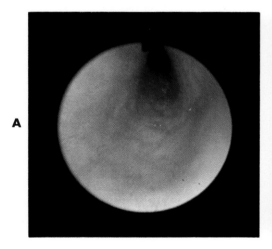
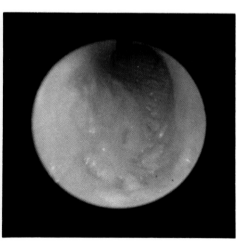 **B**

**Plate 6-16** Mucosal irregularity (fissure effect). The histologic findings were normal, highlighting the fact that an intestinal mucosal disorder cannot be diagnosed based on gross endoscopic examination alone. With further air insufflation, mucosal fissures often are not evident. As shown here, mucosal irregularities may be focal or patchy rather than diffuse. **A,** Relatively smooth proximal descending duodenum. **B,** Mucosal fissures in the distal descending duodenum of the same cat.

# HAIR IN THE DUODENUM

It is not unusual to find hair clumps of various sizes in the upper small intestine of cats. Usually the hair can be easily brushed aside, pushed ahead by the endoscope, or passed. The hair is usually an incidental finding although the presence of large clumps of hair in the stomach or small intestine may suggest the possibility of a gastrointestinal motility disorder. In the rare instance that a tubular hairball actually causes intestinal obstruction, the diagnosis is usually based on the history (ongoing vomiting that may be projectile), abdominal palpation, and survey or barium contrast radiography. Endoscopy is usually not necessary. If endoscopy were undertaken, however, endoscopic findings that would support a complete intestinal obstruction include reflux esophagitis and the pooling of a significant amount of fluid in the stomach and the area of small intestine proximal to the obstruction.

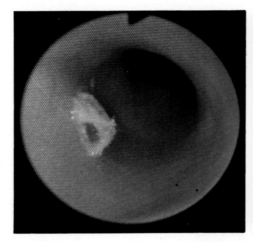

**Plate 6-17** Small clump of hair in the duodenum of a cat with intermittent vomiting (incidental finding).

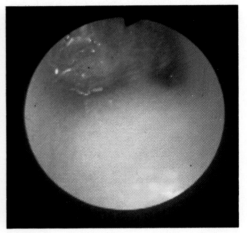

**Plate 6-18** Large tubular hairball (upper aspect in the field of view) that is filling most of the duodenal lumen of a cat with inappetence and intermittent vomiting. Efforts to retrieve the hairball caused it to break apart. The hairball passed uneventfully. The mucosa appeared normal, but histologic examination showed moderate to severe lymphocytic enteritis. The hair material was either an incidental finding or possibly the result of a motility disorder that may have resulted from the inflammatory bowel disease. This case once again emphasizes the importance of histologic examination in establishing a definitive diagnosis.

## DUODENAL PAPILLAE: VARIOUS APPEARANCES

With the use of newer endoscopes that have wide-angle illumination, one or both duodenal papillae of dogs can often be visualized. Sometimes the one papilla (major duodenal papilla) that exists in cats can also be visualized, most often during slow retraction of the endoscope through an air-dilated duodenal lumen at the conclusion of a small bowel examination. The anatomic relationships are described in Chapter 6. Various appearances that can be encountered are shown in Plates 6-19 through 6-24.

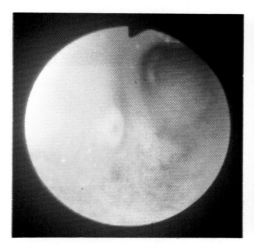

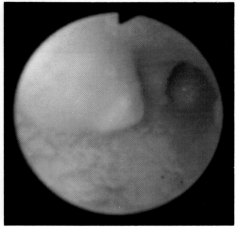

**Plate 6-19** Normal appearance of the major duodenal papilla in a cat (white circular raised structure in the center of the field). Note the bile discharge adjacent to the papilla. The small reddened area (erythema) in the lower right aspect of the field is from endoscope trauma. (The endoscope had already been advanced along the duodenal canal and then retracted.)

**Plate 6-20** Duodenal papilla in a 19-year-old cat (white raised area in the center of the field). The papilla is positioned atop a broad mucosal base. This is an uncommon appearance. The surrounding mucosa appears slightly irregular. The histologic diagnosis was moderate to severe lymphocytic enteritis. The cat had a history of chronic diarrhea.

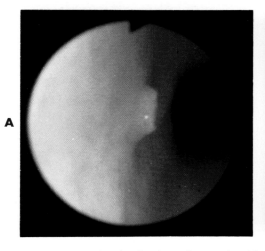

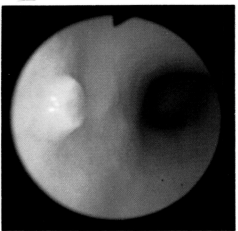

A

B

**Plate 6-21** Major duodenal papilla in a dog. The papilla is slightly raised from the mucosa.
**A,** View from the proximal descending duodenum. **B,** Close-up view.

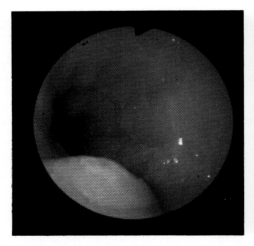

**Plate 6-22** Broad-based major duodenal papilla (7 o'clock position) in a dog.

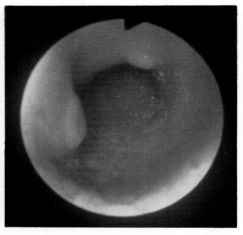

**Plate 6-23** Both major papilla (9 o'clock position) and minor papilla (12:30 position) are visualized in this dog. The minor papilla quite consistently appears as a small, round, slightly raised white structure.

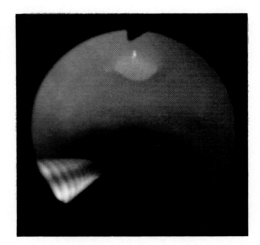

**Plate 6-24** Minor duodenal papilla (12 o'clock position). The surrounding duodenal mucosa appears normal. The shaft of a biopsy instrument is seen in the lower aspect of the field.

## CANINE ILEOCECOCOLIC JUNCTION AND ILEUM: NORMAL APPEARANCES

In many dogs the ileum can be entered with an endoscope, thus providing an opportunity for direct visualization and biopsy. For the ileal orifice to be viewed, the colon must be completely evacuated. Various configurations of the ileal and cecal orifices are shown in Plates 6-25 through 6-28.

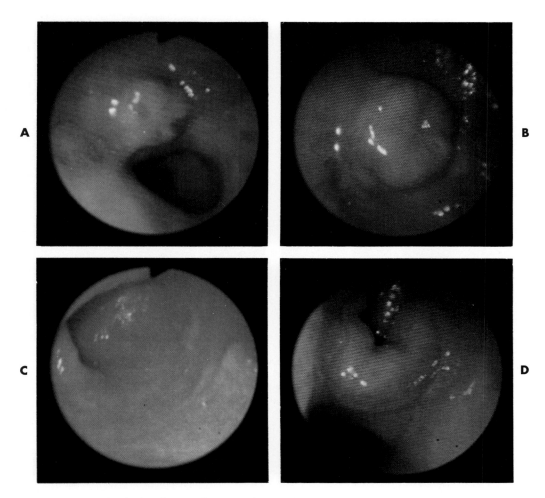

**Plate 6-25** The ileal orifice usually protrudes into the lumen of the terminal ascending colon as a papillary form. **A,** Raised ileocolic junction (just above the center of the field) and cecocolic junction (open area at the lower right in the field of view). The ileal orifice is obscured by a small amount of liquid fecal material. **B,** Close-up of the ileal orifice after the fecal residue has been washed away. The orifice is closed. Note the small depression in the center of the raised valve structure. **C,** Normal ileum. **D,** Ileal orifice (now open) after the endoscope has been retracted from the ileum to the ascending colon. The cecum is at the lower left.

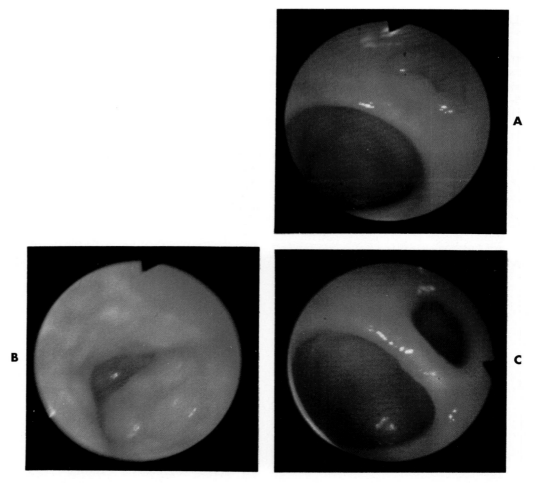

**Plate 6-26 A,** Ileocolic junction (flattened area with a small opening at the 1 o'clock position) and the dilated opening to the cecum (lower left). The endoscope was advanced directly to the ileum. **B,** Normal ileum with light-colored aggregations of lymphoid tissue. **C,** Ileal orifice (upper right) and cecal orifice (lower left) immediately after retraction of the endoscope to the colon.

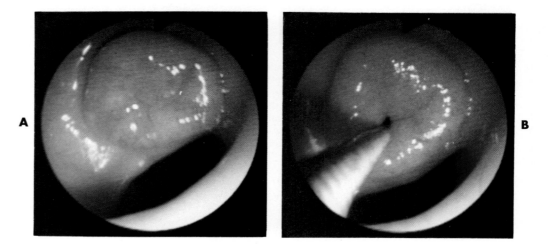

**Plate 6-27** Ileocolic orifice. **A,** In this dog the ileocolic orifice appears as a broad, slightly raised papillary form. The cecal orifice is immediately below. **B,** Because the endoscope could not be advanced through the orifice, a biopsy forceps was passed into the ileum. The endoscope was then advanced over the biopsy instrument to the ileum (See text for a description of the technique.) Alternatively, blind biopsies of the ileum could have been obtained.

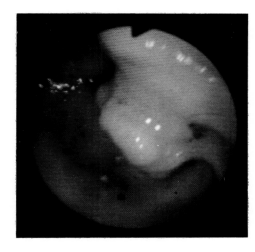

**Plate 6-28** Unusual ileal orifice configuration. In this dog the papillary ileal orifice structure protrudes into the ascending colon at a right angle (center of the field). The cecal orifice is not in view. This ileal orifice angle would be difficult to adjust to a degree suitable for passage of either biopsy forceps or endoscope to the ileum. In some difficult cases it is useful to rotate the patient from left lateral recumbency to dorsal or even right lateral recumbency in order to obtain a more favorable angle of approach to the ileal orifice.

## CANINE INFLAMMATORY BOWEL DISEASE: VARIOUS APPEARANCES

Inflammatory bowel disease is a common cause of vomiting and diarrhea. Histologic examination of intestinal mucosal tissue samples is required for definitive diagnosis. The gross mucosal appearance ranges from normal to mild erythema to varying degrees of mucosal irregularity. Rarely, the mucosa shows marked irregularity with proliferative changes. There is not always a strong correlation between gross appearance and histologic findings. When erythema or mild irregularity alone are seen, histologic appearances can be normal. Sometimes an apparently normal mucosa may reveal histologic evidence of inflammation.

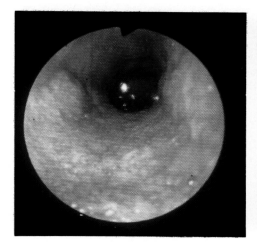

**Plate 6-29** Mild mucosal irregularity and a pronounced grainy appearance of the duodenum in an 8-year-old Doberman pinscher with chronic intermittent vomiting, peripheral eosinophilia, and mild hypoproteinemia (total protein, 5.3 g/dl). The animal had no history of diarrhea. The histologic diagnosis was moderate lymphocytic, plasmacytic, and eosinophilic enteritis. Gastric biopsies were normal.

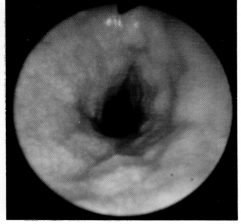

**Plate 6-30** Mild to moderate mucosal irregularity of the duodenum in an 11-year-old English setter with chronic diarrhea, weight loss, and marked panhypoproteinemia (total protein, 3.2 g/dl; albumin, 1.4 g/dl). The histologic diagnosis was moderate to severe lymphocytic, plasmacytic enteritis.

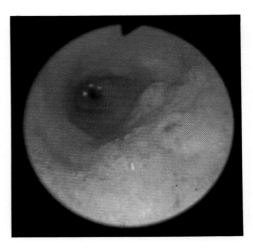

**Plate 6-31** Localized irregularity and proliferative mucosal change (in the forefront of the field) in the descending duodenum of an 11-year-old Siberian husky. The duodenum was grossly normal beyond these lesions. The histologic diagnosis was moderate lymphocytic, plasmacytic duodenitis. Moderate to severe multifocal necrotizing and suppurative, eosinophilic, lymphocytic, and plasmacytic gastritis was found in the antrum and pylorus.

A
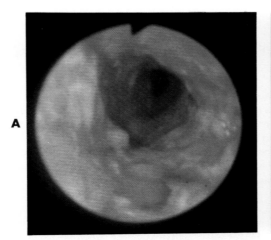

B
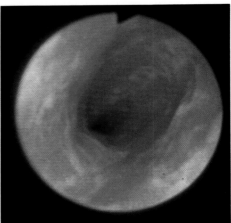

**Plate 6-32** Mild to moderate duodenal mucosal irregularity, erythema, and fibrinous mucoid exudate along the lumenal walls of a 12-year-old Australian shepherd with a 1-year history of intermittent diarrhea. The lamina propria contained a moderate population of plasma cells, and lymphocyte and eosinophil counts were mildly elevated. The fibrinous exudate is indicative of shallow mucosal ulceration or loss of surface epithelium. **A,** Descending duodenum. **B,** Ascending duodenum.

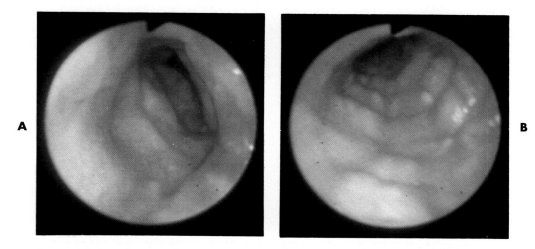

**Plate 6-33** Marked mucosal irregularity of the duodenum of a 14-year-old mixed-breed dog with intermittent vomiting and diarrhea. When air was insufflated, the walls of the duodenum were poorly distensible. **A,** Proximal descending duodenum on entry. Note the superficial erosions with hemorrhage. **B,** Distal descending duodenum during retraction of the endoscope at conclusion of enteroscopy. The histologic diagnosis was moderate lymphocytic, plasmacytic enteritis.

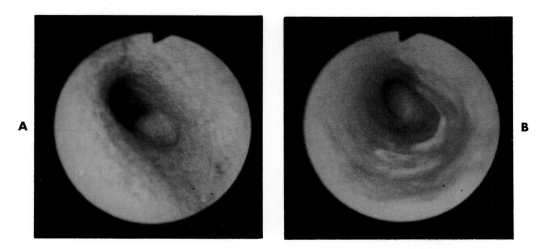

**Plate 6-34** Lymphocytic, plasmacytic enteritis in a basenji with chronic diarrhea. Some basenjis are afflicted with an immunoproliferative enteropathy characterized by diarrhea and intermittent vomiting and inappetence. Gastropathy also occurs in many chronic cases. The gross appearance of the small bowel mucosa varies from mild to marked mucosal irregularity. Histologic evaluation of gastric and intestinal biopsies is necessary for a definitive diagnosis. Diagnostic findings include generalized infiltration of the lamina propria by lymphocytes, plasma cells, and occasionally neutrophils, with blunted and fused villi seen in some cases. **A,** Mild mucosal irregularity and patchy erythema of the proximal descending duodenum. **B,** Grossly normal mucosa at the distal descending duodenum, with a mucoid exudate.

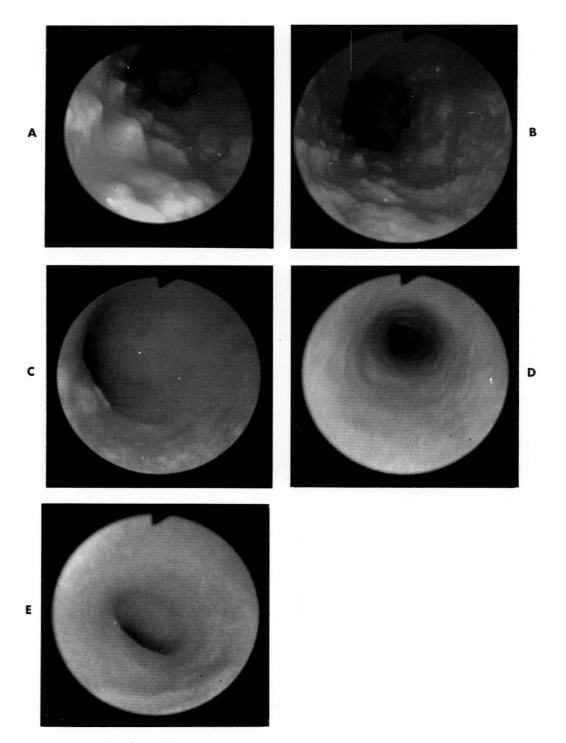

**Plate 6-35** Initial and follow-up endoscopic examinations of a 4-year-old puli with severe inflammatory bowel disease. The animal also had chronic gastritis and colitis. Clinical signs included chronic unrelenting diarrhea, intermittent vomiting, and weight loss. On initial examination, severe mucosal irregularity was seen in the descending duodenum (**A**). Note the degree of hemorrhage (upper half of the field) after two biopsy samples were obtained (**B**). The follow-up examination at 20 months indicated that the animal had responded well to treatment. Alternate-day corticosteroids were still being administered. Grossly, mild erythema is present, but the marked mucosal irregularity has resolved. (**C**) The histologic changes had also improved significantly. At 4-year follow-up, the mucosa of the proximal descending duodenum (**D**) and the distal descending duodenum at the junction between descending and ascending segments (**E**) appears grossly normal. Histologically the mucosa showed only minimal, insignificant inflammatory changes. The dog had been maintained on low-dose every-third-day corticosteroid therapy for the last year. Treatment was discontinued after the 4-year follow-up examination.

## FELINE INFLAMMATORY BOWEL DISEASE: VARIOUS APPEARANCES

In cats—as in dogs—the gross appearance of the mucosa in inflammatory bowel disease can range from normal to varying degrees of mucosal irregularity (Plates 6-36 through 6-42). The mucosa is more likely to have a grossly normal or nearly normal appearance in cats with inflammatory bowel disease.

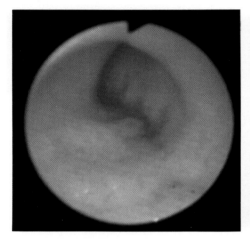

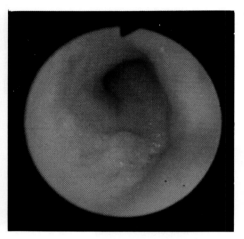

**Plate 6-36** Grossly normal mucosa in a 19-year-old cat with chronic diarrhea as a result of severe lymphocytic enteritis. The procurement of biopsy samples has caused bleeding (center of the field).

**Plate 6-37** Mild mucosal irregularity along the lower wall of the distal descending duodenum in a 16-year-old cat with moderate lymphocytic, plasmacytic, eosinophilic enteritis.

A
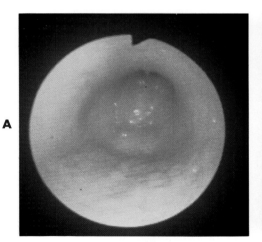

B
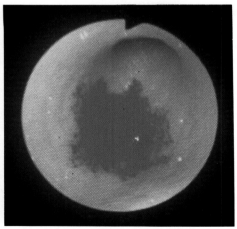

**Plate 6-38 A,** Normal to mildly irregular duodenal mucosa in a 12-year-old cat with chronic intermittent vomiting as a result of severe lymphocytic enteritis. **B,** Hemorrhage after a single biopsy is greater than normal, most likely because of significant disease-related mucosal compromise.

**Plate 6-39 A,** Mucosal irregularity and fissures in a 10-year-old cat with hyperthyroidism and moderate lymphocytic, plasmacytic enteritis. **B,** Marked hemorrhage after two biopsies. A total of five biopsies were obtained from various sites, along the duodenum and jejunum. This degree of hemorrhage would not be expected to occur in normal intestine. Diarrhea, the primary clinical sign, did not respond to methimazole but resolved with prednisone therapy.

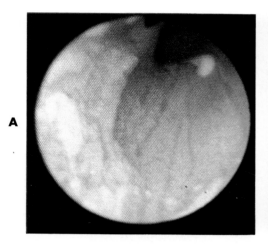
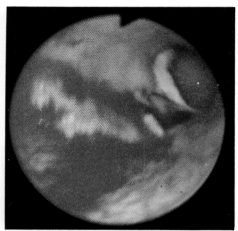

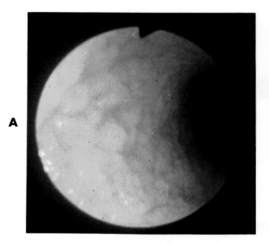
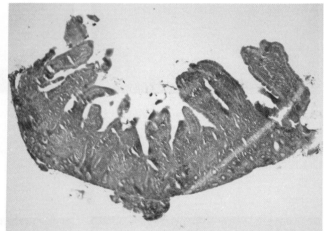

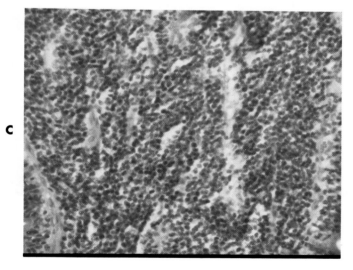

**Plate 6-40 A,** Cobblestone appearance of the mucosa in a 15-year-old cat with chronic vomiting caused by severe lymphocytic enteritis. **B,** Low-power photomicrograph (40). The depth of biopsy extended to the basal lamina propria. The villi are widened, and cell infiltration is increased. **C,** High-power photomicrograph showing sheets of mature small lymphocytes in lamina propria (400). Lymphocytic enteritis is a benign disease in cats and must be differentiated on histologic examination from lymphosarcoma. (Photomicrographs courtesy Stephen J. Engler.)

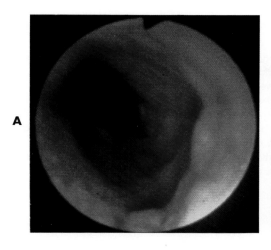
A

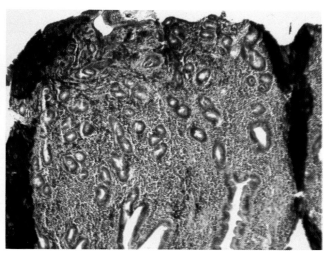
B

**Plate 6-41 A,** Moderate mucosal irregularity with focal erosions (6 o'clock position) in a 12-year-old cat with a 10-month history of unrelenting diarrhea. Large mucosal samples were easily lifted off with biopsy forceps. **B,** Photomicrograph showing a widened and blunted villus with fibrosis and a marked cellular infiltrate (100). (Courtesy Stephen J. Engler.)

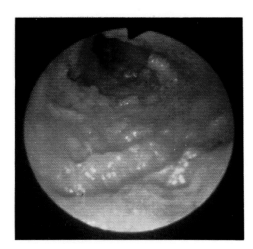

**Plate 6-42** Severe mucosal irregularity (note sizeable troughs) and friability in a 9-month-old cat with ravenous appetite, voluminous cow-pile stools, and weight loss. The animal did not respond to treatment for exocrine pancreatic insufficiency. The histologic diagnosis was moderate to severe lymphocytic, plasmacytic enteritis.

## INTESTINAL LYMPHANGIECTASIA

Lymphangiectasia is a chronic disorder of dogs characterized by marked dilation of intestinal lymphatics and often by a variable inflammatory cell infiltrate in the lamina propria. In most cases the total protein level has decreased moderately to markedly by the time a diagnosis is made. In many but not all cases, the mucosa has a characteristic patchy, milky-white appearance. In some patients gross changes may *only* be noted at exploratory laparotomy. These changes include weblike, milky-white, dilated lymphatic channels in the mesentery and on the serosal surface of the small intestines. The diagnosis of lymphangiectasia is established by histologic examination of the mucosa (biopsies obtained at endoscopy or surgery) or serosal or mesenteric lesions.

**Plate 6-43** Intestinal lymphangiectasia in a Pomeranian with chronic diarrhea and panhypoproteinemia (total protein, 3.6 g/dl). The white discoloration of the duodenal mucosa is due to swollen villi, and the mucosa appears grossly coarsened.

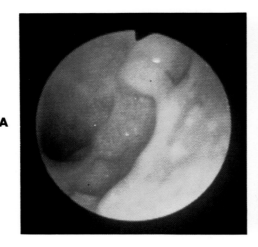

A

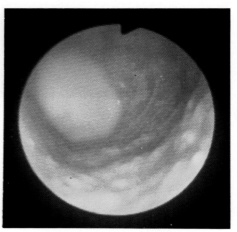

B

**Plate 6-44** Lymphangiectasia in a 3-year-old Doberman pinscher with chronic diarrhea, weight loss, anorexia, and panhypoproteinemia (total protein, 2.4 g/dl). **A,** Mucoid milky exudate along the mucosa of the proximal descending duodenum. **B,** Coarsened ("shaggy") mucosal appearance, whitish tips of swollen villi, and pooled lymph fluid in the distal descending duodenum. The histologic evaluation confirmed the diagnosis of lymphangiectasia.

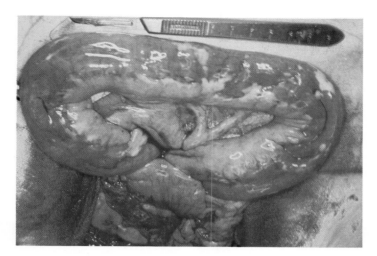

**Plate 6-45** Dilated lymphatic channels involving the serosa and mesentery of a dog with lymphangiectasia.

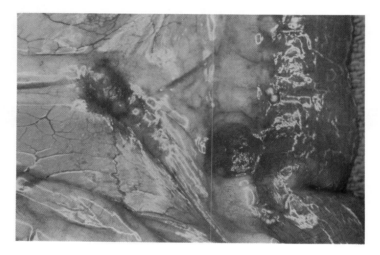

**Plate 6-46** Two obstructing granulomatous lesions (lipogranulomas) as well as dilated lymphatic channels in the mesentery and serosa of a dog with lymphangiectasia.

# ENDOSCOPE-INDUCED MUCOSAL TRAUMA

Depending on the diameter of the endoscope, the diameter of the small intestinal lumen, and the integrity of the mucosa, variable degrees of superficial mucosal trauma can result from an endoscopic procedure. Most often, trauma is minimal, and only minor patches of erythema result. Occasionally, however, the mucosa bleeds or is slightly undermined. This most often occurs when a patient has a significant inflammatory disorder that alters mucosal integrity. Older endoscopes that are less flexible than newer scopes are more likely to cause minor trauma in small patients. Endoscope-induced trauma is rarely a concern. Medication is not necessary to promote healing, and food and water can be administered on a regular postendoscopy schedule.

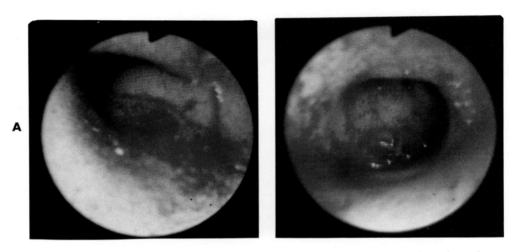

**Plate 6-47** Hemorrhage from endoscope-induced mucosal trauma in a cat with moderate lymphocytic, plasmacytic enteritis. No hemorrhage occurred when the endoscope was first advanced to the small intestinal lumen. **A,** Hemorrhage in the proximal jejunum was first visualized when the endoscope was retracted toward the stomach. Note the mildly grainy appearance of the mucosa. **B,** Descending duodenum at the conclusion of enteroscopy. A 7.9-mm pediatric endoscope was used, and no significant resistance to advance was encountered. Compromised mucosal integrity in this patient most likely predisposed the intestinal mucosa to hemorrhage.

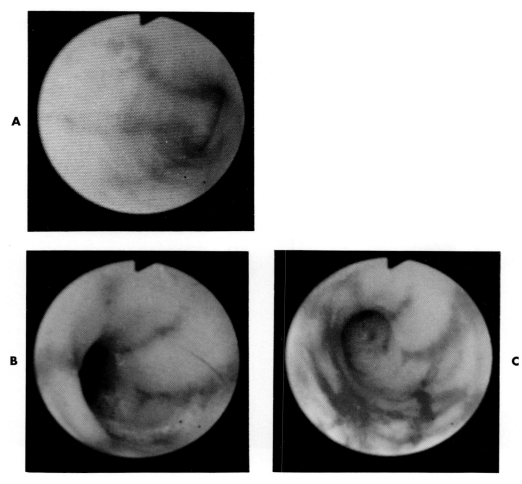

**Plate 6-48** Linear streaks of mucosal trauma in the upper small intestine of a cat with mild lymphocytic, plasmacytic enteritis. This patient was small, and trauma was thought to be related to passage of the endoscope (7.9-mm diameter) through a narrow duodenal canal. **A,** Proximal duodenum. Note the major duodenal papilla at the 11:30 position and the small patch of bile adjacent to it. **B,** More prominent erythematous streaks in the ascending duodenum. A single hair is seen at the 3 o'clock position. **C,** Linear streaks and larger patches of hemorrhage in the distal descending duodenum as visualized at the conclusion of the examination. This area was traumatized by the endoscope tip and by its shaft once the tip was further advanced. No clinical problems resulted from the examination.

## INTESTINAL PARASITES

Intestinal parasites are occasionally encountered during examinations of the upper small intestine. Ascarids are most commonly observed, and they often respond by attempting to move away from the endoscope tip. Upon reaching the small intestine, the endoscopist is often as surprised as the parasite at the unexpected finding. Ascarids can easily be snared with biopsy forceps or foreign body graspers and pulled up through the accessory channel.

As discussed in the text, saline lavage can be performed through polyethylene tubing advanced through the endoscope's accessory channel in an effort to retrieve *Giardia* trophozoites, which can then be identified on microscopic examination.

A           B           C

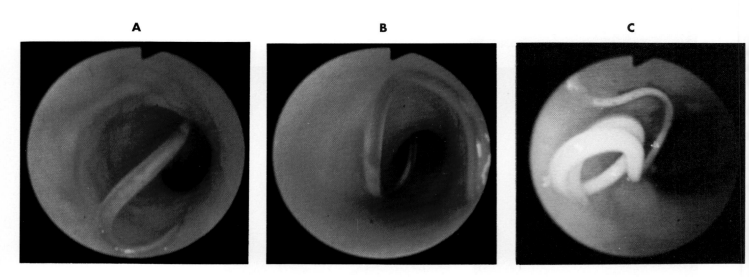

**Plate 6-49** Ascarid infection. **A** and **B,** A single roundworm found in the descending duodenum of a healthy asymptomatic cat during an endoscopy laboratory session. The parasite was actively moving as the endoscope was advanced closer to it. The mucosa appears slightly more irregular in *A* than in *B* because the intestine is slightly more distended with air in *B*. **C,** Roundworm in the proximal descending duodenum of a dog. A small amount of hemorrhage (upper aspect of the field) has occurred because of mucosal trauma from a biopsy instrument that was being maneuvered into position to apprehend the parasite.

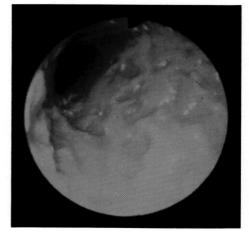

**Plate 6-50** Large mucosal pitting defects represent an unusual duodenal mucosal appearance in a mixed-breed dog with acute giardiasis. The lesions resolved after a course of treatment. A variety of mucosal appearances, ranging from normal to mild mucosal changes to marked irregularity, can be seen in conjunction with giardiasis. Gross changes do not seem to correlate with clinical signs. (Courtesy Michael S. Leib.)

# SMALL INTESTINAL NEOPLASIA

Neoplasia involving the small intestine is much less common than inflammatory bowel disease. Lymphosarcoma and adenocarcinoma are the tumor types most frequently found in the small intestine. Mast cell tumors, leiomyoma, leiomyosarcoma, fibrosarcoma, ganglioneuroma, and carcinoid tumors are encountered somewhat less often.

The likelihood of diagnosing intestinal neoplasia on endoscopic examination is directly related to the area of intestinal involvement and the presence of mucosal involvement. Tumors that more commonly involve the jejunum and ileum often are not amenable to diagnosis unless they are diffuse and these areas can be reached. If the duodenum is involved, a definitive diagnosis can frequently be made. The diffuse type of lymphosarcoma is the most amenable to diagnosis via endoscopy. Every effort must be made to obtain biopsy samples from as deep in the lamina propria as possible in diffuse forms of neoplasia so that an accurate differentiation can be made on histologic examination.

Differentiating benign lymphocytic enteritis (a fairly common type of inflammatory bowel disease in cats) from lymphosarcoma is sometimes difficult, and repeat endoscopic biopsies or abdominal exploratory with full-thickness intestinal biopsies may be required to procure more tissue for analysis. Special immunohistochemical stains performed on endoscopic tissue samples may also be helpful in determining a definitive diagnosis. Masses should be sampled by "digging" as deeply beneath the surface as possible. If only superficial cells are procured, an incorrect diagnosis of fibrous or granulation tissue may be made. Ulcerative lesions are best sampled by taking tissue from an upper wall as it interfaces with intact intestinal lining. Tissue surrounding an ulcer should also be obtained in an effort to differentiate benign from neoplastic ulcer disease.

Despite efforts to obtain adequate-size tissue samples, a neoplastic lesion is sometimes incorrectly diagnosed as benign. The endoscopist should always carefully note gross mucosal appearance. If neoplasia is suspected but a benign disorder is diagnosed, the response to treatment should be carefully evaluated. Failure of the patient to respond may indicate that a malignant disorder is indeed present and further evaluation should be expedited.

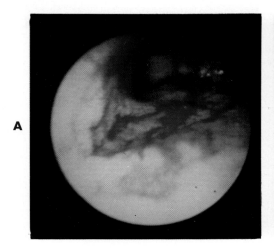 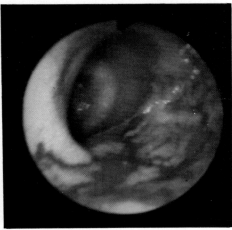

**Plate 6-51** Diffuse lymphosarcoma in the duodenum of an 8-year-old boxer with vomiting, diarrhea, inappetence, and panhypoproteinemia (total protein, 4.6 g/dl). **A,** Mid-descending duodenum. **B,** Distal descending duodenum. Note the mucosal irregularity and the focal color changes from pink to white. The hemorrhage is from the biopsy sites.

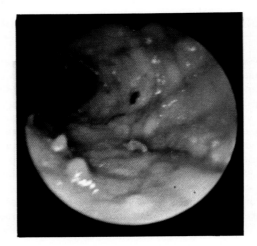

**Plate 6-52** Duodenal lymphosarcoma in a dog with chronic diarrhea and weight loss. Note the single erosion with hemorrhage in the center of the field. Small fragments of food residue are also seen.

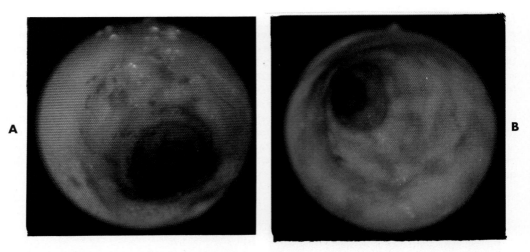

A

B

**Plate 6-53** Duodenal lymphoma in a 5-year-old golden retriever with severe small bowel diarrhea and panhypoproteinemia. **A,** Multiple small erosions with hemorrhage. **B,** Mucosal irregularity with marked patchy erythema. Multiple biopsies confirmed a diagnosis of prolymphocytic lymphosarcoma. (Courtesy Keith P. Richter.)

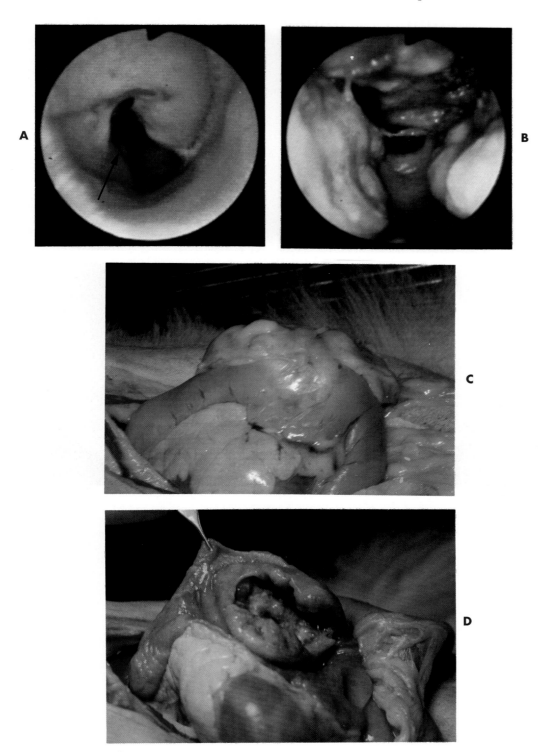

**Plate 6-54** Duodenal adenocarcinoma in a 9-year-old keeshond with vomiting and anorexia. **A,** First endoscopic view of the duodenum immediately beyond the pylorus. A large portion of the intestinal lumen is occluded by the neoplastic mass. The proximal surface of the mass is slightly eroded (area of hemorrhage). The major duodenal papilla is visible *(arrow)*. **B,** View immediately distal to the major duodenal papilla. Almost the entire circumference of the duodenum is effaced by proliferative tissue. Based on the location and extent of the lesion, a poor prognosis was given. Biopsies confirmed a diagnosis of adenocarcinoma. **C,** Appearance at necropsy. **D,** Incised mass at necropsy. The pancreas is immediately adjacent.

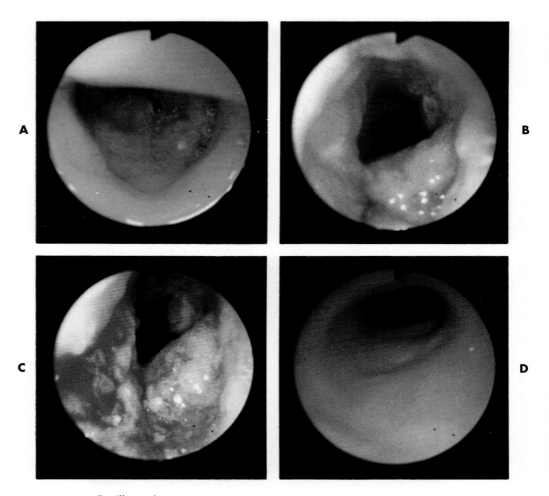

**Plate 6-55** Papillary adenocarcinoma in a 7-year-old dog with anorexia and intermittent vomiting. **A,** Most proximal aspect of the duodenum as seen from the pyloric canal. Note the proliferative tissue in the center of the field. **B,** Full circumferential proliferation of tissue in the proximal descending duodenum. **C,** Same site as in *B,* after a single biopsy from the left side of the field. Note hemorrhage. Multiple tissue samples were eventually obtained. **D,** Grossly normal distal descending duodenum.

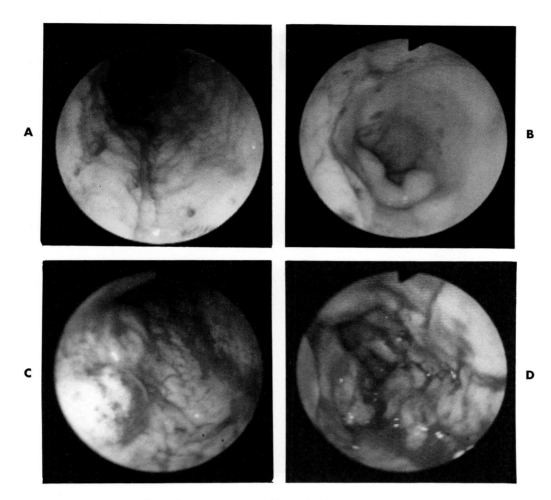

**Plate 6-56** Mast cell neoplasia in an 8-year-old standard poodle with intermittent vomiting and diarrhea. On two separate endoscopy procedures, tissue samples obtained with endoscopic biopsy forceps were *not* diagnostic for the neoplastic disease. The diagnosis was confirmed only by the histologic evaluation of tissues obtained at necropsy. The most diagnostic sections were the small bowel submucosa rather than the mucosa. **A,** Cobblestone mucosal appearance and patchy superficial erosions visualized in the proximal descending duodenum. **B,** Mid-descending duodenum. The mucosa is somewhat smoother, and scattered erosions are present. A Peyer's patch is visualized in the upper right aspect of the field. The distal descending duodenum was grossly normal. Based on the evaluation of multiple tissue samples, the histologic diagnosis was severe lymphocytic and eosinophilic enteritis. The distal duodenum was histologically normal. Initially the animal responded well to corticosteroid therapy, but the response was short-lived. **C** and **D,** Endoscopy was repeated 17 days later. The mucosal irregularity in the proximal duodenum was more severe, and the mucosa bled easily after endoscope contact and the procurement of biopsy samples. The histologic diagnosis was severe granulomatous enteritis. The inflammation was worse, and the character of the inflammatory reaction was changed. Histiocytic cells predominated, and eosinophils were still numerous. Several days after the second endoscopy procedure the dog was euthanized because of ongoing poor response to therapy.

# Chapter 7

# Colonoscopy

**Michael D. Willard**

Colonoscopy is a relatively easy endoscopic proce-dure in dogs and cats. However, not all patients with colonic disease benefit from or need this pro-cedure, even if their disease is chronic. Furthermore, when colonoscopy is indicated, it must be done correctly, or the results may be disappointing or perhaps misleading. This chapter discusses the indications for colonoscopy, the types of procedures available, and the techniques that need to be mastered to use colonoscopy successfully.

## INDICATIONS

Many animals with signs of large bowel diarrhea, such as hematochezia, fecal mucus, or tenesmus, have a self-lim-ited disease or one that can be resolved with symptomatic treatment and supportive care. Colonoscopy is most use-ful in diagnosing infiltrative disorders such as inflamma-tory bowel disease, fungal infections, and neoplasia, as well as anatomic abnormalities such as strictures, intus-susceptions, and masses. Therefore, this procedure is usu-ally performed when clinical or laboratory findings (e.g., significant weight loss, hypoalbuminemia, obstruction) suggest that an animal has a serious disorder, such as in-tussusception, histoplasmosis, or adenocarcinoma, or when the clinical signs and symptoms of large bowel dis-ease fail to respond to appropriate therapeutic trials. In pets that are essentially normal except for large bowel di-arrhea, it is often best to eliminate parasitic disease (e.g., *Giardia*, whipworms), dietary allergy or intolerance, fiber-responsive diarrhea, and *Clostridial* colitis before colonoscopy is considered. These last four conditions are

the more common causes of chronic large bowel dys-function seen in most practice settings and are better di-agnosed by fecal examinations and therapeutic trials than by colonoscopy and biopsy.

Other potential indications for colonoscopy include hematochezia, chronic vomiting (especially in cats), dyschezia, tenesmus, and constipation. Hematochezia (with normal or diarrheic stools) is one of the most com-mon problems in cats with lymphocytic colitis (even when the animals do not have diarrhea) and in dogs with rectal neoplasia. Dogs and cats with coagulopathies are rarely presented with hematochezia as the primary prob-lem, but these disorders should be considered before en-doscopy is performed.

Although vomiting usually suggests the presence of an upper gastrointestinal disease, it may be the predomi-nant sign in cats with inflammation of the ascending colon and/or ileum. Therefore, it is often useful to ex-amine both the *upper* and *lower intestinal tract* in cats with *chronic vomiting*. Dyschezia, tenesmus, and consti-pation are indications for endoscopy when the history and physical examination (which should always include digital rectal examination) eliminate common causes such as anal sac disease, diet, prostatomegaly, perineal hernia, and perianal fistulas. A good digital rectal exam-ination is more sensitive than endoscopy for detecting most of these problems. Animals who have lost weight because of small intestinal disease usually benefit most from gastroduodenoscopy. However, colonoscopy with ileal biopsy may be the only means of endoscopically diagnosing small intestinal disease in some of these patients.

If a patient appears to have generalized colonic disease or the descending colon is obviously affected (e.g., thickened or corrugated rectal mucosa, rectal stricture), rigid colonoscopy (and sometimes proctoscopy) is often adequate for diagnosis. Rigid colonoscopy is easier, quicker, and less expensive than flexible colonoscopy. Rigid techniques also procure larger tissue samples that routinely include generous amounts of submucosa and for this reason are preferred for the evaluation of dense, infiltrative lesions involving submucosal tissue (e.g., schirrotic carcinoma, pythiosis). The advantage of flexible colonoscopy is that it permits examination of the entire colon plus the cecum and ileum (or at least up to the ileocolic valve if the ileum cannot be entered). These areas are not accessible with rigid scopes. I prefer to perform both rigid and flexible colonoscopy in dogs so that I can examine the entire colon and also obtain mucosal biopsy samples from the descending colon using rigid biopsy forceps. With good technique the risk of colonic perforation is *minimal* but may be greater in cats than in dogs. I seldom obtain colonic biopsies with rigid forceps in cats. Consequently no obvious benefit is derived from using both rigid and flexible scopes simultaneously in cats.

Rigid proctoscopy is useful if its limitations are appreciated. The rectal area is the primary site for neoplasms in the colon. Proctoscopy is convenient for evaluating this area, removing polyps, and biopsying deep submucosal masses or strictures. The main drawback to proctoscopy is that only a very limited length of the colon can be inspected. (Figure 7-1).

## INSTRUMENTATION

### Rigid Colonoscopes

Rigid colonoscopy is usually performed with rigid human sigmoidoscopes (Figure 7-2). A scope with the largest diameter and longest length that a patient can accept generally facilitates the most thorough examination. Dogs other than toy breeds typically accept scopes with diameters of 19 to 27 mm. Cats often require sigmoidoscopes with diameters of 11 to 15 mm, but some accept scopes with a diameter of 19 mm or more. The rigid scope can be disposable (i.e., plastic), or it can be made of stainless steel. The scope must have a hinged viewing

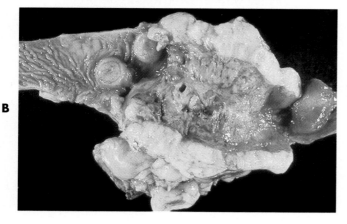

**Figure 7-1 A,** Proctoscopic view of the lower colon in a basenji with hematochezia. A smooth, round polypoid mass is seen. **B,** In this gross view the polypoid mass is obvious, but beyond the polyp is an area of infiltration caused by lymphoma. If a longer scope had been used, this infiltrated area might have been seen and biopsied, thus allowing antemortem rather than postmortem diagnosis.

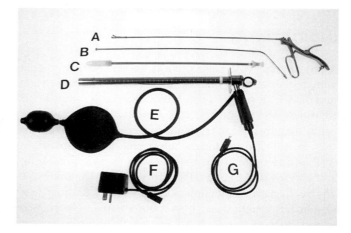

**Figure 7-2** Typical rigid colonoscope with accessories: an alligator biopsy instrument *(A)*, suction tube used to remove debris *(B)*, an obturator that is placed in the sigmoidoscope when the anus is entered *(C)*, a stainless-steel human sigmoidoscope (19-mm diameter, 35-cm length) *(D)*, an insufflation bulb *(E)* attached to the base of the endoscope near to where the light source attaches, a transformer power source that plugs into a wall outlet *(F)*, and a light source *(G)* attached to the bottom of the scope (the light source contains an incandescent bulb).

window that, when closed, seals the scope and keeps insufflated air in the colonic lumen. The endoscopist must be able to open this window and insert biopsy forceps and aspiration cannulas. An obturator with a smooth surface facilitates insertion of the scope into the rectum. It is helpful if the light is emitted at the end of the scope from a 360-degree window or fiberoptic bundle, as opposed to a single bulb that potentially can be covered with feces, thus causing a "blackout." One useful accessory is an aspiration tube that can be inserted through the scope to remove fluid or debris found during the examination. Alternatively, specially made cotton-tipped swabs can be used to clear debris although aspiration tends to be more effective.

## Rigid Proctoscopes

Rigid proctoscopes come in various lengths (e.g., approximately 70 to 130 mm) and diameters (approximately 8 to 25 mm). Operating proctoscopes have an area cut out of the distal wall (Figure 7-3). This cut-out area-allows the clinician to position the instrument so that a mass will protrude into the lumen of the scope. This makes it easier to biopsy or remove the lesion. Most rigid proctoscopes are placed on top of a battery handle (much like an otoscope) although some use transformers that plug into electrical outlets.

## Rigid Biopsy Forceps

High-quality instruments are needed to obtain optimal tissue samples. It should be possible to insert the forceps through the hinged window of the scope and have the tip extend at least 2 or 3 cm beyond the open end of the endoscope. I prefer biopsy forceps with tips that cut and shear the mucosa as opposed to clam-shell biopsy cups that pinch off a piece of tissue (Figure 7-4). The latter

rapidly become dull and then produce substantial tissue artifact. Visualization is enhanced if the tip of the biopsy instrument is at a 30- or 45-degree angle (see Figure 7-4). This biopsy instrument should only be used for sampling soft mucosa. Use on hard materials such as foreign bodies can damage the tip and cause artifact.

## Flexible Colonoscopes

Flexible colonoscopes usually have an outside diameter no greater than 9.8 mm. Smaller outside diameters generally increase the likelihood of entering the ileum. I prefer scopes with a 2.8-mm biopsy channel; the larger channel makes it easier to aspirate debris without plugging up the channel and allows passage of larger flexible biopsy instruments, which in turn obtain larger tissue samples. Colonoscopes that have 2- to 2.5-mm biopsy channels can be used to obtain good tissue samples, but using these scopes requires more care and skill than are necessary with a 2.8-mm channel. Gastroduodenoscopes (i.e., four-way tip deflection plus air, water, and aspiration capability) with a working distance of approximately 1 m are adequate in most dogs. A working length of 1.5 m or longer may be required to reach the ileocolic valve of large dogs. However, a working length greater than 1 m is rarely required if "paradoxic movement" is eliminated (discussed later). If a longer working length is needed, one of the newer veterinary endoscopes should be considered because the larger outside diameter of many flexible human colonoscopes prevents their effective use in the upper gastrointestinal tract of dogs and cats.

Several types of flexible biopsy forceps are available. Forceps with elongated (i.e., ellipsoid) jaws are usually

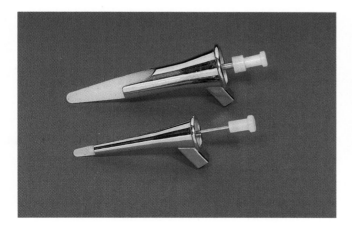

**Figure 7-3** Two rigid proctoscopes, both with an obturator in place. The upper scope is an operating proctoscope with a cut-out area through which the obturator is seen.

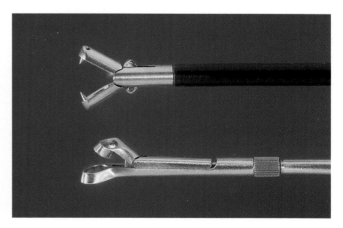

**Figure 7-4** Tips of two alligator biopsy forceps. The upper instrument is a clam-shell type in which the edges of the upper and lower jaws meet, edge on edge. The lower one has a smaller upper punch that fits into a lower, larger cup; thus this instrument shears the tissue much as a pair of scissors does. The lower tip is also at a 30-degree angle, which facilitates observation during the biopsy process.

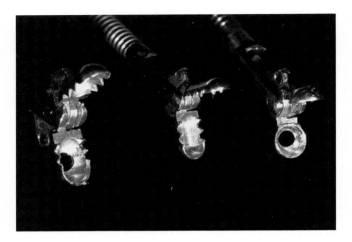

**Figure 7-5** Three types of flexible biopsy forceps. To the far left is the tip of a 2.8-mm ellipsoid forceps with alligator (i.e., serrated) jaws and fenestrated cups. In the middle is the tip of a 2-mm ellipsoid alligator-jaws forceps without a fenestrated cup. To the far right is the tip of a 2-mm round forceps with fenestrated cups. Note the difference in size between the 2.8-mm and 2-mm forceps. The 2.8-mm forceps allows the endoscopist to obtain a tissue sample that is often larger than the size of the sample that can be procured by the other forceps.

preferable to those with round jaws (Figure 7-5). I prefer forceps with fenestrated and serrated cups. Some clinicians like to have at least one set of forceps with a needle or blade in the middle. The needle helps maintain the position of the forceps while the operator attempts to push it against the mucosa at an acute angle. However, forceps with a needle or blade are not needed in most cases. (See Chapter 10 for further discussion of endoscopic biopsy instruments.)

## PATIENT PREPARATION

As mentioned previously, multiple *fecal examinations* for parasites and ova (especially whipworms and *Giardia* organisms) are usually performed *before* an animal is prepared for *endoscopy*. Likewise, if the clinician wishes to culture for pathogens (e.g., *Salmonella Campylobacter* species), perform fecal cytology (e.g., look for *Clostridium* spores), or assay for *Clostridium perfringens* enterotoxin, fecal samples should be obtained before enemas or lavage solutions are administered. Flexible colonoscopy requires rigorous patient preparation for at least two reasons:

1. All of the colon will be visualized, and it is harder to reliably clean the ileocecocolic valve area than the descending colon.
2. Large debris cannot be aspirated as well with flexible scopes as with rigid scopes.

The patient should *not* be fed (water is acceptable) for at least *24 hours* (preferably *36 hours*) before the procedure.

Lavage solutions are optimal for removing food and feces from the alimentary tract. These isosmotic solutions produce an osmotic diarrhea that washes particulate matter out of the colon. Several protocols may be used. In one protocol a product such as GoLYTELY or COLYTE is administered through a gastric or nasoesophageal tube during the afternoon before the procedure. The animal is given the solution in a dose of 25 to 30 ml/kg (11 to 13.5 ml/lb). A minimum of two doses are administered at least 2 hours apart. Because large volumes of solution may be necessary, the clinician and staff must watch carefully to ensure that gastric dilation or torsion does not occur in dogs whose conformation predisposes them to these problems. A third and sometimes a fourth dose of the isosmotic solution is administered the morning of the procedure. The animal also usually receives one warm water enema (discussed later) on the morning of the procedure, at least 2 hours before endoscopy is performed. Another method for using lavage solutions is to administer 22 ml/kg/hr (10 ml/lb/hr) by continuous drip via a nasoesophageal tube for 4 hours before the procedure. In addition to lavage solutions some clinicians use an osmotic cathartic (such as magnesium citrate). If magnesium citrate is used, it is administered before the lavage solution, usually at a dose of 25 ml/kg (11 ml/lb). The bottle of magnesium citrate should be opened several hours before use to allow the cathartic to "de-fiz," thereby reducing the likelihood of vomiting and discomfort. The combination of a lavage solution and an osmotic cathartic results in the best colonic preparation and minimizes artifacts induced by enema tubes. Some clinicians also administer cisapride to facilitate passage of the lavage solutions through the intestinal tract.

Colonic lavage is an excellent means for preparing any animal for colonoscopy, but it is particularly important in several situations:

1. When colonoscopy is to be performed in a large animal. (It is difficult to clean out the intestinal tract of large animals using enemas alone.)
2. When it is important to enter the ileum.
3. When an animal has severe rectal pain for which multiple enemas are inappropriate.

However, lavage solutions do have potential disadvantages. First, they are more expensive than enemas, and large volumes are required in some animals. In addition, administration requires several orogastric intubations, (which can be difficult to achieve in animals with an aggressive temperament). Other complications associated with lavage solutions are possible.

Enemas may be administered instead of lavage solutions. Although enemas cost less than the lavage solution, it is easy to end up with a poorly prepared animal and/or multiple mucosal artifacts if the enemas are administered improperly. Therefore the patient should also be fasted for *at least 36* hours before the procedure. Hypertonic phosphate enema solutions should *never* be used. Rather, at least two or three generous warm water enemas should be administered the night before and again the morning of the procedure.

In medium-sized dogs, at least 1 L of water should be used for each enema. Dogs weighing more than 32 kg (70 lb) may accept twice that amount. To administer the enema, the clinician carefully inserts a well-lubricated enema tube as far into the dog's colon as it will easily go (at least to the level of the last rib). The tube is then repeatedly and gently inserted and withdrawn as water is administered by gravity flow to help loosen feces that is adhering to the colonic mucosa. If resistance is encountered, the tube should not be forcibly advanced or traumatic mucosal hemorrhages will occur (Figure 7-6). Water often exits the rectum while the dog is receiving the enema because the colon has been filled to capacity. This is not a problem as long as the fluid is entering via gravity flow and the dog is not vomiting or demonstrating obvious abdominal pain. The night before the procedure a laxative such as bisacodyl should be administered in a dose of 5 mg in small dogs or cats and 10 to 15 mg for medium- to large-sized dogs. If the colon is adequately prepared, clear, undiscolored water should be evacuated after the last enema. Although this technique is usually more than adequate for preparing the descending colon for examination, it is unreliable for cleansing the ascending and transverse colon and the ileocolic valve area.

The procedure for administering enemas must be modified for *cats*. In normal-sized cats (2.7 to 4.1 kg; 6 to 9 lb) each enema uses 50 to 60 ml of warm water or approximately 20 ml/kg (9 ml/lb). This water is administered through a 10-14 French flexible male urinary catheter attached to a 60-ml syringe. The water should be administered less aggressively than in dogs (i.e., over 1 to 2 minutes) because overfilling the colon may cause vomiting. It is harder to adequately prepare a feline colon with enemas than it is to prepare a canine colon, probably because cats absorb much of the enema fluid and their feces can adhere more tightly to the mucosa.

If proctoscopy is being performed, one or two enemas may be administered shortly before the procedure to evacuate the rectum. If necessary, the animal can be anesthetized and the feces removed digitally with a gloved hand.

## RESTRAINT

Colonoscopy can be performed with manual restraint, sedatives, or general anesthesia. Most patients should receive at least a sedative or an analgesic (e.g., acetylpro-

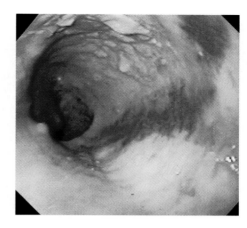

**Figure 7-6** Endoscopic view of a canine colon. Note the linear erythematous lesion (right side of the field), which is extending parallel to the lumen. This is an iatrogenic lesion caused by an enema tube. Note that the colon contains quite a bit of mucus and feces and thus was not as well prepared as it could have been.

mazine, ketamine, xylazine), especially if flexible colonoscopy is planned. Narcotics should be *avoided* because they may cause spasm and make it difficult to enter the ileum. Chemical restraint allows the endoscopist to work without having to deal with unexpected movement from the patient.

General anesthesia allows the most careful and complete examination, especially when the cecum and ileum are to be examined. When these structures are to be viewed, it may be necessary to advance the scope into the colon with a modest amount of pressure and/or substantial inflation of the colon, both of which can cause noticeable discomfort to awake animals. Ill animals and those with suspected intussusception may be manually held (left lateral recumbent or standing position) during the examination. (Note that abdominal ultrasonography is the preferred method for evaluating animals for intussusception, but flexible endoscopy is also useful for finding intussusceptions into the colon.) Biopsy specimens can usually be obtained from the descending colon (not the rectum or anus) in a conscious animal without causing obvious pain. If proctoscopy is being performed to examine a patient for anal or rectal lesions, general anesthesia is indicated because biopsies (frequently deep ones) may need to be obtained from sensitive areas.

## POSITIONING

For *rigid colonoscopy,* the animal should be placed in a *right lateral recumbent* position so that any fluid left in the colon from the bowel cleansing or entering the colon from the ileum pools in the dependent ascending colon. The animal can be placed on a tilt table

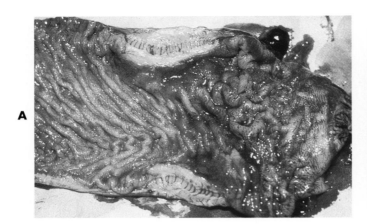 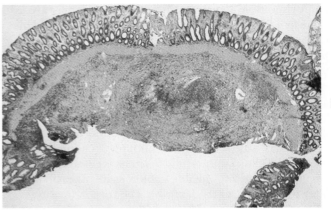

**Figure 7-7 A,** Gross view of the rectal area of a dog that had a rectal adenocarcinoma. No evidence of mucosal disease is seen; only the submucosa is thickened. **B,** Microscopic view of a similar infiltrative lesion. The biopsy specimen was obtained with a rigid biopsy forceps. The darkened areas in the submucosa are the diagnostic areas. If the tissue sample had not included these areas (i.e., if the sample had been obtained with flexible forceps), the diagnosis would have been chronic active proctitis instead of pythiosis. (From Nelson RW, Couto CG, editors: *Essentials of small animal internal medicine*, St. Louis, 1992, Mosby.)

with the head slightly lower than the anus. With this positioning, fluids in the colonic lumen flow toward and pool in the transverse colon, away from the descending colon which is being examined. For *flexible colonoscopy,* the *left lateral recumbent* position allows any fluid entering the colon from the ileum to flow away from this area and into the transverse and descending colon. This position also prevents abdominal viscera from being dorsal to the ileocolic valve area and collapsing it, thereby making it difficult to distend and examine this area. Animals undergoing proctoscopy may be positioned in almost any position that is convenient to the clinician.

## PROCEDURE

### Rectal Digital Examination

A digital rectal examination should *always* be performed before an instrument is inserted into the rectum. Anal lesions are easy to miss during colonoscopy because it is hard to adequately distend and inspect this area. More importantly, lesions may weaken the rectal wall, making perforation likely if the tip of the scope is advanced into a blind sac. Finally, the endoscopist often encounters a vestibule-like dilation of the lumen just past the anus and then must rediscover the continuation of the colonic lumen. It is particularly easy for the tip of a scope (especially a flexible one) to become trapped

in a mucosal fold at this site. It is sometimes easier to continue into the colonic lumen if a digital rectal examination is performed immediately before the scope is inserted into the anus. This examination seems to help straighten out the rectal area so that the instrument can be more easily inserted into the colonic lumen.

### Rigid Proctoscopy and Biopsy

Proctoscopy is the best endoscopic technique for locating and examining rectal and anal lesions. The scope and obturator are first lubricated and then gently inserted as far as possible into the anus. If substantial *resistance* is encountered, the endoscopist should stop advancing the scope, remove the obturator, and identify the cause. If obvious mucosal thickening is seen or a submucosal mass is suspected, biopsy specimens should be obtained from the submucosa as well as the mucosa (Figure 7-7).

Obtaining adequate samples of submucosal lesions can be difficult. Use of rigid biopsy forceps with the tip diverted at a 30- to 45-degree angle is preferred. For this purpose it is helpful to have available an older biopsy instrument that is not used for delicate mucosal biopsies. The forceps tip should be pushed into the mass or thickening, and pressure should be maintained as the jaws are slowly closed. The endoscopist needs to be sure that the tissue sample contains both mucosa and submucosa but not muscle or serosa. At least one and preferably two appropriate specimens should be obtained. Proctoscopes sometimes

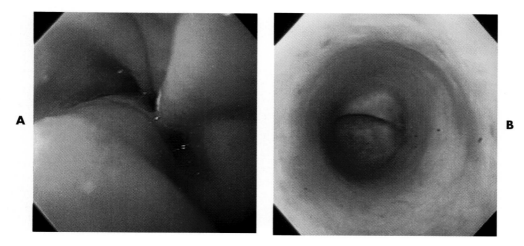

**Figure 7-8 A,** Endoscopic view of normal colonic mucosa before air has been insufflated into the lumen. Because only tissue folds can be seen, the surface of the mucosa cannot be adequately evaluated. **B,** The colonic lumen has been distended with air. Note the smooth surface of the mucosa and how the lumen can be visualized for some distance.

stretch the mucosa so that the necessary deep biopsy cannot be performed. In such cases the endoscopist may have to remove the proctoscope and blindly guide the tip of the biopsy instrument into the mass or thickening with a finger. Only the thickened area should be biopsied or the rectum may be perforated.

## Rigid Colonoscopy

Sterilization of rigid endoscopes and biopsy forceps is usually not as crucial in veterinary medicine as in human medicine. However, measures must be taken to avoid transmitting infections between patients. Enzymatic cleaners promote the removal of fecal matter, which facilitates sterilization. Plasma sterilization (e.g., hydrogen peroxide plasma sterilization) is optimal, but appropriate glutaraldehyde solutions (e.g., Cidex Plus) are satisfactory. However, detergents and disinfectants need to be cleared from the scope before use to avoid producing iatrogenic mucosal lesions. Most rigid instruments may be sterilized in an autoclave, but care must be taken to avoid damaging plastic parts or dulling sharp cutting edges.

Rigid colonoscopy is performed by inserting the well-lubricated tip of a disinfected endoscope (with the obturator in place) 2 to 3 inches into the anus. The obturator is then removed, and the hinged glass window over the front of the scope is closed to establish an air-tight seal. Initially, the colonic lumen is usually collapsed (Figure 7-8). Therefore, the endoscopist must insufflate air into the colonic lumen while observing through the window. Insufflation is continued until the colonic lumen is distended and smooth with no mucosal folds that may hide

lesions (see Figure 7-8). The normal colon should inflate readily unless gas is escaping out the anus. The endoscope is then advanced slowly into the distended lumen, with the tip of the scope maintained in the center of the lumen. *The lumen should always be visualized as the endoscope is advanced.* The scope should *never* be blindly pushed into the colon. Following these suggestions helps prevent perforations and allows excellent observation of the mucosa.

Normal colonic mucosa should be smooth and pink, and it should not bleed or become hyperemic when the endoscope rubs against it gently. Depending on the angle of view, submucosal blood vessels normally can be seen (Figure 7-9). Small "holes" or indentations representing the sites of lymphoid follicles may be observed in the mucosa near the rectum (Figure 7-10). Once the endoscope has been advanced as far as possible into the colon, it is slowly withdrawn as the colon is inflated, and the mucosa is examined again. The rectal area is difficult to keep inflated; therefore it is easy to miss polyps, tumors, and submucosal strictures unless a careful examination is conducted.

If the colonic lumen does not readily open as air is insufflated, the endoscopist must resist the urge to blindly and forcefully push the scope ahead. Either a lesion (e.g., intramural or extramural mass or infiltration) is obstructing passage, or the colonic mucosa is "tacky" and is causing one side of the lumen to adhere to other side (possibly because of modest amounts of somewhat dry, tenacious mucus). In the latter situation the air insufflated into the colon escapes around the scope and out the anus because the pressure required to

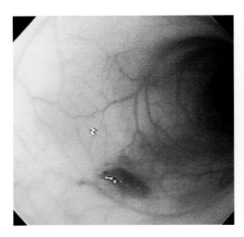

**Figure 7-9** Endoscopic view showing submucosal blood vessels in a normal canine colon.

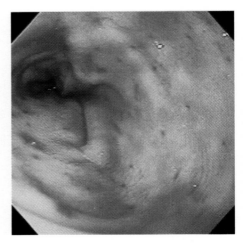

**Figure 7-10** Endoscopic view of normal canine rectal mucosa. A biopsy procedure has caused a slight amount of bleeding. This blood serves to highlight the small mucosal indentations that mark the sites of solitary lymph follicles.

separate the mucosa is greater than the pressure generated by the insufflated air. Two maneuvers may be tried in such patients. During one type of maneuver, an assistant can tightly hold the anus around the endoscope so that the insufflated air cannot escape. Alternatively, the scope can be carefully advanced between the two sides of the colonic mucosa to pry them apart. In the latter maneuver, the endoscopist must view the mucosa while advancing the scope to avoid perforating the colon. The two sides of the mucosa should part easily. Suction should be applied carefully to remove excessive fluid, mucus, or fecal debris. Colonic mucosa should not be suctioned into the tip of the aspiration channel because the suction force may produce red spots that later may be mistakenly attributed to spontaneous lesions.

## Biopsy with Rigid Equipment

After the colonic mucosa has been examined, the scope should be advanced as far as possible. At this point the hinged window is opened so that the lumen deflates. Folds of mucosa should then appear (Figure 7-11). If mucosal folds are not seen, the tip of the endoscope should be repeatedly advanced and retracted a few millimeters to create folds. Then the edge of a mucosal fold is grasped with a rigid alligator biopsy instrument (Figure 7-11), and the instrument is gently moved back and forth a few millimeters. The mucosa, but not the entire colonic wall, should move. If the entire colonic wall moves, too deep a "bite" has been taken (i.e., the mus-

cular tunics have been grasped). If this occurs, the tissue should be released and another attempt made. When an appropriate sample has been grasped, sufficient pressure is applied to sever the mucosal sample from the colon. Depending on the sharpness of the forceps, a gentle tug may be needed to free the sample. A hard pull should *never* be necessary. If there is some doubt about whether excessive traction is needed to free the sample, the sample should be released and another site tried. It is always better to take a smaller than desired piece than to obtain a large piece that causes a perforation. When rigid biopsy forceps are used, the colon should not be reinflated after the biopsy procedure is started, because a site that was biopsied too deeply may rupture when air pressure builds up in the colonic lumen. In addition, an enema should *never* be administered shortly after this procedure. Mild hemorrhage is expected after mucosal biopsy, but the bleeding should stop spontaneously without a problem. If a mucosal biopsy procedure is performed properly, the risk of perforation is minimal in dogs weighing more than 4.5 kg (10 lb).

After the first tissue sample is obtained, the tip of the scope is withdrawn 2 or 3 inches and another sample is obtained. This process is repeated until four or five tissue specimens have been acquired. It is almost never appropriate to obtain only one or two pieces of tissue; lesions can be sporadic and therefore may be missed if too few samples are taken (Figure 7-12). For example, I had one case in which the diagnosis was apparent in only one of five mucosal samples. Biopsy specimens should be obtained from obvious lesions (e.g., strictures, growths, ul-

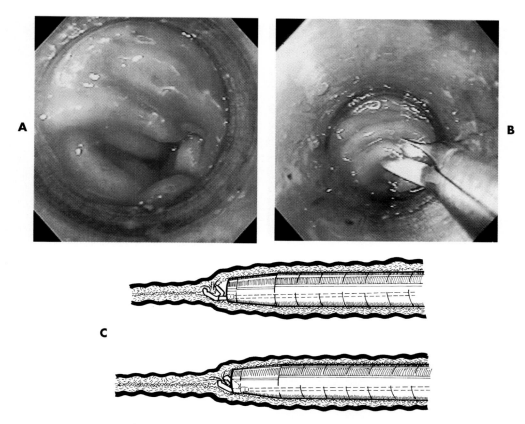

**Figure 7-11 A** Normal colonic mucosa as seen through a rigid endoscope after air has been released by opening the hinged window. **B,** One of the folds has been grasped by the tip of an alligator biopsy forceps. Note that the 30-degree angle of the tip permits easy visualization of the tissue being biopsied. **C,** Diagramatic representation of **B.** The edge of one of the mucosal folds has been grasped with the forceps. Note how mucosa can be grasped without including muscular tunics (i.e., thick dark line).

cers, discolorations) as well as nearby areas that do not appear abnormal. This approach makes it possible to determine if inflammation at the site of a gross lesion is the cause or the effect of an ulcer or stricture.

Whenever a rigid biopsy instrument is used, the tissue sample should always be examined for muscle or serosa. The sample should contain pink mucosa and hopefully a smaller area of submucosa that is off-white in color and contains small blood vessels (Figure 7-13). If submucosa is present, a full-thickness mucosal sample has been obtained. However, a relatively hard piece of reddish tissue is probably smooth muscle. Finding smooth muscle does not mean that the colon has been perforated, but it does mean that the biopsy was too deep and perforation is possible. The tip of the endoscope should be withdrawn from the area of excessively deep biopsy, and the biopsy procedure should be completed. Then the animal should

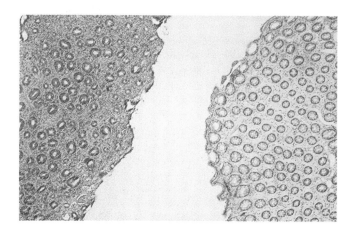

**Figure 7-12** Photomicrograph of two pieces of feline colonic mucosa obtained within centimeters of each other. The tissue on the left clearly has a much greater cellular infiltrate than the one on the right. However, on gross examination the tissue samples appeared the same. This shows the need to take *multiple* biopsies from the colon.

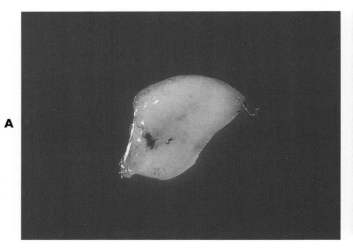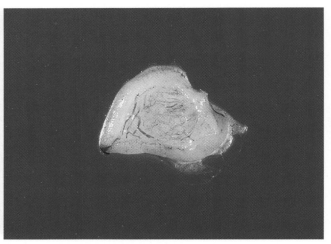

A    B

**Figure 7-13** A, Mucosal surface of a colonic biopsy specimen obtained with rigid forceps. B, Submucosal surface of the same biopsy. The blood vessels in the whitish submucosa show that this sample has a full thickness of mucosa plus a small amount of submucosa.

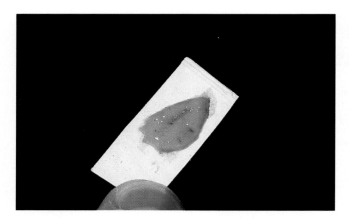

**Figure 7-14** Colonic mucosa obtained with rigid biopsy forceps. The biopsy specimens are laid out on paper, ready to be fixed in formalin.

be closely observed for 24 hours; preferably, radiographs should also be obtained. Pneumoperitoneum *confirms* perforation, which should be closed *immediately* via celiotomy. Colonic perforations occasionally seal spontaneously, but waiting to see if this will occur is risky.

Colonic mucosa is more resistant to artifacts than duodenal or ileal mucosa, but it still must be treated carefully. The tissue is carefully retrieved from the jaws of the biopsy instrument and placed on paper or sponge with a needle. Two needles are used to unfold the sample and smooth it out so that it lies flat, mucosal side up (Figure 7-14). After all samples are taken, the paper or sponge with the samples is turned upside down and

placed in formalin. In this manner it is possible for the histopathologist to obtain perfect cross sections of the mucosa and to evaluate the mucosa from lumen to submucosa.

In rigid colonoscopy, flexible biopsy forceps may be used instead of rigid ones. Although flexible biopsy forceps are safer, their use is rarely necessary except perhaps in cats. Using flexible biopsy instruments with a rigid scope eliminates the major benefit of rigid colonoscopy in that the tissue sample is rarely as good as one obtained with rigid forceps. Furthermore it is harder to direct the flexible forceps through the rigid scope.

### Flexible Colonoileoscopy

Most flexible scopes can be cleaned and disinfected with solutions that have been approved for this purpose by the manufacturer (e.g., Enzol Enzymatic Detergent, Cidex Plus). The manufacturer's recommendations for cleaning an instrument should always be followed. Flexible endoscopes should not be subjected to excessive heat (e.g., autoclaving). As mentioned previously, disinfectants and enzymatic cleaners used on the scopes and accessories must be removed before the equipment is inserted into a patient.

For flexible colonoscopy the endoscopist inserts the tip of the scope into the rectum and then insufflates air. As the tip of the scope is advanced (aiming for the center of the lumen), the endoscopist examines the mucosa and lumen. The endoscope is advanced to its most orad limit and then slowly withdrawn so that the mucosa can be examined more carefully. Then once again the scope is advanced to its orad-most limit, and biopsy samples

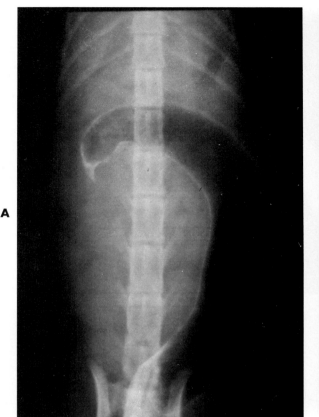 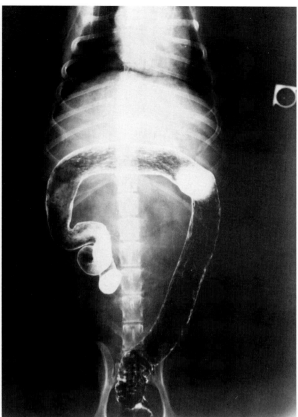

**Figure 7-15 A,** Radiograph obtained subsequent to barium enema of a normal feline colon. The expected morphology is seen. The cecum is a blind pouch at the most orad end of the colon. (Courtesy Linda J. Konde.) **B,** Following a barium enema in a dog, the radiograph shows a "typical" shape of the colon. Notice the difference in the shape and size of the canine and feline cecums.

are obtained as the instrument is progressively withdrawn.

Although most cats and many dogs have a relatively straight descending colon (Figure 7-15), some have a more convoluted path (Figure 7-16). The splenic flexure (Figure 7-17) is the orad-most part of the descending colon and is the area where the descending colon turns and becomes the transverse colon. To enter the transverse colon, the endoscopist must divert the tip of the scope in the direction of the lumen and then carefully advance the tip using a blind "slide-by" technique. When this technique is used, the tip of the scope usually lightly pushes against the colonic wall and visualization is lost for 1 to 2 cm because the lens is too close to the mucosa (Figure 7-18). The same technique can be used to enter the ascending colon or negotiate unexpected bends in the descending colon.

In cats the transverse and ascending sections of the colon usually merge together into one "shepherd's crook" (Figure 7-15). Only rarely can the mucosa of this section be carefully examined because the tight bend makes it impossible for the endoscope tip to stay in the center of the lumen. The endoscopist typically performs a blind slide-by from the descending colon up to the ascending colon and immediately finds the cecum and ileocolic valve. The feline cecum is a blind pouch that sometimes is not perceived as being a blind sac (Figure 7-19). The ileocolic valve is often comparatively small and may be obscured by matter entering the colon from the ileum. If this valve is not seen, the endoscopist may keep pushing the tip of the scope into the cecum, thinking it is the continuation of the colonic lumen. It may help to flex the tip of the scope to near maximum and then push it cranial for approximately 1 cm (a "walking stick" maneuver). This is an attempt to put more distance between the tip of the scope and the ileocolic valve, which allows the endoscopist a panoramic view instead of a close-up view in which structures are out of focus. Alternatively, withdrawing the tip of the scope into the descending colon and then reinserting it into the ascending colon sometimes allows visualization of the ileocolic valve. With this technique the endoscopist may be able to pass flexi-

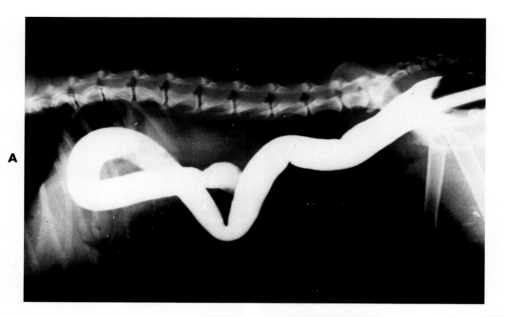

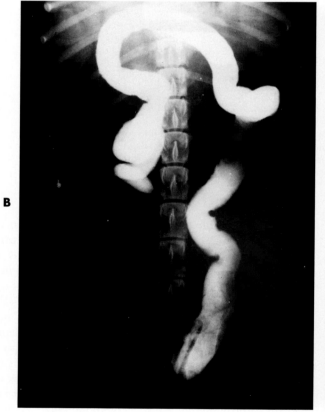

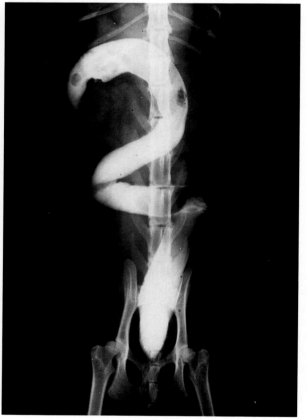

**Figure 7-16** Lateral (**A**) and dorsoventral (**B**) views subsequent to the administration of a barium contrast enema in a dog with a markedly convoluted colon. Passing an endoscope through some of these "unexpected" turns could be difficult. Radiograph taken in conjunction with a barium enema in a cat that has a similarly convoluted colon (**C**).

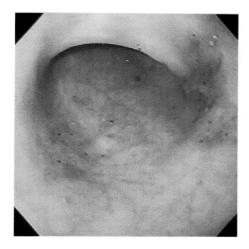

**Figure 7-17** When the tip of the scope approaches the splenic flexure, the colonic lumen disappears dorsally as the colon bends nearly 90 degrees.

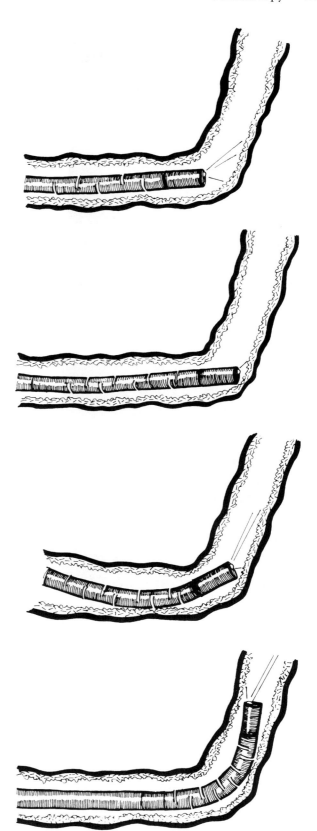

ble biopsy forceps through the ileocolic valve and blindly obtain ileal biopsies (Figure 7-20).

Substantial manipulation may be required to negotiate the bends that sometimes occur in the canine descending colon (see Figure 7-16). Some cats also have redundant colons. Such bends may make it difficult to pass the endoscope up to the ileocolic valve and can also make paradoxic movement more likely when the endoscopist tries to advance the scope through the colonic lumen. *Paradoxic movement* refers to finding that the tip of the scope either stays in the same place or starts backing up as more insertion tube length is passed into the patient (Figure 7-21). This phenomenon becomes more likely as the ileocolic valve is approached. If paradoxic movement is occurring, the endoscopist must first ensure that the insertion tube is well lubricated. Then the endoscope tip is repeatedly advanced and retracted carefully while the entire scope is gently rotated (as opposed to forcing the tip of the instrument forward into the lumen). Withdrawing the scope several inches after dilat-

**Figure 7-18** Diagrammatic representation of the "slide-by" technique. In the top panel the tip of the scope is approaching the splenic flexure. In the second panel from the top, the tip of the scope is so close to the wall of the colon that visualization is lost. As the tip of the scope is then deflected upward, it stays so close to mucosa that visualization remains lost (third panel) until the tip makes the bend and the center of the lumen is seen again (bottom panel).

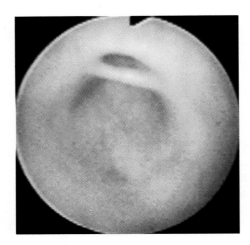

**Figure 7-19** Endoscopic view of the ileocecocolic valve area of the cat. The ileocolic valve is the slit at the 12 o'clock position. The cecum is the blind pouch into which the colon ends.

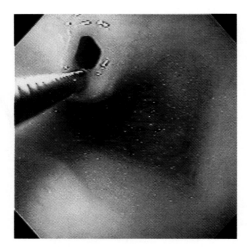

**Figure 7-20** Endoscopic view of the ileocolic valve area of a cat. A flexible biopsy instrument has been passed into the ileum to blindly obtain ileal biopsies.

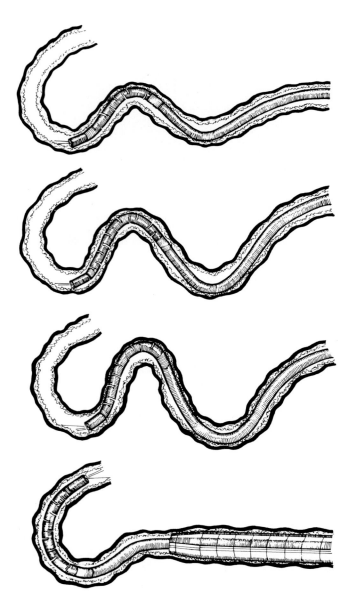

**Figure 7-21** Diagrammatic representation of "paradoxic movement" in a dog's colon. In the top panel the endoscope is in a colon that has a somewhat more convoluted path than normal. As more of the insertion tube is advanced into the colon (second and third panels), the colon is bowed out laterally by the insertion tube instead of having the endoscope tip advance into the colonic lumen. In the bottom panel the flexible scope has been passed through the lumen of a rigid scope that was previously advanced as far as possible into the colon. In this manner, much of the paradoxic movement is eliminated, and feeding the insertion tube into the colon results in forward movement of the endoscope tip.

ing the colonic lumen with air sometimes straightens out the insertion tube and makes it easier to advance the tip of the endoscope.

If paradoxic movement is still occurring, rigid and flexible scopes may be used simultaneously. First the descending colon is examined with a rigid colonoscope, advancing the scope as far as possible into this section of the colon. Next, the flexible scope is passed through the rigid endoscope and into the colon (see Figure 7-21). This should eliminate most paradoxic movement and give the endoscopist more control of the tip of the scope during attempts to enter the cecum and ileum. The flex-

ible scope must not be pulled forcefully into the rigid scope or the flexible instrument may be damaged by the edge of the open end of the rigid scope.

When the tip of the scope approaches the canine ileocolic valve, careful observation is necessary or the valve

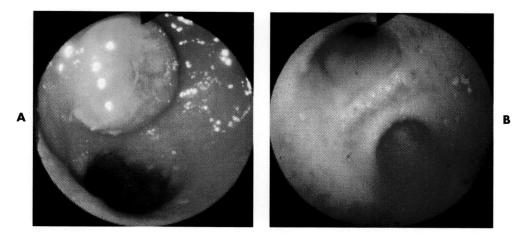

**Figure 7-22 A,** Endoscopic view of the ileocecocolic valve area in a normal dog. The mush-roomlike structure is the ileocolic valve, and the opening is the cecocolic valve. **B,** Endoscopic view of the ileocecocolic valve area in another normal dog. In this case the ileocolic valve is diffi-cult to distinguish from the cecocolic valve. (From Willard MD: Endoscopy case of the month, *Vet Med* 88;108, 1993.)

may be bypassed and the tip of the scope may enter the cecum. If the area is clean, it is possible to see both the ileocolic valve (which often resembles a small intussus-ception) and the cecocolic valve (Figure 7-22). Occa-sionally the ileocolic valve simply appears as another opening adjacent to the cecocolic valve. However, this portion of the colon tends to be less well prepared be-cause mucus and debris entering from the ileum may cover and hide the ileocolic valve. In this situation the only hint of the ileocolic valve may be a "ledge" of tis-sue to one side of what appears to be the continuation of the colonic lumen (but which is really the cecal lumen) (Figure 7-23). If the endoscopist enters the cecum, think-ing it is the colon, the lumen will make additional bends that cannot be negotiated with the tip of the scope. No attempt should be made to vigorously push the tip of the scope past one of these "bends" or the cecum may be perforated. Therefore, if it seems difficult to pass the scope any farther into the "colon," the endoscopist should withdraw the tip several centimeters, flush water into the lumen, aspirate to remove debris, and check again for the ileocolic valve. If the working length of the scope has seemingly been exhausted during an attempt to enter the cecum, the endoscope should be retracted several centimeters and air should be aspirated to par-tially collapse the lumen. This may shorten the distance to the cecocolic (or ileocolic) valve.

## Retroflexed View of Anus

When a flexible scope is used to examine rectal lesions, a retroflexed view (Figure 7-24) is often necessary. If avail-able, a rigid proctoscope is often better for examining this site. Depending on the diameter of the scope; only dogs weighing 9 to 14 kg (20 to 30 lb) or more usually have

colonic lumens large enough to perform this maneuver. The scope is advanced approximately 5 to 10 cm past the rectum, the lumen is maximally distended with air, and then the tip is maximally deflected up (usually 210 de-grees). The tip should now be directed caudally, back at the anus. This allows the rectal area to be examined un-less the lumen does not distend because of air leakage.

## Biopsy with Flexible Instruments

Many of the same principles apply for biopsy procedures performed with rigid or flexible instruments. The major difference is that the risk of perforation is extremely un-likely with flexible biopsy. After the ileum and cecum have been examined, *multiple tissue samples* should be obtained, regardless of how normal the tissues appear. Mucosal biopsy samples are primarily obtained for histopathologic evaluation. However, *Salmonella* organ-isms sometimes can be cultured from tissue samples when they cannot be grown from feces. At least two samples for histopathologic examination should be ob-tained from each of the following: ileum, cecum, as-cending colon, transverse colon, high descending colon, and lower descending colon. The endoscope should be advanced as far as desired into the patient (e.g., the ileum), and samples should be taken from the different areas as the scope is progressively withdrawn. It is often advantageous to partially collapse the colonic lumen be-fore the mucosa is grasped with biopsy forceps (Figure 7-25). When the lumen is maximally inflated, the mu-cosa is "stretched," and a relatively "thin" mucosal sample, perhaps without submucosa, is usually ob-tained. When the lumen is partially collapsed, the for-ceps often take a larger, deeper sample that typically in-cludes submucosa. Although the colon should not be

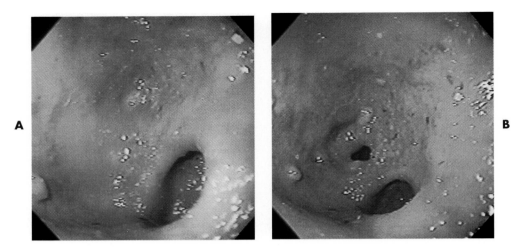

**Figure 7-23 A,** Endoscopic view of a poorly prepared ileocecocolic valve area in a dog. The one obvious opening may be mistaken for the continuation of the colon. **B,** Some of the mucus and other debris have fallen away from the opening of the ileocolic valve, revealing the opening to the left of the cecocolic valve.

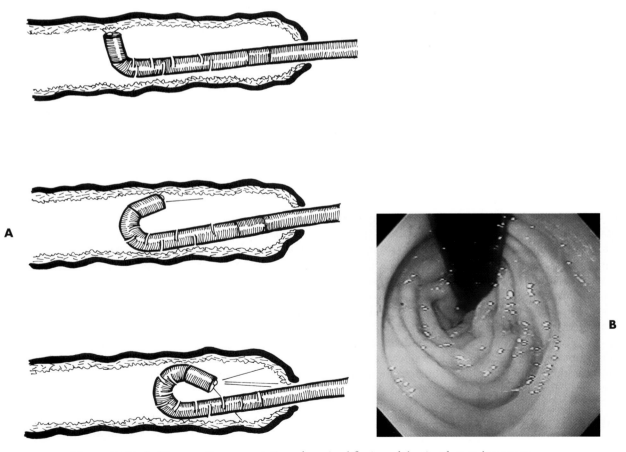

**Figure 7-24 A,** Diagramatic representation of maximal flexion of the tip of an endoscope to view the rectum. The progression is from top to bottom. **B,** Endoscopic view of a normal canine rectum obtained using this retroflex maneuver.

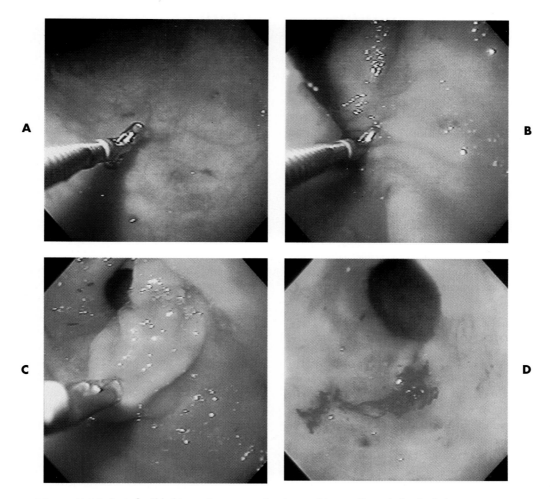

**Figure 7-25 A,** A flexible biopsy instrument is advanced into a distended colonic lumen through a flexible colonoscope. **B,** The colonic lumen is partially collapsed, and the instrument is pushed into the mucosa. **C,** The jaws of the biopsy instrument are closed, and the biopsy instrument is withdrawn into the scope. **D,** A small amount of bleeding is normal after such a biopsy.

reinflated after the biopsy procedure is initiated with a rigid instrument, it is safe to reinflate the colon after biopsy specimens are obtained with flexible forceps. I prefer to obtain biopsy tissue samples with a flexible scope only in areas that are inaccessible to rigid scopes.

Care must be taken in advancing a biopsy instrument through a maximally deflected scope (e.g., when obtaining a retroflexed view or when the tip is in the cecum or

ileum). In this situation it is easy to damage the biopsy channel and have water leak into the insertion tube. If the endoscopist encounters undue resistance when trying to insert the biopsy instrument while the tip of the scope is flexed, the flexion of the tip should be relaxed (even if visualization is lost) and the biopsy instrument should be gently inserted until it is just past the area of resistance. Then the tip may be flexed back to its previous position.

## POSTPROCEDURE CARE

The patient is recovered from anesthesia and may usually be sent home later that day without waiting for the histopathology report. The animal's next bowel movement often contains a little blood, but bleeding from the biopsy procedure is expected to stop spontaneously within 2 to 3 hours (usually within 1 hour). The animal should be rechecked if it becomes nauseous, anorexic, or depressed or if it has continued, unexpected bleeding from the anus. Such complications are very rare. Antibiotics are *not* needed before, during, or after colonoscopy, except in the rare case in which the risk of systemic infection is great. An example of such a condition is a cat with suspected suppurative cholangitis-cholangiohepatitis secondary to inflammatory bowel disease. Analgesics are almost never needed after the procedure, unless deep submucosal biopsy specimens have been taken from rectal lesions.

### Mucosal Cytology

Cytologic examination can diagnose histoplasmosis, protothecosis (Figure 7-26), some neoplasms, and occasionally amoebic infections, but it is inconsistent and unreliable for diagnosing most inflammatory bowel diseases except perhaps eosinophilic infiltrates. (Note that pythiosis often has concurrent eosinophilic mucosal infiltrates.) Specimens for mucosal cytologic evaluation may be obtained in four ways:

1. The rectal mucosa may be scraped with a flat spatula. This sampling, which may be done in conscious animals, is especially useful if the rectal mucosa is thickened or corrugated.

2. A cytology brush may be passed through the endoscope and rubbed against a lesion. The brush is then retrieved and rubbed against a microscope slide. This technique is used primarily for focal lesions beyond the reach of a spatula.
3. A gloved finger may be used to scrape clean mucosa.
4. A small (i.e., approximately 1-mm diameter) mucosal sample may be obtained endoscopically and then squashed between two microscope slides.

Fecal cytology, not mucosal cytology, is used to help diagnose *Clostridial* and *Campylobacter* colitis.

## UNPREPARED COLONS

In rare instances the colon cannot be properly prepared before an examination. For example, a rectal stricture may prevent adequate cleansing, or the administration of lavage or enemas may not be possible because of an animal's temperament or financial or client constraints. Although inadequate preparation prevents a thorough evaluation and greatly increases the chances of missing significant lesions, a minimal examination can be performed and random biopsies can be obtained. Sometimes enemas may be administered to anesthetized patients. If that is not possible, the endoscopist may insufflate air and try to advance the tip of a flexible scope between the feces and the colonic wall. This works best if the feces are relatively firm and do not adhere to the colonic wall. If a rigid scope is used, an attempt may be made to aspirate soft feces with a large-bore aspiration tube. Alternatively, a rigid scope may be carefully advanced under direct vision into the feces, thereby impacting feces into the scope lumen. The scope is then withdrawn, and the feces is expelled using the obturator. This process is repeated as necessary. This method of cleansing the colon is not recommended, but it can be used when no other alternatives are possible.

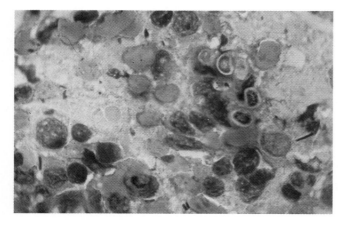

**Figure 7-26** Cytologic preparation of colonic mucosa from a dog with protothecosis. The prototheca are the dark, bean-shaped structures with clear areas around them.

### REFERENCES

Burrows CF: Evaluation of a colonic lavage solution to prepare the colon of the dog for colonoscopy, *J Am Vet Med Assoc* 195:1719, 1989.

Church EM, Mehlaff CJ, Patnaik AK: Colorectal adenocarcinoma in dogs: 78 cases (1973–1984), *J Am Vet Med Assoc* 191:727, 1987.

Clinkenbeard KD, Cowell RL, Tyler RD: Disseminated histoplasmosis in cats: 12 cases (1981–1986), *J Am Vet Med Assoc* 190:1445, 1987.

Clinkenbeard KD, Wolf AM, Cowell RL et al: Canine disseminated histoplasmosis, *Compend Cont Educ* 11:1347, 1989.

Dennis JS, Kruger JM, Mullaney TP: Lymphocytic/plasmacytic colitis in cats: 14 cases (1985–1990), *J Am Vet Med Assoc* 202:313, 1993.

Dimski DS, Buffington CA: Dietary fiber in small animal therapeutics, *J Am Vet Med Assoc* 199:1142, 1991.

Durante L, Zulty JC, Israel E et al: Investigation of an outbreak of bloody diarrhea: association with endoscopic cleaning solution and demonstration of lesions in an animal model, *Am J Med* 92:476, 1992.

Holt PE, Lucke VM: Rectal neoplasia in the dog: a clinicopathological review of 31 cases, *Vet Rec* 116:400, 1985.

Jergens AE: Inflammatory bowel disease, In August JR, editor: *Consultations in feline internal medicine,* Philadelphia, 1994, WB Saunders.

Jonas C, Mahoney A, Murray J et al: Chemical colitis due to endoscope cleaning solutions: a mimic of pseudomembranous colitis, *Gastroenterology* 95:1403, 1988.

Jones BD: Personal communication, 1995.

Leib MS, Matz ME: Diseases of the large Intestine, In Ettinger SJ, Feldman EC, editors: *Textbook of veterinary internal Medicine,* Philadelphia, 1995, WB Saunders.

Miller RI: Gastrointestinal phycomycosis in 63 dogs, *J Am Vet Med Assoc* 186:473, 1985.

Nelson RW, Stookey LJ, Kazacos E: Nutritional management of idiopathic chronic colitis in the dog, *J Vet Intern Med* 2:133, 1988.

Otto CM, Dodds WJ, Greene CE: Factor 12 and partial prekallikrein deficiencies in a dog with recurrent gastrointestinal hemorrhage, *J Am Vet Med Assoc* 198:129, 1991.

Reinemeyer CR: Feline gastrointestinal parasites. In Kirk RW, Bonagura JD, editors: *Current veterinary therapy XI,* Philadelphia, 1992, WB Saunders.

Richter KP: Lymphocytic plasmacytic enterocolitis in dogs, *Semin Vet Med Surg (Small Anim)* 7:134, 1992.

Santoro MJ, Chen YK, Collen MJ: Polyethylene glycol electrolyte lavage solution-induced Mallory-Weiss tears, *Am J Gastroenterol* 88:1292, 1993.

Sherding RG, Johnson SE: Intestinal histoplasmosis. In Kirk RW, Bonagura JD, editors: *Current veterinary therapy XI,* Philadelphia, 1992, W.B. Saunders Co.

Spach DH, Silverstein FE, Stamm WE: Transmission of infection by gastrointestinal endoscopy and bronchoscopy, *Ann Intern Med* 118:117, 1993.

Strombeck DR, Guilford WG: Infectious, parasitic, and toxic Gastroenteritis. In Strombeck DR, Guilford WG, editors: *Small animal gastroenterology,* ed 2, Davis, Calif., 1990, Stonegate.

Tams TR: Irritable bowel syndrome, In Kirk RW, Bonagura JD, editors: *Current veterinary therapy XI,* Philadelphia, 1992, WB Saunders.

Twedt DC: Canine *Clostridium perfringens* diarrhea, *Proc Waltham/OSU Symp* 17:28, 1993.

Wilcock B: Endoscopic biopsy interpretation in canine or feline enterocolitis, *Semin Vet Med Surg (Small Anim)* 7:162, 1992.

## COLOR PLATES    PAGES 236-245

### CANINE COLITIS
**Plate 7-1,** p. 236 Hemorrhage associated with moderately severe eosinophilic colitis
**Plate 7-2,** p. 236 Hyperemia associated with eosinophilic colitis
**Plate 7-3,** p. 236 Mucosal hemorrhage associated with purulent colitis
**Plate 7-4,** p. 237 Generalized hyperemia secondary to severe lymphocytic-plasmacytic colitis

### FELINE COLITIS
**Plate 7-5,** p. 237 Hemorrhage associated with severe lymphocytic-plasmacytic colitis
**Plate 7-6,** p. 237 Lymphoid follicles
**Plate 7-7,** p. 238 Hemorrhage associated with suppurative colitis
**Plate 7-8,** p. 238 Numerous hemorrhages in a cat with renal and colonic amyloidosis

### MYCOTIC COLITIS
**Plate 7-9,** p. 238 Histoplasmosis with hyperemia and ulceration
**Plate 7-10,** p. 239 Histoplasmosis, special stain

**Plate 7-11,** p. 239 Pythiosis with diffuse and intense hyperemia
**Plate 7-12,** p. 239 Phytiosis with an associated rectal stricture
**Plate 7-13,** p. 239 Pythiosis, ileococolic valve area

### STRICTURES AND OBSTRUCTIONS
**Plate 7-14,** p. 240 Partial stricture in descending colon of a cat
**Plate 7-15,** p. 240 Partial obstruction of descending colon of a basenji with abdominal lymphoma
**Plate 7-16,** p. 241 Complete rectal obstruction of a German shepherd dog
**Plate 7-17,** p. 241 Partial stricture near the rectum

### ILEOCECOCOLIC VALVE REGION
**Plate 7-18,** p. 241 Whipworms in the cecum and descending colon
**Plate 7-19,** p. 242 Unexplained mucosal hemorrhage of ileocolic valve
**Plate 7-20,** p. 242 Cecocolic intussusception
**Plate 7-21,** p. 242 Ileocolic intussusception

**Plate 7-22,** p. 242 Open ileocolic valve in a cat (congenital abnormality)

### NEOPLASIA
**Plate 7-23,** p. 243 Adenocarcinoma in mid-descending colon—canine
**Plate 7-24,** p. 243 Poorly differentiated sarcoma—canine
**Plate 7-25,** p. 243 Lymphosarcoma—feline
**Plate 7-26,** p. 244 Benign epithelial polyps with underlying submucosal carcinoma—feline
**Plate 7-27,** p. 244 Rectal polyp
**Plate 7-28,** p. 244 Rectal polyp, retroflexed view
**Plate 7-29,** p. 244 Multiple benign rectal polyps
**Plate 7-30,** p. 245 Multiple benign polyps and severe mucopurulent colitis
**Plate 7-31,** p. 245 Multiple benign polyps
**Plate 7-32,** p. 245 Large mass at the ileocolic area in a Scottish terrier (diagnosis not determined)
**Plate 7-33,** p. 245 Small benign polyp

## CANINE COLITIS

The endoscopic appearance of colitis varies substantially between and within patients. Obvious changes may include hyperemia, hemorrhage (either spontaneous or in response to gentle abrasion from the endoscope), a roughened (i.e., granular) appearance to the mucosal surface, discoloration, and erosions. However, many animals with substantial mucosal inflammatory infiltrates have *no* grossly observed changes or only *minimal* changes that cannot confidently be declared to represent disease. Therefore biopsies should be obtained in *every* animal that undergoes endoscopy. I prefer to use both rigid and flexible endoscopes in all but the smallest dogs. The flexible scope is used to evaluate and biopsy the cecum, ileum, ascending colon, transverse colon, and the part of the descending colon that is beyond the reach of the rigid scope. The rigid endoscope is used to obtain biopsy specimens from the descending colon at three to five sites. Both gross lesions and relatively normal-appearing mucosa should be biopsied, with at least two samples taken from each site. In my practice, inflammatory bowel disease (e.g., lymphocytic-plasmacytic colitis or eosinophilic colitis) is a rare cause of large bowel signs in dogs, but fiber-responsive disease, dietary intolerance or allergy, and *Clostridial* colitis are common.

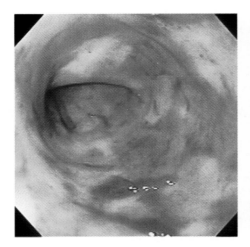

**Plate 7-1** Hemorrhage into the lumen of the colon of a cocker spaniel with moderately severe eosinophilic colitis.

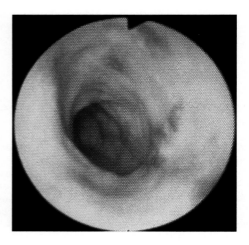

**Plate 7-2** Hyperemic colonic mucosa in a dog with eosinophilic colitis.

**Plate 7-3** Mucosal hemorrhage in the descending colon (**A**) and ileocecocolic valve area (**B**) in a schnauzer with purulent colitis. This animal's clinical signs did not respond to sulfasalazine. The only response was to metronidazole.

**A**

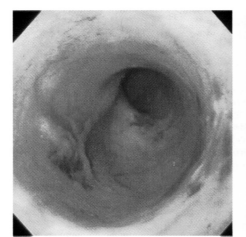

**B**

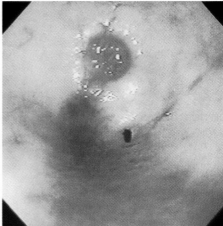

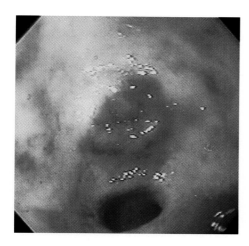

**Plate 7-4** Ileocolic valve area (cecocolic valve at the 6 o'clock position and the ileocolic valve in the center) in an 11-year-old schnauzer with chronic, large bowel disease. Endoscopy demonstrated hyperemic mucosa throughout the colon. The histopathologic evaluation revealed severe lymphoplasmacytic colitis, which was well controlled with prednisolone.

## FELINE COLITIS

In my practice, lymphocytic-plasmacytic colitis is a very common cause of hematochezia with or without diarrhea in cats. The most common endoscopic finding is either a normal colon or spontaneous hemorrhage.

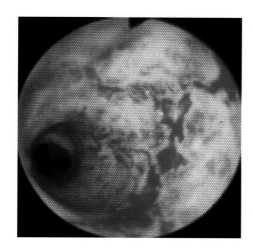

**Plate 7-5** View of the colon in a 12-year-old domestic shorthair cat with chronic hematochezia, diarrhea, and weight loss. Severe lymphocytic-plasmacytic colitis was diagnosed. The hemorrhage is spontaneous; that is, it was seen as the endoscope was advanced, before the tip of the scope had touched the mucosa.

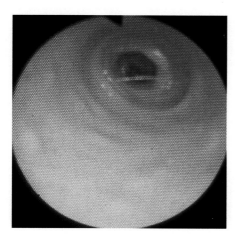

**Plate 7-6** Lymphoid follicles (nodules) in a 2-year-old cat with a history of chronic hematochezia but no diarrhea.

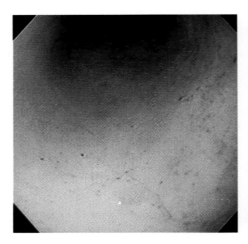

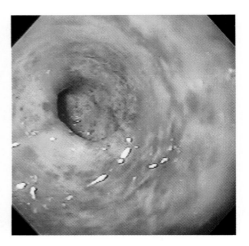

**Plate 7-7** Areas of hemorrhage ("freckles") in the colon of a 6-year-old cat with chronic weight loss, diarrhea, and fever. Examination of biopsy specimens revealed marked, suppurative colitis.

**Plate 7-8** This 11-year-old Abyssinian cat had renal failure due to amyloidosis. The animal developed bloody diarrhea and tenesmus. Endoscopy revealed countless hemorrhages throughout the mucosa, especially near the rectum. Biopsy specimens showed moderate amyloidosis in the mucosa with minimal inflammation. Infectious organisms could not be cultured from the feces.

## MYCOTIC COLITIS

Histoplasmosis is probably the most common fungal infection of the canine colon. The feline colon is very rarely affected. Although this infection often causes a severe, bloody diarrhea with hypoproteinemia and weight loss, it may also be present in dogs with no obvious evidence of colonic disease. Occasionally, histoplasmosis is limited to a focal area in the colon. In most cases the organism may be found in the mucosa. However, if a report of granulomatous colitis or pyogranulomatous colitis is received, special stains and/or recuts should usually be requested in case the fungus was initially missed.

Pythiosis is a fungal infection that was once seen primarily in the southeastern United States. However, with increased travel by dogs this disorder is now found in much of this country today. Pythiosis may be seen in any portion of the alimentary tract, but the pylorus, ileocecocolic valve area, and rectal area are commonly affected. The lesion is initially submucosal with mild secondary mucosal changes. Partial strictures are common. With time the mucosa may be severely affected. Biopsy samples *must* include the submucosa because the hyphae are rarely present in the mucosa.

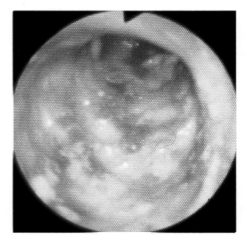

**Plate 7-9** Colon of a Labrador retriever with severe histoplasmosis. Marked hyperemia and obvious ulceration (light areas) are present. (From Leib MS: *Vet Med* 86:917, 1991.)

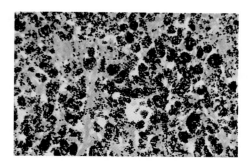

**Plate 7-10** Special staining of mucosa from the colon in Plate 7-9 reveals black dots, with each dot representing a yeast cell.

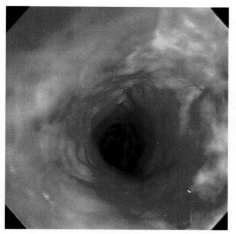
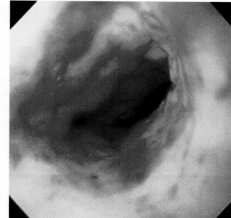

**Plate 7-11** Colon of a mixed-breed dog with severe, widespread pythiosis. Obvious, intense, diffuse mucosal hyperemia is present.

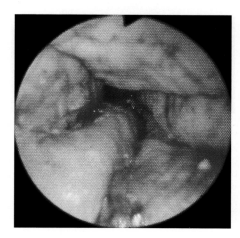
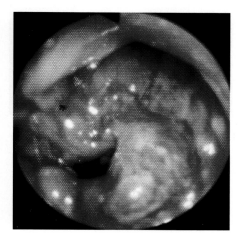

**Plate 7-12** Endoscopic view of the rectum of a dog with a partial rectal stricture caused by a pythiosis granuloma.

**Plate 7-13** Ileocecocolic valve area in a dog with weight loss and profuse bloody stools. The mucosa is very darkened and rough. *Pythium insidiosum* had invaded the mesenteric vessels and caused ischemic necrosis of the area.

# STRICTURES AND OBSTRUCTIONS

An attempt should be made to differentiate strictures and obstructions as *mucosal, intramural* (submucosal), or *extramural* (i.e., outside the colon but pushing into it). This task cannot always be accomplished endoscopically although certain signs may help distinguish the different types. Extramural lesions are often associated with a smooth, relatively normal mucosa. Intramural lesions may have a similar appearance but more commonly display some secondary mucosal irritation and hyperemia. Mucosal disease causing a stricture is usually obvious because it is characterized by an irregular, roughened, highly inflamed mucosa.

Colonic strictures are relatively uncommon whereas rectal strictures occur more frequently. Congenital obstructions may occasionally be seen in young animals, primarily at or near the rectum. A presumptive diagnosis can usually be made based on the history and physical examination. However, biopsy samples should be obtained if the diagnosis is in doubt. In such cases the biopsy must include submucosal tissue. Obstructions may also be due to cicatrix, especially in older dogs and cats. Such obstructions usually occur at or near the rectum. Treatment consists of rectal ballooning or dilation by other means. Surgery should be performed only if dilation methods fail.

Inflammatory strictures may occur in association with inflammatory bowel disease, fungal infections, or perianal fistulas. It is imperative to obtain deep biopsy samples from the stricture (as well as mucosal biopsies of surrounding tissues that appear normal) to differentiate inflammatory from neoplastic causes.

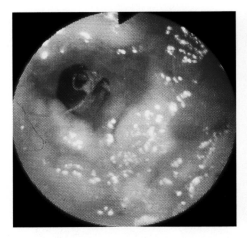 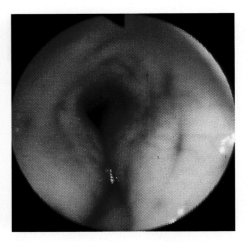

**Plate 7-14** Partial stricture of the descending colon in a cat, caused by eosinophilic colitis. Note the extremely roughened mucosa.

**Plate 7-15** Partial obstruction of the descending colon in a basenji with abdominal lymphoma. Note how the colon appears to be compressed (much as would occur if the organ were held between a thumb and forefinger). The texture of the mucosa appears relatively normal.

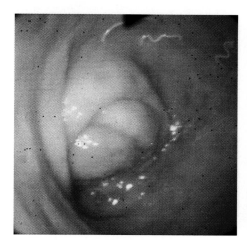

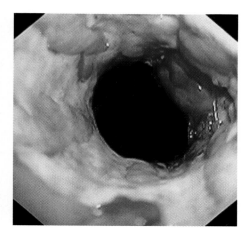

**Plate 7-16** Complete obstruction of the rectum in a German shepherd. The obstructing granuloma appeared to be caused by *Blastomyces dermatitides*. In addition, whipworms are attached to the surface of the rectum. (From Allen D, editor: *Small animal medicine*, Philadelphia, 1991, Lippincott.)

**Plate 7-17** Partial stricture near the rectum in a 6-year-old Chesapeake Bay retriever. Notice the cobblestone-like areas and the failure of the lumen to open as widely as expected. The examination of biopsy specimens revealed a chronic ulcerative process with changes suggestive of but not diagnostic for neoplasia.

## ILEOCECOCOLIC VALVE REGION

Examination of the ileocecocolic valve area can only be done with a flexible endoscope. Although most colonic disorders may be diagnosed by examining the descending colon with a rigid scope, the diagnosis of several diseases requires examination of the ileocecocolic valve region.

A 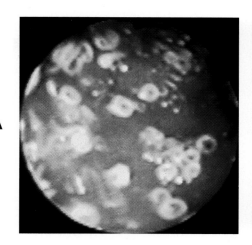   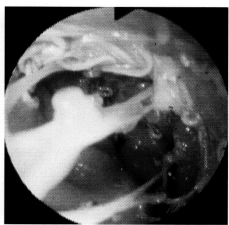 B

**Plate 7-18 A,** Whipworms in the cecum of a dog. **B,** Whipworms in the descending colon of a dog. Whipworms are relatively common in some parts of the United States. It is clearly preferable for dogs to be treated for these parasites before endoscopy, even if fecal examinations have been negative for ova. Whipworm ova are relatively heavy and sink in flotation solutions that are not properly made. Furthermore these helminths may shed intermittently. Occasionally they are found endoscopically.

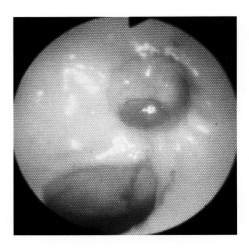

**Plate 7-19** Area of obvious hemorrhage in the ileocolic valve of a dog with persistent hematochezia. The biopsy specimens revealed mucosal hemorrhage but no inflammation. The animal's problem resolved with a change in diet.

**Plate 7-20 A,** Tubular mass in the colonic lumen. This cecocolic intussusception was so long that at first it was believed to be an ileocolic intussusception. The distinction could be made only when the valve area was reached and a normal ileocolic valve was seen. (From Willard MD: Endoscopy case of the month, *Vet Med* 88:108, 1993.) **B,** The curved, reddish tubular mass is an intussuscepted cecum. The surrounding colon is dark brown because of the presence of mucus.

**A** 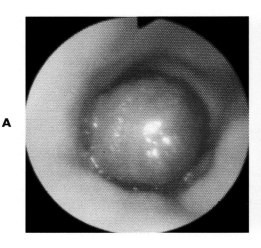   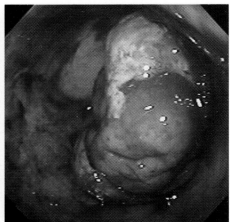 **B**

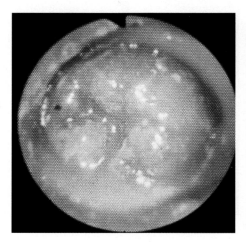

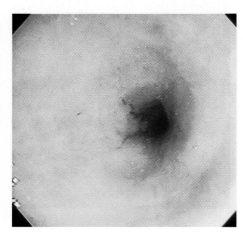

**Plate 7-21** End-on view of an ileocolic intussusception. Because this mass was seen in the descending colon, it had to be an intussuscepted ileum instead of a cecum. Furthermore an opening in the front of the mass corresponds to the lumen of the ileum.

**Plate 7-22** Ileocolic valve of a young cat (obtained as a stray) with intractable diarrhea. No cecum is seen. The ileocolic valve is simply a large opening at the distal end of the colon. It was possible to advance 60 cm of a 9.4-mm-diameter endoscope into the cat's rectum without difficulty. This apparently congenital defect was thought to allow severe small intestinal bacterial overgrowth.

# NEOPLASIA

Benign and malignant neoplasms of the canine gastrointestinal tract most commonly develop in the rectal area, although they are occasionally seen throughout the length of the canal. The most common clinical sign is usually hematochezia, but dyschezia and constipation from obstruction also occur. It is particularly important to differentiate benign polyps from cancers. For this to be done reliably, it is crucial to obtain large, deep biopsies that include the submucosa whenever possible. A reactive, polypoid growth may overlie a malignancy. Benign and malignant lesions cannot be differentiated based on size or appearance. Polyps may be singular or multiple, large or small. If the digital rectal examination reveals a hard, firm mass, an infiltrative disorder is likely, but malignancy still must be differentiated from inflammation.

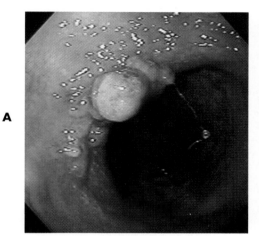

A

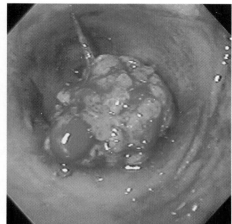

B

**Plate 7-23 A,** An old English sheepdog with a small polyp and adjacent roughened colonic mucosa. This polyp and several smaller lesions were adenocarcinomas. **B,** Large polypoid mass in the mid-descending colon of a poodle. This was an adenocarcinoma.

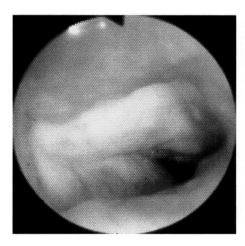

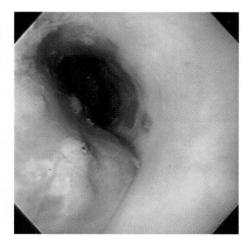

**Plate 7-24** Colon of a mixed-breed dog with signs of large bowel disease. Note the sharply demarcated area that is much lighter in color than the rest of the colon. When biopsied, this area was much firmer and more difficult to sample than the rest of the colonic mucosa. The discolored area was a poorly differentiated sarcoma.

**Plate 7-25** Large sessile mass (6 to 12 o'-clock position in the field of view) in a 6-year-old mixed-breed cat with signs of large bowel disease. Note the erosions on the surface of the mass. The histopathologic examination revealed lymphosarcoma.

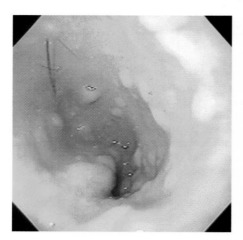

**Plate 7-26** Benign epithelial polyps caused by an underlying submucosal carcinoma in an 11-year-old cat with a history of vomiting that had become especially severe over the previous two to three weeks. After gastroduodenoscopy was done, it was discovered that the colon had not been prepared. Nevertheless, colonoscopy was performed. The opening near the bottom of the field of view (6 o'clock-position) is the ileocolic valve. Numerous nodules are seen despite the copious amounts of fecal material.

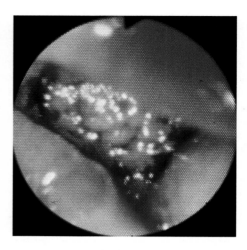

**Plate 7-27** Rectal polyp seen with a flexible endoscope placed just inside the rectum. Because the rectum could not be distended with air, the view is partial and inferior.

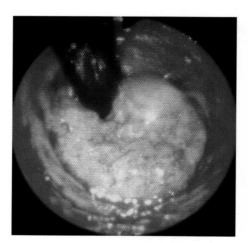

**Plate 7-28** Retroflexed view of the polyp shown in Plate 7-27. Note how much better the lesion can be examined from this position.

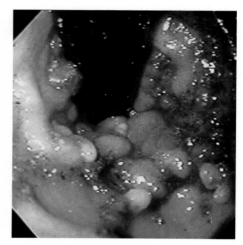

**Plate 7-29** Retroflexed view of the rectum of a dog with multiple benign polyps. Refer to Figure 7-24, **A** for a schematic representation of the retroflex maneuver in the lower colon and rectum.

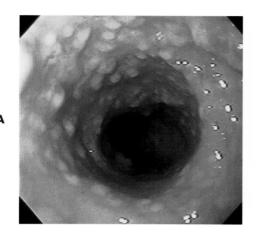

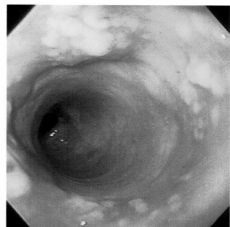

**Plate 7-30** A, Extreme irregularity in the distal colon of a dachshund. The protrusions are multiple benign polyps. B, Farther orad in the same colon the area of gross irregularity ceases, and the colon appears smooth and normal as the scope is advanced. This condition responded transiently to steroid enemas, but surgical resection was necessary to eliminate the clinical signs.

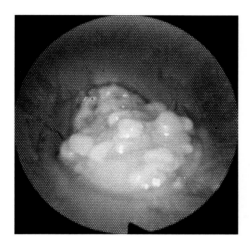

**Plate 7-31** Rectum of a dog with multiple benign polyps as viewed through an operating proctoscope.

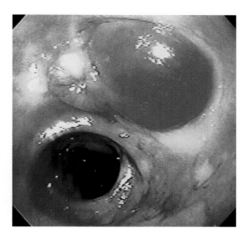

**Plate 7-32** Large mass at the ileocolic valve in a Scottish terrier. The dog was being examined prior to surgery for a benign rectal polyp, and the presence of other masses was not suspected. Mucosal biopsy through the flexible scope was not diagnostic. The client did not allow the examiners to determine what this mass was.

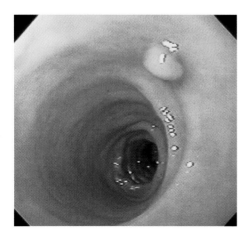

**Plate 7-33** Small benign polyp in the descending colon of the dog in Plate 7-32.

# Chapter 8

# Endoscopic Removal of Gastrointestinal Foreign Bodies

**Todd R. Tams**

Foreign bodies in the upper gastrointestinal tract are encountered frequently in clinical practice. In many instances these objects pass through the gastrointestinal tract uneventfully with minimal or no symptoms being exhibited by patients. However, foreign bodies occasionally become impacted in the esophagus, stomach, or intestinal tract or are freely movable but trapped within the stomach. In such cases some method of removal is required. Until the late 1970s rigid esophagoscopy under general anesthesia was the procedure of choice for retrieving esophageal foreign bodies. Into the early 1980s surgical removal via gastrotomy and enterotomy was the standard therapy for foreign bodies of the stomach and intestinal tract, respectively. Improvements in flexible fiberoptic endoscopes and the development of foreign body grasping forceps, retrieval baskets, and polypectomy snares for use with endoscopes, however, have clearly made endoscopic retrieval the current procedure of choice for dealing with retained esophageal and gastric foreign bodies. Physicians and veterinarians who are skilled in endoscopy have become adept at retrieving foreign bodies of various sizes and shapes. Today it is uncommon for patients with a foreign body in the esophagus, stomach, or colon to undergo surgical removal.

A classic monograph on the management of foreign bodies of the upper airway and esophagus in humans was published in 1937 (Jackson and Jackson). This monograph was based on 3266 cases in which a rigid endoscope was used. Subsequently little material appeared in the literature until the late 1970s, when scattered reports described the successful retrieval of foreign bodies from humans using flexible endoscopes. This chapter presents current information regarding guidelines and detailed techniques for the endoscopic removal of foreign bodies. The information is based on my personal experiences as well as those of other veterinary endoscopists.

## ANATOMIC CONSIDERATIONS

Foreign bodies become impacted in the gastrointestinal tract at both normal anatomic and pathologic points of narrowing. The major factors in determining whether a foreign body will pass uneventfully or be retained are its size and configuration (e.g., rough versus smooth edges, presence or absence of projections, and width). Once the pointed objects (e.g., needles, wishbones) are beyond the oropharynx, they occasionally become lodged in the pyriform processes. These areas can be seen with an endoscope but are best evaluated with a laryngoscope.

The four areas of physiologic narrowing in the esophagus are the area of the upper esophageal sphincter, the thoracic inlet, the heart base area, and the distal esophagus just proximal to the gastroesophageal junction.

Most foreign bodies become impacted in one of the latter three areas in dogs and cats. A variety of foreign bodies can be involved, but in my experience bones are the most common objects found in the esophagus. Although a sharp object has the potential to perforate into the aorta at the level of the aortic arch or to pierce through the esophagus into the chest cavity, such situations are extremely rare. If *blunt* objects fail to pass through the esophagus spontaneously, the presence of an esophageal motility disorder or a pathologic area of narrowing (e.g., benign or malignant esophageal stricture) should be suspected.

Many foreign bodies that enter the stomach pass through the remainder of the gastrointestinal tract without difficulty. However, large smooth objects (e.g., rocks, balls, lead sinkers), nonpliable materials (e.g., leather, or plastic), and objects with sharp or irregular edges may be retained in the stomach because they are either too large to pass through the pylorus or their sharp edges become impacted in the antrum, pylorus, or cardia. A tubular hairball or other material may be retained because of a gastric motility disorder rather than its size or configuration.

Other points of anatomic narrowing in the gastrointestinal tract include the angles of the duodenum, ileocecal valve, and anus. Pathologic abnormalities in the intestine, such as strictures, tumors, and areas of prior surgical intervention, predispose to impaction by foreign bodies.

## TYPES OF FOREIGN BODIES

Foreign bodies should be characterized as sharp or dull, pointed or blunt, and toxic or nontoxic. If the objects are visible radiographically, their length and width should be measured and the likelihood of their passing through the gastrointestinal tract without the need for endoscopic or surgical intervention should be clinically assessed. The configuration and physical makeup of an object, as well as its location, help determine whether endoscopic removal is feasible. An attempt should be made as early as possible to retrieve objects impacted in the esophagus. Most bones, fishhooks, and other objects retained in the esophagus can be successfully removed with endoscopy. Sewing needles are most commonly ingested by kittens or young cats, and frequently the alimentary tract is capable of passing these objects without incident. If possible, the clinician should determine whether any significant length of thread was attached to the ingested needle because this would increase the potential for a dangerous sequela of intestinal plication if the needle were to become impacted at the pylorus with the thread moving progressively down the intestine.

The ability of the alimentary tract to pass sharp objects such as needles is thought to be attributable to reflex mural relaxation of the intestinal musculature. Axial flow in the intestinal lumen, combined with slowing of peristalsis and reflex relaxation, tends to facilitate passage around the numerous curves of the intestinal tract. In some cases the objects actually turn around so that the sharper end trails rather than leads. Once in the colon, foreign objects often become covered by fecal material, which protects the bowel wall.

Although I have observed numerous clinical cases in which needles have successfully traversed the intestinal tract, I have also evaluated animals with peritonitis caused by foreign body perforation of the intestinal wall. In several cases, needles passed as far as the descending colon before migrating through the bowel wall and into the abdominal cavity. Because the retrieval of needles from the stomach with flexible endoscopic instrumentation is a quick and relatively easy procedure, early intervention is currently my treatment of choice rather than the more conservative but uncertain "wait and see" approach.

## PATIENT PROFILES

Although foreign body ingestion is certainly more common in young animals than middle-aged to older animals, the possibility of a foreign body–related disorder must always be considered in any animal with suggestive signs. Most commonly, foreign bodies are ingested during a foray through garbage ("dietary indiscretion") or when an animal is playing (e.g., whole or partial sections of toys chewed and eaten, balls swallowed suddenly after being caught in flight, fishhooks and needles ingested during an inquisitive investigation). Dogs that chew rocks occasionally swallow partial or whole rocks, which may then become retained in the gastrointestinal tract. In some instances an animal ingests an object for no readily apparent reason. Included in my case files are such examples as an ingested 11-cm potato nail (see Plate 8-21, C), a rigid patch of leather ingested by a cat (see Plate 8-15), and an accumulation of ingested pine needles that caused gastric impaction in a cat (see Plate 8-20). These and many other interesting cases were successfully managed by endoscopy-guided retrieval.

Our physician counterparts encounter two dissimilar patient population profiles when dealing with foreign bodies. In most instances, ingestion of foreign bodies occurs in children, particularly between 1 and 5 years of age, who swallow objects accidentally. Most of these foreign bodies tend to be small, blunt, and nontoxic (e.g., coins, small toys) and pass without intervention. In contrast, five groups of adults have been identified as being prone to ingest foreign bodies or to suffer from impaction of food boluses. These five groups include persons with preexisting esophageal disease (e.g., stricture, diverticulum, motility disorder, neoplasia), alcoholics, psychopaths, mentally retarded, handicapped persons, and prisoners. Older adults (greater than 60 years) are much more likely to have food bolus foreign bodies. Young adults (less than 40 years) are more likely to ingest true foreign bodies (inorganic objects). It is not uncommon for prisoners and persons with psychiatric disorders to intentionally swallow a foreign body as a manipulative measure. The resulting hospital admission period with endoscopic therapy is preferable to prison or institutionalization. Prisoners often ingest sharp objects such as razor blades or bedsprings encased in toilet paper or tissue paper to protect the mouth and tongue during swallowing. Once these materials have been ingested, hospital surveillance usually becomes mandatory.

## CLINICAL SIGNS

Presenting symptoms resulting from a gastrointestinal foreign body vary, often depending on the area of lodgment. Clinical signs related to foreign body impaction in the esophagus are often acute and usually include salivation, which may become bloody, and regurgitation. Odynophagia, dysphagia, forceful retching, and anorexia may also occur. Occasionally an esophageal foreign body remains undetected for a number of days. Chronic signs usually include depression, anorexia, salivation, and regurgitation. Clinical evidence of an esophageal foreign body complication, such as esophageal perforation with resultant pleuritis, mediastinitis, and pyothorax, may also be present. Other potential sequelae include esophageal stricture, diverticula, and severe esophagitis.

Gastric foreign bodies are commonly associated with partial or complete outlet obstruction with accompanying characteristic symptoms. If the foreign object is freely movable, vomiting may occur only intermittently and, especially if the object is small, there may be many days when the animal displays no clinical signs whatsoever. Large foreign bodies are usually associated with frequent vomiting, and signs are usually most pronounced when the foreign body lodges in the antrum. Occasionally a tubular hairball lodges in the pyloric canal, causing complete outflow obstruction and frequent vomiting (see Plate 5-94). The presence of a gastric foreign body may also cause inappetence or complete anorexia, malaise, and nonspecific mild abdominal tenderness. The combination of pain and fever suggests perforation, which may be associated with signs of peritonitis or which may be walled off with minimal or no abdominal signs evident. Toxic foreign objects may cause other clinical signs such as seizures (e.g., seizure activity related to lead toxicity resulting from the retention of a lead sinker in the gastrointestinal tract). Small

disk batteries used as an energy source for watches, hearing aids, and cameras contain alkali, such as potassium hydroxide, and the heavy metals mercury and cadmium. Toxicity depends on the leakage of these substances from their casings, the duration of contact with the mucosa, and the inherent toxicity of the chemicals themselves. Endoscopic or surgical removal of a toxic foreign body is mandatory if the object remains in the stomach for longer than 24 hours or if it lodges in the intestinal tract.

Sometimes the clinical signs that are exhibited seem incongruous with the type or size of foreign body present. For example, I have seen dogs (usually small breeds) become completely anorectic as a result of a small gastric foreign body such as a peach pit. The appetite predictably returns to normal as soon as the foreign body is removed. In other cases some foreign bodies that have been present for weeks to months cause minimal or no clinical signs.

## DIAGNOSTIC EVALUATION

The diagnosis of a retained foreign body may be readily apparent from the history. For example, an owner may have observed the garbage foray during which a bone was ingested, a section of a toy may be missing, or fishing line attached to a hook may be observed dangling from a pet's mouth. In other cases no specific contributory historical information is available. In yet other cases the client may deny any possibility of foreign body ingestion.

Survey radiographs of the thorax and abdomen should be the first study performed because radiopaque objects can easily be localized in most cases. Cervical soft tissue radiographs are also obtained if an esophageal foreign body is suspected. Lateral films of the neck are particularly important for detecting bone fragments impacted in the cervical esophagus. Esophageal dilation anterior to a foreign body may be seen. Thoracic radiographs should be carefully evaluated for evidence of esophageal perforation, including pneumomediastinum or pleural effusion. *More than one foreign body may be present; hence it is very important to evaluate survey radiographs carefully for evidence of additional foreign bodies that may be less obvious than an easily recognized radiopaque object.*

Radiolucent foreign bodies pose a significant diagnostic challenge. Stomach size is important in the assessment of radiolucent gastric foreign bodies. Gastric distension is a finding compatible with a long-standing gastric foreign body. Increased width of a localized portion of the stomach, attributable to an inability of the stomach to collapse in the involved segment, is seen with foreign bodies of lesser duration. The presence of gas may help outline a foreign body. A negative contrast gastrogram is useful in cases of suspected radiolucent foreign body (Figure 8-1). Fish bones, plastic, and wood are not radiopaque. A negative contrast agent such as air will *not* mask foreign bodies as barium tends to do. Some foreign bodies may be composed of both radiopaque and radiolucent materials. As a result their size may be underestimated on survey radiographs.

Foreign bodies are sometimes identified unexpectedly during routine endoscopy undertaken to evaluate patients with unexplained inappetence or vomiting. Often survey radiographs are unrevealing in these patients, and contrast studies to look for a radiolucent foreign body are not performed. Occasionally, when clients have significantly limited financial means, endoscopy is performed as a preliminary diagnostic step to avoid the expense of radiographs in patients with chronic intermittent vomiting. This is sometimes a reasonable approach, especially when patients have chronic signs and the findings of the history and physical examination are not diagnostic. Such patients are highly likely to require endoscopy with biopsy at some point, regardless of the radiographic findings. If a foreign body is found during diagnostic endoscopy, an attempt can be made to remove the object. If the foreign body cannot be removed, the patient can be taken to surgery while still under anesthesia. When a foreign body is removed, gastric and small intestinal biopsies still should be obtained in animals with *chronic* vomiting in order to investigate for concurrent problems. Sometimes a foreign body may not pass spontaneously because the patient has a motility disorder or an inflammatory disease with a secondary motility disorder. In such cases it is best to be thorough.

## OVERVIEW OF TREATMENT OF INGESTED FOREIGN BODIES

Once a foreign body has been localized, the clinician must decide whether to observe for its passage or remove the object endoscopically or surgically. Most esophageal and gastric foreign bodies are amenable to endoscopic retrieval. As a rule, any foreign object retained in the esophagus should be removed as soon as possible; if this cannot be done, the object should at least be advanced to the stomach. Esophageal perforation is uncommon but is always a risk, especially when a sharp or pointed object is involved.

In most cases an esophageal foreign body does not have to be removed as a true "emergency" procedure. Exceptions include foreign body impaction in the proximal esophagus that is causing respiratory distress because of tracheal compression, and a wedged sharp object such as a bone that is causing significant patient distress. These situations may be evidenced by groaning, copious salivation, or forceful gagging. If rapid intervention is not required, the patient should be stabilized as needed with intravenous fluids, antibiotics, and pain medications (e.g., oxymorphone or morphine plus a

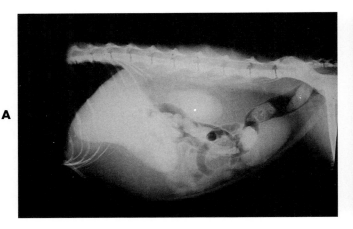
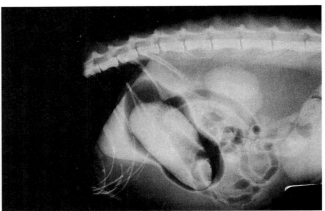

**Figure 8-1** A, Lateral abdominal radiograph from a 10-year-old cat with intestinal lymphoma. The animal was also positive for feline immunodeficiency virus. The cat was presented because of a gradually decreasing appetite, recent onset of intermittent vomiting, and occasional episodes of nonproductive retching. Abdominal palpation revealed a doughy mass in the region of the stomach. **A,** Radiograph showing a distended stomach and a soft tissue/fluid opacity. The small intestine and colon are normal. **B,** Gastrogram taken after 40 mL of air was injected into the stomach through a small feeding tube. A large mass density within the lumen of the stomach is consistent with a gastric trichobezoar. This simple procedure allowed rapid confirmation that a foreign body was present in the stomach. The trichobezoar was removed surgically (this mass was too wide to consider endoscopic retrieval). (From Tams TR: Gastrointestinal symptoms. In Tams TR, editor : *Handbook of small animal gastroenterology,* Philadelphia, 1996, WB Saunders)

transdermal fentanyl patch if ongoing pain is anticipated), and a thorough radiographic assessment should be completed. Ideally endoscopy should be undertaken within 4 to 12 hours of presentation. Endoscopy is indicated as the initial procedure of choice for all esophageal foreign bodies. If endoscopic equipment is not available, the patient should be referred to an appropriate facility.

Sharp or pointed objects, such as pieces of plastic, needles, and safety pins, should be removed from the stomach endoscopically. As discussed previously, needles frequently pass through the gastrointestinal tract uneventfully, but early removal is recommended because of the increased potential for complications with such objects and the high success rate of endoscopic retrieval. Rounded or blunt gastric foreign bodies often pass spontaneously; therefore, if significant clinical signs such as frequent vomiting are not present, such patients may be managed conservatively with close observation and radiographic surveillance for 3 to 7 days. If signs of obstruction develop, surgical intervention is indicated.

Some foreign bodies can be successfully retrieved from the upper small intestine endoscopically, but if an object becomes impacted to any degree, it is usually quite difficult to grip it firmly enough with foreign body graspers to move it. An enterotomy is then required. Although some animals can retain gastric foreign bodies for long periods of time with minimal untoward effects, it is always best to remove objects retained for a prolonged period (greater than 2 to 3 weeks) to avoid chronic mucosal damage.

Endoscopic foreign body removal has numerous advantages over other means of treatment. The procedure is minimally invasive and not appreciably time-consuming. In my experience, endoscopic foreign body retrieval generally requires 5 to 15 minutes once anesthesia is induced. Especially troublesome objects may require up to an hour, but endoscopy is still less expensive and less invasive than surgery. Patients are often discharged within 4 hours to 2 days of the procedure. Endoscopy allows for rapid intervention when sharp objects or valuable prized possessions such as jewelry or coins are ingested. Rather than rely on observation and radiographic surveillance in such clinical situations, the clinician can use endoscopic equipment to quickly retrieve the object in question. The main limiting factor with endoscopy is the necessity for general anesthesia.

Foreign bodies that are not likely to be removed endoscopically include corncobs, large rocks (bigger than the rocks shown in Plate 8-21, *A*), large hard rubber balls (e.g., Superball), and sometimes heavy objects such as lead sinkers. Problems with retrieval of foreign objects are related to their size in relation to the width of the grasping range of pronged foreign body retrieval instruments, the diameter of basket and snare instruments, the weight or surface texture of the foreign body, and the *grasping strength and quality* of the foreign body retrieval instruments being used. Smooth objects are sometimes difficult to grasp firmly enough for retrieval through the narrow areas of the lower and upper esophageal sphincters.

## INSTRUMENTATION

A variety of instruments are available for foreign body retrieval. A laryngoscope and forceps (e.g., Kelly clamp, sponge forceps) should be immediately available for removing pharyngeal foreign bodies and any object that is difficult to pull through the upper esophageal sphincter with standard prong-type endoscopic grasping instruments. Until the 1970s the rigid endoscope was always used for retrieving esophageal foreign bodies. Today, however, the flexible endoscope is the instrument of choice because visualization and maneuverability are greatly enhanced. In some cases it might be best to use a flexible endoscope in conjunction with a rigid scope. Areas such as the stomach and duodenum, which are inaccessible to a rigid endoscope, can easily be reached with a flexible endoscope as long as it has sufficient length. Nonetheless, it is still advantageous to have several rigid scopes of different lengths and diameters available for selected esophageal bone foreign body cases and for possible use as an overtube for the flexible endoscope.

A variety of foreign body forceps are available for use with flexible endoscopes. The diameter of the working channel of the endoscope limits to some degree the type and size of grasping instruments that can be used. Larger, sturdier instruments made by some manufacturers require a 2.8-mm or larger working channel. Pediatric endoscopes that are less than 8 mm in diameter usually have a 2-mm channel. In my experience, a majority of gastric and esophageal foreign bodies can be successfully retrieved with instrumentation that can be used through a 2-mm channel.

Two-, three-, and four-pronged grasping instruments are most commonly used for foreign body retrieval. A *sturdy* two-pronged instrument (Figure 8-2) is adequate for grasping many foreign objects and can be used with a pediatric endoscope that has a narrow working channel. *Sturdy* three-pronged (tripod) graspers usually require a 2.8-mm channel. Sheathed four-pronged graspers can be purchased (e.g., Microvasive, Watertown, Mass) for use through small working channels, but these instruments do not tend to be as durable. Alligator-jaw forceps (Figure 8-3) are particularly useful for grasping smooth flat objects. Rat-tooth forceps (Figure 8-4) have excellent gripping power and are especially useful for retrieving heavy cloth objects such as large socks or towels.

Polypectomy snares are the most versatile instruments for removing foreign bodies (Figure 8-5). The snare loop

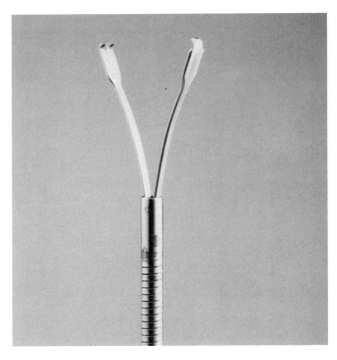

**Figure 8-2** Two-pronged grasping forceps. The width between the grasping teeth (when fully separated) is approximately 1.4 cm. This is a versatile instrument because of its grasping teeth and long arms, as well as the adequate space between the grasping ends when the arms are fully extended. (Courtesy Olympus America, Inc., Melville, N.Y.)

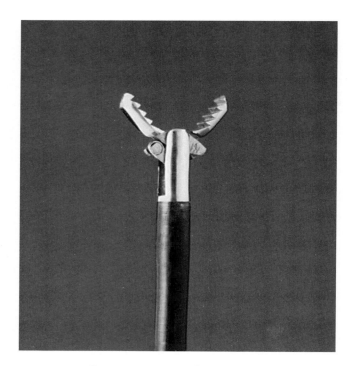

**Figure 8-3** Alligator-jaw grasping forceps. (Courtesy Olympus America, Inc., Melville, N.Y.)

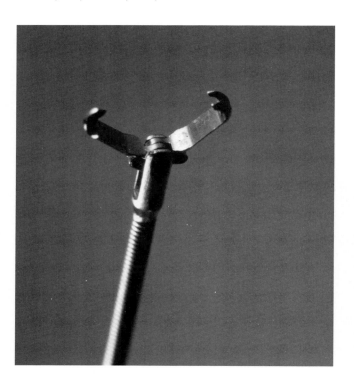

**Figure 8-4** Sharp (rat-tooth) grasping forceps with an opening width of 4.7 mm. This instrument requires a 2.8-mm instrument channel. (The two-prong instrument shown in Figure 8-2 can be passed through a 2-mm instrument channel.) The grasping strength of the rat-tooth forceps is excellent, and the instrument is particularly suited for retrieving heavy cloth (e.g., socks, towels) and other pliable or relatively thin objects. (Courtesy Olympus America, Inc., Melville, N.Y.)

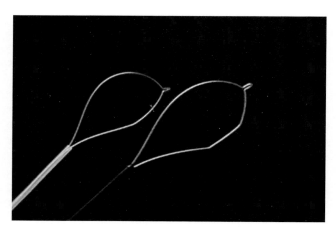

**Figure 8-5** Oval (*left*) and crescent (*right*) grasping snares. (Courtesy Olympus America, Inc., Melville, N.Y.)

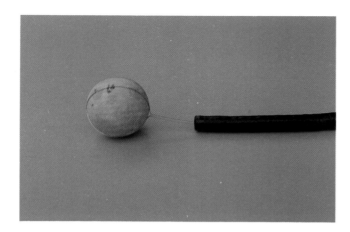

**Figure 8-6** Snare technique used to remove a hard, smooth-surfaced ball from the stomach. A prong-type instrument would be inadequate for grasping this object.

can be extended around an object to provide a much stronger grasp than can sometimes be achieved by the single end grasp applied by a pronged instrument. Round objects with a smooth surface (e.g., balls) are much more easily grasped with a snare than with a pronged instrument, which typically slips off the object as the prongs are closed around it (Figure 8-6). Basket retrievers (Figure 8-7) are less commonly required but are helpful in extracting smooth, rounded objects. Standard endoscopic biopsy forceps generally are not useful for removing foreign bodies other than thin, light objects. In fact, it is strongly advised that endoscopic biopsy instruments *not* be used for foreign body retrieval because such use may damage the forceps or cause the edges to become more dull and thus less effective for procuring adequate-size tissue samples.

Experienced endoscopists have personal preferences regarding the types of grasping instruments they like to use in certain situations. My own advice to veterinarians who are purchasing foreign body retrieval instrumentation is to obtain *high-quality* sturdy instruments that are "built to last." Lower quality instruments may cost less, but they tend to be somewhat less effective and less durable. Significant *frustration* often results from the use of *lower quality* instruments! I advise having a minimum of two types of instruments: a two-prong grasper with long arms (see Figure 8-2) and a snare loop instrument (see Figure 8-5). Once experience has been gained, an endoscopist can successfully retrieve a majority of gastric foreign bodies with one of these two instruments. My next preference would be a rat-tooth instrument (see Figure 8-4) if my endoscope working channel can accommodate an instrument of this size. Finally, I would add a basket instrument. Occasionally a basket is slightly more effective than a single snare loop for retrieving a smooth-edged foreign object.

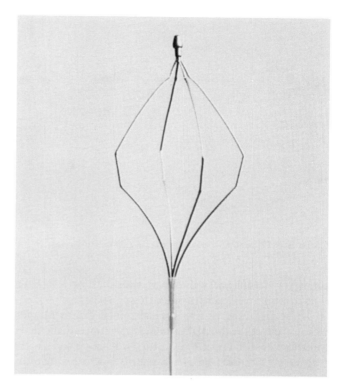

**Figure 8-7** Basket-type grasping forceps. (Courtesy Olympus America, Inc., Melville, N.Y.)

An *overtube* is an extremely useful ancillary instrument for protecting the esophageal mucosal when sharp or pointed foreign bodies must be removed. This tube fits over the endoscope, and sharp objects are drawn into its lumen before the endoscope and tube apparatus are withdrawn from the patient. Overtubes may be purchased commercially, or they can be made from tubing. The inner diameter of an overtube should be approximately 2 mm larger than the outside diameter of the endoscope. The end should be beveled smooth to facilitate passage and to prevent mucosal trauma from sharp edges. An endotracheal tube or rigid endoscope can also be employed as an overtube. For use in the stomach, an overtube should be 50 to 60 cm long; a shorter tube usually suffices in the esophagus.

The tube is first passed over the endoscope to the level of the control handle (Figure 8-8). The endoscope is then inserted in the usual manner, and the overtube is advanced as needed. The inner walls of the overtube should be well lubricated to allow easy passage of the endoscope through it. When a foreign body is being withdrawn, the overtube remains in position beyond the tip of the endoscope, thereby protecting the mucosal surface (Figure 8-9). An overtube can be useful even if a sharp object cannot be completely drawn into its lumen. Because it has a wider diameter than the endoscope, the overtube serves to maintain better dilation at the lower

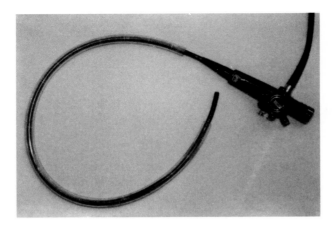

**Figure 8-8** Overtube in position on a flexible endoscope.

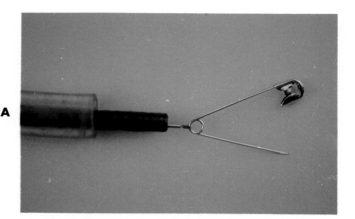

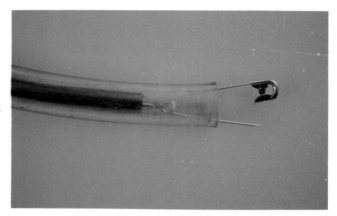

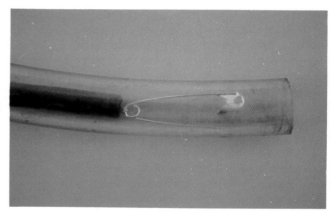

and upper esophageal sphincters, thus making it less difficult to pull an object through these orifices.

Use of an overtube has several minor disadvantages. With an overtube in place, it may be more difficult to read the measure markings on the endoscope so that the total length of insertion is not readily apparent. A more troublesome problem is that the overtube may interfere with torquing of the endoscope, which makes thorough scanning in the stomach somewhat more difficult. Therefore, when dealing with a gastric foreign body, the endoscopist should usually complete the diagnostic evaluation portion of the procedure before using the overtube.

In my experience it has been rarely necessary to use an overtube in retrieving foreign bodies from animals. The most significant advantage provided by an overtube has been in facilitating passage of wide foreign bodies through the narrow areas of the lower and upper esophageal sphincters.

## ENDOSCOPIC REMOVAL OF ESOPHAGEAL FOREIGN BODIES

Safe extraction of an esophageal foreign body requires an adequate preliminary evaluation and the selection of proper equipment, including appropriate grasping forceps or snare. An overtube, laryngoscope, and curved grasping forceps should also be readily available in case their use becomes necessary. Patient evaluation includes a thorough physical examination to check for problems directly related to the foreign body, such as dyspnea, gagging, bloody saliva, fever, and dehydration, and for problems that may complicate the use of general anesthesia, such as preexisting cardiac or renal disease. Analgesia must be provided to enhance patient comfort. Leukocytosis with a left shift is present in some cases of long-standing bone impaction (more than 3 to 4 days) and is likely attributable to secondary infection in damaged esophageal mucosa. Fermentation of retained food

**Figure 8-9** Example of the usefulness of an overtube in the removal of a sharp foreign body. **A,** An opened safety pin is grasped firmly at the blunt end with a forceps instrument before withdrawal into an overtube. **B,** The endoscope and safety pin is being pulled into the overtube. **C,** The safety pin has been totally withdrawn into the overtube. Use of this technique keeps the sharp point of the safety pin from coming into contact with mucosa. The overtube and endoscope can be safely withdrawn at the same time.

material also takes place. Cervical and thoracic radiographs are carefully reviewed to determine foreign body conformation and location and to look for evidence of esophageal perforation. If pleural fluid is present, the chest should be tapped to obtain a sample for cytology, Gram stain, and culture and sensitivity studies. Pyothorax is best managed with the placement of a chest tube for drainage and lavage. Once the patient is stabilized, a thoracotomy is done as soon as possible, either alone or in conjunction with endoscopy to remove the foreign body and to evaluate and repair the esophageal wall. In my experience, it is rare for even bone foreign bodies that have been lodged in the esophagus for several days to weeks to cause complete esophageal perforation.

As with any type of esophagogastroduodenoscopy procedure the patient is maintained under general anesthesia in a left lateral recumbent position. In this position the esophagus lies above the aorta. The endotracheal tube is especially important in preventing tracheal compression as a large foreign body is pulled retrograde through the esophagus and in preventing aspiration of any object that might be inadvertently dropped in the pharynx during retrieval. The endoscope should be passed under direct visual guidance through the pharynx and upper esophageal sphincter to avoid striking any foreign body material that may be present in the proximal esophagus and subsequently may damage the mucosa. As the endoscope is advanced, the esophageal mucosa should be carefully evaluated for any foreign body–related damage. For enhanced visualization, air should be insufflated to distend the esophageal walls, but the patient's respiratory status must be carefully monitored while this is done. Air may be forced around an impacted foreign body and into the stomach, which can lead to significant gastric distension with resultant respiratory compromise. Cats and small dogs are most at risk. The distension should be relieved as quickly as possible. In most cases this can be done by periodically passing the endoscope around the foreign body and into the stomach so that the air can be suctioned. Air insufflation to a perforated esophagus can also result in acute respiratory signs. The anesthetist is advised to monitor both respiratory character and degree of gastric distension during the procedure.

Successful extraction of a foreign body requires adequate visualization, a firm grasp of the object, and removal with minimal force to avoid further damage. The endoscope tip should not be used as a "ramming rod" to dislodge or advance an object because significant damage could be incurred to the endoscope. Once freed, most objects can be pulled back to the tip of the endoscope. The endoscope and foreign body are then gently removed simultaneously. Undue force should *never* be exerted. Gentle manipulation is the rule. If possible, pointed objects such as bones and needles should be withdrawn with the pointed edge trailing. If a sharp end is positioned proximally, the grasping prongs can sometimes be used to cover it (e.g., toothpick or needle), thus protecting the esophageal mucosa, or the object can be advanced to the stomach and repositioned so that the

sharp end trails. This latter technique works well when irregular pieces of a material such as plastic are involved. Alternatively, objects with sharp or irregular edges can be removed with the aid of an overtube to prevent mucosal damage. After an esophageal foreign body is removed, the entire esophagus should be inspected for damage, and the stomach should be examined for the presence of any foreign material. Some degree of mucosal laceration usually occurs at the site of bone impaction in the esophagus. The extent of damage should be carefully evaluated, and appropriate medication (see next section) should be instituted after the procedure.

The most commonly encountered esophageal foreign bodies in dogs are bones and fishhooks. Techniques for their removal are discussed in detail in the following sections. Rigid sections of plastic may also become impacted, and these objects behave similarly to bones. Esophageal foreign bodies are encountered much less commonly in cats, but the management principles are identical.

## Esophageal Bone Foreign Bodies

Bones are usually not dislodged easily once they become impacted in the esophagus. Wishbones are an exception, especially if the furcular process of the bone is positioned cranially. Usually one or both of the furcular rami of the bone have a sharp edge (caused by trauma during ingestion) that impales the esophageal mucosa during transit (see Plate 8-1). Once the edge becomes wedged into the esophageal wall, the wishbone is unlikely to pass. The bone is usually easily removed simply by grasping the furcular process with a pronged instrument, pulling it directly to the endoscope tip, and simultaneously retrieving the endoscope and bone as a unit.

Chicken, pork, or rib bones are usually difficult to dislodge. Often a bone has been lodged for several days or more before a definitive diagnosis of esophageal obstruction is made. In most cases some degree of mucosal laceration acts as an anchoring site. Spasm of esophageal muscle may also prevent movement of the bone.

As the bone is approached, an accumulation of foam, saliva, and bits of food is usually seen just proximal to the foreign body. The area should be suctioned and lavaged through the endoscope to obtain as clear a view as possible of the foreign body and the points of lodgment. If chunks of food are present, lavage and suction may need to be performed through an overtube. Air insufflation can be attempted in an effort to distend the walls of the esophagus away from the bone, but impingement of sharp edges into the mucosa often prevents this from being a useful maneuver. If possible without causing further damage to the mucosa or a perforation, the endoscope should be eased around the foreign body so that the esophagus distal to the obstruction can be examined. Occasionally a mild stricture or diverticulum is identified and can be implicated as an underlying cause of the foreign body obstruction. The endoscope or a bougie can be used to dilate a stricture. Excess air should be suctioned from the stomach before the endoscope is retracted to the foreign body site.

The bone must be dislodged from the site of impingement before it can be retrieved. With the endoscope tip positioned proximal to the bone, a sturdy pronged grasping instrument is passed through the scope and advanced to the bone. A firm grasp is applied to an available prominence, and an attempt is made to retract the bone toward the endoscope tip. A grooved area around a prominence is an ideal place to grasp because it may be easier to effectively anchor the prongs. The esophageal wall must not be included in the grip of the prongs. If the bone does not move in response to this initial effort (as is often the case), several procedures can be attempted. As stated previously, the endoscope tip should not be used to forcefully push against the foreign body, or the scope may be damaged. An overtube can be used, however, to apply caudally directed force under direct visualization. Any force should be carefully applied. The goal at this juncture is to first disengage the bone from the esophageal wall so that it can be freely moved. Caudal force followed by grasping and pulling in short interchangeable motions may help free the foreign body. If a rigid esophagoscope is used, a rigid grasping instrument can be passed through it to the bone. Once a firm purchase is obtained, an attempt is made to twist the bone back and forth in short motions to disengage it from the wall. Standard flexible grasping forceps cannot be used effectively in this manner. Rigid grasping forceps can also be passed alongside a flexible endoscope.

Another method that I have used successfully is to pass one or more pilling bougies (see Chapter 4) alongside the endoscope shaft to a point just beyond the distal bone tip. The base of the bougie section is then drawn back and hooked against the bone so that it is possible to apply more retraction force than can be generated with the foreign body graspers alone. A narrow bougie can sometimes be used to pry an impacted bone away from the mucosa by sliding the tip gently between the bone and the esophageal perforation. If it is apparent that a sharp lower end of a bone is deeply wedged into the mucosa, caudally directed force should not be applied. Doing so may cause a wall. If esophageal spasm is considered a significant problem, glucagon may be administered intravenously (0.05 mg/kg [0.11 mg/lb], not to exceed a total dose of 1 mg) to promote relaxation. Once freed, the bone and endoscope are retracted simultaneously, with the bone preferably pulled snugly against an overtube. The overtube helps maintain dilation of the upper esophageal sphincter, thereby improving the likelihood of pulling the bone through the sphincter area without having it dislodge from the grasper. If the bone

does dislodge at the sphincter area, forceps can be used to regrasp and retrieve it the final distance.

If a foreign body cannot be retrieved in a retrograde manner, an attempt should be made to advance it to the stomach. Bones are usually decalcified by gastric juices, and the remaining fragments pass through the intestinal tract without incident. If a bone is firmly wedged in the distal esophagus at the time of presentation, it may be best to direct all efforts at advancing it to the stomach rather than risking any problems by pulling it retrograde.

The esophageal wall is invariably damaged from bone impaction and subsequent retrieval efforts. Most lacerations heal uneventfully, and when careful endoscopic technique is used, surgical intervention is rarely necessary. The mucosa should be carefully inspected once the bone is removed. The degree of damage is usually directly related to the time the foreign body was lodged and can be worsened by retrieval efforts. If significant erosive damage has occurred, the patient is treated for 5 to 7 days with a liquid sucralfate suspension for topical protective effect (1 g per 30 kg [66 lb] qid), a histamine$_2$ (H$_2$)-receptor blocker to decrease the acidity of any gastric contents that may be refluxed to the esophagus (e.g., famotidine 0.5 mg/kg [0.23 mg/lb] intravenously twice daily or 0.5 to 1.1 mg/kg [0.23 to 0.5 mg/lb] taken orally twice daily), and an antibiotic such as amoxicillin or a cephalosporin. Sucralfate is available in suspension form, or alternatively it can be mixed into solution by dissolving a tablet in 15 to 30 ml of lukewarm water. H$_2$-receptor blockers do not decrease gastric acid levels enough to prevent digestion of a bone that may have been advanced from the esophagus to the stomach instead of being removed retrograde. If the patient has no evidence of infection (e.g., pyrexia, leukocytosis with left shift, mediastinitis, pneumonia), corticosteroids are used (e.g., prednisone 0.5 mg/kg [0.23 mg/lb] twice daily for 3 days and then tapered over the next 7 to 10 days) to decrease fibroblastic response and stricture formation. Although no proof exists that corticosteroids are absolutely effective in this regard, their antiinflammatory effect is still likely to be of some benefit to the patient. Pain relief may also be necessary in some cases, and its thoughtful use should not be overlooked (e.g., oxymorphone, morphine, transdermal fentanyl patch).

Water is generally offered 12 hours after bone removal, and soft food can be offered at 18 to 24 hours. If esophageal perforation is a possibility, thoracic radiographs should be obtained immediately and at 12 and 24 hours after bone removal and compared with preprocedure films. Pneumomediastinum, pneumothorax, or pleural fluid may be present if esophageal perforation has occurred. Most patients are discharged from the hospital 1 to 4 days after a foreign body has been removed.

If the esophageal mucosa has been severely damaged, periodic endoscopic surveillance during the first 1 to 3 weeks after a bone has been removed is recommended to evaluate the esophagus for stricture formation (see Plate 8-2). Once-weekly examination is usually adequate. If damage has been particularly severe, the first examination should be done at 3 to 5 days. If a stricture occurs, it should be treated according to the guidelines presented in Chapter 4.

## Fishhook Esophageal Foreign Bodies

Veterinarians are occasionally presented with dogs or cats that have swallowed a fishhook. The diagnosis is generally straightforward because the client usually has either observed the hook being swallowed or has seen fishing line dangling from the animal's mouth. Because most animal owners recognize the gravity of the situation, they tug on the fishing line in an effort to pull the hook out. Unfortunately this usually embeds the hook into the esophageal or gastric mucosa.

Most patients are presented within several hours of ingestion of the hook. Signs of discomfort are usually minimal, and because the esophageal lumen is not significantly occluded in most cases, signs consistent with obstruction are rarely exhibited. Cervical and thoracic radiographs are obtained to identify the position of the hook, and general anesthesia is induced in preparation for esophagoscopy.

At first it may be difficult to visualize a hook that is embedded in the cranial esophagus because this section of the esophagus expands just caudal to the upper esophageal sphincter (Figure 8-10). A hook in this location can easily be bypassed by a standard forward-viewing endoscope as it is passed through the sphincter. This problem usually occurs only if the hook is not attached to any fishing line that can be followed from the oral cavity (someone has already erred in yanking the line free during a misguided attempt to retrieve the hook). With knowledge of the fishhook's location based on radiographs the endoscopist should perform a thorough full circumferential examination of the proximal esophagus if the hook is not seen on first view. A laryngoscope and curved forceps may be useful for dislodging the hook if it is difficult to maneuver a flexible endoscope into proper position in this area.

Fishhooks that are located beyond the most cranial aspect of the esophagus are easily found at esophagoscopy. Little or no debris is usually present around the site of impingement. The depth of esophageal wall penetration should be estimated, and if a treble hook is involved, the number of hooks that are embedded should be determined. If the depth of penetration is *shallow,* two-pronged graspers can be used to grab the curved portion just beyond the stem. The hook is then rotated outwardly by deflecting the tip of the endoscope. A technique that I

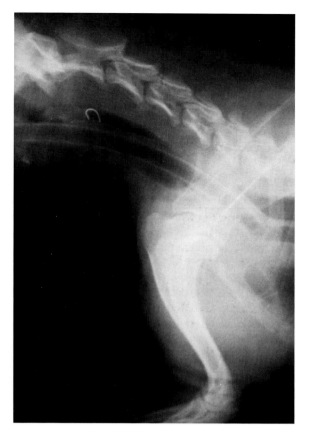

**Figure 8-10** Radiograph showing a small fishhook located just caudal to the upper esophageal sphincter. The hook was not visible with a forward-viewing endoscope until the tip of the scope was angled considerably to provide a view of the area just beyond the sphincter. The barb and most of the curved portion of the hook were embedded in the mucosa, leaving only the straight section in the lumen. Initially the hook was difficult to find. This radiograph was taken to reconfirm the location. Note air in the esophagus from previous endoscope insufflation. Once located, the hook was successfully removed.

have used successfully when a hook is embedded more deeply is to grasp the hook firmly, align it snugly against the tip of the endoscope or an overtube, and then forcefully thrust it in a *caudal* direction, thus wrenching the hook and barb away from the esophageal wall and into the lumen. This maneuver causes a usually insignificant small tear in the inner wall. Once the hook is free in the lumen, it can be easily pulled retrograde. Air is insufflated through the endoscope, and the upper esophageal sphincter is traversed with minimal difficulty in most cases. If there is concern about a hook becoming snagged in the esophagus or upper esophageal sphincter, an overtube should be used.

If a hook cannot be freed from the esophageal wall, a thoracotomy is necessary. This approach is usually necessary when hook and barb have penetrated the outer wall of the esophagus. The hook can be removed endoscopically after the surgeon cuts the end of the hook free from the esophageal wall. With this approach the surgeon does not have to incise the esophageal wall, thus minimizing chances of postoperative complications, particularly esophageal dehiscence.

## GASTRIC FOREIGN BODIES

Many types of gastric foreign bodies can be removed using endoscopic techniques. As stated previously, all retained foreign bodies should be removed, especially if they are large, long, sharp, or potentially toxic. If minimal or no significant clinical signs are manifest and a foreign object is small and nontoxic, an observation period of up to several weeks is reasonable to allow for possible spontaneous passage. Objects retained for longer than 2 weeks should be removed. If significant clinical signs (e.g., persistent vomiting, dehydration, inappetence) are present, a foreign body should be removed as soon as possible.

An *abdominal radiograph* should be obtained shortly before the induction of anesthesia to reconfirm the position of the foreign body. Foreign body location as identified on radiographs made 1 hour or more earlier may no longer be the same. If the foreign body has been in the stomach for only a short time, it may have even exited the stomach and traversed a portion of the intestinal tract by the time endoscopy is begun if a period of several hours has elapsed between radiographs and the induction of anesthesia for endoscopy (Figure 8-11). Failure to recognize that the foreign body has moved may result in undertaking the unnecessary risk of anesthesia. An inexperienced endoscopist may spend a considerable amount of time searching the stomach for an already departed foreign body while feeling concern that lack of experience is causing the difficulty in locating the foreign body when in fact the object has moved beyond the stomach. Even experienced generalists and specialists have made the mistake of not repeating radiographs shortly before the induction of anesthesia to reconfirm the location of the foreign object. Once this error is made, it is rarely repeated!

The key to successful retrieval of a gastric foreign body is to obtain as firm a grip as possible and to maintain the object in proper alignment for retrograde movement from the stomach through the lower esophageal sphincter to the esophagus, cranially along the esophagus, and through the upper esophageal sphincter. The stomach should be as empty of food as possible so that the foreign body can be easily located. The stomach should be thoroughly examined for the presence of any foreign material that may not have been identified on radiographs. Failure to examine the fundus and cardia carefully using the retroflexion maneuver (see Chapter 5)

**A**

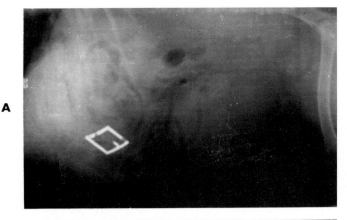

**B**

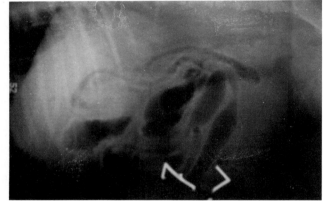

**Figure 8-11 A,** Radiograph showing a buckle in the pylorus of a cocker spaniel that ingested the end of a belt. Endoscopic examination of the stomach was begun 4 hours after this radiograph was obtained. Belt fragments were identified in the stomach and removed, but the buckle could not be found during a thorough examination of the stomach and duodenum. **B,** Radiograph made 5 hours after the previous radiograph, while the dog was still under anesthesia. The buckle had separated into two main sections, both of which were in the small intestine beyond the duodenum and the reach of the endoscope. Both buckle sections passed uneventfully through the remainder of the intestinal tract. Had this radiograph been made immediately before endoscopy, the procedure could have been avoided.

may result in a small foreign body wedged in this area being missed (Figure 8-12). If food or debris is present and difficulty is experienced in finding the foreign body, the patient should be rotated from the left lateral to dorsal recumbent position and then to the right lateral position, if necessary, to shift and separate the gastric contents. This may need to be repeated one or more times during the procedure if a particularly slippery foreign body is dropped back into the food or debris after it has been grasped. With the patient in the left lateral recumbent position, foreign bodies usually migrate to the fundus or body, which is in a dependent position. Objects with irregular surfaces that are wedged in the antrum usually remain there despite positioning changes.

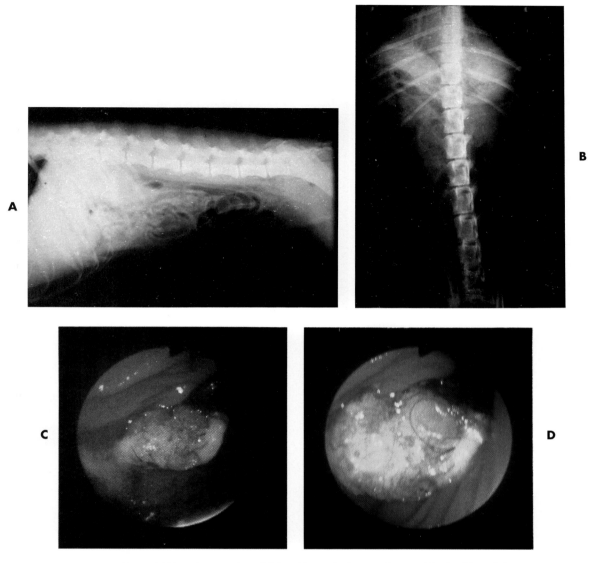

**Figure 8-12** Lateral (**A**) and ventrodorsal (**B**) radiographs from a 6-year-old mixed-breed dog with a 6-week history of intermittent vomiting. No radiographic abnormalities are seen. The complete blood count, biochemical profile, and urinalysis were normal. **C,** Endoscopic view of the fundus and cardia with the tip of the scope in retroflexion. A plastic foreign body with an irregular surface was found superficially impaled in the mucosa. The foreign body could not be seen with a standard forward view from the gastroesophageal junction, and the body and antrum were normal. Failure to perform a retroflexion maneuver would have resulted in an incorrect diagnosis. The endoscope shaft is faintly visible at the 1 o'clock position. **D,** Close-up view of the foreign body. It was pried away from the mucosa with a two-pronged grasper and then retrieved.

Once a foreign body is firmly grasped, it is pulled to the endoscope tip. The scope and foreign body are then retracted as a unit (Figure 8-13). Having an assistant present to control the grasping instrument, retraction of the endoscope shaft, or both while the endoscopist controls tip deflection may be helpful. However, once proper experience is gained, the endoscopist can often easily perform the entire procedure alone. An endoscopist working alone can maintain the foreign body in position against the endoscope tip by bending the pliable stem of the grasping instrument at the point where it exits the working channel port while using the thumb on the handle to hold the prongs in a closed position around the foreign body (Figure 8-14). The left hand is then used to withdraw the endoscope shaft.

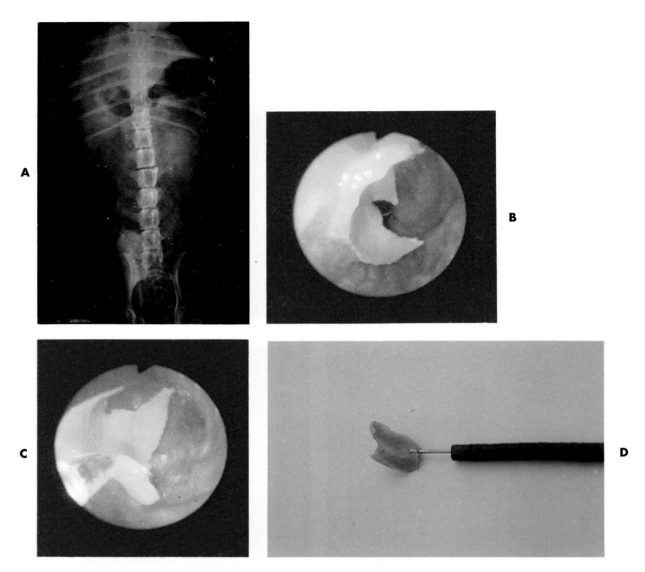

**Figure 8-13 A,** Ventrodorsal radiograph showing a radiodense object in the antral region of the stomach in a 10-year-old terrier with a 3-week history of intermittent vomiting that was only partially responsive to metoclopramide therapy. **B,** Retroflexion view of the gastric body. A small section of the endoscope shaft is visible in the center of the field, beyond the foreign object. When the dog was placed in the left lateral recumbent position, the foreign body migrated to a dependent area of the gastric body. **C,** Forward view of the foreign object in the gastric body. The object has been grasped with a two-pronged instrument. Note that the sharp ends will be trailing as the object is pulled into the esophagus. **D,** Grasping technique used during the procedure. The object was a piece of plastic from a large toy.

The greatest difficulties encountered in removing a gastric foreign body involve successfully pulling it through the gastroesophageal junction without dropping it back into the stomach and traversing the upper esophageal sphincter. When the foreign body is initially approached in the stomach, its size and configuration should be carefully studied to determine the best way to grasp it for both the strongest grip (look for grooves or prominences on which an anchored grip can be obtained) and easiest direction for removal. For example, although a long bone can be easily grasped horizontally along its shaft, it could not be pulled in a horizontal position through the lower or upper esophageal sphincter if it is longer than the width of these areas. It would be best to grasp such a foreign body at the blunter end, with the sharper end trailing, so that the bone (or other object)

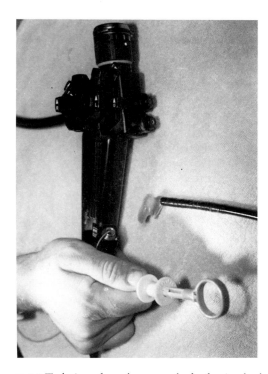

**Figure 8-14** Technique for solo removal of a foreign body. The right hand holds the endoscope at the lower end of the control housing while maintaining the shaft of the grasping instrument in position. This keeps the grasped object in position against the endoscope tip. The thumb maintains the prongs in a closed position with upward pressure on the handle of the grasping instrument.

can be removed in a longitudinal position. Objects that are flat (e.g., coins) or that have irregular surfaces or narrow projections can usually be grasped without difficulty. In contrast, considerable skill and patience may be required to achieve a firm grip on objects that are smooth or slippery either because of their physical makeup or because of an accumulation of gastric or duodenal fluid on their surface. Time allotted for careful maneuvering to apply a firm grip of an object at a favorable position or angle for successful retrieval is well spent.

If difficulty is experienced in retracting a foreign body through the lower esophageal sphincter, the endoscope tip should be deflected approximately 30 to 40 degrees (the normal angle between esophagus and stomach) as the foreign body is pulled toward the cardia and locked in this position. This often facilitates the maneuvering of a large or irregular object through the curve at the gastroesophageal junction. Failure to do this when attempting to pull a large foreign body through the junction may result in the object being dropped during a number of attempts before it ever reaches the esophagus. Problems involving traversing the upper esophageal sphincter are dealt with according to guidelines presented in the section on esophageal foreign bodies.

An overtube can also be used to maintain dilation of the lower esophageal sphincter so that the foreign body may slip through more easily as it is held snugly against the overtube during the retraction of the endoscope, overtube, and foreign body as a unit. If multiple small pieces of foreign material (e.g., fragmented chunks of Tupperware, plant material) need to be removed, procedure time can be shortened by inserting an overtube into the stomach and removing the objects through this tube with the endoscope. The endoscope can be returned quickly to the stomach each time it is removed. Furthermore, esophageal mucosa and sphincters undergo less when this method is used.

Hairballs (trichobezoars) can sometimes be removed endoscopically with a foreign body forceps or snare, especially if the hairball has a tubular shape and can be easily grasped at either end for retrieval in one section (see Plate 5-94). Large trichobezoars that fill much of the stomach cannot be removed with endoscopic methods because they are usually oblong and quite hard, and the entwined hair prevents fragmentation of the mass into smaller sections that are more suitable for removal. These large trichobezoars should be removed surgically. A case involving an esophageal hairball in a cat is presented in Plate 8-8.

Once a foreign body has been successfully retrieved, the entire stomach and proximal duodenum must be thoroughly inspected for any remaining foreign material before the procedure can be considered complete. Even when radiographs suggest that only one foreign body is present, there may be more. This may involve either radiolucent material or several pieces of radiodense objects that may have been stacked when the radiographs were made, giving the appearance of a single isolated object. Stacked objects can potentially separate at any time before endoscopy and scatter to different sites in the stomach (see Plate 8-14).

It is not commonly necessary to administer gastric mucosal protectant agents (e.g., sucralfate) or $H_2$-receptor blockers to animals that have had a retained gastric foreign body. The stomach mucosa usually heals quickly, and clinical signs directly related to the foreign body generally abate as soon as the object has been removed. Food and water can usually be resumed within 8 to 12 hours after the procedure is completed.

## DUODENAL FOREIGN BODIES

Duodenal foreign bodies are more difficult to remove than are gastric foreign bodies because foreign bodies retained in this area often become wedged and there is limited space for maneuvering. In addition, an overtube usually cannot be used in the small intestine because of difficulty encountered in advancing the tube around the angulus and through the pylorus. If a foreign body is found, an attempt is made to grasp it. If the object slides freely with minimal resistance, it is retracted to the stomach and repositioned, if necessary, for retrieval through the esophagus. Glucagon (0.05 mg/kg [0.23 mg/lb] not to exceed a total dose of 1 mg) can be administered intravenously to relax the pylorus and duodenum so that bothersome contractions are minimized. This may improve visualization and help decrease resistance in pulling the foreign body retrograde. String foreign bodies that are found in the small intestine may be grasped and *gently* tugged, but if resistance is encountered, further traction should not be applied or a perforation may occur farther down the intestinal tract. Surgical exploration is indicated.

## RECTAL FOREIGN BODIES

Retained rectal foreign bodies are an uncommon problem in dogs and cats. Foreign bodies that successfully traverse the upper gastrointestinal tract usually become encased in fecal material in the colon and are passed uneventfully through the anus. Occasionally an object with a sharp point, such as a needle, impacts the colonic mucosa and becomes wedged there or even passes completely through the colonic wall into the abdomen. Bone fragments may become impacted in the colonic mucosa and cause partial- or full-thickness lacerations. A thermometer may inadvertently be passed completely into the rectum or accidentally broken off inside during attempts to retrieve it. Occasionally an animal is the unfortunate victim of malicious intent in having a foreign object advanced through the anus to the rectum. Because of sphincter spasm, these objects may not be passed out spontaneously in due course.

If a rectal foreign body is suspected, a rectal examination may reveal its presence and also provide important information about rectal damage, hemorrhage, and pain. A survey radiographic assessment of the abdomen is necessary to determine the location of the object and to check for signs of perforation. If evidence of perforation is found, surgical intervention is required.

If no evidence supports the presence of perforation, colonoscopy should be performed under general anesthesia using either rigid or flexible endoscopic equipment. If the foreign body is in the transverse or ascending colon, a flexible endoscope must be used. Bones in the descending colon or rectum can most safely be removed through a rigid scope, which is used both for visualization and as an overtube, thus protecting the mucosa from damage as the bone fragments are retrieved. Foreign body graspers or polypectomy snares are the most versatile instruments for removing foreign bodies, but a clamp such as a sponge forceps may be required if the object is large and resistance is met in the distal rectum and anal sphincter area. After the foreign body has been removed, the entire rectum and colon should be inspected for lacerations.

## COMPLICATIONS OF ENDOSCOPIC FOREIGN BODY REMOVAL

Complications rarely occur with endoscopic retrieval of foreign bodies. Potential complications include perforation, hemorrhage, worsened impaction of a foreign body, and respiratory problems (pyothorax, pneumomediastinum, pneumothorax) related to an esophageal foreign body.

The veterinary literature contains few reports detailing the success and complication rates for endoscopically managed foreign body cases. In my most recent experience with 80 carefully reviewed foreign body ingestion cases, an overall successful removal rate of 86% was achieved with endoscopic management. No significant complications occurred in this series. More data need to be collected to predict the frequency of complications and the success rates. However, based on experience to date it is clear that endoscopy can be used safely and effectively in the management of the majority of foreign body ingestions in dogs and cats. Once proper skills are developed, endoscopy can be successfully used to extract foreign bodies in almost any type of practice setting.

### REFERENCES

Altman AR, Gottfried EB: Intragastric closure of an ingested open safety pin, *Gastrointest Endosc* 24:294, 1978.
Brady PG: Endoscopic removal of foreign bodies. In Silvis SE, editor: *Therapeutic gastrointestinal endoscopy,* New York, 1985, Igaku-Shoin.
Burk RL, Ackerman N: The abdomen. In Burk RL, Ackerman N, editors: *Small animal radiography and ultrasonography,* Philadelphia, 1996, WB Saunders.
Dunkerly RC et al: Fiberendoscopic removal of large foreign bodies from the stomach, *Gastrointest Endosc* 21:170, 1975.
Fossum TW et al: *Small animal surgery,* St Louis, 1997, Mosby.
Jackson C, Jackson CL: *Diseases of the air and food passages of foreign body origin,* Philadelphia, 1937, WB Saunders.
Rogers BHG et al: An overtube for the flexible fiberoptic esophagogastroduodenoscope gastroduodenoscope, *Gastrointest Endosc* 28:256, 1982.
Roudebush P, Jones BD, Voughan RW: Medical aspects of esophageal disease. In Jones BD, editor: *Canine and feline gastroenterology,* Philadelphia, 1986, WB Saunders.
Sanowski RA: Foreign body extraction in the gastrointestinal tract. In Sivak MV, editor: *Gastroenterologic endoscopy,* Philadelphia, 1987, WB Saunders.
Tams TR: Diseases of the esophagus. In Tams TR, editor, *Handbook of small animal gastroenterology.* Philadelphia, 1996, WB Saunders.
Vizcarrondo FJ, Brady PG, Nord HJ: Foreign bodies of the upper gastrointestinal tract, *Gastrointest Endosc* 29:208, 1983.
Webb WA, McDaniel L, Jones L: Foreign bodies of the upper gastrointestinal tract: current management, *South Med J,* 77:1083, 1984.
Zawie DA: Medical diseases of the esophagus, *Compend Contin Ed Pract Vet* 9:1146, 1987.

# ESOPHAGEAL FOREIGN BODIES

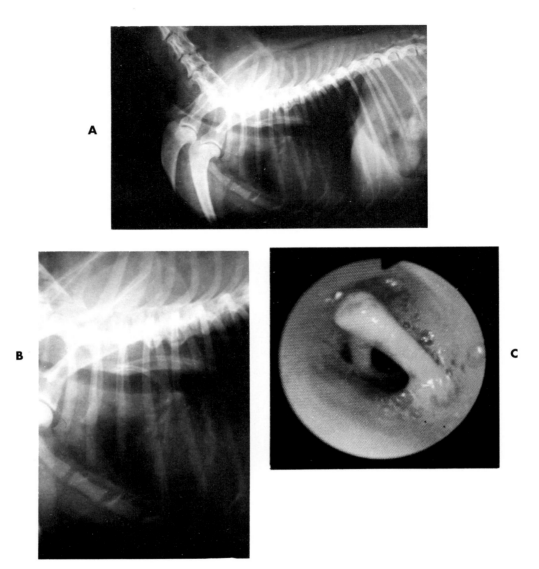

**Plate 8-1** Bone foreign body (wishbone) in the esophagus of a 3-year-old male Pomeranian. The bone had been swallowed 2 days previously. Clinical signs included periodic gagging and regurgitation of food shortly after eating. The dog was bright, alert, and responsive when admitted to the hospital as a referral for endoscopy. **A,** Lateral thoracic radiograph showing a wishbone lodged over the base of the heart with the furcular rami directed caudally. No radiographic signs of esophageal perforation are present. **B,** Close-up view highlighting the position of the bone. **C,** Clearly visualized bone on first approach with the endoscope. The furcular process is at the 11 o'clock position. The shorter furcular ramus is embedded sufficiently in the esophageal mucosa (4 o'clock position) to prevent further passage of the bone toward the stomach. The exact site of impingement is obscured by foam. A small area of mucosal damage is seen at the 12 o'clock position.

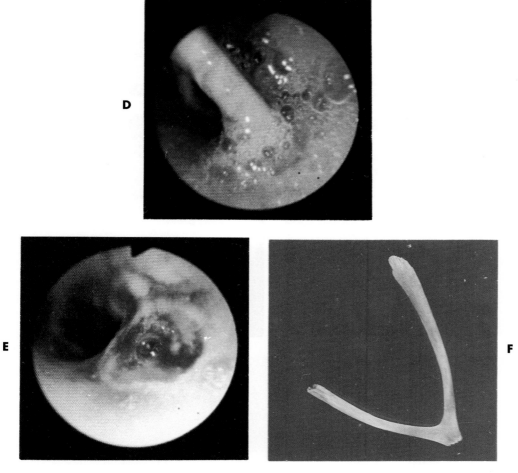

**Plate 8-1—cont'd** D, Close-up view at the site of impingement. The bone was easily retrieved by grasping the junction area of the furcular process and ramus with a two-pronged instrument. No resistance was encountered when the bone was pulled cranially to a position against the endoscope tip, and no impedance was met at the upper esophageal sphincter. **E,** Site of focal mucosal damage in the esophagus where the bone was embedded. A lesion of this degree would be expected to heal uneventfully. The dog was treated with cimetidine and a liquid preparation of sucralfate for 4 days after the procedure. The animal had no abnormal clinical signs after the bone was removed. **F,** Wishbone foreign body. The shorter ramus with the sharp tip was embedded in the mucosa.

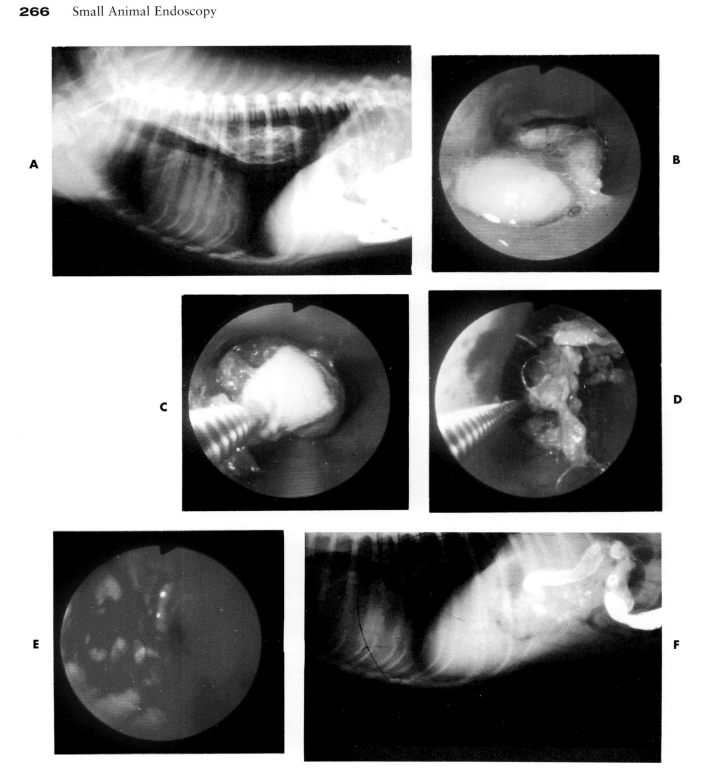

**G** 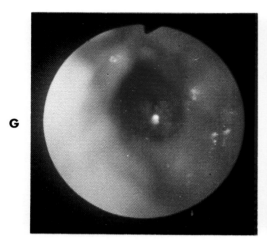 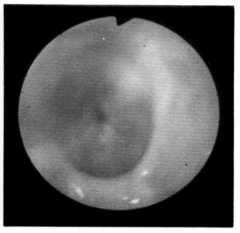 **H**

**Plate 8-2** Esophageal bone foreign body in a 2-year-old West Highland terrier. The dog was found on the kitchen table swallowing a chicken bone wrapped in paper towel. The dog was presented on a referral basis for endoscopy on the eighth day after ingestion when serial radiographs at the referring hospital showed that the bone had remained lodged in the esophagus. The complete blood count showed leukocytosis (23,000 cells/mm$^3$) with a left shift (2500 band cells). The dog was not febrile. **A,** Lateral thoracic radiograph showing dilation of the lower esophagus with increased density in the lumen. Barium was administered to highlight the features of the foreign body. The radiograph showed no evidence of esophageal perforation. **B,** Endoscopic view in the esophagus as the foreign body was approached. The light-colored material is paper towel. A putrid odor emanated from the esophageal lumen, and the mucosa was quite friable. Note the hemorrhage (upper aspect of the field) that occurred after gentle mucosal contact by the endoscope. **C,** Section of paper towel being removed with foreign body graspers (two-prong instrument). The initial part of the procedure involved removing the moistened paper towel in chunks so that the areas of bone impingement could be more carefully assessed and as firm a grip as possible could be applied to the bone with the graspers. The endoscope was removed each time a section of paper was freed. The bone can be seen under the paper. **D,** Appearance of the bone once it was uncovered. Note the surrounding mucosal erythema. The shaft of the grasping instrument is in view, extending to the distal point of impingement. Despite the presence of numerous potential grasping sites at the proximal end of the bone (note irregular prominences that are ideal for grasping), the bone could not be moved to any degree when traction was applied at the proximal end. In addition, small fragments were easily broken from the bone when it was firmly grasped, making it extremely difficult to maintain an effective grip. The distal end of the bone was gripped, and alternate cranial and caudal forces were applied in an effort to dislodge the bone. When these efforts failed, a rigid plastic overtube was used to push the bone into the stomach. Once dislodged by the overtube, the bone was easily advanced through the gastroesophageal junction. The bone was left in the stomach for digestion. **E,** Appearance of the esophagus immediately after the bone was dislodged and advanced to the stomach. Note the full circumferential erosive damage and hemorrhage. The gastroesophageal junction is closed (slightly to the right of center). A postprocedure radiograph showed no evidence of esophageal perforation. **F,** A 48-hour postprocedure radiograph showing no increased density in the area of the distal esophagus. A small amount of food is present in the stomach, but no bone is seen. Postprocedure treatment included cimetidine, metoclopramide (to reduce the potential for gastroesophageal reflux), and amoxicillin. Sucralfate was not available when this case was managed, but its use in this clinical situation would currently be recommended. Soft food was initially offered 24 hours after the procedure. **G,** Follow-up esophagoscopy to evaluate for stricture formation 8 days after the foreign body was removed. Full circumferential narrowing of the lumen has occurred at the foreign body site. A 9-mm endoscope was easily passed through without contacting the walls. The gastroesophageal junction is closed (slightly above and to the right of center). The dog was completely asymptomatic. Prednisone therapy (1.1 mg/kg/day [0.5 mg/lb/day] for 10 days and then gradually decreased) was initiated to decrease the potential for further stricture formation. In retrospect, prednisone could have been started sooner. **H,** Follow-up esophagoscopy at 41 days after foreign body removal. The foreign body site is well healed, and clinically insignificant mild narrowing (ring formation) is present in the distal esophagus. The gastroesophageal junction is closed. Prednisone use was discontinued after a total of 5 weeks.

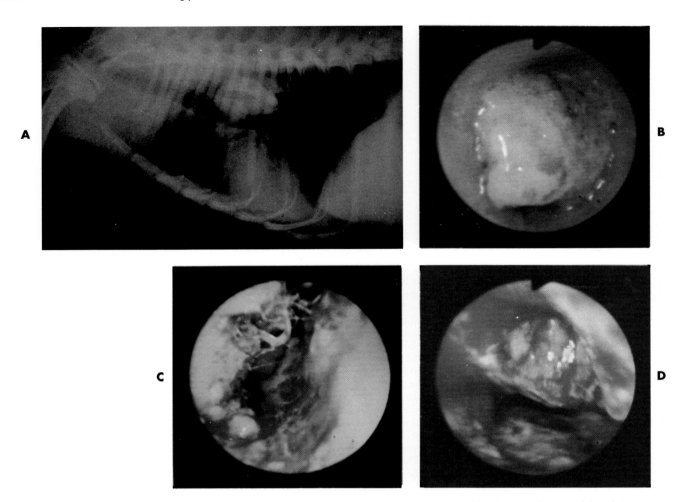

**Plate 8-3** Esophageal pork bone foreign body in a 4-year-old 6-kg (13.2-lb) mixed-breed dog (6 kg). The owner had given the bone to the dog as a treat; 1 hour later the animal began having frequent gagging episodes. Radiographs were not made at the referring hospital until 3 days (second presentation of the patient) after bone ingestion. The radiographs showed a bone density in the esophagus, and the dog was referred for endoscopy. Clinical signs included intermittent gagging, salivation, nausea, and regurgitation shortly after eating. The appetite remained normal. **A,** Lateral thoracic radiograph showing a large irregular bone lodged in the esophagus at the heart base. **B,** First endoscopic view of the bone. Saliva and foam were accumulated around the bone, making it difficult to sustain a firm grip. The bone was tightly wedged. **C,** Erosions and hemorrhage of the esophageal wall, which began once the bone was pried away with pilling bougies. The endoscope tip has been passed beyond the proximal aspect of the bone. When all efforts to dislodge the bone failed (both pulling and pushing forces at the proximal end), two large pilling bougies (32 and 36 FR) were *gently* passed singly around the bone. This helped pry one end of the bone away from the esophageal wall. The bases of both bougies were then retracted against the distal border of the bone to apply cranially directed force. Simultaneously traction was applied at the cranial end using a two-pronged grasper passed through the endoscope. (Alternatively a snare could have been used.) This dislodged the bone, and it was retrieved through the mouth using the grasping instrument. **D,** Site of lodgment immediately after the bone was removed. Note the grooved (lacerated) area in the uppermost aspect of the field. If a rigid instrument had been used to force the bone caudally, an edge of the bone could have been forced through the wall of the esophagus. The animal was treated with injectable cimetidine, ampicillin, and prednisone (0.8 mg/kg/day [0.35 mg/lb] initially), intravenous fluids, sucralfate suspension, and meperidine (the dog seemed to be in a great deal of pain after the procedure). Morphine or oxymorphone would be used if the case were managed today.

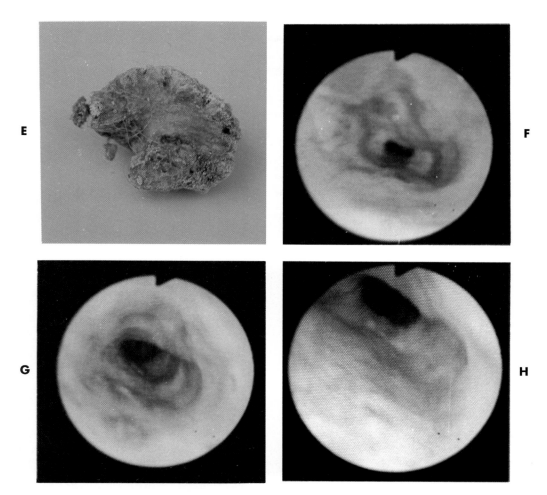

**Plate 8-3—cont'd E,** Retrieved pork bone. **F,** View on esophagoscopy at 3-day follow-up. The integrity of the esophageal walls has improved dramatically (i.e., the walls distended readily on air insufflation). **G,** At 7-day follow-up the dog was completely asymptomatic. The esophageal mucosa was healed. Mild erythema was still evident, but the esophagus was healing well with no evidence of stricture formation. All medications except prednisone were discontinued. **H,** At 14-day follow-up the dog was completely asymptomatic, and the esophageal mucosa was healed. Mild erythema was still evident, and small follicular changes were observed (sometimes seen in conjunction with healing esophageal lesions). The prednisone was gradually tapered. Recovery was uneventful.

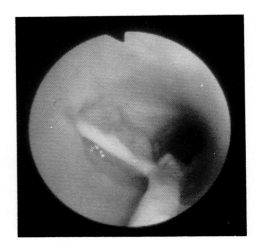

**Plate 8-4** Endoscopic view of a small chicken rib bone lodged in the esophagus of a 1-year-old poodle. The bone had been present in the esophagus for 30 days before endoscopy. Clinical signs included gagging and intermittent salivation. Despite the owner's belief that the dog had ingested a bone, it was treated after an initial examination for a collapsing trachea. No improvement occurred, and survey radiographs were made several weeks later. The radiographs failed to clearly show an esophageal foreign body, probably because of the thin nature of the bone. Contrast studies were not performed. A change in antibiotics failed to effect improvement of the suspected respiratory condition, and when the owner still insisted that a bone was "lodged in the dog's throat," the animal was referred for endoscopy. The owner's diagnosis was correct, and the bone, which was located at the thoracic inlet, was successfully retrieved at endoscopy. (Courtesy Dennis A. Zawie.)

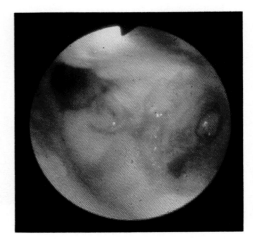

**Plate 8-5** Esophageal perforation (3 o'clock position) in a dog, caused by a bone foreign body. Note the mucosal damage surrounding the perforation site. The dog had pleural effusion caused by pyothorax and died before treatment could be instituted. As a point of clinical interest, the esophagus was examined endoscopically after the dog died. Esophagoscopy should not be attempted if there is an esophageal perforation, because of the strong potential for life-threatening complications. (Courtesy Dennis A. Zawie.)

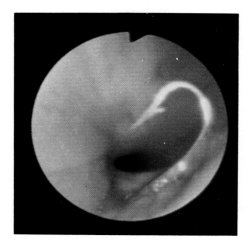

**Plate 8-6** Fishhook in the thoracic esophagus of a 3-year-old mixed-breed dog. The owner had attempted to retrieve the hook by pulling on the attached fishing line. Both the hook and the stem became embedded in the thoracic mucosa. When the hook could not be freed with two-pronged foreign body graspers, a uterine biopsy punch was advanced alongside the endoscope to grasp the stem of the hook. With distally directed movement the hook was forced away from the mucosa. It was difficult to position the rigid instrument in the exact spot necessary to grasp the hook without also grasping the mucosa in the cups of the biopsy instrument. Once dislodged, the hook was retrieved without difficulty.

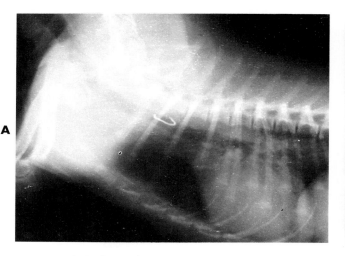

A

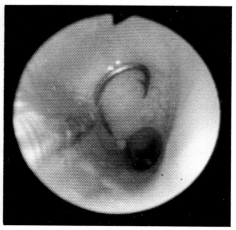

B

**Plate 8-7** A, Radiograph showing a fishhook in the thoracic esophagus of a dog. B, The hook was dislodged using a two-pronged grasping instrument. The hook was then turned around (maneuver shown in this photograph) and finally grasped at the curved base for retrieval. Removing a hook in this direction minimizes the chance of impaling the upper esophageal sphincter as the foreign body is pulled through.

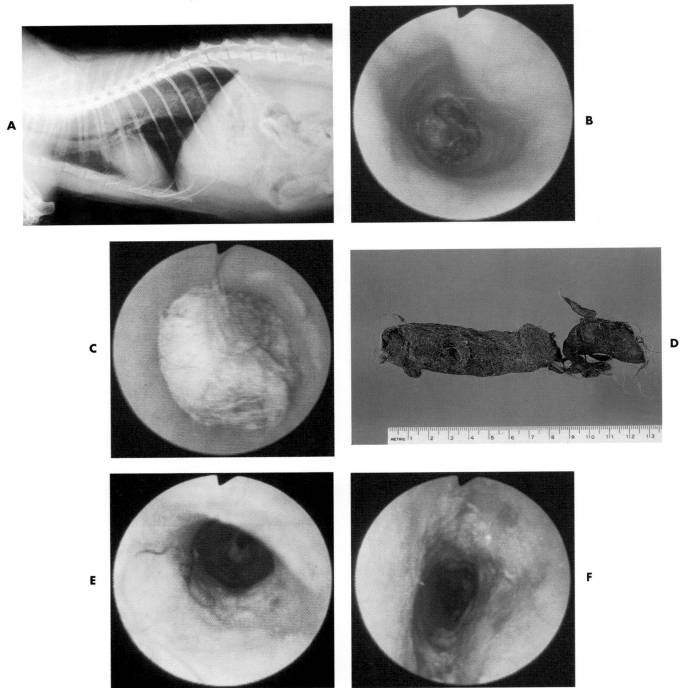

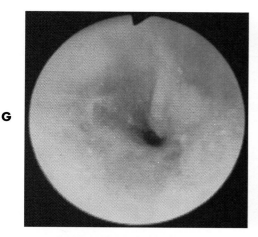 G
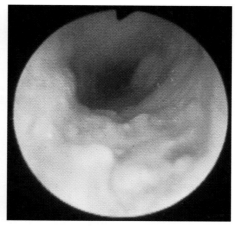 H

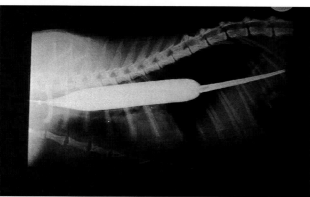 I

**Plate 8-8** Esophageal foreign body with subsequent development of esophagitis and later a severe esophageal stricture in a 6-year-old Maine coon cat. The history included an acute onset of respiratory distress and salivation. The cat was presented as an emergency patient. **A,** Lateral thoracic radiograph demonstrating a long area of increased opacity in the dorsocaudal thorax (later confirmed to be a hairball) and ventral deviation of the trachea. The cardiac silhouette was normal, and no evidence of pleural effusion was seen. Early on, cardiac disease (cardiomyopathy and heartworm disease), bronchial disease, and pleural effusion were excluded.
**B,** Esophagoscopy confirmed a diagnosis of esophageal foreign body (hairball). The cranial edge of the hairball can be seen from the cervical esophagus. **C,** Close-up view of the hairball, which was found to be so tightly wedged in the esophagus that it could not be advanced toward the stomach to any degree. As expected, attempts to pull the hairball cranially were futile. (Small fragments were pulled off as graspers were used to pull on the hairball.) Gastrotomy was performed to remove the hairball through the stomach. Forceps were advanced from the stomach into the esophagus to pull the hairball back into the gastric body. **D,** Retrieved hairball. Smaller fragments of the hairball were in the lower stomach (not pictured). **E,** Endoscopic appearance of the esophagus immediately after the hairball was removed. A full-circumference thin layer of hair adhered to the esophageal mucosa along much of the esophagus. Based on the rough texture of the hair and the likelihood that gastric acid and activated enzymes accompanied the hairball into the esophagus, it was considered very likely that esophagitis had developed. **F,** Patchy excoriated areas of esophageal mucosa observed after some of the hair residue was gently scraped and washed away from the esophageal walls (thoracic esophagus). **G,** Eroded and inflamed mucosa of the lower esophagus at the gastroesophageal junction. Immediate treatment for esophagitis included sucralfate suspension, famotidine, metoclopramide, and prednisone. The possibility that an esophageal stricture might develop over the following 7–14 days was a concern because vomiturition of a large hairball is a known risk factor for esophageal strictures in cats. Follow-up endoscopic examinations were planned to evaluate for this possibility. **H,** Esophagus at 5 days after surgery. The mucosa was quite irregular and friable. At 9 days the esophagus had narrowed, and at 12 days a stricture prevented the advancement of a 7.9-mm endoscope beyond the mid-thoracic esophagus. The cat had begun to regurgitate shortly after eating. Medical management for esophagitis had been continuously administered. Balloon dilation procedures were initiated to resolve the stricture. (See Chapter 4 for a complete description of management of esophageal strictures.) **I,** Fully distended 20-mm balloon dilator in the thoracic esophagus. Contrast material was added to sterile water to enhance visualization of the balloon (for photographic purposes). Multiple balloon procedures were required to resolve the stricture in this cat. This was one of the most difficult to manage esophageal strictures in my case series. Six years later the cat was doing extremely well and had no signs of an esophageal disorder.

## GASTRIC FOREIGN BODIES

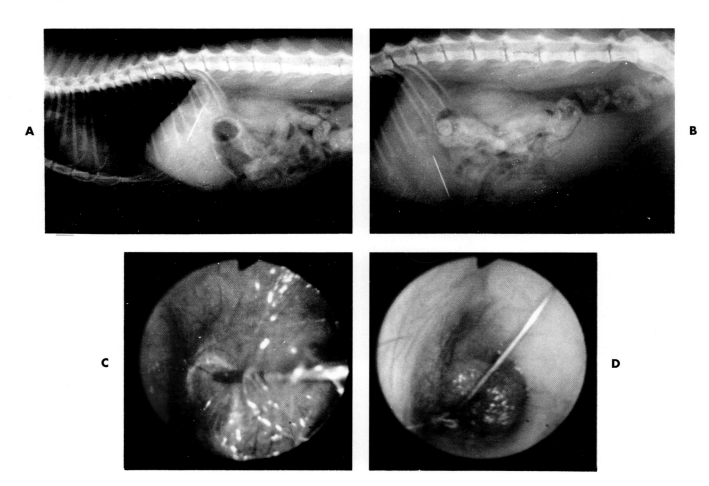

**Plate 8-9** Sewing needle foreign body in a 4-year-old cat. The owner saw the cat swallow the needle and approximately 8 inches of attached thread 30 minutes before presentation. **A,** Radiograph showing the needle surrounded by soft tissue dense material in the stomach. **B,** Radiograph obtained 4 hours later, immediately before anesthetic induction for endoscopy, to determine the current position of the needle. The needle is located in the antral region of the stomach. **C,** First endoscopic view in the antrum. A hairball fills much of the field, and the needle can be seen extending from the center of the field to the 3 o'clock position. **D,** The needle, thread (7 o'clock position), and remaining hair are visualized after much of the hair was removed as the initial step of the procedure. The pyloric orifice is obscured by the hair.

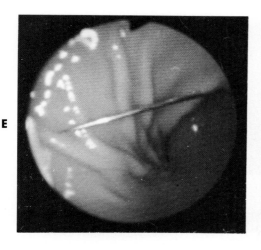

E

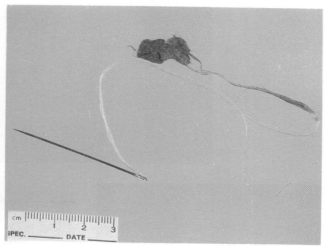

F

**Plate 8-9—cont'd E,** The needle has been repositioned in the distal gastric body (the angulus extends from the 2:30 position toward the center of the field). This was done so that the point of the needle could be enclosed completely within the teeth of the grasping instrument. This alleviates any opportunity for the needle point to impale the gastric or esophageal mucosa during retrieval. Once grasped, the needle and thread were removed within seconds. An overtube could have been used but was not considered necessary. **F,** Needle, thread, and an attached clump of hair.

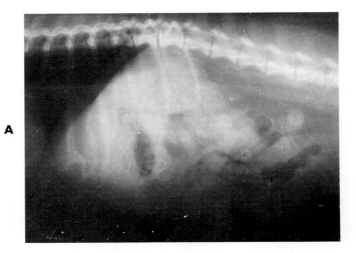

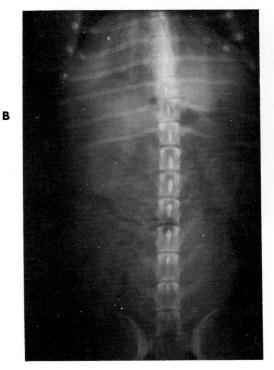

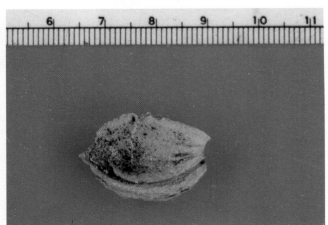

**Plate 8-10** Peach pit gastric foreign body in an 8-year-old dachshund with an 8-day history of complete anorexia and two known episodes of vomiting. The owner considered it likely that the dog had swallowed a peach pit. **A,** The lateral view suggested the possibility of a small foreign body in the antral-pyloric region. **B,** The ventrodorsal radiograph was unremarkable. Because the owner was convinced that a foreign body had been ingested, endoscopy was considered the most useful procedure. **C,** A peach pit was found in the stomach, unattached to the mucosa, and was removed by grasping it longitudinally. It would have been quite difficult to pull the object horizontally through the esophageal sphincters.

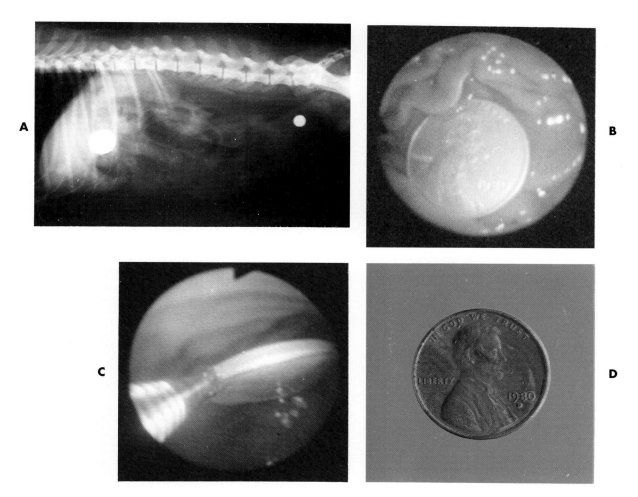

**Plate 8-11** Coin foreign body in the stomach of a 10-year-old poodle. At the time of referral for endoscopy the coin had been in the stomach for 2 weeks. Other than an occasional episode of vomiting, no gastrointestinal signs were present. **A,** Abdominal radiograph showing a single coin in the stomach. A small unidentified radiodense object is also present in the descending colon. **B,** A 1980 penny was found in the gastric body. **C,** The coin was freely movable and easily grasped with a two-pronged instrument. **D,** The retrieved coin.

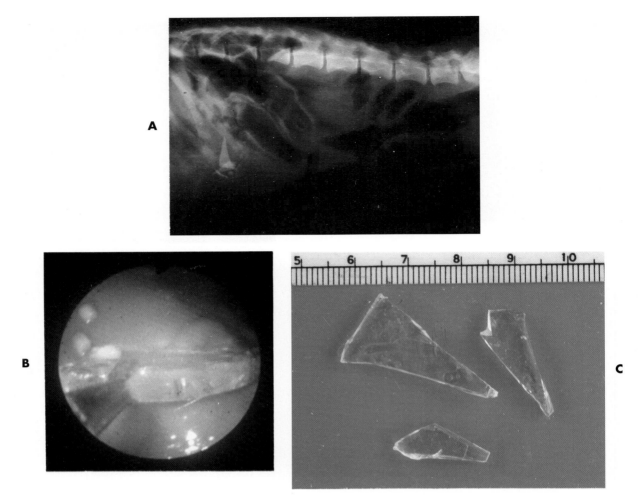

**Plate 8-12** Glass fragments in the stomach of a young German shepherd. The dog had under-gone surgery for an intussusception 36 hours previously. While exercising freely in the intensive care room, the dog jumped on a countertop, and in an effort to lick baby food from an open jar knocked it to the floor where it shattered. The dog then ingested both baby food and glass frag-ments from the floor. **A,** Abdominal radiograph showing glass fragments in the stomach. En-doscopy was performed shortly after the glass was ingested. **B,** The pieces of glass were each grasped and retrieved individually using a two-pronged grasper. During retrieval they were held closely against the tip of the endoscope, and the mucosa of the esophagus and esophageal sphincters was not damaged. An overtube could have been used to provide greater mucosal pro-tection but was considered unnecessary. **C,** Retrieved glass fragments.

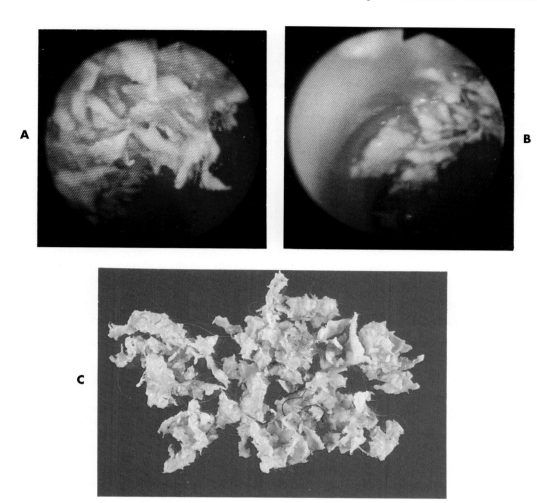

**Plate 8-13** Multiple Tupperware fragments in the antrum of a 7-year-old Labrador retriever with persistent vomiting for 4 days. **A,** Multiple Tupperware fragments wedged together in the antrum. The pyloric orifice is obscured by the foreign objects. Several of the fragments were impaled in the antral mucosa, thus preventing most of the conjoined material to move elsewhere in the stomach. Fragments were removed individually using a two-pronged grasper. **B,** Endoscopic view of the antrum after much of the foreign material was removed. The pyloric orifice is at the lower end of the field (6 o'clock position). **C,** Multiple retrieved Tupperware fragments. It is highly unlikely that this material would have passed spontaneously out of the stomach. No further vomiting occurred after the endoscopic procedure was completed.

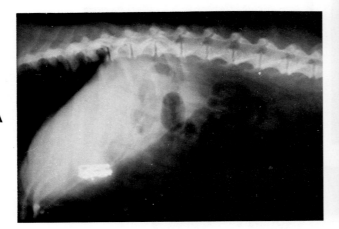

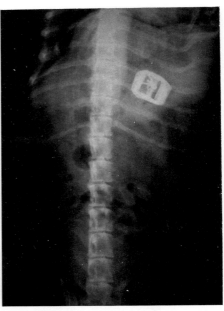

**Plate 8-14** Three buckle foreign bodies in the stomach that appeared radiographically to be a single foreign body. The patient was a 5-year-old basset hound with a single episode of vomiting and no known recent history of foreign body ingestion. A buckle foreign body was seen on radiographs. The owner elected not to pursue treatment unless significant clinical signs developed. **A** and **B,** Lateral and ventrodorsal abdominal radiographs made *3 months* later when the dog was referred for endoscopy. A buckle-shaped object is best appreciated on the ventrodorsal view. The dog had not vomited in 3 months and had a normal appetite. The owner had finally decided to have the foreign body removed on the recommendation of the referring veterinarian. **C,** First endoscopic view of the stomach at the start of the procedure. A buckle is clearly in view. The buckle was retrieved longitudinally with a two-pronged grasper without resistance. **D,** Endoscopic view during immediate subsequent examination of the stomach. A portion of a second buckle is seen in the upper left aspect of the field. This photograph represents a retroflexion view of the fundus and cardia. The endoscope shaft can be seen faintly at the 1 o'clock position. A third buckle was subsequently found and retrieved. **E,** The three retrieved buckles as they appeared after being in the stomach for at least 3 months. Apparently the buckles were stacked at the time radiographs were obtained but separated between the time of radiography and endoscopy. *After a foreign body is removed, the esophagus and stomach must always be carefully inspected before the procedure can be considered completed.* Failure to do so in this case would have resulted in two buckles being left in the stomach.

C

D

E

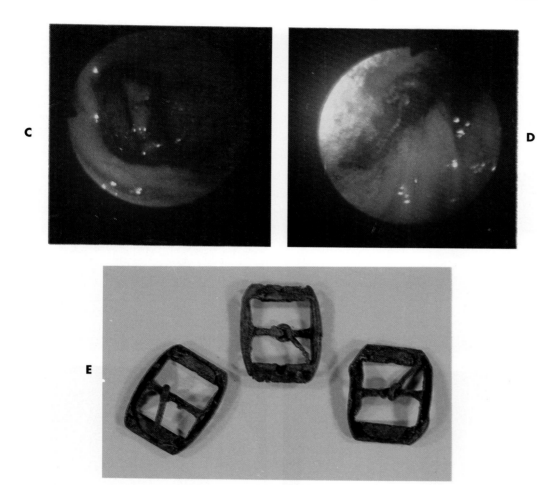

**Plate 8-14—cont'd** For legend see opposite page.

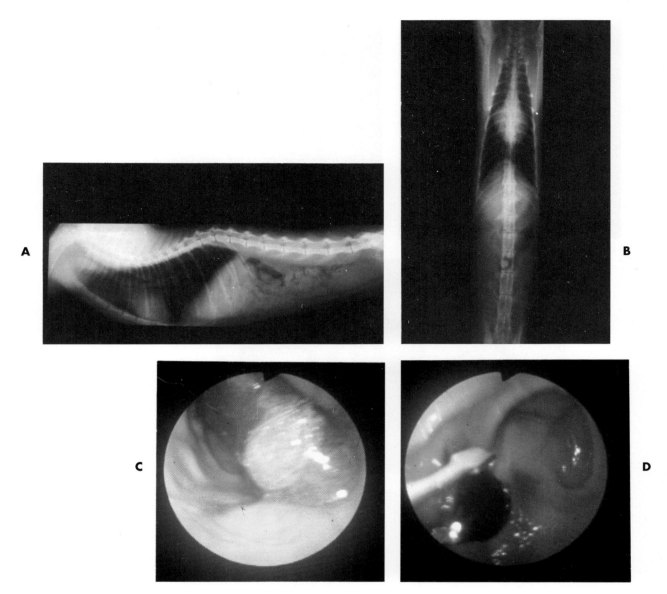

**Plate 8-15** Rigid leather patch in the stomach of a 1-year-old cat with a 6-week history of vomiting. Interestingly, the vomiting always occurred between 5:00 and 7:00 AM and was limited to one to two episodes per day. Multiple treatments had been tried empirically without benefit. The cat was referred for a diagnostic workup. **A** and **B**, Lateral and ventrodorsal abdominal radiographs. On close inspection a square foreign body was identified. On the ventrodorsal view much of the foreign body overlies the junctional area of the first and second lumbar vertebrae so that only a corner of the foreign body is visualized to the right of the second lumbar vertebra. **C**, Foreign body as it appeared on initial approach. It was wedged between the distal body and the antrum at the angulus. **D**, The object was grasped at two corners using a two-pronged instrument. In this view the stomach is distended, and the angulus is at the 1 to 3 o'clock position. Once the foreign body was grasped, it was apparent that it might be difficult to pull such a nonpliable object through the esophageal sphincters.

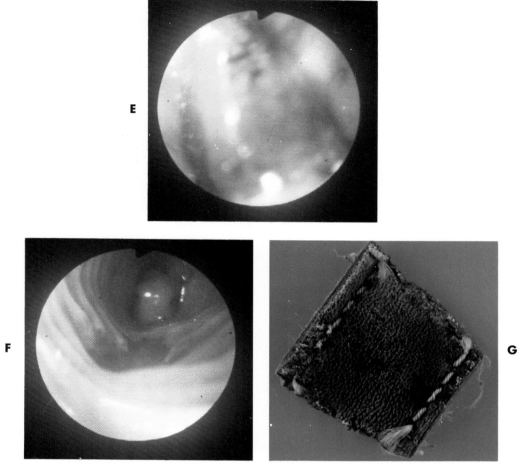

**Plate 8-15—cont'd** E, Typical blurred view of a foreign body as it is held in position against the endoscope tip during retrieval. The object was pulled smoothly from the stomach into the esophagus by maintaining the endoscope tip at a 30-degree angle (the natural gastroesophageal angle). However, a sharp corner of the object impaled the wall of the distal esophagus and caused the object to become wedged. The object was pushed caudally and gently rotated using the endoscopic graspers. Once freed, the object was gradually retracted against minimal resistance through the remaining esophagus and upper esophageal sphincter. F, Site of foreign body impingement in the esophageal wall (torn reddened area in center of field). A small area of stomach is seen protruding into the lower esophagus (upper aspect of the field). The use of an overtube would have provided more mucosal protection by dilating the esophagus to a greater degree than was possible with the endoscope alone. The esophageal laceration was expected to heal uneventfully. Cimetidine and sucralfate were administered for 5 days. The animal had no abnormal clinical signs after the procedure. G, The foreign object was a rigid piece of leather, an unusual type of foreign body to be swallowed by a cat!

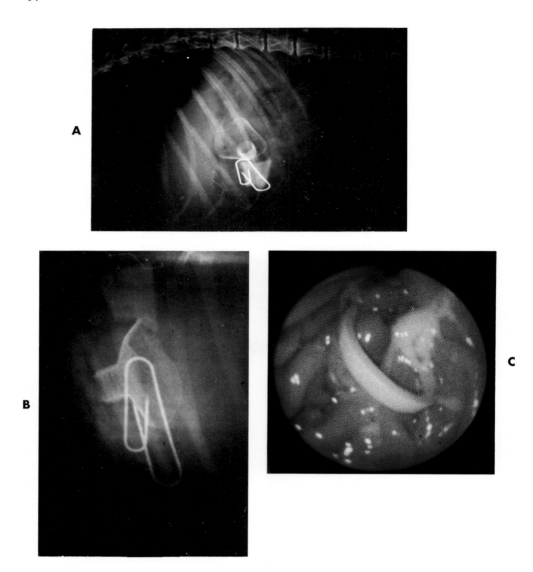

**Plate 8-16** Multiple foreign bodies in the stomach of a 14-year-old poodle cross (8 kg [17.5 lb]) with a 6-day history of intermittent vomiting. When different types of objects are identified on radiographs, the possibility that the objects may be grouped together in some way as a conglomeration should be considered. When foreign bodies are composed of both radiodense and radiolucent materials, the total size of the foreign material may be underestimated. **A,** Survey abdominal radiograph showing four different types of radiodense foreign objects in the stomach. A paper clip can be readily identified, and the faintly visible object cranial to it is most likely a piece of wire. The paper clip and wire could potentially traverse the gastrointestinal tract, but it is unlikely that the other two objects, based on their shape, could pass through the pylorus of an 8-kg (17.5-lb) dog. Endoscopic retrieval was planned. **B,** Close-up a radiograph made just before endoscopy. The paper clip is clearly visualized, and the other object appears to be (but in fact was not) the base of a broken light bulb. The trapezoid-shaped object and wire are dorsal. **C,** First endoscopic view in the gastric body. The tip of the paper clip is to the left of center (9 o'clock position). A rubber band is in the foreground, with other unidentifiable material beyond it. The paper clip, rubber band, a group of small twigs, and a small amount of string were all hooked together and retrieved as a single group (see F).

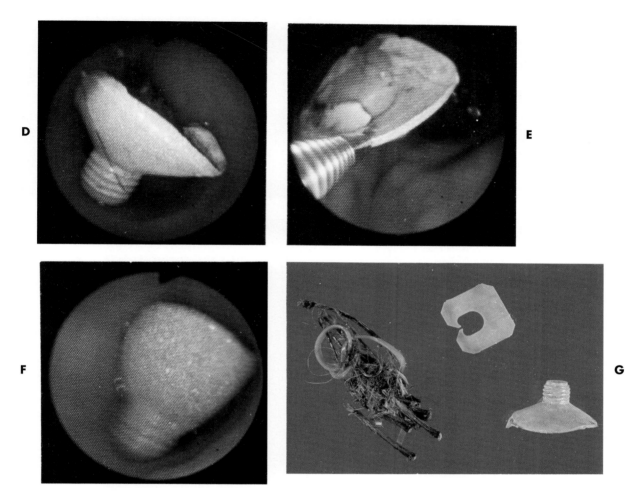

**Plate 8-16—cont'd D,** The object with the screw top as it appeared when wedged in the antrum. Attempts to grasp the threaded area were unsuccessful. (The object was too slippery to maintain a grip.) **E,** Once the rim of the object was grasped, it was pulled away from the antrum into the gastric body. **F,** Appearance of the object wedged just caudal to the *upper* esophageal sphincter. It was difficult to pull the foreign body through the sphincter using the two-pronged graspers. Sponge forceps were used to retrieve it the final distance. **G,** The irregular object was actually the rim of a Nutrical tube. Much of the retrieved material shown here was not radiographically visible (including the wrapper clip). The wire and trapezoid-shaped radiodense object are not shown.

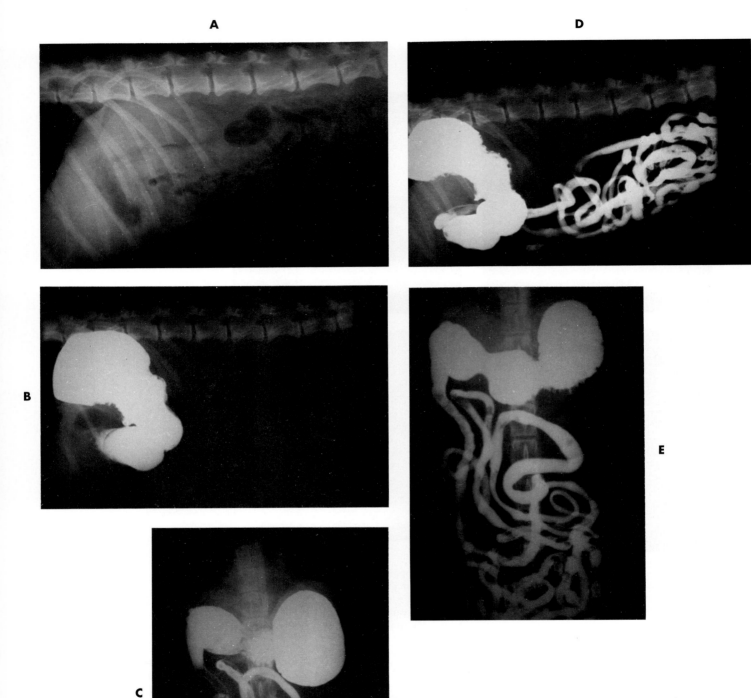

**Plate 8-17** Large (3.7-cm diameter) rounded plastic foreign body in the stomach of a 12-year-old Great Dane/German shepherd dog cross. **A,** Lateral (shown here) and ventrodorsal survey abdominal radiographs were unremarkable. Because the owner strongly suspected that the dog had ingested the plastic object, a barium series was performed next. A negative-contrast gastrogram is more useful for identifying a radiolucent object in the stomach (barium tends to mask a foreign body), but an intestinal study was desired as well; hence the use of barium. **B** and **C,** Start of the barium series. **D** and **E,** Radiographs obtained at 15 minutes. Note the circular configuration in the pyloric antral area and the beaklike projection just above it in the lateral view.

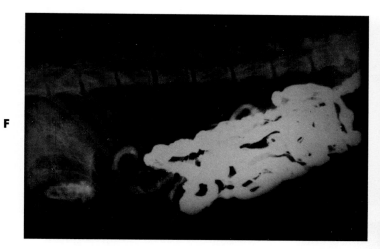

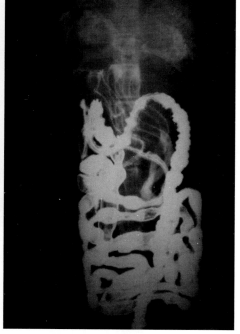

**Plate 8-17—cont'd** F and G, Radiographs taken at two hours. Only a small amount of residual barium is in the stomach. Barium is retained around what appears to be a foreign object in the pyloric antrum. Endoscopy was done shortly after the 2-hour radiographs were obtained. **H,** The foreign body, with barium in and around it, was found freely movable in the distal gastric body. A two-pronged instrument was used to grasp an edge of the rim. No significant resistance was encountered until the object was pulled against the upper esophageal sphincter. **I,** Position of the foreign body in the cranial esophagus after the grip was lost at the upper esophageal sphincter. **J,** The object was grasped and rotated, and several more unsuccessful attempts were made to pull it through the upper esophageal sphincter using the endoscopic graspers. A curved clamp was then passed alongside the endoscope to grasp the object and retrieve it the final distance. When clamps are used, care must be taken *not* to grasp mucosa along with the object. The esophagus and stomach were subsequently reexamined, and no evidence of mucosal damage was found. **K,** The object was the plastic base of a yogurt popsicle push-up (3.7-cm diameter).

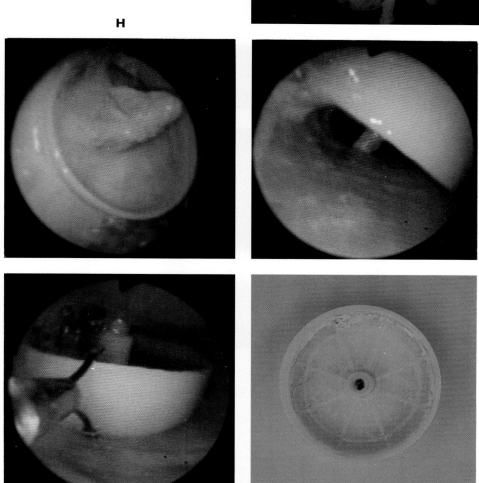

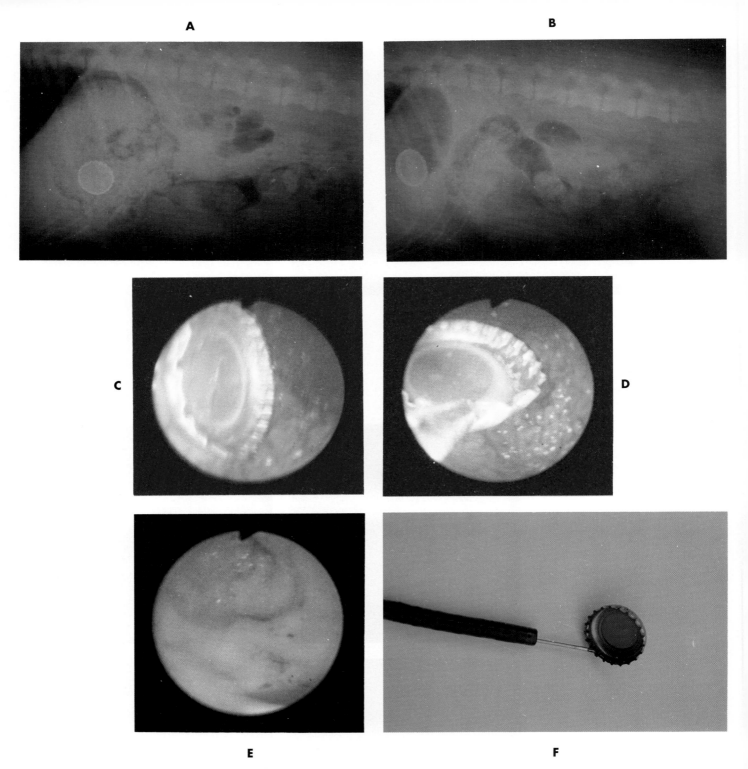

**Plate 8-18** Bottle cap foreign body in the stomach of a 3-year-old English springer spaniel. The owner saw the dog ingest the cap and immediately took the animal to an emergency clinic.
**A,** Lateral abdominal radiograph confirming the presence of a bottle cap and food in the stomach. Vomiting was induced, and a large volume of food was produced. **B,** Radiograph taken 90 minutes after vomiting was induced. The bottle cap was still in the stomach. The dog was referred for endoscopic foreign body retrieval. **C,** Endoscopic view of the bottle cap in the gastric body. The cap was initially found adhering to one of the antral walls. Strong antral contractions made it difficult to grip the cap firmly enough to pull it out of the antrum. Once the cap was freed from the antrum, it fell to the fundus (patient in left lateral recumbent position). It was then grasped and placed in the gastric body so that it could be aligned for retrieval. **D,** Bottle cap as it was pulled toward the endoscope tip. No significant resistance was encountered as the cap was pulled through the esophageal sphincters. **E,** Superficial erosions of antral mucosa from contact with the rim of the bottle cap. The pyloric orifice is at the 12 o'clock position. **F,** Best method of grasping a bottle cap with an endoscopic retrieval instrument. Bottle caps can be easily retrieved by firmly gripping the rim. It is extremely difficult to apply a firm grip on the top surface.

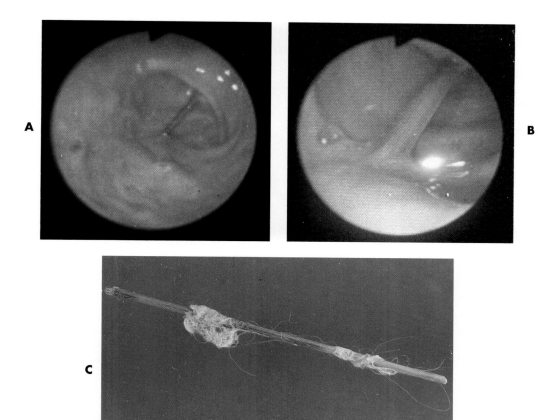

**Plate 8-19** Gastric perforation by a stick foreign body in a 10-year-old schnauzer with a 5-week history of intermittent vomiting, inappetence, and weight loss. The animal had no known history of foreign body ingestion. Survey abdominal radiographs were unremarkable. **A,** View from the proximal gastric body. Mild generalized erythema and superficial patchy erosions are present. A foreign object is observed impaled in the gastric wall at the junction of the gastric body and antrum (opposite the angulus). The angulus fold extends from the 12 to 3 o'clock position. **B,** Close-up of the foreign body as it passes through the gastric wall. When gently manipulated with a grasping instrument, the object could not be moved. At laparotomy the wooden object was found extending through the duodenum and impaling the body wall. The object and a section of duodenum were removed, and the dog recovered uneventfully. **C,** The wood foreign body was thought to be a food stick. The owner considered it likely that construction personnel working at the house 5 to 6 weeks previously had not disposed of the stick properly. The dog weighed only 5 kg (11 lb).

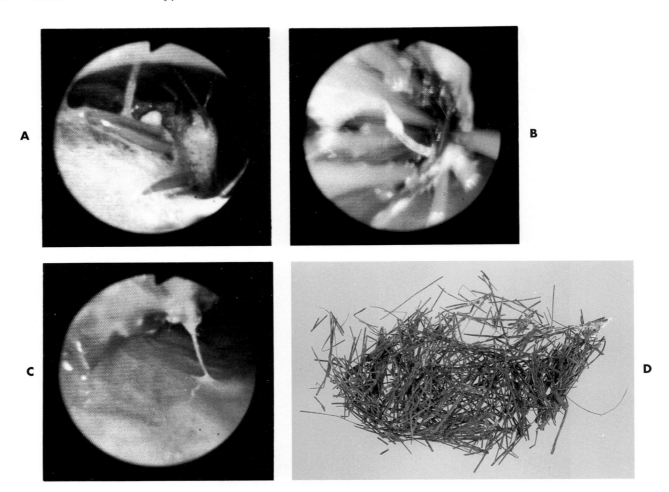

**Plate 8-20** Large accumulation of pine needles in the stomach of a 3-year-old cat. The cat had a history of intermittent hematemesis for 24 hours. Financial constraints prohibited radiography. Because the owner had observed the cat ingest pine needles, endoscopy was considered the procedure of choice. **A,** First view as the stomach was entered. Amazingly the stomach was impacted with pine needles. **B,** View in the mid-gastric body. During a tedious procedure the pine needles were removed in clumps using a four-pronged grasper. Because of cost, gastrotomy was not an option. **C,** Section of the gastric body wall after a number of pine needles had been removed. Note the superficial erosive damage of the mucosa. The cat was discharged several hours after the procedure was completed, and sucralfate and famotidine were administered for 5 days. The animal had no further clinical signs. **D,** Pine needles.

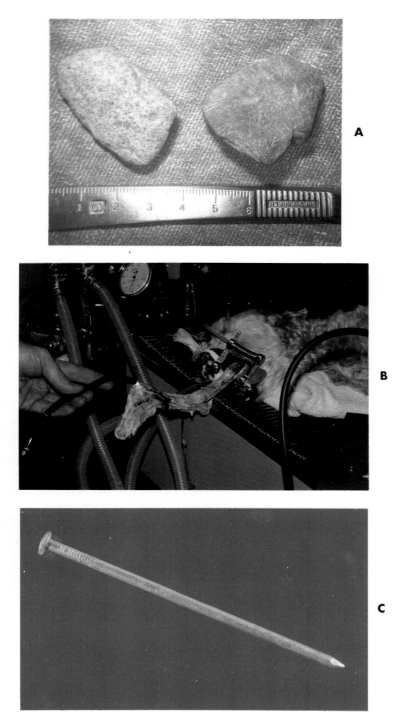

**Plate 8-21** In addition to the foreign bodies described in the previous plates, other types of objects can be removed under endoscopic guidance. Several interesting examples are shown here. **A,** Two rocks retrieved with a two-pronged grasper (see Figure 8-2) from a golden retriever with a 6-day history of anorexia but no vomiting. **B,** Endoscopy-guided retrieval of a sock from a 5-year-old cocker spaniel cross. The sock had been in the stomach for 6 days. A two-pronged grasper was used. A rat tooth grasper (see Figure 8-4) is also excellent for retrieving heavy cloth or pliable objects. Socks are most easily removed in stretched rather than bunched configuration. **C,** An 11-cm potato nail removed from the stomach of a dog. The nail was grasped at the head using a two-pronged instrument. (Courtesy David S. Bruyette.)        *Continued*

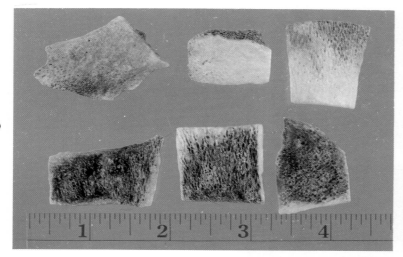

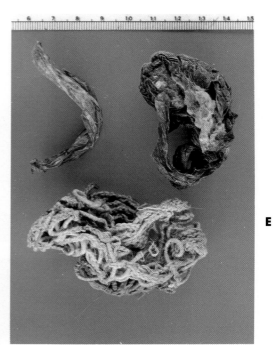

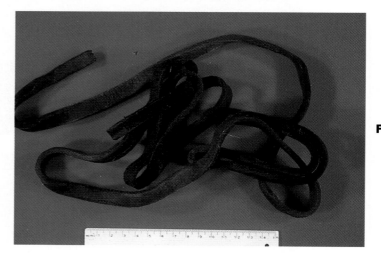

**Plate 8-21—cont'd** D, Multiple bone chips. E, Plastic and cord wrappings of a roast removed from the stomach of a dachshund. Frequent episodes of vomiting during a 10-hour period shortly after this material was ingested failed to eject the foreign objects. F, A 5-foot-long leather leash ingested by a young Labrador retriever as it was sitting in the back of its owner's car en route to a park for a run. The dog ingested the entire leash while it was hooked to its collar, leaving only the hook on the collar. The leash was ingested in two sections. Both segments were retrieved under endoscopic guidance using a two-pronged grasper. The segments were grasped at the free ends.

## DUODENAL FOREIGN BODIES

Duodenal foreign bodies are often difficult to retrieve endoscopically (see text). In some cases, however, endoscopy is a valuable diagnostic procedure for confirming suspected foreign bodies, assessing mucosal damage, and determining *early* in the clinical course whether or not surgery is indicated. The small intestines of animals that have *fragmented* gastric foreign bodies should always be examined carefully, as far as the endoscope can reach, to check for the presence of additional fragments.

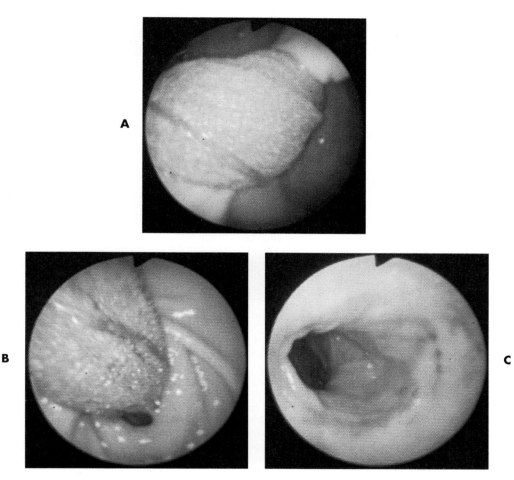

**Plate 8-22** Gastric and intestinal foreign body (panty hose) in a 10-month-old Doberman with a history of acute severe vomiting for 2 days. Clinical signs were consistent with a high intestinal obstruction. Survey abdominal radiographs suggested but did not definitively identify small bowel obstruction. Endoscopy was done to confirm clinical suspicions before proceeding to exploratory surgery. Also, if a foreign body was present, an attempt could be made to remove it via endoscopy. **A,** A section of pantyhose was found in the gastric body and is shown here extending around and beyond the angulus fold (center of field from 1 to 7 o'clock position). A blade of grass is seen on the material. **B,** View at pylorus. A long section of panty hose extended beyond the pylorus and along the small bowel. The endoscope was advanced to the mid-descending duodenum. Attempts to retract the panty hose toward the stomach failed. The foreign material was removed surgically. Recovery was uneventful. **C,** An important endoscopic finding in this patient was esophagitis. Bilious fluid was pooled in the thoracic esophagus (not shown here), and significant inflammation and erosive injury were present at the gastroesophageal junction. The junction area is open. Esophagitis should be considered in any animal that has persistent vomiting. Esophagitis is also a relatively common sequela of vomiting associated with intestinal foreign bodies, especially high intestinal obstructions and linear foreign bodies. It no doubt causes pain, as it does in humans. Treatment for esophagitis should be instituted for animals with these problems, whether or not endoscopy is performed.

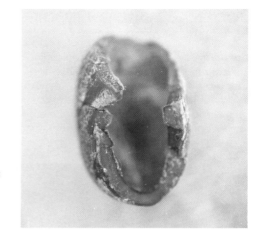

**Plate 8-23** One half of a hollow rubber ball removed through an enterotomy of the proximal jejunum in a cat with persistent vomiting. The diagnosis was made during an endoscopic examination. When it was recognized that the ball was not freely movable, surgery was performed. The open end had been facing proximally.

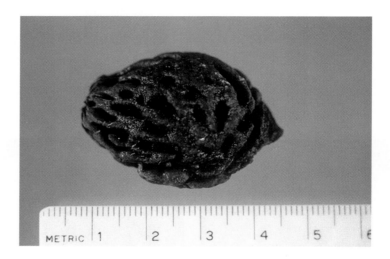

**Plate 8-24** Nectarine pit foreign body removed from the mid-jejunum of a 10-kg (22-lb) dog with a history of intermittent vomiting (one to two episodes per week) for 1 year. The animal had no history of weight loss or inappetence. The dog was presented because of an acute onset of persistent vomiting of two days' duration. Other than evidence of dehydration, the findings of baseline tests were unremarkable. Abdominal radiographs were also unremarkable. The animal had a minimal response to intravenous metoclopramide (constant rate infusion). Endoscopy was performed to evaluate the stomach and small intestine. The findings included bilious fluid accumulation in the esophagus and stomach, which suggested either a motility disorder (unlikely because of the minimal response to metoclopramide) or an obstruction in the small bowel. The endoscope was advanced to the jejunum, and a nectarine pit was found, firmly lodged in the mid-jejunum. Although it was not possible to remove the foreign body via endoscopy, the endoscopic examination played an extremely important role in establishing the diagnosis. In most similar cases, survey abdominal radiographs would be helpful in establishing a diagnosis, but no radiographic signs of obstruction whatsoever were seen in this patient. The animal recovered uneventfully from surgery. NOTE: The owner reported that she had seen the dog ingest the nectarine pit 1 year earlier (at the time the intermittent vomiting began). The nectarine pit remained in the stomach for a year until it spontaneously passed into the small intestine, at which time the acute frequent vomiting began.

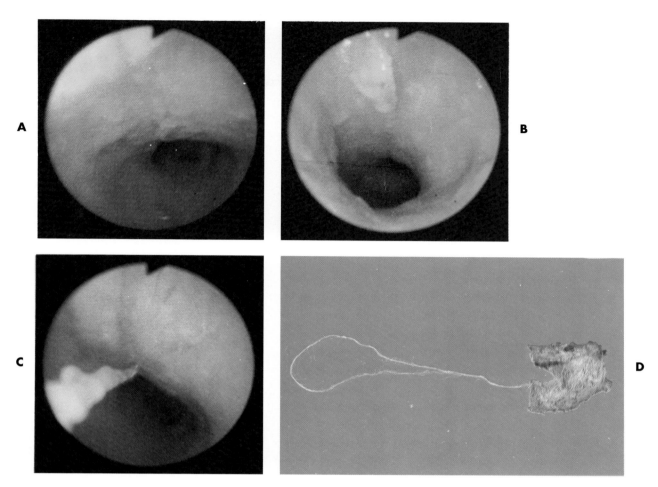

**Plate 8-25** String attached to an irregular foreign object in the duodenum of a 2-year-old bull-terrier. There had been intermittent vomiting for 10 days. Gastroscopy revealed numerous leatherlike foreign objects that were removed endoscopically. The duodenum was then routinely examined for the presence of foreign material. **A,** On close examination of the duodenal lumen, a thin linear streak of yellow fluid was detected (extending from the 12 o'clock position to the center of the field) on the intestinal wall. **B,** Close-up view suggesting the presence of a threadlike or string foreign body along the wall. **C,** A biopsy forceps instrument was advanced through the endoscope and used to grasp a small area where fluid had accumulated. As the instrument was retracted, the thin linear foreign material was pulled away from the wall. The string was firmly attached to something further distal in the intestine. With *gentle* retraction force, the string could not be moved. A laparotomy was then performed. **D,** The string material is attached to an irregular and stiff piece of material. The foreign body was found wedged along the duodenal wall but was not causing a significant degree of obstruction. Failure to perform a careful duodenal examination after the gastric foreign bodies had been retrieved would have resulted in the small intestinal object being missed.

Chapter 9

# Endoscopy in Nondomestic Species

## Colin F. Burrows and Darryl J. Heard

The principles of and indications for endoscopy in exotic (nondomestic) species are similar to those in dogs and cats. A standard 110-cm by 10-mm gastroscope works well in most species although a 1.6- or even 3-m-long endoscope is invaluable in large snakes, birds, big cats, and the larger mammals. Compared to dogs and cats, reptiles and many birds (particularly raptors and fish eaters) have a more distensible and accessible esophagus. Thus small esophageal diameter is not necessarily a contraindication to upper gastrointestinal endoscopy. We have, for example, used a standard 110-cm by 9-mm gastroscope to perform upper gastrointestinal endoscopy successfully in lizards and tortoises weighing as little as 0.5 kg (1 lb).

## INDICATIONS

Indications for endoscopy in exotic species reflect the signs of diseases unique to that group. In snakes and lizards, for example, the most common indications are prolonged anorexia and regurgitation. Endoscopy is commonly indicated in tortoises with anorexia and diarrhea; birds with anorexia, regurgitation, and radiographic evidence of an upper gastrointestinal foreign body; and mammals with regurgitation, anorexia, vomiting, and diarrhea.

## RESTRAINT AND PATIENT PREPARATION

Endoscopy is best performed under general anesthesia in most species although in crocodiles and alligators it can be performed using either a zolazepam/tiletamine combination (Telazol) or a muscle relaxant (e.g., succinylcholine) (Bennett, 1991) and appropriate bite block (i.e., a piece of 2- by 4-inch board) with a hole drilled through it or a section of hard plastic tube with an appropriate diameter. Isoflurane is the inhalant anesthetic of choice in most species.

Preparation for upper gastrointestinal endoscopy usually entails only an overnight fast. Lower gastrointestinal endoscopy requires adequate cloacal or colonic lavage. In mammals, visualization of the colonic mucosa is enhanced by the appropriate administration of enemas and an oral colonic lavage solution the day before the procedure. In some species this is a daunting task that requires heavy sedation or anesthesia to allow administration of the lavage solution via a stomach tube. Primates can often be induced to drink a colonic lavage solution if it is mixed with juice or flavored sugar water (e.g., KoolAid). In preparing nondomestic species for endoscopy, veterinarians should always work closely with keepers or handlers because these individuals know their charges and are often extremely innovative.

## REFERENCES

Bennett RA: A review of anesthesia and chemical restraint in reptiles. *J Zoo Wildlife Med* 22:282, 1991.
Schumacher J et al: Inclusion body disease in boid snakes. *J Zoo Wildlife Med* 25:511, 1994.

# ENDOSCOPY IN REPTILES

## SNAKES

The most common indication for endoscopy in snakes is prolonged anorexia and repetitive regurgitation; diarrhea is an uncommon indication. Endoscopy is best performed in a relaxed anesthetized snake that is stretched out as straight as possible. In snakes the stomach is located about two thirds of the distance between the mouth and tail. This means that large snakes need to be stretched out over at least two examination tables placed end to end. Other than mucus-secreting glands in the mouth that moisten the oral cavity and lubricate food, the proximal portion of the reptile gastrointestinal tract does not appear to possess many mucus-secreting glands. Therefore it is important to continually lubricate the endoscope as it is inserted. However, the gastrointestinal tract is lined with mucus epithelial cells. This lining becomes sticky and "grabs" the scope, which makes advancement difficult.

Because the proximal esophagus in snakes is very thin, underlying organs and vessels can be readily identified. Tan- to yellow-orange-colored esophageal tonsils are distributed throughout the length of the esophagus in boids (pythons and boas). In snakes infected with boid inclusion body disease (a retrovirus) these esophageal tonsils contain numerous lymphocytes and other white cells that may have diagnostic inclusions (Schumacher et al., 1994). The distal esophagus is slightly thicker and often more vascular than the proximal part of the organ. It is also difficult to distinguish the point at which this part of the esophagus changes into the true stomach. The snake has no obvious lower esophageal sphincter, but the endoscopist should be aware that the esophagus can contract and form rings that resemble sphincters, even in the anesthetized animal.

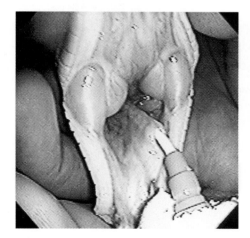

**Plate 9-1** Oral cavity of an emerald tree boa *(Corallus canina)*. The animal was undergoing upper gastrointestinal endoscopy as part of an evaluation for chronic regurgitation, a common problem in wild-caught emerald tree boas and green tree pythons *(Chondropyton viridis)*. The snake has been intubated. Note how much farther forward the glottis is in snakes than in mammals. This anatomic configuration allows snakes to breath as they swallow large prey.

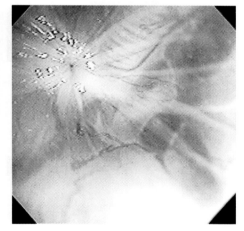

**Plate 9-2** Proximal esophagus of an emerald tree boa. The esophagus is very thin and transparent but appears to be extremely tough. The trachea and submucosal blood vessels are readily seen.

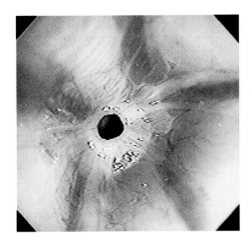

**Plate 9-3** Esophageal constriction ring in an emerald tree boa. The endoscopist can reduce such rings by gentle air insufflation as the tip of the endoscope is moved distally.

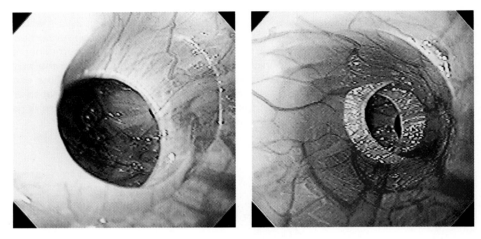

**Plate 9-4** Esophageal constriction rings in the mid-esophagus of an emerald tree boa. Blood vessels are readily apparent.

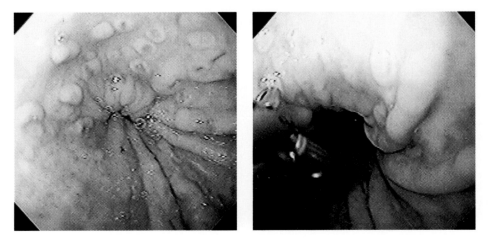

**Plate 9-5** Esophageal tonsils in an emerald tree boa. Biopsy specimens should be obtained from these nodules as the endoscope is passed distally.

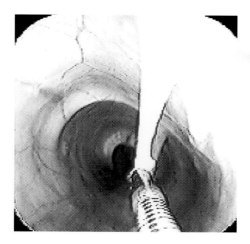

**Plate 9-6** Mid-esophagus in a Burmese python *(Python molurus biuittatus)*. Despite its apparent thinness the esophageal mucosa of snakes can and should be biopsied.

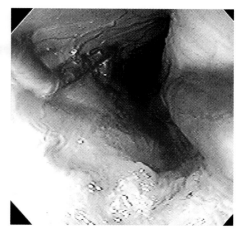

**Plate 9-7** Jugular vein seen through the thin and transparent esophageal wall in a Burmese python.

A

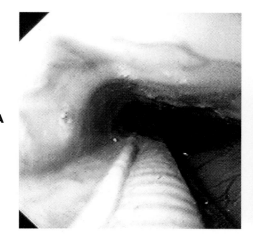

B

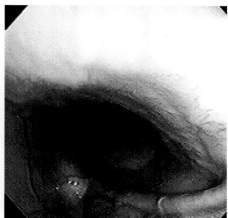

**Plate 9-8** Thin, transparent esophageal wall in an albino boa constrictor *(Boa constrictor)*. A, Adjacent trachea (6 o'clock position). B, Jugular vein.

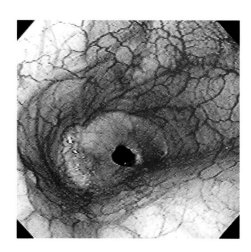

**Plate 9-9** The esophageal mucosa in some snakes, as in the mid-esophagus of this albino boa, can be highly vascular. This is not necessarily a sign of inflammation or disease.

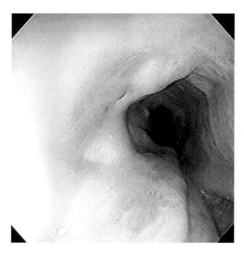

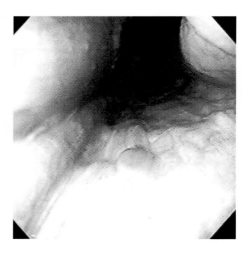

**Plate 9-10** Esophageal lymphoid nodules in some snakes, as in this boa, appear yellow-brown in color.

**Plate 9-11** In this Burmese python the esophageal tonsils are orange in color and very prominent. No abnormality was noted on biopsy specimens.

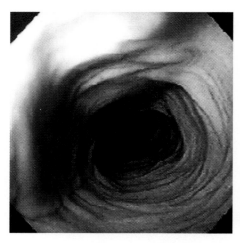

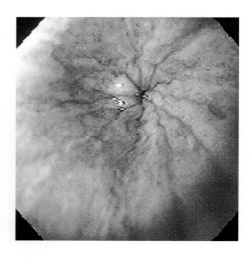

**Plate 9-12** The distal esophagus in most snakes, as in this indigo snake *(Drymarchon corais couperi)*, is thicker than the rest of the esophagus, and submucosal vessels are usually absent.

**Plate 9-13** Gastroesophageal junction (lower esophageal sphincter) in an indigo snake. Although this looks like a constriction ring, gastric mucosa was evident when the tip of the scope was advanced.

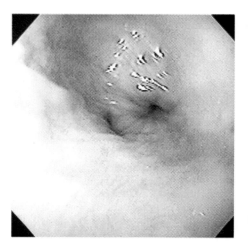

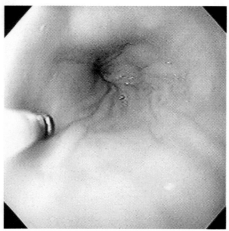

**Plate 9-14** Distal esophagus or proximal stomach in an emerald tree boa. Examination of a biopsy specimen later revealed that this was the distal esophagus.

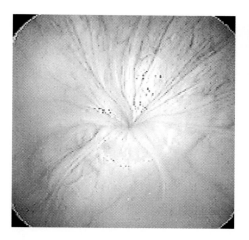

**Plate 9-15** Distal esophagus in a 3.3-m-long 140-lb female Burmese python. A 3-m video-endoscope was used, approximately 2 m from the animal's mouth. The endoscope was passed through the apparent sphincter (a ring of esophageal constriction) with minimal air insufflation.

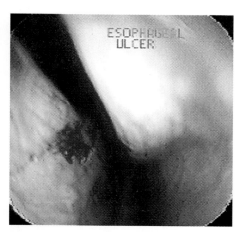

**Plate 9-16** Esophageal ulcer (9 o'clock position) in a clinically normal Burmese python. The cause of the ulcer was not determined. Biopsy of the lesion revealed only mild inflammatory changes.

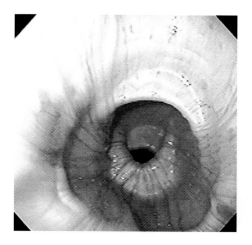

**Plate 9-17** Distal esophagus in a Burmese python. Note the many esophageal "rings" and the orange-colored esophageal lymph aggregates.

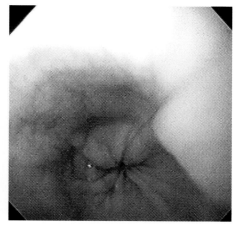

**Plate 9-18** Gastroesophageal junction in an emerald tree boa. At first, this looked like an esophageal ring, but rugal folds were seen when the endoscope was passed through the opening.

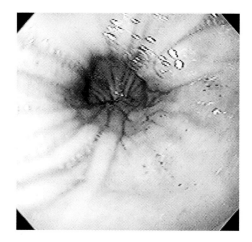

**Plate 9-19** Proximal stomach in an emerald tree boa, beyond the ring in Plate 9-18. Rugal folds can be seen running distally. Small red spots (right and lower right) are gastric erosions that on biopsy were found to be associated with plasmacytic, lymphocytic gastritis.

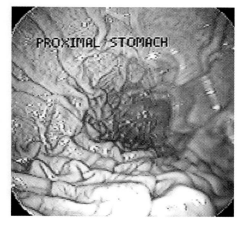

**Plate 9-20** Proximal stomach in a female Burmese python. The snake was 3.5 m long and weighed 5.4 kg (120 lb). The stomach was located 2.5 m from the mouth. The examination was performed with a 3-m videoendoscope.

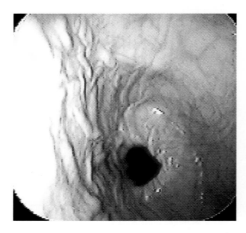

**Plate 9-21** Antrum of a Burmese python. Note the open pylorus.

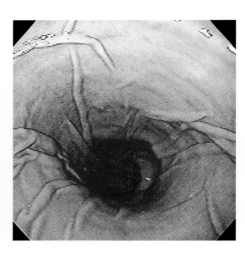

**Plate 9-22** Distal stomach in an albino boa. Rugal folds run at various angles, and a hint of flexure (incisura) is present.

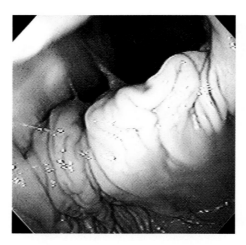

**Plate 9-23** Gastric flexure in a python. Some snakes appear to have a curved stomach, almost like mammals with the equivalent of an incisura.

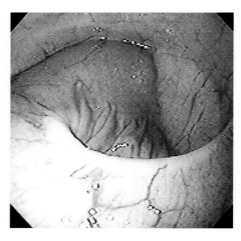

**Plate 9-24** Junction between the proximal and distal stomach in an albino boa. Note the gastric flexure and "incisura."

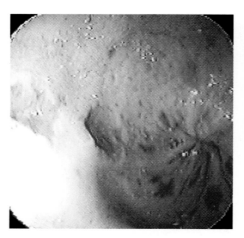

**Plate 9-25** Multiple gastric ulcers in a Burmese python. The animal had bacterial pneumonia and had been anorexic for several months. Examination of biopsy specimens revealed a plasmacytic, lymphocytic gastritis.

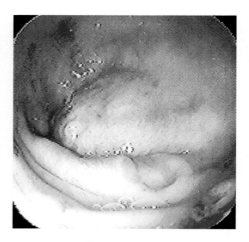

**Plate 9-26** Follow-up endoscopy in the python shown in Plate 9-25 after 4 weeks of treatment with antibiotics, ranitidine, and sucralfate. The ulcers were diminished in size and number and appeared to be healing. The snake was eventually euthanized because of a cardiac mass. At autopsy the stomach was normal.

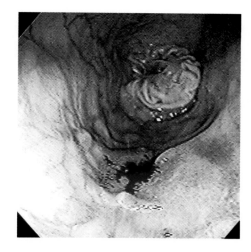

**Plate 9-27** Bleeding gastric ulcer in an albino boa. In addition, the mucosa in the distal stomach is also partially invaginated. This occurs when the endoscope is withdrawn too abruptly. The mucosa adheres to the tip of the instrument and is pulled forward as the scope is withdrawn.

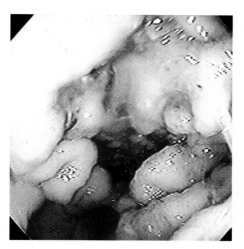 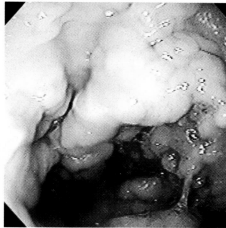

**Plate 9-28** Granulomatous gastritis in a boa constrictor. The snake was presented with a 4-month history of regurgitation and a 3-month history of anorexia. Examination of biopsy specimens revealed pyogranulomatous gastritis. At autopsy a large granuloma was found to be causing gastric outlet obstruction.

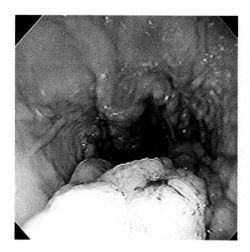 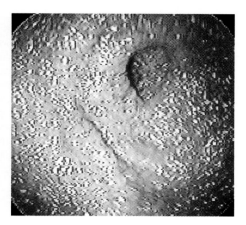

**Plate 9-29** Bleeding granulomatous ulcer in the snake described in Plate 9-28.

**Plate 9-30** Proximal duodenum in a Burmese python. Duodenoscopy can only be performed in large snakes such as this 2.9-m-long specimen. The multiple white dots are reflected light from individual villi. The duodenal flexure can be seen in the distance.

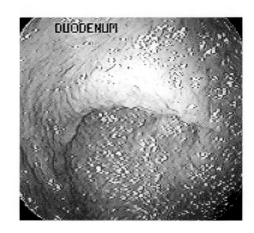

**Plate 9-31** Duodenal flexure (middle of the field) in the snake described in Plate 9-30.

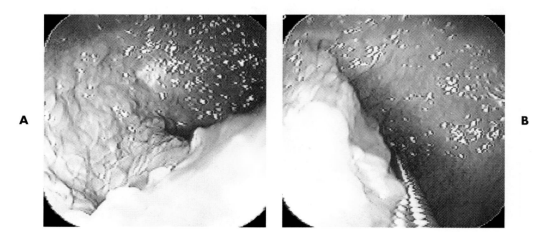

A                                                                                        B

**Plate 9-32 A,** Close-up of the duodenal mucosa in a Burmese python. The villi appear more flattened than those in mammals. **B,** The biopsy revealed a mild plasmacytic, lymphocytic infiltrate. This is the same snake with gastric ulcers and plasmacytic, lymphocytic gastritis described in Plates 9-25 and 9-26.

## TURTLES AND TORTOISES

Endoscopy in turtles and tortoises is relatively straightforward. The exceptions are sea turtles, in which the esophagus is lined with keratinized backward-pointing spines and the distal esophagus has a sharp right-angled bend that must be negotiated blindly. In contrast, the gastrointestinal tract of tortoises is readily accessible: the esophagus is distensible, the stomach is similar to that of mammals, and the endoscope can be easily passed into the proximal intestine. Using a 9-mm-diameter gastroscope, the endoscopist can perform a thorough upper gastrointestinal examination in tortoises as small as 6 inches in length. However, the lower gastrointestinal tract is much more difficult to evaluate. Tortoises have a cloaca that is readily examined and is usually kept clean by urine. The cloaca is separated from the rectum and colon by an extremely tight sphincter through which it is almost impossible to pass an endoscope.

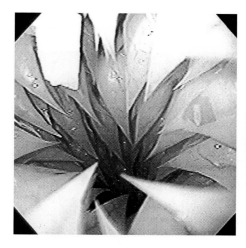 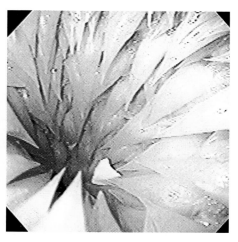

**A**

**B**

**Figure 9-33 A,** Backward-pointing keratinized spines in the esophagus of a loggerhead sea turtle *(Caretta caretta)*. The function of these spines is controversial, but they are believed to prevent the escape of ingesta. They function as a baleen in whales, allowing them to expel water without losing food. **B,** Close-up of the turtle esophagus.

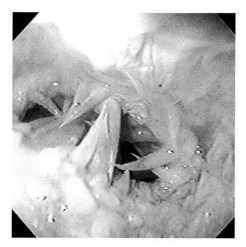 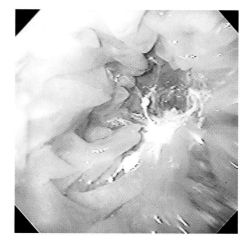

**Plate 9-34** Distal esophagus in a Kemp's or Atlantic Ridley sea turtle *(Lepidochelys kempii)*. The spines become smaller in the distal esophagus. The spines are quite mobile; although they look like they could damage the endoscope, they rarely (if ever) cause any problems. An endoscope has been passed more than 50 times in various sea turtles without incurring any damage.

**Plate 9-35** Anatomic differences exist between turtle species. For example, the spines in the gastroesophageal junction of a hawksbill sea turtle *(Eretmochelys imbricata)* are rounder and shorter than those in the turtle shown in Plate 9-34.

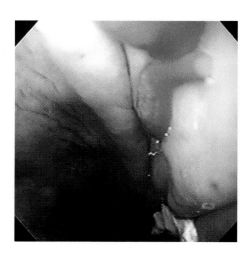

**Plate 9-36** Flukes in the stomach of a hawksbill sea turtle. The stomach of sea turtles often harbors a wide variety of parasites.

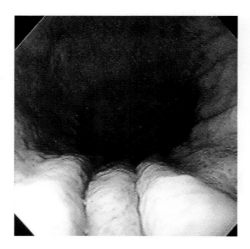

**Plate 9-37** Stomach of a Kemp's or Atlantic Ridley sea turtle. The surface has a reticulated appearance, but mucosal folds are almost always evident.

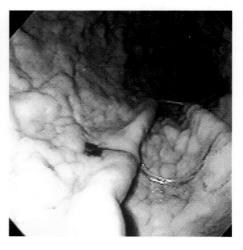

**Plate 9-38** Gastric ulcer in a loggerhead sea turtle. Ulcers are a common finding in the stomach of sick turtles. These lesions may be associated with the stress of disease and restraint, or other factors may be involved. Appropriate stains of histologic sections of biopsy specimens have revealed large populations of mucosal bacteria.

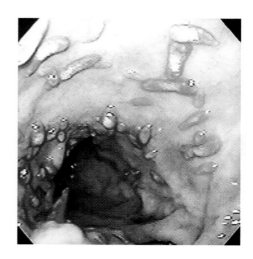

**Plate 9-39** Nematode parasites in the stomach of a loggerhead sea turtle.

**Plate 9-40** Large numbers of nematode parasites in the stomach of a Kemp's or Atlantic Ridley sea turtle. The parasites appeared to be submucosal but very mobile.

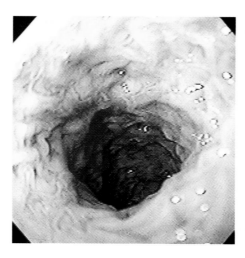

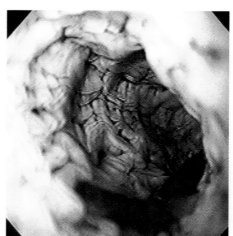

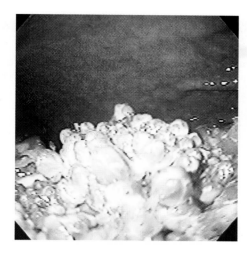

**Plate 9-41** Gastric mucosa of an African spurred tortoise *(Geochelone sulcata)*. The mucosa seems to lack folds, but this appearance may be due to overdistension. The animal had eaten broccoli 6 hours previously.

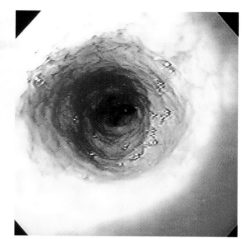

**Plate 9-42** Proximal small intestine of a spurred tortoise. The mucosa appears hyperemic. Histologic examination of a biopsy specimen revealed chronic enteritis.

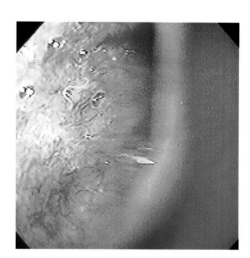

**Plate 9-43** Proximal small intestine of a radiated tortoise *(Geochelone radiata)*. A small nematode parasite is attached to the mucosa (upper left at the 11 o'clock position).

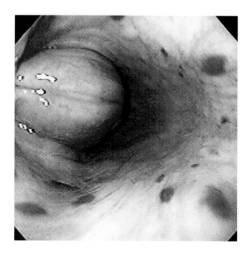

**Plate 9-44** Cloaca of a female radiated tortoise. The protruding mucosa with an apparent slit is the urogenital ridge. The slit leads to the uterus.

## CROCODILES AND ALLIGATORS

Endoscopy in crocodilians is perhaps easier than in any other nondomestic species. Crocodilians have a distensible esophagus and stomach and a duodenum that can be readily entered and examined.

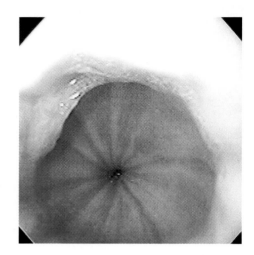

**Plate 9-45** Distal esophagus and gastroesophageal junction of an American alligator *(Alligator mississippiensis).*

**Plate 9-46 A,** Gastric foreign body (bezoar of nutria hair) in a Chinese alligator *(Alligator sinensis).* Many attempts were made to remove the accumulation of hair with retrieval forceps, but only small pieces were removed each time. **B,** The repeated passage of the endoscope caused erythema of the gastroesophageal junction. The bezoar was eventually removed by an enterprising student who volunteered to remove it manually.

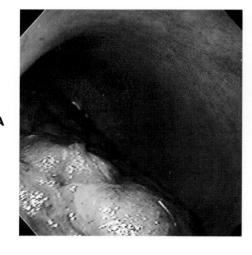

A

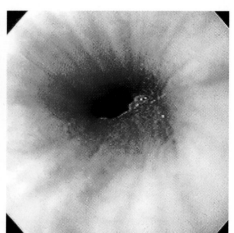

B

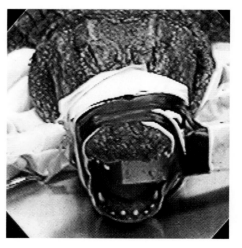

**Plate 9-47** A tough bite block (in this case a piece of 2- by 4-inch board) and plenty of strong tape are essential to protect both the endoscope and the endoscopist, when crocodilians are being examined.

# ENDOSCOPY IN MAMMALS

The same basic principles apply to endoscopy in nondomestic mammals as in dogs and cats. Primates are the easiest of all species to evaluate endoscopically. They have a short esophagus, usually a wide-open pylorus, and a wide duodenum. Endoscopy in the large cats, wolves, and bears is similar to that in dogs and cats. A long endoscope (1.8 to 3 m) is required for a complete evaluation in these animals. Endoscopy is difficult in small mammals such as ferrets and rabbits because the anatomy of their oropharynx does not allow enough distension for the passage of an endoscope. However, endoscopic examination can be performed in small mammals if a 3- or 5-mm-diameter bronchoscope is used.

# PRIMATES

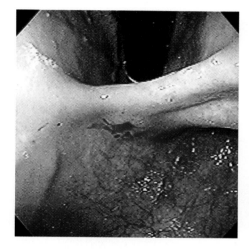

**Plate 9-48** Incisura and fundus of a capuchin monkey *(Cebus apella)* that was presented for the evaluation of repeated regurgitation. No esophageal disease was found. The hemorrhagic spot (center of the field) is the site of a mucosal biopsy.

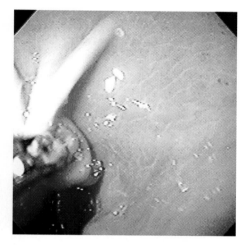

**Plate 9-49** Gastric biopsy in a capuchin monkey.

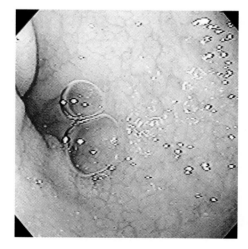

**Plate 9-50** Stomach of an orangutan *(Pongo pygameus)* presented for the evaluation of stunted growth, hypoproteinemia, and eosinophilia.

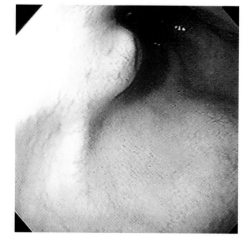

**Plate 9-51** Proximal duodenum of the orangutan in Plate 9-50. Note the prominent pancreatic papilla in the upper center of the field of view. This papilla is seen in all primates.

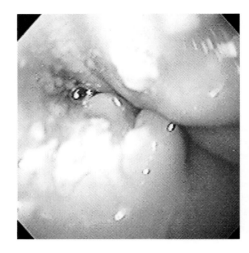
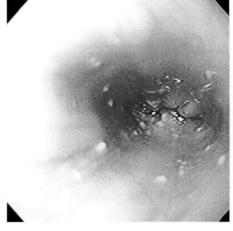

**Plate 9-52** Esophagus of an orangutan approximately 9 months after treatment with chronic prednisone and antibiotic therapy for moderate to severe eosinophilic colitis. The white plaques were secondary to overgrowth with *Candida albicans*, and the animal was determined to have *Candida* esophagitis.

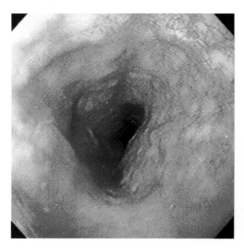

**Plate 9-53** Descending colon in a capuchin monkey with signs of large bowel diarrhea. The animal was later determined to have plasmacytic, lymphocytic colitis.

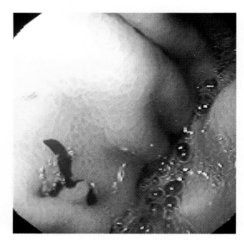

**Plate 9-54** Stomach of a black howler monkey *(Alouatta caraya)*. These animals are leaf eaters and have a large stomach. The reticulated pattern is normal in this species.

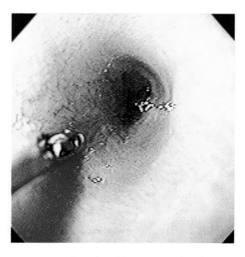

**Plate 9-55** Duodenal biopsy in a howler monkey.

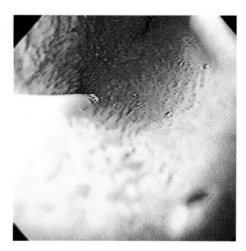

**Plate 9-56** Duodenal aspiration in a howler monkey. The tip of the aspiration tube can be seen at the lower left in the field of view. Individual villi are visible. Microscopic examination of the aspirated fluid revealed infection with *Giardia*.

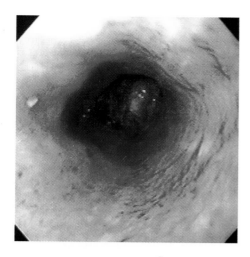

**Plate 9-57** Severe esophagitis in a stump-tailed macaque *(Macaca aetoides)*. The animal had a hiatal hernia with chronic acid reflux into the esophagus. Everted gastric mucosa can be seen in the distal esophagus.

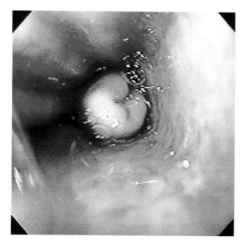

**Plate 9-58** Invagination of the gastric mucosa into the esophagus of the macaque described in Plate 9-57. The animal responded well to treatment with cisapride, sucralfate, and omeprazole.

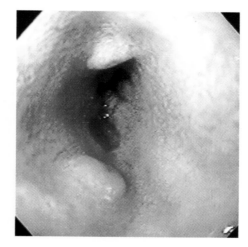

**Plate 9-59** As seen in this macaque, primates often have two separate and distinct pancreatic papillae.

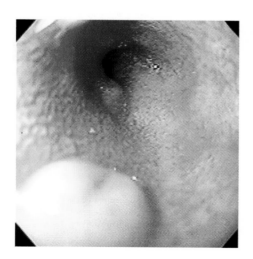

**Plate 9-60** Bile flowing from the common pancreatic and bile duct opening (7 o'clock position) in a macaque.

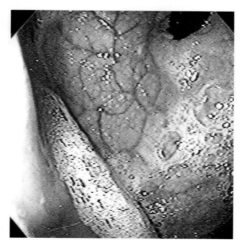

**Plate 9-61** Fundus in a siamang *(Hylobates syndactylus)*. This gibbon species appears to have a highly vascular stomach. Note the endoscope entering the stomach (top right in the field of view).

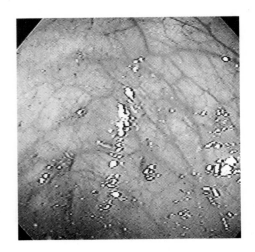

**Plate 9-62** Colon of a siamang. Prominent submucosal vessels can be seen. Histologic examination of a biopsy specimen revealed plasmacytic lymphocytic colitis.

# RABBITS AND FERRETS

Rabbits and ferrets can be difficult to examine endoscopically because they have a narrow caudal oropharynx that restricts passage of an endoscope. We now use a 4-mm video-bronchoscope to perform upper gastrointestinal endoscopy in these species.

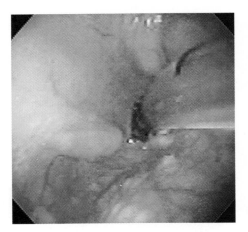

**Plate 9-63** Tonsillar hypertrophy in a ferret *(Mustela putorius furo)* presented with a chronic history of dysphagia, regurgitation, and vomiting.

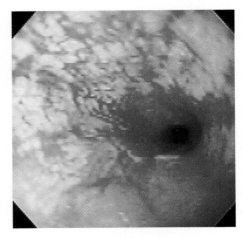

**Plate 9-64** The ferret described in Plate 9-63 had a hyperemic esophagus with white plaques on the surface, very reminiscent of the *Candida albicans* infection shown in Plate 9-52. However, smears of the material showed only dead epithelial cells, and the fungal culture was negative. Histologic examination of a biopsy specimen revealed esophagitis. It was later determined that these white plaques may be a normal finding in some ferrets and are composed of squamous keratinization (Collins BR: Personal communication, July, 1996).

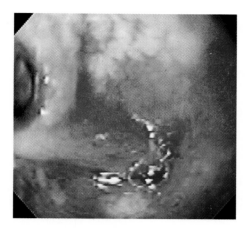

**Plate 9-65** Biopsy of the esophageal mucosa in the ferret described in Plates 9-64 and 9-65. The stomach of this animal appeared normal, but histologic examination of a biopsy specimen revealed gastritis and large numbers of organisms that were compatible with *Helicobacter mustelae*. The animal improved dramatically after symptomatic therapy with sucralfate and cisapride and antibiotic therapy for the *Helicobacter* infection.

# BEARS

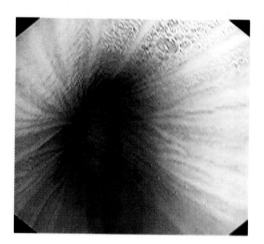

**Plate 9-66** Esophagus of a black bear *(Ursus americanus)*. Some gastric reflux is seen. The esophagus in bears has longitudinal folds.

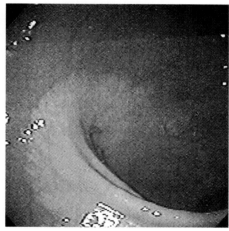

**Plate 9-67** Stomach of a black bear. A distinct line of demarcation is seen between the glandular and antral portions. A similar line is present in the stomach of a pig.

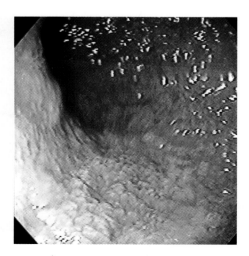

**Plate 9-68** Small intestinal mucosa of a black bear.

## CARNIVORA

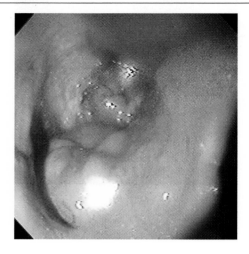

**Plate 9-69** Ileocolonic junction in a maned wolf *(Chrysocyon brachyurus).* The animal appears to have two separate ileocolonic sphincters. Biopsy forceps were easily passed through each orifice, and samples of ileal mucosa were obtained from each. Whether this is a normal finding in this species is not known. The cecal orifice can be seen on the left. The animal was presented because of diarrhea and hematochezia. Histologic examination of a biopsy specimen revealed plasmacytic, lymphocytic colitis.

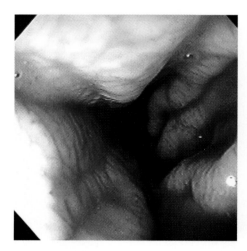

**Plate 9-70** Colon in the maned wolf described in Plate 9-69.

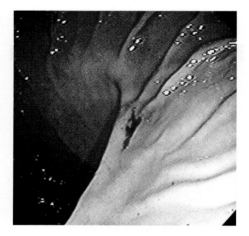

**Plate 9-71** Bleeding gastric ulcer in a lion *(Panthera leo)* who had vomiting and neurologic signs. Postmortem, the animal's brain showed signs of meningoencephalitis. No histologic evidence of gastritis or *Helicobacter* infection was found, but a urease test on a biopsy specimen was positive.

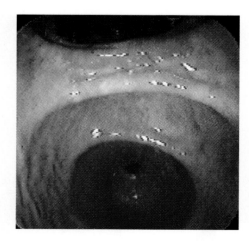

**Plate 9-72** Gastric hyperemia in a lion presented because of anorexia and vomiting. The animal had severe eosinophilic plaques in its oral cavity.

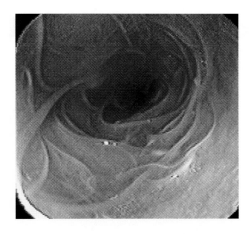

**Plate 9-73** Marked roundworm *(Toxascaris)* infection, which was an incidental finding in the small intestine of the lion described in Plate 9-72.

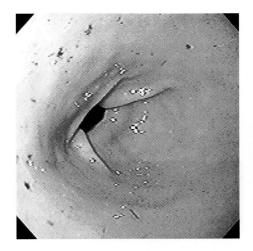

**Plate 9-74** Antrum of a jungle cat *(Felis chaus)* with gastric erosions caused by a ball of nylon ripped from a play toy (see Plate 9-75).

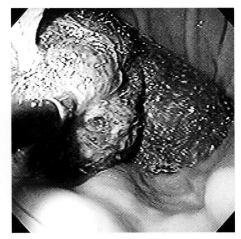

**Plate 9-75** Ball of nylon being retrieved from the stomach of a jungle cat *(Felis chaus)*.

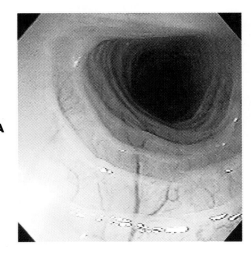

A

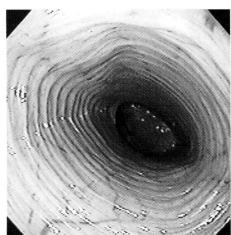

B

**Plate 9-76** The esophagus in the larger members of the cat family contains herring-bone folds identical to those in the domestic cat. **A,** Esophagus in a western cougar *(Felis concolor)*. Submucosal blood vessels are a normal finding in this species. **B,** Similar findings in a lion.

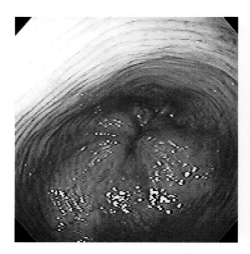

**Plate 9-77** Reflux esophagitis and a bulging lower esophageal sphincter in a 7-month-old male lion with a hiatal hernia.

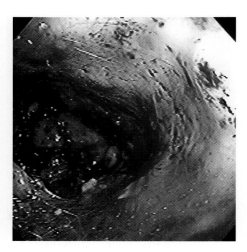

**Plate 9-78** Erosive gastritis and ulceration in a 15-year-old western cougar. The animal had not been fed for 24 hours, but food was still present in the stomach, suggesting delayed gastric emptying. The stomach was shown to be heavily infected with *Helicobacter*. The animal was asymptomatic for its gastric disease and was actually presented for the insertion of an artificial joint into an arthritic knee.

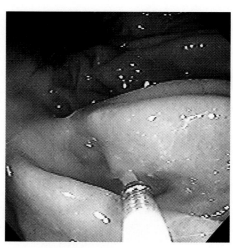

**Plate 9-79** Cougar shown in Plate 9-78. It is difficult if not impossible to regularly treat large cats with oral medication. An attempt was made to ameliorate the animal's gastritis by inserting sucralfate suspension directly into the stomach via a catheter placed through the biopsy channel of the endoscope.

# BIRDS

Flexible endoscopy is useful in the diagnosis and management of conditions of the crop, esophagus, proventriculus, and ventriculus. Indications for the endoscopic examination of birds include anorexia, hypophagia, dysphagia, regurgitation, and abnormal swelling in the cervical or anterior thoracic region.

A standard 9-mm-diameter gastroscope can only be used in birds larger than a macaw. A 7-mm-diameter gastroscope or a 3- or 4-mm bronchoscope can be used in smaller birds. Maneuverability is limited in smaller birds, and bronchoscopes lack the air and water systems that are usually necessary in upper gastrointestinal endoscopy.

Endoscopy should only be performed in the relaxed anesthetized patient. Isoflurane anesthesia appears to be the safest technique. Dorsal recumbent or lateral positioning affords adequate examination. It is not necessary to tilt the body. The head and neck should be extended, and the endoscope should be inserted gently. The endoscope is advanced along the proximal esophagus and then into the crop (except in ratites, which have no crop). The crop and esophagus may contain excess mucus that impairs visualization of the lumen and walls. Air insufflation and irrigation can help clear the view. The endoscope is withdrawn from the crop and next is inserted into the proventriculus and ventriculus. The small intestine can then be examined in larger species.

See Chapter 17 for a complete discussion of *rigid* endoscopy in avian species.

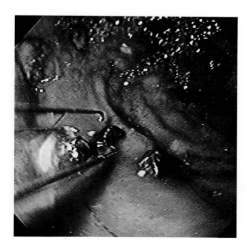

**Plate 9-80** Retrieval of foreign bodies (lead fishing weights) from the proventriculus of a turkey vulture *(Cathartes aura)*. The bird was presented with neurologic signs and a high blood lead concentration.

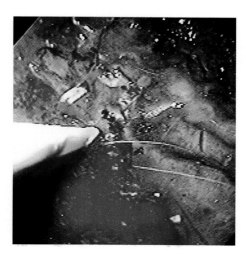

**Plate 9-81** Gastritis (proventriculitis) in a turkey vulture.

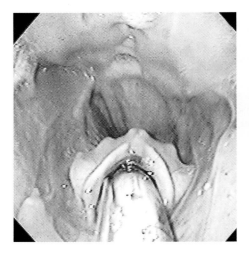

**Plate 9-82** Oral cavity of a young ostrich *(Struthio camelus)*. The trachea has been intubated.

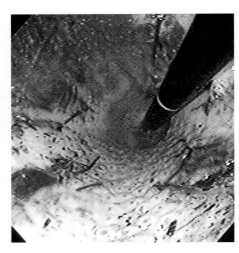

**Plate 9-83** Retroflexion of the endoscope tip (J maneuver) in an ostrich, revealing the proximal proventriculus. The small, raised structures with red dots are gastric glands.

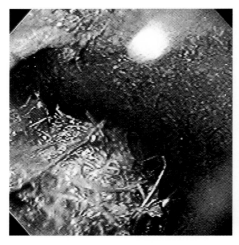

**Plate 9-84** Impaction of the proventriculus in the bird shown in Plate 9-83.

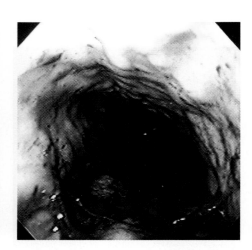

**Plate 9-85** Proventriculus in an emu *(Dromaius novaehollandiae)*.

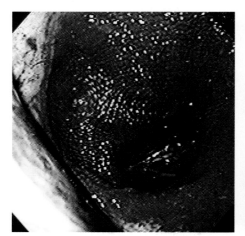

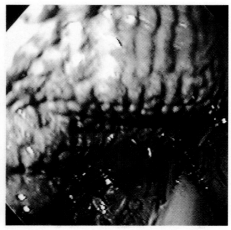

**Plate 9-86** Ventriculus in an emu. The wall is lined by a protein secretion (koilin) that is stained green by refluxed bile pigments from the duodenum. This is a normal finding in this species.

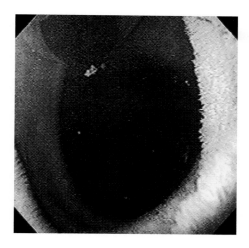

**Plate 9-87** Cloaca of an emu. This structure is usually filled with fluid (urine) and is lined with fingerlike structures that resemble villi.

**A** 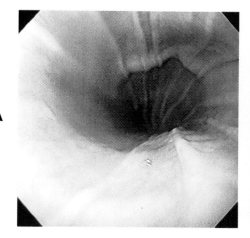 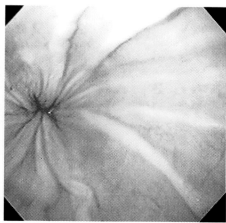 **B**

**Plate 9-88 A,** Esophagus of a common loon *(Gavia immer)*. The esophagus of these fish-eating birds contains longitudinal folds that run the length of the organ and allow distension when a fish is swallowed. This species has no crop. **B,** Gastroesophageal junction of a loon.

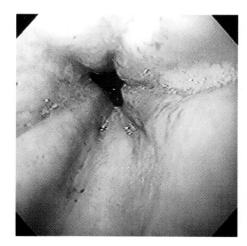

**Plate 9-89** Proventriculus of a loon. The green color is from refluxed bile.

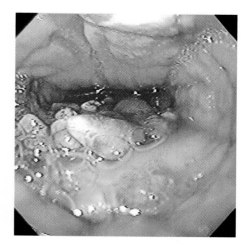

**Plate 9-90** Distal ventriculus of a loon. The organ contains a number of small pebbles that presumably help in digestion.

# Chapter 10

# Endoscopic Biopsy Specimen Collection and Histopathologic Considerations

**Albert E. Jergens and Frances M. Moore**

Dramatic advances in endoscopic techniques have revolutionized the visualization and biopsy of parenchymal organs in small animals. Endoscopy facilitates direct, minimally invasive examination of mucosal and serosal surfaces and permits tissues to be obtained for histologic and cytologic examination or fluids to be procured for laboratory evaluation. The evaluation of endoscopic biopsy material is extremely helpful in establishing a diagnosis, prognosis, and therapeutic approach for many small animal diseases. Sequential biopsy results may be useful in monitoring the response to therapy or progression of the disease process. In our experience the expanding use of gastrointestinal tract endoscopy has significantly increased the number of biopsy specimens for histologic review.

An inherent limitation of biopsy specimens obtained by endoscopic techniques is their small size. Pathologists now have the task of examining multiple, minute, often poorly oriented tissue specimens that are prone to a variety of handling and/or processing artifacts. This is particularly true of small intestinal biopsy specimens, which often contain only villus and superficial subvillus lamina propria for histologic evaluation. In addition, pathologists must be able to recognize the wide range of normal mucosal cellularity in intestinal mucosal biopsies. Furthermore, the interpretation of these specimens is often subjective (even for commonly diagnosed disorders such as inflammatory bowel disease) and relies heavily on the experience and bias of the individual pathologist. These considerations are important if a meaningful correlation of abnormal histology and intestinal function is to be made.

This chapter provides the following:

1. A brief discussion of practical matters relating to endoscopic biopsy
2. A summary of endoscopic accessories available to the clinician
3. Technical comments on the handling and processing of biopsy specimens
4. Succinct morphologic descriptions of disease entities diagnosed most often by endoscopic biopsy

Standardized terminology for describing endoscopic abnormalities and their correlation with histologic findings is also included. Emphasis is placed on the evaluation of biopsy specimens from the alimentary tract of dogs and cats.

## PRACTICAL CONSIDERATIONS FOR ENDOSCOPIC BIOPSY

Endoscopic examination with the procurement of biopsy specimens is very useful in the diagnosis of many gastrointestinal mucosal disorders. However, endoscopy merely serves as an *adjunctive* procedure, one that complements the information gained from a careful history, a thorough physical examination, and selected laboratory and radiographic studies. Endoscopic biopsy detects morphologic rather than functional disease. It does not detect abnormal gastrointestinal motility, gastrointestinal secretory disorders, and subcellular defects such as brush border enzyme deficiencies (Strombeck, Guilford, 1990a). A variety of clinical disorders characterized by primary or secondary gastrointestinal signs but no significant changes in tissue morphology are commonly encountered (Box 10-1).

For the veterinarian the decision to perform endoscopic biopsy is made after salient clinicopathologic parameters have been considered, and the procedure has been discussed with the client. Patient status, procedural time, costs, and inherent risks should all be considered. Once endoscopic biopsy is deemed appropriate, careful consideration should be given to the instrumentation needed for optimal specimen collection. For example, which organs are being sampled? Biopsy of the esophagus often requires a suction biopsy capsule instrument whereas mucosal biopsy of the stomach, small intestine, and colon is best performed with pinch biopsy forceps. Another consideration is the concept of focal versus diffuse mucosal disease. Localized lesions, including ulcers, solitary masses, and malignant strictures, require very precise and directed biopsy (often at the periphery of normal- and abnormal-appearing tissue) to confirm a diagnosis. In contrast, generalized mucosal disorders, such as inflammatory bowel disease, chronic gastritis, and diffuse

neoplasia, may be diagnosed with random biopsy specimens obtained from the affected organs. Lastly, the nature of the suspected lesion (e.g., superficial versus deep mucosal disease) influences not only instrument selection but also biopsy technique. Neoplastic lesions are best sampled deeply, often in the same site, to obtain diagnostic tissue. In these instances, superficial biopsy specimens should be avoided because such tissues contain necrotic surface debris and superficial cells that can obscure the correct diagnosis.

## DESCRIPTION OF THE MUCOSA

A thorough and systematic examination of mucosal structures should precede all biopsy procedures. (Excellent descriptive summaries of normal endoscopic mucosal examinations are provided elsewhere in this book.) Standard terminology is used to describe endoscopic abnormalities, including the size and location of intraluminal masses, strictures, and ulcers, as well as their association with normal structures. Additional criteria for mucosal assessment are listed in Box 10-2, (Roth et al, 1990a; Jergens, 1993).

Consistent endoscopic terminology has been proposed to aid in lesion description and the formulation of a definitive diagnosis (Leib, 1989). *Erythema* denotes mucosal redness, which may be the sign of a pathologic condition or a normal physiologic response to excessive insufflation or blood flow changes associated with anesthesia. *Friability* describes the ease with which the mucosa is damaged by contact with the endoscope or biopsy instrument. Alterations in surface texture are described as increased *granularity*. Granularity of the small intestinal mucosa may be influenced by gland height and crypt depth as the light of the endoscope reflects off these structures. (Roth et al, 1990a). *Mass lesions* are commonly seen with infiltrative mucosal dis-

---

| **Box 10-1** | Gastrointestinal Diseases Unaccompanied by Significant Histopathologic Lesions |
|---|---|

Motility abnormalities
Irritable bowel syndrome
Brush border defects
Intestinal bacterial overgrowth
Secretory diarrheas
Food intolerance
Permeability defects

---

| **Box 10-2** | Endoscopic Criteria for Mucosal Assessment |
|---|---|

Degree of erythema
Tissue friability
Mucosal granularity
Mass lesions
Erosions and ulcers
Stricture
Luminal distension
Visibility of submucosal vessels

eases (inflammatory disorders, malignant neoplasia, benign polyps) and may be pedunculated or sessile. As previously noted, masses should be biopsied deeply to avoid misdiagnosis. If diffuse neoplasia is suspected, multiple deep biopsy specimens should be obtained from both normal- and abnormal-appearing mucosa within the lamina propria.

Gastrointestinal *ulceration* or *erosion* is defined as an endoscopically visible breach in mucosal integrity associated with active hemorrhage. *Ulcers* are typically solitary, crateriform, well-circumscribed lesions that extend deeply into the mucosa and contain central fibrinous exudate. *Erosions* are discrete, superficial mucosal defects without raised margins or necrotic centers. Ulcers and erosions are characteristic of inflammatory and neoplastic lesions (Roth et al, 1990a; Jergens et al, 1992a). Erosive lesions should be biopsied directly. Ulcerative lesions are best biopsied by obtaining specimens from the ulcer rim where it comes into contact with adjacent tissue. Mucosal specimens from tissues surrounding an ulcer should also be procured to characterize benign from malignant ulcer disease. Figure 10-1 highlights these abnormal endoscopic mucosal appearances.

Miscellaneous endoscopic observations should also be noted. Inadequate distension following air insufflation may be seen with extraluminal compression, strictures, infiltrative diseases, and severe fibrosis secondary to chronic inflammation. Normal submucosal blood vessels may not be visualized because of mucosal edema, the accumulation of exudate (blood, mucus, necrotic debris), and the infiltration of inflammatory or neoplastic cells. Gross pitting of the duodenal mucosa has been associated with acute *Giardia* infection in the dog (Leib, 1989). A characteristic milky-white appearance to the mucosa or a milky exudate within the intestinal lumen may be seen in dogs with lymphangiectasia. In all instances, mucosal abnormalities should be observed as the endoscope is advanced *forward* to avoid misinterpretation as a result of operator-induced trauma. A written description of the endoscopic observations should be recorded on an endoscopy procedure form or directly into the medical record itself. Videotaped or photographic records may also be kept.

## INSTRUMENTATION FOR SPECIMEN COLLECTION

The selection of appropriate biopsy instrumentation is influenced by the type of endoscope used (rigid versus flexible) and the range of equipment available for specimen collection. Practical endoscopic accessories include pinch biopsy forceps, suction biopsy capsule, cytology brushes, and aspiration catheters for acquiring duodenal fluid. In most clinical situations, mucosal biopsy specimens obtained using flexible endoscopic techniques are required for definitive diagnosis. The relative merits of endoscopic accessories are discussed in the following sections.

## Pinch Biopsy Forceps

Pinch forceps are most commonly used to obtain representative mucosal specimens from the gastrointestinal tract. These small, flexible forceps with opposing 2- to 3-mm cups on their distal end are passed through the operating channel of the endoscope. Biopsy cups may be smooth or serrated, standard or fenestrated, and they may come with or without a central needle (Figure 10-2). Fenestrated forceps are reported to cause less crush artifact and yield larger biopsy specimens than nonfenestrated models (Golden, 1993). Forceps with a central needle may be helpful in "seating" biopsy cups in the mucosa of narrow tubular organs such as the esophagus and small intestine. Both multiple-use and disposable forceps provide directed mucosal biopsy under endoscopic guidance. Six to 10 tissue specimens from each organ are generally adequate for histologic review. Specimens containing epithelium and superficial lamina propria are procured with pinch forceps by means of tissue avulsion (Figure 10-3).

The technique for obtaining biopsy specimens using pinch forceps is similar in all regions of the gastrointestinal tract. The procedure may be performed by a single endoscopist; alternatively an assistant may open and close the biopsy jaws as instructed by the endoscopist. If possible the endoscope tip is positioned directly in front of and perpendicular to the area to be biopsied (Figure 10-4). (This may not be possible in small feline patients with narrow lumens that limit endoscopic maneuverability.) The pinch biopsy instrument is passed through the operating channel and extended beyond the tip of the endoscope, the jaws are opened, and the instrument is advanced into the mucosa using forward pressure. Larger, deeper, and more diagnostically significant specimens are obtained by applying pressure at the time of biopsy (Danesh et al, 1985). Larger forceps also yield better quality specimens. Adequate forward pressure is evidenced by displacement of the tissue away from the endoscope and gentle "bowing" of the biopsy instrument shaft. The jaws of the forceps are then closed firmly, the instrument is retracted to the endoscope tip, and a firm steady tug is then used to tear a tissue sample free. The forceps instrument is withdrawn from the operating channel, and the tissue specimen is carefully removed from the open jaws of the forceps for processing. Specimens may also be used to make touch imprints for cytologic evaluation.

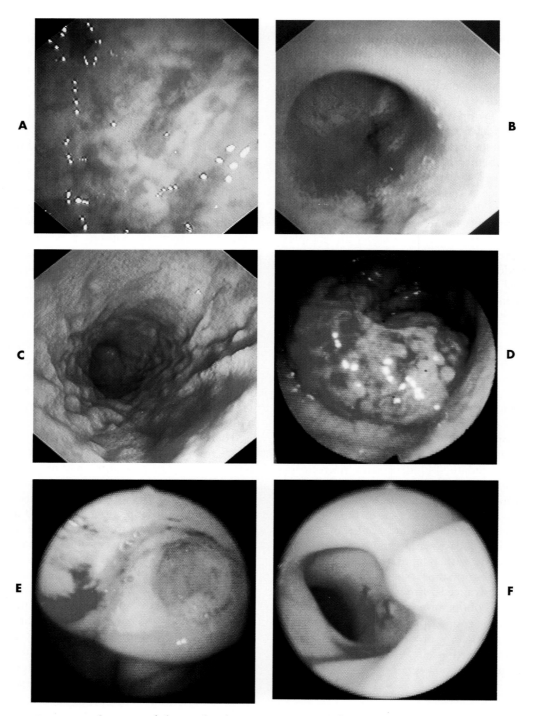

**Figure 10-1** Spectrum of abnormal endoscopic appearances of mucosa in dogs and cats. **A,** *Erythema:* patchy gastric mucosal erythema in a 6-year-old Yorkshire terrier. **B,** *Friability:* increased hemorrhage from the duodenal mucosa after endoscopic biopsy in a 2-year-old Maltese. **C,** Granularity: marked mucosal irregularity of the duodenum in a 6-year-old mixed-breed dog. **D,** *Mass:* large focal granuloma in the descending colon of a 7-year-old domestic longhair cat. **E,** *Ulcer:* focal ulcer along the angulus in a 2-year-old setter mix. **F,** *Erosions:* multiple linear erosive lesions along the lateral duodenal mucosa in a cat with eosinophilic enteritis. (Courtesy Claire Andreason, Ames, Iowa.)

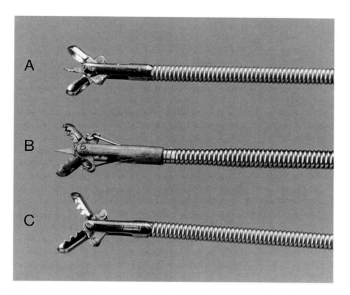

**Figure 10-2** Biopsy cups with pinch forceps. Standard forceps with a central needle (**A**), serrated-jaw forceps with a central needle (**B**), and serrated-jaw forceps without a central needle. (From Jergens AE: Gastrointestinal endoscopic biopsy techniques. In August JR, editor: *Consultations in feline internal medicine*, ed 3, Philadelphia, 1997, WB Saunders.)

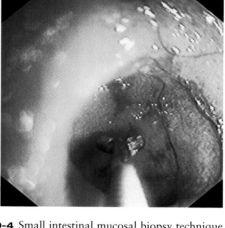

**Figure 10-4** Small intestinal mucosal biopsy technique using pinch forceps. Note the perpendicular placement of biopsy forceps at an intestinal flexure site.

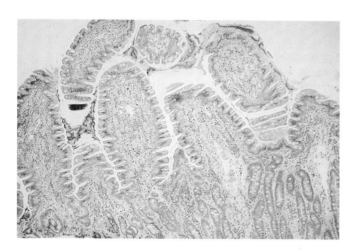

**Figure 10-3** Small intestinal biopsy specimen procured with pinch forceps from a healthy dog. Note the excellent quality of this specimen, as evidenced by numerous intact villi, perpendicular orientation of crypts to surface epithelium, and inclusion of deeper lamina propria tissue (hematoxylin-eosin stain).

## Suction Biopsy Capsule

The Multipurpose Suction Biopsy Instrument (Quinton Instrument Co., Seattle, Wash.) allows relatively large mucosal specimens to be obtained safely and rapidly from accessible regions of the gastrointestinal tract (Figure 10-5). Although the instrument is most commonly used for nondirected biopsy of the esophagus and descending colon, it may also be positioned under endo-scopic guidance. This biopsy instrument employs negative pressure, applied by the operator using a syringe and measured by a vacuum gauge, to pull mucosa into the biopsy capsule where a blade cuts the tissue sample. The instrument is removed from the patient, the capsule is opened, and the biopsy specimen is retrieved from the blade apparatus. Tissue samples obtained by suction biopsy techniques typically contain full-thickness mucosa, including the muscularis mucosae (Figure 10-6). The Quinton biopsy instrument is no longer manufactured, but used instruments may be obtained from some endoscopic equipment retailers.

## Cytology Brushes and Catheters

Disposable guarded cytology brushes are useful for obtaining cell specimens. These brushes are passed through the endoscope's operating channel under direct guidance and are protected from contamination by an outer sheath (Figure 10-7). Once the area to be sampled is identified, the brush is extended from its sheath, rubbed vigorously against the mucosa or surface of the lesion, and then retracted into the operating channel. Next the brush cytology instrument is removed from the endoscope. Superficial cells and cellular debris are then rolled or rubbed on microscopic slides, air dried, stained with a Giemsa-type stain (Diff-Quik); and examined microscopically for evidence of inflammation, neoplasia, or infectious agents (Jones, 1990). Alternatively, touch cytology may be performed by transferring a mucosal

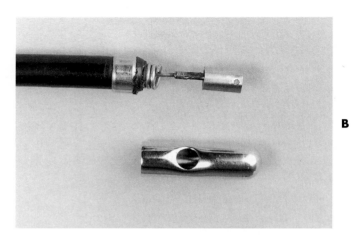

**Figure 10-5 A,** Multipurpose Suction Biopsy Instrument (Quinton Instrument Co., Seattle, Wash.) assembled and ready for use. Components include operating handle with pull wire attached *(A)*, vacuum gauge for recording pressure *(B)*, flexible tubing enclosing the pull wire and connecting to the biopsy capsule *(C)*, and biopsy capsule *(D)*. **B,** Close-up of opened biopsy capsule with exposed blade apparatus. (From Jergens AE: Gastrointestinal endoscopic biopsy techniques. In August JR, editor: *Consultations in feline internal medicine,* ed 3, Philadelphia, 1997, WB Saunders.)

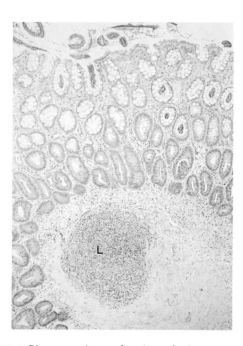

**Figure 10-6** Biopsy specimen of canine colonic mucosa obtained with a suction biopsy instrument. Note that full-thickness mucosa and underlying muscularis mucosa have been procured. A lymphoid aggregate *(L)* is also present (hematoxylin-eosin stain).

specimen from the biopsy forceps to a glass slide with a needle and then gently touching the specimen onto the slide so that a cytologic imprint is obtained.

Recent studies in humans have confirmed the clinical utility of brush cytologic samples in the diagnosis of upper gastrointestinal malignancies and infections. (Behmard,

Sadeghi, Bagheri, 1978; Shroff, Nanivadekar, 1988; Debongie et al, 1994). Endoscopic exfoliative cytology is simple to perform, is less invasive than biopsy, and provides a rapid diagnosis. The paucity of published data describing the use of endoscopically obtained cytologic samples in small animal is noteworthy. One small study reported good correlation of cytologic and histopathologic findings in 55 dogs diagnosed with benign mucosal inflammation and lymphoid malignancy involving the duodenum (Tobey, Willard, Krehbiel, 1988). Unfortunately, comparative data for gastric and colonic specimens were not reported.

In a more extensive investigation, brush and touch cytologic specimens were obtained by endoscopic examination of the stomach (n = 49), small intestine (n = 47), and colon (n = 18) in 44 dogs and 14 cats (Jergens, Andreasen, Hagemoser, 1997). All cytologic smears were blindly reviewed and objectively graded for inflammatory cellularity, cellular atypia, bacterial organisms, hemorrhage, and background mucus and debris. In each case a cytologic diagnosis was rendered and compared with the histologic findings. Excellent correlation was observed. For detecting abnormalities, the examination of endoscopically obtained cytologic specimens was found to have a sensitivity and specificity of, respectively, 100% and 92% for the stomach, 93% and 93% for the small intestine, and 88% and 88% for the colon. A similar diagnosis was made for both cytologic and histologic specimens determined to be normal or to have lymphocytic-plasmacytic inflammation, mixed inflammation, eosinophic inflammation, and lymphoid malignancy (Figure 10-8). Brush cytology was most useful in detect-

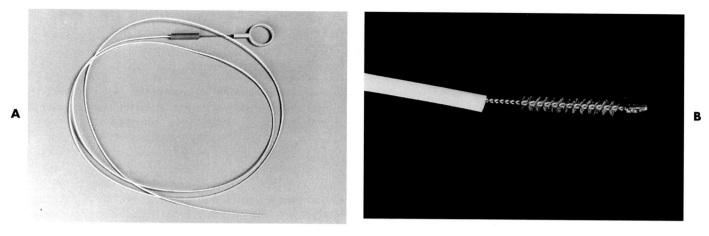

**Figure 10-7 A,** Disposable guarded cytology brush. **B,** Close-up of brush extended beyond its protective sheath.

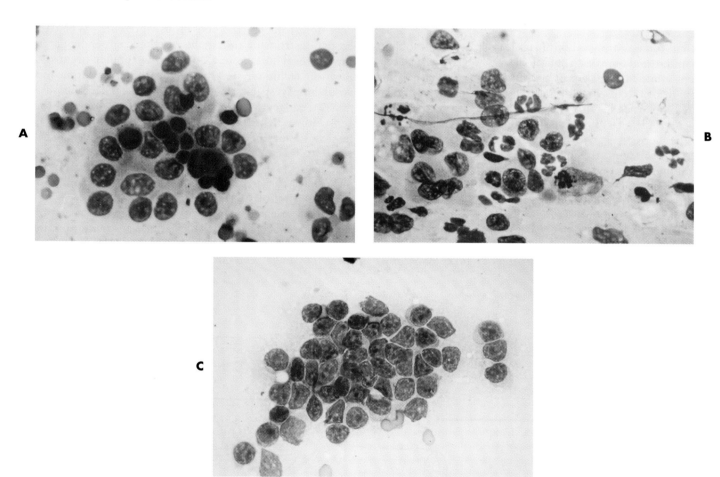

**Figure 10-8** Gastrointestinal endoscopic exfoliative cytology preparations. **A,** Brush cytologic specimen obtained from the small intestine of a dog with moderate (grade 5 to 6) lymphocytic enteritis. Note the numerous small lymphocytes embedded within the duodenal epithelia. **B,** Touch cytologic specimen obtained from the small intestine of a dog with moderate (grade 5 to 6) suppurative enteritis. Numerous neutrophils and occasional eosinophils have infiltrated the duodenal epithelia. **C,** Brush cytologic specimen obtained from the duodenum of a cat with alimentary lymphosarcoma. Note the fairly homogenous population of medium-sized lymphoblasts with multiple and prominent nucleoli. A Giemsa-type stain (Diff-Quik) was used on all specimens.

ing lamina propria cellular infiltrates; touch cytology was more likely to detect acute mucosal inflammation as evidenced by increased numbers of neutrophils. These results indicate that exfoliative cytology is a useful and reliable adjunct to endoscopic biopsy. Nevertheless, endoscopic cytology is probably underutilized as a diagnostic tool for primary gastrointestinal disease.

Catheters may be used to aspirate duodenal fluid. This fluid may then be examined for *Giardia* trophozoites (Pitts, Twedt, Mallie, 1983) or cultured in patients with suspected intestinal bacterial overgrowth. For example, sterile, disposable 4.5-French (1.52-mm outer diameter) polyethylene tubing (Intramedic Polyethylene Tubing, Becton, Dickinson & Co., Parsippany, N.Y.) may be passed through the operating channel of the endoscope to collect duodenal contents.

## Rigid Forceps

Rigid forceps are used with rigid proctoscopes to obtain semidirected biopsies from the descending colon. The forceps come in a variety of styles that differ mainly in the length of the instrument and the type and angulation of the biopsy head. With jaws open the rigid forceps instrument is advanced through the endoscope, and the mucosa to be biopsied is gently grasped. Light backward traction is used to "tent" the mucosa away from the submucosa, and the mucosa is out as the forceps jaws are closed.

The risk of colonic perforation is increased when rigid forceps are used. Furthermore these rigid instruments can obtain tissue specimens from only the distal colon. Their routine use by inexperienced operators in the procurement of colonic biopsy specimens is *not* recommended. (See Chapter 7 for further discussion of rigid colonoscopy.)

## TECHNICAL CONSIDERATIONS FOR ENDOSCOPIC BIOPSY

### General Comments

Endoscopists commonly obtain six or more directed biopsy specimens when a mucosal lesion is discovered on endoscopic examination. Even when no gross mucosal abnormalities are observed, multiple random specimens should be submitted from each area sampled to avoid submitting specimens that are inadequate for complete microscopic evaluation. This practice enhances the likelihood that several areas of mucosa will be available for histopathologic review. The morphologic information that can be obtained from such evaluation depends on the depth of the tissue, the total volume of tissue obtained, and the orientation of the biopsy specimen. As previously noted, specimen quality is significantly influenced by forceps size and biopsy pressure. When the biopsy instrument cannot be oriented perpendicular to the mucosal surface (e.g., in narrow tubular organs), a push-off technique may be used to obtain a larger mucosal biopsy specimen (Gowen, 1986). The mucosa is grasped tangential to the mucosal surface, and the forceps biopsy instrument (or the endoscope with forceps held stationary in place) is then advanced 4 to 5 cm aborally to tear off a strip of tissue from the mucosal surface (Figure 10-9). Samples obtained with this technique are usually larger but not as deep as those obtained by avulsion (pull-off) techniques.

Proper orientation of biopsy specimens is as important as specimen size. To achieve the best orientation, the pathologist or a technician manipulates the specimens after they have been embedded in paraffin. Paraffin em-

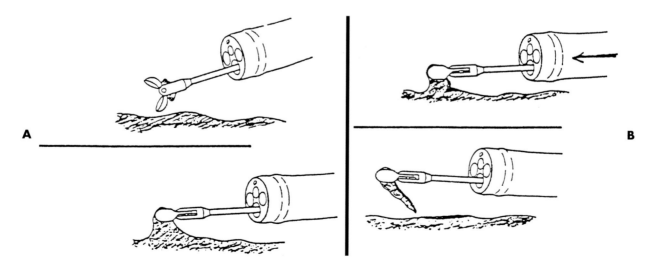

**Figure 10-9** Push-off technique for procuring larger mucosal biopsy specimens. **A,** A pinch biopsy forceps positioned tangentially to the mucosal surface. **B,** The instrument advanced aborally to tear off a linear strip of mucosa. (From McGowen GF: An improved technique of endoscopic biopsy in the upper gastrointestinal tract, *Gastrointest Endosc* 32:59, 1986.)

bedding of each biopsy specimen *singularly* also increases the likelihood that at least several tissues will be suitably oriented for microscopic examination. Serial sections placed in several rows on a single slide are then evaluated. With careful orientation, expert serial sectioning, and the avoidance or recognition of mechanical artifacts yield biopsy specimens of consistent quality that correlate well with the mucosal appearance in vivo.

## Biopsy Specimen Handling

Endoscopic biopsy specimens are small, fragile pieces of tissue that are subject to extensive handling and processing artifact from the moment of collection to the microtome sectioning of the paraffin-embedded tissue. The artifactual changes can be minimized if special care is exercised in procuring and handling the specimen once it is obtained by the biopsy forceps. The fresh specimen should be gently teased from the forceps with a needle and placed on lens paper, cucumber slice, or specially designed biopsy sponge presoaked in formalin. Commercial cassettes with precut "sponges" can be used for the submission of endoscopic biopsy specimens (Figure 10-10). Multiple biopsy specimens can be placed on a sponge. The sponge is then covered with a second formalin-wetted sponge to form a "sandwich," and the sponges are placed directly in the cassette. The entire cassette is immersed in 10% buffered formalin for submission to the laboratory.

Alternatively, cucumber slices can be an excellent medium for the submission of endoscopic biopsy specimens. Mucosal biopsy tissue samples are placed on thin slices of cucumber (preserved in alcohol), which are then deposited in formalin containers and submitted for processing (Figure 10-11). At the laboratory the cucumber slices are removed from the formalin. Then smaller cucumber sections containing one to three biopsy specimens are trimmed away and placed on their side in the processing cassette (e.g., perpendicular to the cassette surface to optimize tissue orientation after sectioning), and the tissues are embedded in paraffin. The specimens do not have to be removed from the cucumber slices prior to embedding because the microtome can readily cut through the vegetable material. This technique minimizes specimen handling at the laboratory and consistently yields well-oriented tissues of high diagnostic quality. The cucumber technique works best for institutions with an in-house pathology service. The protocol for the preparation of cucumber slices is presented in Box 10-3.

Attempts to *reorient* specimens on biopsy sponges or cucumber slices prior to formalin fixation should be *avoided*. Specimens should not be allowed to "sit" on cucumber or sponge surfaces for extended periods because air drying contributes to tissue artifact. In addition, the exposed samples may adhere tightly to the sponge or cucumber and thus may be damaged when later removed by the pathology service. Samples from specific sites (e.g., stomach, duodenum, colon) should be placed in *separate containers* and *appropriately labeled*. The endoscopist should note the number of specimens obtained from each site, relevant endoscopic observations, and salient historical and clinical data on the *histopathology form*.

## Tissue Artifacts

A variety of artifacts may interfere with the accurate interpretation of endoscopic biopsy specimens. In formalin

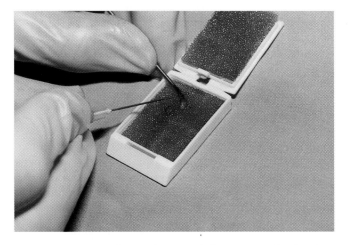

**Figure 10-10** Use of a needle to carefully remove a duodenal biopsy specimen from pinch forceps. Multiple specimens are then placed on formalin-soaked biopsy sponges. (From Jergens AE: Gastrointestinal endoscopic biopsy techniques. In August JR, editor: Consultations in feline internal medicine, ed 3, Philadelphia, 1997, WB Saunders.)

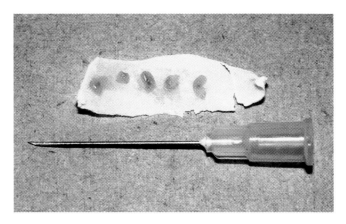

**Figure 10-11** Multiple gastric biopsy specimens may be placed on cucumber slices prior to tissue processing. This minimizes specimen handling at the pathology laboratory.

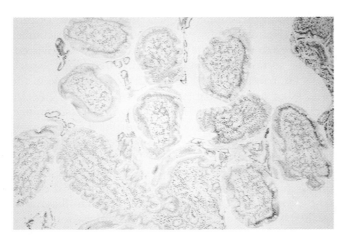

**Figure 10-12** Poor-quality small intestinal biopsy specimen. Note that the specimen consists of villus tips only, without underlying subvillus lamina propria and associated structures. This type of tissue artifact may be caused by poor biopsy technique or a specimen rolling over during fixation. (hematoxylin-eosin stain).

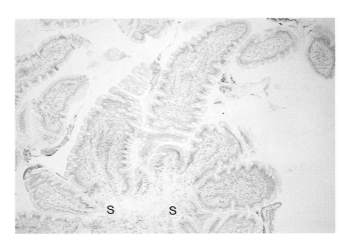

**Figure 10-13** Small intestinal tissue sample showing significant squeeze artifact at the base of specimen *(S)*. Artifacts of this type are sometimes difficult to avoid, even with good biopsy technique (hematoxylin-eosin stain).

---

**Box 10-3   Cucumber Paper Preparation**

1. Slice a firm cucumber as thinly as possible, avoiding seed areas.
2. Place cucumber slices in 95% ethanol for 3 days; change ethanol daily.
3. Then store the cucumber slices in 95% ethanol in a refrigerator.
4. Blot excess ethanol from the surface of a cucumber slice before placing biopsy tissue on the "cucumber paper," leaving the villi (or surface epithelia) pointed upward.
5. Do not allow the cucumber slices to dry out completely; biopsy specimens adhere less well to dry cucumber and may float off in formalin.

From Swan RW, Davis HJ: The biopsy-cucumber unit, *Obstet Gynecol* 36:803, 1970.

the mucosa of the gastrointestinal biopsy has a tendency to roll over the submucosa, making precise orientation of the specimens difficult. Multiple samples are embedded in the same paraffin block, and 6 μm sections are shaved from the block until the section obtained represents the largest specimen of each of the tissues. Many of the sections are oblique, and if the mucosa has significant rollover artifact, the surface of some specimens may be the only tissue available for microscopic examination. Hence some small intestinal biopsy sections may consist of villi only (Figure 10-12). In these instances it is not possible to evaluate the subvillus lamina propria with its comple-

ment of mucosal glands (e.g., crypts) and proprial cellular populations. Other sections may be devoid of surface epithelium, creating the false impression of an ulcer.

Squeeze artifacts created at the margins of biopsy specimens (Figure 10-13) are evidenced by the "telescoping" of mucosal glands, the expression of mucosal glands from underlying lamina propria into the area of the lumen, and the "streaming" of chromatin. To some extent these changes are unavoidable. Good biopsy technique (especially avoiding rapid closure of the biopsy forceps during tissue procurement) and gentle handling of specimens after biopsy can minimize the effects of these artifacts. *Streaming chromatin artifact is enhanced in tissues with malignant lymphoma. If lymphoma is the suspected diagnosis, the endoscopist should be particularly gentle with the specimen prior to fixation, and additional samples of the suspect lesion should be obtained to maximize the chance that a diagnostic specimen is procured.*

## Tissue Fixation and Stains

Fixation in 10% neutral buffered formalin is adequate for routine histologic examination of biopsy specimens. Glutaraldehyde fixation is optimal for specimens that are to be examined by electron microscopy. Immunohistochemical studies of certain antigens may require tissue that has been snap frozen in liquid nitrogen or preserved in fixatives other than formalin (e.g., alcohol).

Standard tissue-staining methods using hematoxylin and eosin provide excellent tissue detail for routine microscopic examination. Special stains may be used to highlight certain infectious agents. A variety of silver im-

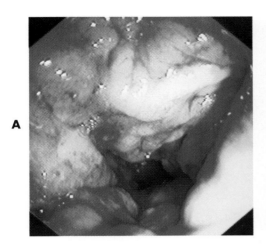
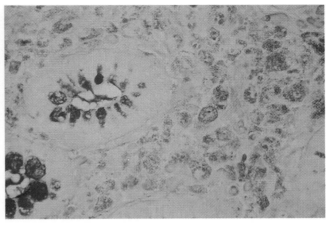

**Figure 10-14 A,** Histiocytic ulcerative colitis in a 7-month-old boxer with hematochezia. The colonic mucosa displays marked granularity, and the colonic wall is poorly distensible.
**B,** Colonic biopsy specimen showing a diffuse infiltrate of foamy macrophages within the lamina propria. Within their cytoplasm the macrophages contain material that is positive (purple) for periodic acid–Schiff (PAS) stain.

pregnation methods and Giemsa staining have been employed to identify *Helicobacter* organisms in gastric biopsy specimens.* The fluorescent, acridine orange dye can also be used for this purpose. Fungi can be identified in sections stained with periodic acid–Schiff reagents (PAS) or evaluated by silver techniques (e.g., Gomori's methanamine silver stain). Bacteria can be assessed in Gram-stained sections of tissue. Finally, PAS stain highlights colonic mucus and histiocytes in histiocytic ulcerative colitis of boxer dogs (Figure 10-14).

Immunoperoxidase methods have been applied to endoscopic biopsy tissues for a variety of purposes. Antibodies to intermediate filaments may be useful in determining the cell of origin for some gastrointestinal tumors. Immunoglobulin and lymphocyte antibodies have been used to identify cellular populations in normal dogs and in dogs with gastrointestinal inflammation, including inflammatory bowel disease (Figure 10-15), (Jergens et al, 1996a).

## CORRELATION OF ENDOSCOPIC AND PATHOLOGIC FINDINGS

The premise for recommending endoscopic biopsy is that histopathologic examination of tissue specimens will hopefully confirm a specific diagnosis, thereby facilitating therapy for the animal's clinical signs. Endoscopy allows direct mucosal visualization and the opportunity to acquire targeted biopsy specimens from grossly ab-

*Weber, Hasa, Sautter, 1958, Radin et al, 1990; Handt et al, 1991; Heilmann, Borchard, 1991; Lee et al, 1992; Otto et al, 1994.

normal tissues. The clinical significance of endoscopic observations and their correlation with histologic findings has been the subject of recent investigations. One investigation found that approximately two thirds of cases with endoscopic lesions had histologic abnormalities, including inflammatory infiltrates (Roth et al, 1990a). Excess mucosal granularity and friability were associated with histologic abnormalities in 82% of cases. In the absence of other endoscopic findings, mucosal erythema held the least predictive value for histologic abnormality in this study. A separate report similarly found mucosal lesions (granularity, friability, erosions or ulcers) during endoscopy in 52% of dogs and 42% of cats with the histologic infiltrates of inflammatory bowel disease (Jergens et al, 1992b). Mucosal erythema was frequently observed in these animals but may have been influenced by physiologic mechanisms or the effects of anesthesia.

Endoscopic observations do *not* always correlate with histopathologic findings. In one study, 96.5% (56 of 58) tissues assessed as normal endoscopically were microscopically normal, but up to 26.8% of tissues assessed as abnormal endoscopically were also microscopically normal (Roth et al, 1990a). Possible reasons for endoscopic-microscopic discordance include the failure to obtain representative biopsy tissue, the presence of artifactually induced lesions, the failure to recognize histologic lesions and the inability to distinguish mild histologic changes from normal tissue (Roth et al, 1990a; van der Gaag, 1994). Obvious clinical signs are frequently present in animals lacking both endoscopic and histologic abnormalities. These patients may have functional defects such as motility disturbances, secretory diarrheas, and permeability defects (Hall, 1994).

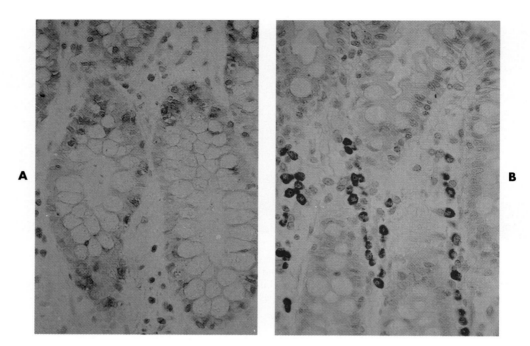

**Figure 10-15** Immunohistochemical stains of canine colonic biopsy specimens. **A,** Specimen from a healthy dog stained for pan-T (CD3) antigen. The numerous positive-staining T cells within the epithelium of the colonic glands are intraepithelial lymphocytes. **B,** Specimen from a dog with inflammatory bowel disease, stained for cells that contain immunoglobulin A (IgA). Note the intense eosinophilic intracytoplasmic staining and the tendency of these IgA cells to reside as cords of cells within the colonic lamina propria.

## DIAGNOSTIC UTILITY OF ENDOSCOPIC BIOPSY

Gastrointestinal endoscopy is an excellent means for examining the esophageal, gastric, duodenal, jejunal (depending on patient size and endoscopic length), colonic, and rectal mucosa. Mural lesions in these sites and mucosal and mural lesions of the distal duodenum and jejunum are inaccessible by this technique. Alternatively, ileal mucosa may be biopsied via retrograde ileoscopy when diffuse intestinal disease is suspected or adequate proximal intestinal biopsies cannot be obtained. Gastrointestinal endoscopy with the procurement of biopsy specimens is particularly well suited for diagnosing mucosal inflammatory lesions, determining the causes of gastrointestinal ulceration or erosion, and detecting alimentary tract neoplasia.

### Noninfectious Inflammatory Lesions

Inflammatory lesions are found in the majority of endoscopic biopsy specimens. If infectious agents, protozoa; or nematodes are documented in animals with these microscopic lesions, the inflammatory changes are attributed to the identified pathogen. However, similar lesions found unassociated with a defined cause are often at-

tributed to inflammatory bowel disease.* Inflammatory bowel disease is a clinical syndrome characterized by chronic gastrointestinal signs in which clinical signs often resolve with dietary and antiinflammatory treatment. Inflammatory bowel disease in dogs and cats most likely encompasses disease processes that have diverse causes but have in common gastrointestinal symptoms and inflammatory lesions apparent in endoscopic biopsy specimens.

The *microscopic* findings in *inflammatory bowel disease* consist of minimal to pronounced cellular infiltrate of the stomach and intestine accompanied by mucosal epithelial and glandular immaturity and varying degrees of mucosal architectural disruption. No standard microscopic grading system has been established for the lesions in inflammatory bowel disease. We use a grading system based on the extent of architectural disruption and mucosal epithelial changes (Jergens et al, 1992a, 1992b, 1996a). The severity of the lesion grade by this system is inconsistent with the extent of clinical signs, but the grading scheme may be less subject to interobserver variation. In our gradation

*Hayden, Van Kruiningen, 1982; Tams, 1986; Tams 1989; Jacobs et al, 1990; Strombeck, Guilford, 1990b; Roth et al 1990b; Feinstein, Olsson, 1992, Jergens et al, 1992b.

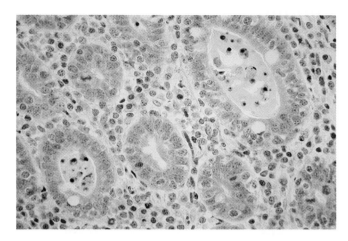

**Figure 10-16** Severe inflammatory bowel disease in the small intestine of a dog. Lymphocytic, plasmacytic cellular infiltrates are accompanied by marked epithelial and glandular alterations. Note that multiple crypts are dilated and contain proteinaceous and degenerate cellular debris (hematoxylin-eosin stain).

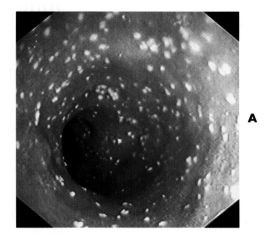

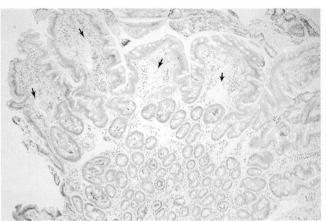

**Figure 10-17** Intestinal lymphangiectasia in a 14-year-old Afghan hound. **A,** Endoscopic appearance of the proximal duodenal mucosa. Note the miliary, raised white structures present along the duodenal mucosal surface. These structures are grossly dilated central lacteals filled with chylomicron-rich material. **B,** Duodenal biopsy specimen from the same dog. Note the shortened intestinal villi, which contain dilated central lacteals *(arrows)*. Mild lymphocytic, plasmacytic infiltration and edema within the lamina propria are also present (hematoxylin-eosin stain).

scheme, *mild* lesions are those with no mucosal architectural disruption, glandular necrosis, immaturity, or fibrosis of the lamina propria. *Severe* inflammatory bowel disease is manifested by architectural distortion of the mucosa (e.g., extensive ulceration, necrosis, and glandular loss or severe glandular hyperplasia or fibrosis of the lamina propria [Figure 10-16]). *Moderate* lesions have microscopic changes of severity between the two extremes. Note that in this grading scheme no attempt is made to quantitate the number of inflammatory cells within the lamina propria. Rather, inflammatory cell types are included in the pathologist's report using standard classification schemes, including lymphocytic-plasmacytic, eosinophilic, suppurative, and granulomatous enterocolitis based on the predominance of the cells present. In our experience, neutrophils are often observed in inflammatory bowel disease lesions of the feline colon. Globule leukocytes are also commonly observed in these lesions in cats but less frequently in dogs. The reason for these apparent species differences remains undetermined.

The utility of this grading scheme may be the consistency of the observations between pathologists. Gradation of lesions by this and other methods has shown poor correlation between microscopic lesions and the severity of clinical signs. In addition, more detailed quantitative assessment of lamina proprial inflammatory cells in cases of inflammatory bowel disease by morphometric analysis has not defined categories of microscopic lesions that can predict the clinical severity of disease or the likely response to therapy. Inflammatory bowel disease largely remains a diagnosis of exclusion that is substantiated by the remission of gastrointestinal signs in response to appropriate medical therapy.

Endoscopy can be useful in documenting cases of intestinal lymphangiectasia associated with protein-losing enteropathy. The most severe lesions of this disorder frequently involve the jejunum and therefore are often inaccessible to endoscopic procedures. However, lacteal dilation, one of the key microscopic lesions of protein-losing enteropathy, may be observed in the duodenum of affected animals (Figure 10-17). The extent of lacteal dilation seen with this disorder is generally more severe than that seen with inflammatory bowel disease unassociated with protein-losing enteropathy. Ruptured lacteals and serosal lymphatics with associated lipogranulomatous mucosal and serosal enteritis are other hallmarks of protein-losing enteropathy.

## Infectious Inflammatory Lesions

Viral diseases often involve the digestive tract of small animals, but the diagnosis of these infections is seldom based on an assessment of endoscopic biopsy specimens. Canine and feline parvoviral enteritis is characterized by severe architectural disruption of the small intestinal mucosa with loss of mucosal glands and villi and regeneration of the remaining glands. Rarely, intranuclear viral inclusions are seen. Dogs with distemper may have intracytoplasmic and intranuclear inclusions within gastric and intestinal mucosa. Distemper inclusions may be found unassociated with mucosal damage.

With the exception of *Salmonella* organisms (Ikeda et al, 1986; Dow et al 1989) and *Campylobacter* organisms (Blaser et al, 1980; Fox, Krakowka, Taylor, 1985; Fox, Claps, Beaucage, 1986; Fox et al, 1988), pathogenic bacteria are infrequently documented causes of gastroenteritis in small animals. Small intestinal bacterial overgrowth may be associated with enteritis and is often found secondary to exocrine pancreatic insufficiency. Bacterial overgrowth does not result in specific histologic lesions, and a definitive diagnosis is only made after duodenal fluids have been cultured. Enteritis associated with adherent gram-positive cocci (identified in one case as *Streptococcus durans*) has been noted in two dogs in which the organisms were found in close association with villus epithelium in endoscopic biopsy specimens (Jergens et al, 1991).

Significant attention has recently been given to *Helicobacter* species as a cause of gastritis in dogs and cats.[*] The pathogenicity of gastric *Helicobacter* infection is controversial. Part of the confusion is the recent taxonomic recategorization of *Gastrospirillum* species as *Helicobacter heilmannii*. *Gastrospirillum* species are recognized as normal gastric flora in many species, including dogs and cats. The significance of these bacteria in gastric biopsy specimens is disputable. Some authors have suggested a causal relationship between *H. heilmannii* and gastritis in dogs and have compared the disease to *Helicobacter pylori*-associated gastritis in humans. The pathogenicity of *H. heilmannii* in dogs and cats remains to be proved. *Helicobacter felis*, which is morphologically distinct from *H. heilmannii*, has also been associated with gastritis in cats and dogs. The problem in determining the significance of *Helicobacter* in gastric biopsy specimens in dogs and cats is in distinguishing the normal resident *Helicobacter* organisms from those of pathologic significance. Quantitation of the organisms is difficult *(H. felis)* or impossible *(H. heilmannii)*. The pathogenicity of *H. heilmannii* has been inferred based

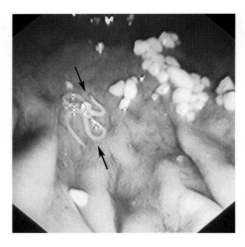

**Figure 10-18** Multiple *Physaloptera* nematodes *(arrows)* lying on the gastric mucosa in a dog. These nematodes may cause the chronic vomiting and histologic lesions of lymphocytic, plasmacytic gastritis.

on the response of clinical signs to antibacterial therapy. Current research may elucidate the role of *Helicobacter* organisms in the pathogenesis of gastritis in dogs and cats.

Intestinal coccidiosis is predominately an infection of puppies and kittens. Cryptosporidiosis has been rarely found, except in immunosuppressed animals or animals that are stressed with concurrent disease problems (Green, Jacobs, Prickett, 1984; Kukushuma, Helman, 1984; Turnwald et al, 1988). However, it is now being identified more often as animals with diarrhea are routinely being tested for this parasite. Some of the nematodes that infect dogs and cats may be found on endoscopic examination (Figure 10-18). Fungal infections are uncommonly diagnosed in endoscopic biopsy specimens of the gastrointestinal tract. Rare cases of phycomycosis in the stomach and histoplasmosis and cryptococcosis of the intestines have been observed in our experience. On rare occasions, prototheca may also be found within intestinal biopsy specimens from dogs with chronic gastrointestinal signs.

## Gastrointestinal Ulceration or Erosion

Gastrointestinal ulceration or erosion may be associated with a variety of primary digestive and systemic disorders. In our experience the most common causes are gastrointestinal neoplasia, nonsteroidal antiinflammatory drugs, and inflammatory bowel disease. In general, gastrointestinal erosion or ulceration is seen more frequently in dogs than in cats. Erosive lesions are more common than ulcers, and both ulcerations and erosions occur more often in the antral and pyloric regions of the stomach than in the proximal intestine (Figure 10-19).

[*]Weber, Hasa, Sautter, 1958; Radin et al, 1990; Heilmann, Borchard, 1991; Lee et al., 1992; Handt et al., 1994; Otto et al, 1994; De Novo, Magne, 1995; Magne, 1995.

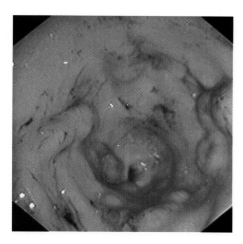

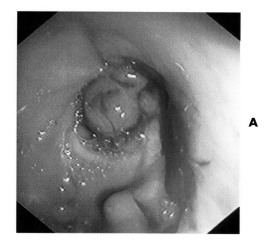

**Figure 10-19** Multiple gastric erosions observed in the antrum of a 12-year-old miniature schnauzer with a history of chronic vomiting. Note the linear appearance and superficial nature of these mucosal defects.

Ulcers vary in microscopic appearance, depending on their aggression and stage of development. Acute gastric lesions begin as erosions with superficial necrotic debris, neutrophilic infiltrates, and loss of mucosal architecture. More chronic ulcers are characterized by a base and sides composed of granulation tissue of varying thickness and maturity that is intermingled with a mixed inflammatory cellular infiltrate and overlaid by necrotic surface debris. Excellent biopsy technique is required to differentiate *benign* from *malignant* causes of gastrointestinal ulcers and erosions. Biopsy samples should be obtained from the rim rather than the pit of the ulcer to avoid superficial inflammation and fibrinous exudate that may cloud diagnostic interpretation. Brush cytology is an extremely useful adjunct to histopathologic examination when alimentary neoplasia is suspected as the cause for gastrointestinal ulceration or erosion.

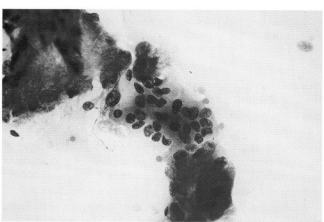

**Figure 10-20 A,** Large gastric polyp causing pyloric outflow obstruction and postprandial vomiting in a 12-year-old miniature poodle. **B,** Endoscopic brush cytology confirmed the presence of a homogenous population of benign epithelial cells suggestive of an adenomatous polyp. Surgical removal of the polyp was curative.

## Neoplasms

Gastrointestinal mucosal neoplasia can be diagnosed by endoscopy and biopsy. Gastric and intestinal polyps are commonly seen. Villous adenomatous polyps are found in the stomach and large bowel and frequently form pedunculated masses that project into the lumen, often "downstream" from the point of mucosal attachment (Figure 10-20). These lesions are characterized by mucosal glandular hyperplasia that is frequently accompanied by varying degrees of mucosal epithelial atypia, especially in large bowel polyps (Moulton, 1978). Invasion of the submucosa is the hallmark of malignancy in these lesions. Submucosal invasion is often difficult to determine because of disorientation of the biopsy specimens caused by their irregularity. Frequently the stalk cannot be thoroughly examined mi-croscopically to assess the completeness of excision. However, the majority of gastrointestinal polyps in small animals are benign.

Leiomyomas and leiomyosarcomas of the digestive tract are difficult to diagnose by endoscopic techniques. Because these tumors arise within the wall (e.g., tunica muscularis) of gastrointestinal organs, representative biopsy specimens are not routinely procured. However, leiomyosarcomas may be accompanied by overlying mucosal ulceration, and deep mucosal biopsy of the mass may be productive.

Gastrointestinal adenocarcinomas often ulcerate and induce reactive fibroplasia, resulting in stiff, noncompliant regions of the stomach or intestine (Figure 10-21). In cats, stricture is a common sequela of distal small intestinal adenocarcinoma (the *napkin-ring lesion*). Gastric carcinoma is often recognized by the effect of asso-

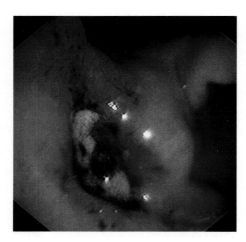

**Figure 10-21** Focal gastric ulceration along the angulus in an 11-year-old dog with adenocarcinoma. Multiple deep mucosal biopsies obtained with pinch forceps from the ulcer rim and adjacent gastric mucosa confirmed the diagnosis.

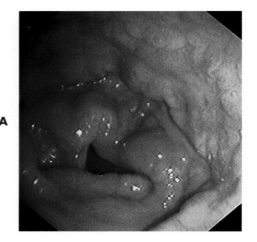

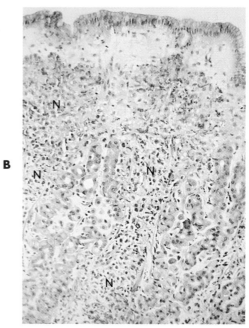

**Figure 10-22 A,** Lymphosarcoma involving the gastric antrum and pylorus in an 8-year-old Labrador retriever with chronic vomiting and weight loss. Note the severe granularity to the gastric mucosa. **B,** Gastric biopsy specimen showing cords of neoplastic lymphocytes *(N)* infiltrating within gastric mucosa. The gastric glands are greatly reduced in number (hematoxylin-eosin stain).

ciated desmoplasia on the pliability of the stomach. During gastroscopy and endoscopic biopsy the endoscopist may note a stiff, noncompliant feel to the gastric mucosa. In contrast, gastric lymphoma does not induce this fibroblastic reaction[45] (Moulton, 1978). Gastric carcinoma is rare in cats compared to dogs. Consequently, a large mucosal gastric mass in a cat is much more likely to be *lymphoma* than gastric carcinoma (see Plate 5-81).

Malignant lymphoma is the most common neoplastic condition of the gastrointestinal tract diagnosed by endoscopy (Figure 10-22). Low-grade, small, lymphocytic malignant lymphoma is common in older cats and may be difficult to distinguish from lymphocytic, plasmacytic enteritis (Mahony et al, 1995; Brodey, 1966; Carpenter, Andrews, Holzworth, 1987). Tissues infiltrated with malignant lymphoma tend to be fragile and prone to extensive squeeze artifact. *Multiple* biopsy specimens should be taken from any lesion suspicious for malignant lymphoma to maximize the chances of obtaining a specimen sufficiently free of artifact for evaluation. In contrast to the fibroblastic reaction seen in intestinal adenocarcinoma, malignant lymphoma causes a mass lesion that is often associated with dilated, ulcerated regions of the intestine and soft pliant lesions within the gastric mucosa. Mesenteric lymph nodes are often infiltrated with malignant lymphoma, as are the spleen and liver. The large granular form of malignant lymphoma is a unique variant that occurs in cats and often involves the digestive tract. In this form of lymphoma the lesions are composed of large lymphocytes and lymphobasts with variably sized, slightly eosinophilic granules. The granules within the lymphocytes are larger and more eosinophilic than the granules commonly observed in granular lymphocytes of other species.

In dogs and cats, intestinal mast cell tumors occur much less frequently than malignant lymphoma. On gross examination the tumors tend to resemble malignant lymphoma. The affected intestinal segment is thickened and dilated, often with an ulcerated surface. Eosinophils may accompany intestinal mast cell tumors in dogs but are seldom seen in cats. Giemsa staining may reveal metachromatic granules with neoplastic mast cell tumors in dogs but is frequently negative in cats. As is the case with malignant lymphoma, other organs and structures, especially regional lymph nodes, may be infiltrated by neoplastic mast cells.

We have observed three cases of an unusual, progressive lesion of uncertain etiology in cats. Vomiting and anorexia are the primary clinical signs. The intestinal wall and mesenteric lymph nodes of the affected animals are infiltrated or replaced by an infiltrate of eosinophils, fewer scattered mast cells, fibroblasts, and capillaries alternating with regions of dense collagen. The few mast cells within the lesion have normal morphologic features. Unfortunately the lesions frequently are not amenable to resection, and clinical signs are persistent. The infiltrative character of the lesions resembles that of a neoplasm, but the lesion's heterogeneous nature suggests a nonneoplastic process. A similar lesion has been recently described and diagnosed as an unusual form of intestinal mast cell tumor in cats (Howl, Petersen, 1995).

## THE FUTURE

The histopathologic applications of gastrointestinal endoscopy are continually expanding. Exfoliative cytology from biopsy specimens and duodenal aspirates is being used with greater frequency to deliver rapid, clinically relevant diagnostic information. The evaluation of cytologic specimens may provide initial prognostic information in patients with significant mucosal disease and may also indicate the need for additional tests such as culture of duodenal secretions when bacterial overgrowth is suspected. Preliminary studies performed at the senior author's institution show good correlation between brush cytologic impressions and histopathologic findings in dogs and cats with gastrointestinal inflammation of varied causes.

A variety of new diagnostic techniques are now being applied to endoscopic biopsy specimens. *Helicobacter*-associated gastritis in companion animals may now be diagnosed by polymerase chain reaction analysis of gastric mucosal biopsies. Investigators have recently described an image analysis method for analyzing cellular populations in normal and pathologic duodenal biopsy specimens (Jergens et al, 1996a). Other studies have utilized ocular morphometry and immunohistochemistry to evaluate immunoglobulin-containing cells and T cells in colonic biopsy specimens from healthy dogs (Jergens, Gamet, Bailey, 1995a, 1995b) and from dogs with inflammatory bowel disease (Jergens et al, 1996b). New diagnostic modalities, especially those in the areas of immunohistochemistry and molecular biology, are likely to be applied to endoscopic specimens in the future.

## REFERENCES

Behmard S, Sadeghi A, Bagheri SA: Diagnostic accuracy of endoscopy with brushing cytology and biopsy in the upper gastrointestinal lesions, *Acta Cytol* 22:153, 1978.

Blaser MJ et al: Reservoirs for human campylobacteriosis, *J Infect Dis* 141:665, 1980.

Brodey RS: Alimentary neoplasms in the cat: a clinicopathologic survey of 46 cases, *Am J Vet Res* 27:74, 1966.

Carpenter JL, Andrews LK, Holzworth J: Tumors and tumor-like lesions. In Holzworth J, editor: *Diseases of the cat. Medicine and surgery,* Philadelphia, 1987, WB Saunders.

Danesh BJZ et al: Comparison of weight, depth, and diagnostic adequacy of specimens obtained with 16 different biopsy forceps designed for upper gastrointestinal biopsy, *Gut* 26:227, 1985.

Debongnie JC et al: Touch cytology: a quick, simple, screening test in the diagnosis of infections of the gastrointestinal mucosa, *Arch Pathol Lab Med* 118:1115, 1994.

DeNovo RC, Magne ML: Current concepts in the management of *Helicobacter*-associated gastritis, *Proc 13th ACVIM Forum* 57, 1995.

Dow SW et al: Clinical features of salmonellosis in cats: six cases (1981-1986), *J Am Vet Med Assoc* 194:1464, 1989.

Feinstein RE, Olsson E: Chronic gastroenterocolitis in nine cats, *J Vet Diagn Invest* 4:293, 1992.

Fox JG, Claps M, Beaucage CM: Chronic diarrhea associated with *Campylobacter jejuni* infection in a cat, *J Am Vet Med Assoc* 189:455, 1986.

Fox JG, Krakowka S, Taylor NS: Acute-onset *Campylobacter*-associated gastroenteritis in adult beagles, *J Am Vet Med Assoc* 187:1268, 1985.

Fox JG et al: *Campylobacter jejuni virgula coli* in commercially reared beagles: prevalence and serotypes, *Lab Anim Sci* 38:262, 1988.

Golden DL: Gastrointestinal endoscopic biopsy techniques, *Vet Clin North Am Small Anim Pract* 8:239, 1993.

Gowen GF: An improved technique of endoscopic biopsy in the upper gastrointestinal tract [Letter], *Gastrointest Endosc* 32:59, 1986.

Green CE, Jacobs GJ, Prickett D: Intestinal malabsorption and cryptosporidiosis in an adult dog, *J Am Vet Med Assoc* 197:365, 1990.

Hall EJ: Small intestinal disease—is endoscopic biopsy the answer? *J Small Anim Pract* 35:408, 1994.

Handt LK et al: *Helicobacter pylori* isolated from the domestic cat: public health implications, *Infect Immun* 62:2367, 1994.

Heilmann KL, Borchard F: Gastritis due to spiral shaped bacteria other than *Helicobacter pylori:* clinical, histological and ultrastructural findings, *Gut* 32:137, 1991.

Hayden DW, Van Kruiningen HJ: Lymphocytic-plasmacytic enteritis in German shepherd dogs, *J Am Anim Hosp Assoc* 18:89, 1982.

Howl JH, Petersen MG: Intestinal mast cell tumor in a cat: presentation as eosinophilic enteritis, *J Am Anim Hosp Assoc* 31:457, 1995.

Ikeda JS et al: Characteristics of *Salmonella* isolated from animals at a veterinary medical teaching hospital, *Am J Vet Res* 47:232, 1986.

Jacobs G et al: Lymphocytic-plasmacytic enteritis in 24 dogs, *J Vet Intern Med* 4:45, 1990.

Jergens AE: Endoscopic examination of the gastrointestinal tract, *Proc 11th ACVIM Forum* 896, 1993.

Jergens AE, Andreasen CB, Hagemoser WH: The use of endoscopic cytology in the diagnosis of gastrointestinal disease, *J Vet Intern Med* 11:115, 1997.

Jergens AE, Gamet Y, Bailey TB: Morphometric evaluation of immunoglobulin-containing cells and T cells in the canine colon, *J Vet Intern Med* 9:190, 1995a.

Jergens AE, Gamet Y, Bailey TB: Morphometric evaluation of T cell subsets in colonic mucosa of healthy dogs, *Vet Pathol* 32:587, 1995b.

Jergens AE et al: Colonic immune cell populations in canine inflammatory bowel disease, *J Vet Intern Med* 10:158, 1996b.

Jergens AE et al: Idiopathic inflammatory bowel disease associated with gastroduodenal ulceration-erosion: a report of nine cases in the dog and cat, *J Am Anim Hosp Assoc* 28:21, 1992a.

Jergens AE et al: Immunohistochemical characterization of immunoglobulin-containing cells and T cells in the colonic mucosa of healthy dogs, *Am J Vet Res* 59:552, 1998.

Jergens AE et al: Idiopathic inflammatory bowel disease in dogs and cats: 84 cases (1987–1990), *J Am Vet Med Assoc* 201:1603, 1992b.

Jergens AE et al: Morphometric evaluation of IgA- and IgG-containing cells and T cells in duodenal mucosa from healthy dogs and from dogs with inflammatory bowel disease or nonspecific gastroenteritis, *Am J Vet Res* 57:697, 1996a.

Jergens AE et al: *Streptococcus* villous adherence in two dogs with gastrointestinal disease, *J Am Vet Med Assoc* 98:1950, 1991.

Jones BD: Endoscopy of the lower gastrointestinal tract, *Vet Clin North Am Small Anim Pract* 20:1229, 1990.

Kukushuma K, Helman RG. Cryptosporidiosis in a pup with distemper, *Vet Pathol* 21:247, 1984.

Lee A et al: Role of *Helicobacter felis* in chronic canine gastritis, *Vet Pathol* 29:487, 1992.

Leib MS: Gastrointestinal endoscopy: endoscopic and histologic correlation, *Proc 7th ACVIM Forum* 784, 1989.

Magne ML: Treatment of gastric *Helicobacter* in companion animals. *Proc 13th ACVIM Forum* 60, 1995.

Mahony OM et al: Alimentary lymphoma in cats: 28 cases (1988–1993), *J Am Vet Med Assoc* 207:1593, 1995.

Moulton JE: Tumors of the alimentary tract. In Moulton JE, editor: *Tumors in domestic animals*, Los Angeles, 1978, University of California Press.

Otto G et al: Animal and public health implications of gastric colonization of cats by *Helicobacter*-like organisms, *J Clin Microbiol* 32:1043, 1994.

Pitts RP, Twedt DC, Mallie KA: Comparison of duodenal aspiration with fecal flotation for diagnosis of giardiasis in dogs, *J Am Vet Med Assoc* 182:1210, 1983.

Radin MJ et al: *Helicobacter pylori* gastric infection in gnotobiotic beagle dogs, *Infect Immun* 58:2607, 1990.

Roth L et al: Comparisons between endoscopic and histologic evaluation of the gastrointestinal tract in dogs and cats: 75 cases (1984–1987), *J Am Vet Med Assoc* 196:635, 1990a.

Roth L et al. A grading system for lymphocytic plasmacytic colitis in dogs, *J Vet Diagn Invest* 2:257, 1990b.

Shroff CP, Nanivadekar SA: Endoscopic brushing cytology and biopsy in the diagnosis of upper gastrointestinal tract lesions: a study of 350 cases, *Acta Cytol* 32:455, 1988.

Strombeck DR, Guilford WG: Gastrointestinal endoscopy. In Strombeck DR, Guilford WG, editors: *Small animal gastroenterology*, Davis, Calif, 1990a, Stonegate.

Strombeck DR, Guilford WG: Idiopathic inflammatory bowel disease. In: Strombeck DR, Guilford WB, editors: *Small animal gastroenterology*, Davis, Calif, 1990b, Stonegate.

Tams TR: Chronic canine lymphocytic plasmacytic enteritis. *Comp Contin Educ Pract Vet* 9:1184, 1987.

Tams TR: Chronic feline inflammatory bowel disorders. Part 1. Idiopathic inflammatory bowel disease, *Comp Contin Educ Pract Vet* 8:1184, 1986.

Tobey JC, Willard MD, Krehbiel JD: Comparison of cytologic and histopathologic evaluations of duodenal biopsies, *Proc Am Coll Vet Path* 6, 1988.

Turnwald GH et al: Cryptosporidiosis associated with immunosuppression attributable to distemper in a pup, *J Am Vet Med Assoc* 192:79, 1988.

van der Gaag I: The role of biopsy in the diagnosis of gastrointestinal conditions in small animals, *Veterinary Annual* (34):141, 1994.

Weber AF, Hasa O, Sautter JH: Some observations concerning the presence of spirilla in the fundic glands of dogs and cats, *Am J Vet Res*, 677, 1958.

# Chapter 11

# Endoscopic Placement of Gastrostomy and Jejunostomy Tubes

**Keith Richter**

The provision of nutritional support to dogs and cats that are unable or unwilling to eat is an important aspect of their overall medical care. The benefits of nutritional support have been well reviewed (Wheeler, McGuire, 1989; Abood, Buffington, 1992). Because force-feeding can be difficult or impossible in most patients, endoscopically placed enteral feeding tubes have become popular. These tubes provide access for the delivery of calories, specific nutrients, vitamins, minerals, electrolytes, water, and medications. Enteral feeding requires an adequately functioning gastrointestinal tract; otherwise parenteral feeding must be used. The feeding tubes most commonly placed under endoscopic guidance are *percutaneous endoscopic gastrostomy (PEG) tubes* and *percutaneous endoscopic jejunostomy (PEJ) tubes.* PEG tube placement is one of the most common indications for upper gastrointestinal endoscopy in humans, with approximately 75,000 PEG procedures performed annually in the United States.

## INDICATIONS

Generally, PEG tubes are placed in animals that are unable or unwilling to eat but otherwise have normal gastroin-testinal function. Indications for PEG tube placement in 97 cases, including patients in my own series and those reported by others (Armstrong, Hardie, 1990; Bright et al, 1991), are summarized in Table 11-1. In these series, esophageal disease was the most common indication for tube placement in dogs (58%), whereas hepatic disease was the most common indication in cats (47%).

Indications for PEJ tube placement include disorders of gastric emptying, vomiting caused by gastric disease, gastroesophageal reflux, and pancreatitis. These diseases require that nutrients be delivered directly into the jejunum to allow proper utilization and prevent exacerbation of the underlying disease.

## Advantages of PEG Tubes

Endoscopic placement of feeding tubes has several advantages over other methods of tube placement. The *advantages* of PEG tubes over nasogastric tubes include the following:

1. Gruels of commercial canned food prepared with a blender can be delivered through PEG tubes. (In contrast, specialized liquid food must be used with the smaller diameter nasal feeding tubes.)

**Table 11-1**  Indications for Percutaneous Endoscopic Gastrostomy Tube Placement in 97 Animals

| Disorder | Total animals (N = 97) | Dogs (N = 40) | Cats (N = 57) |
| --- | --- | --- | --- |
| Hepatic disease | 27 (28%) | 0 (0%) | 27 (47%) |
| Esophageal disease | 28 (29%) | 23 (58%) | 5 (9%) |
| Megaesophagus | 16 (16%) | 13 (33%) | 3 (5%) |
| Stricture | 5 (5%) | 4 (10%) | 1 (2%) |
| Foreign body | 4 (4%) | 4 (10%) | 0 (0%) |
| Laceration | 2 (2%) | 2 (5%) | 0 (0%) |
| Neoplasia | 1 (1%) | 0 (0%) | 1 (2%) |
| Oronasal disease | 27 (28%) | 13 (33%) | 14 (25%) |
| Cranial nerve deficits | 3 (3%) | 3 (8%) | 0 (0%) |
| Anorexia | 8 (8%) | 0 (0%) | 8 (14%) |
| Miscellaneous | 4 (4%) | 1 (3%) | 3 (5%) |

From Armstrong PJ, Hardie EM: Percutaneous endoscopic gastrostomy: a retrospective study of 54 clinical cases in dogs and cats, *J Vet Intern Med* 4:202, 1990; Bright RM et al: Percutaneous tube gastrostomy for enteral alimentation is small animals, *Compend Contin Educ Pract Vet* 13:15, 1991; Richter K: Unpublished data, 1988-1991.

2. Because PEG tubes do not traverse the lower esophageal sphincter, gastroesophageal reflux is less likely.
3. PEG tubes can be placed easily in patients with megaesophagus.
4. PEG tubes are better tolerated by patients and better accepted by clients for home use.
5. PEG tubes allow better access in animals with maxillary or nasal disorders.
6. PEG tubes allow oral feeding to be resumed with the tube still in place.

A disadvantage of pharyngostomy tubes is the potential for laryngeal dysfunction. In fact, it is now recommended pharyngostomy tubes *not* be used. Advantages of PEG tubes over surgically placed tubes include reduced anesthetic time, reduced tissue trauma in a potentially debilitated patient, and reduced cost.

The *disadvantages* of endoscopically placed tubes include the need for an endoscope, specialized tubes, and an initial anesthetic procedure. Furthermore, depending on the type of tube used, a second anesthetic procedure may be required to remove a PEG tube.

### Contraindications

Contraindications for PEG tube placement include intolerance of general anesthesia, a nonfunctional gastrointestinal tract, and disorders that require PEJ tubes. Relative contraindications include coagulopathies and any condition or lesion that would interfere with contact between the stomach and the abdominal wall (e.g., se-vere ascites, abdominal masses, splenomegaly, previous gastropexy).

### EQUIPMENT

The placement of PEG or PEJ tubes requires a flexible endoscope and a special feeding tube. Either homemade tubes or commercial kits designed for use in humans can be used. I prefer commercial kits because they are easier to use and come preassembled. In addition, the commercial tubes are made of biocompatible silicone or polyurethane and therefore can function longer in the body. Although commercial kits are more expensive than homemade tube kits, the difference in cost is not significant for most clients who approve placement of a feeding tube. Various PEG tube commercial kits are shown in Figures 11-1 through 11-7. Tubes with an 18- through 24-French diameter are suitable for use in cats and in dogs of any size. Commercial PEG tube kits and their manufacturers are listed in Table 11-2. These kits differ in the design of the internal retention device, the material used (silicone versus polyurethane), and the placement method (push versus pull method).

Tubes intended to be placed with the pull method have a tapered end with a preattached wire loop. The tapered end can be pulled through the body wall with the aid of an endoscopically placed long suture that is attached to the preattached wire loop. Tubes intended to be inserted with the push method have a tapered end that can be pushed across the body wall

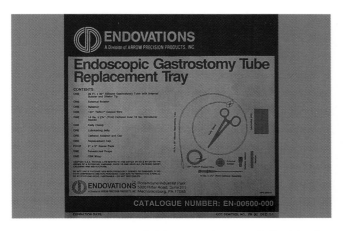

**Figure 11-1** PEG kit intended for use in humans (Ballard Medical).

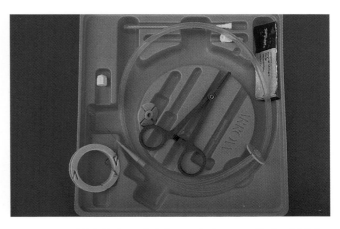

**Figure 11-2** PEG kit intended for use in humans (Ballard Medical).

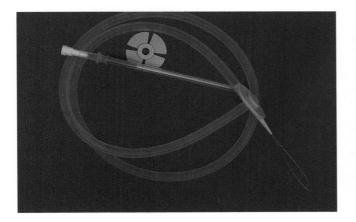

**Figure 11-3** PEG kit intended for use in humans (Ballard Medical).

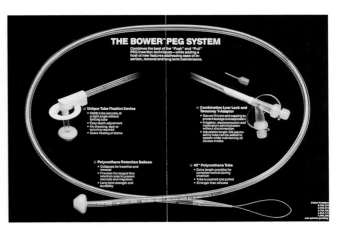

**Figure 11-4** PEG kit intended for use in humans (Corpak).

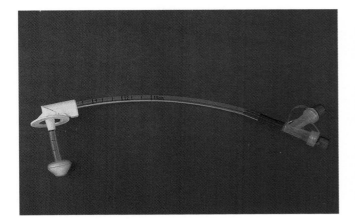

**Figure 11-5** PEG kit intended for use in humans (Corpak).

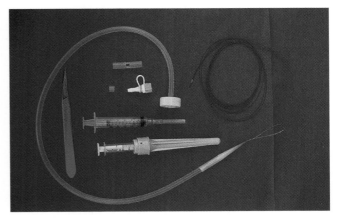

**Figure 11-6** PEG kit intended for use in humans (Bard).

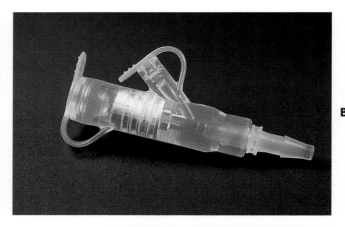

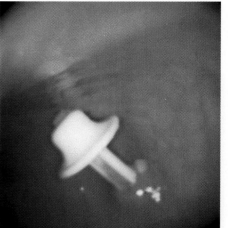

**Figure 11-7 A,** Custom PEG kit for veterinary use (Medical Innovations Corp., a division of Ballard Medical Products). The kit includes an 18-French pull PEG tube with a custom-attached bumper, a looped placement wire, an introducer needle with over-the-needle catheter, a retention disk, and a feeding adaptor. **B,** Close-up of the feeding adapter. **C,** Endoscopic view after placement of the internal bumper of the PEG tube shown in *A*. Note that the inner bumper needs to be pulled closer to the gastric mucosa for proper placement. (See 11-8 through 11-12 and 11-32, *A* for correct positioning of the bumper against the gastric mucosa.)

over an endoscopically placed guide wire. The end of the tube that is to remain in the stomach has a fixation device usually referred to as the *internal bumper* or *retention disk*. The design of the internal bumper varies with the manufacturer (Figures 11-7 through 11-12). Depending on the design, the tube can be removed either percutaneously with steady traction or with the aid of an endoscope.

Homemade tubes using a French–de Pezzer mushroom-tip catheter (Bard Urological Catheter, CR Bard Inc., Murray Hill, N.J.) have been described (Bright and Burrows, 1988; Debowes, Coyne, Layton, 1993). The homemade tube kits are very simple. Therefore, the description of PEG placement technique presented in this chapter focuses on commercial kits. (See texts cited in the reference list for details on the placement of homemade catheters.)

PEJ tubes are usually specially constructed devices designed to be placed percutaneously through an existing PEG tube with the aid of an endoscope. Jejunal feeding can also be accomplished by placing a nasojejunal tube under endoscopic guidance. The nasojejunal tube can be any 5- to 8-French tube of sufficient length (depending on patient size) to reach the proximal jejunum.

## TECHNIQUE FOR PEG TUBE PLACEMENT AND USE

### Tube Placement

Before anesthesia is induced, the animal is prepared by clipping an area caudal to the last rib on the left side. The area should be large enough to allow sterile placement of the tube at this site. After general anesthesia is induced, the animal is placed in the *right lateral recumbent* position (the opposite of the recumbency used in most endoscopic procedures).

An oral speculum is placed, and the lubricated endoscope is inserted into the stomach. The stomach is briefly examined to ensure that no obvious underlying gastric abnormality is present. The stomach is maximally insufflated with air (an assistant may need to apply external pressure to the cervical esophagus to prevent the escape of air) so that the gastric wall

**Table 11-2**  Commercial Kits for Percutaneous Endoscopic Gastrostomy Tubes and Low-Profile Feeding Buttons Designed for Use in Humans

| Manufacturer | Location | Trade name | Phone number |
|---|---|---|---|
| Applied Medical Technology | Cleveland, Ohio | Stick PEG* <br> One-Step Button‖ | 800-869-7382 |
| Ballard Medical | Draper, Utah | MIC PEG Kit† <br> PEG Tube Replacement Tray§ <br> (formerly Endovations) | 800-255-4848 |
| Bard | Billerica, Mass. | Ponsky PEG Tray <br> Ponsky-Gauderer PEG Tray <br> Others <br> The Button‡ | 800-826-2273 |
| Cook | Bloomington, Ind. | PEG Tube | 800-826-2380 |
| Corpak | Wheeling, Ill. | Bower PEG Kit* (distributed <br> by Mila: 888-645-2468) <br> Corpak Button‡ | 800-323-6305 |
| Ross Products | Columbus, Ohio | Sacks-Vine Gastrostomy Kit <br> Stomate Low Profile Kit‡ | 800-544-7495 |
| Novarz Nutrition <br> (previously Sandoz) | Minneapolis, Minn. | Compat PEGs <br> Gastro-Port‡ | 800-999-9978 |
| Kendall, Sherwood, Davis, <br> and Geck | Mannsfield, Mass. | EntriStar* | 800-325-7472 |
| Surgitek | Racine, Wisc. | Surgi-Peg* <br> Surgitek Button‡ | 800-558-9494 |

*These devices can be removed percutaneously with positive traction and without the aid of an endoscope.
†Ballard Medical will make custom kits for veterinarians that are less expensive than the kits designed for humans.
‡Low-profile feeding button.
§The Gastrostomy Tube Replacement Tray made by Ballard Medical (formerly Endovations) is suitable for initial placement and is less expensive than the tube marketed for initial placement.
‖Placement of this low-profile feeding button can be the initial procedure.

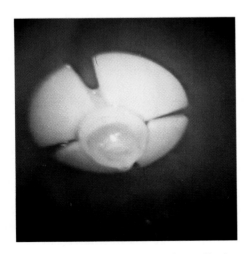

**Figure 11-8** Internal bumper of a PEG tube (Ballard Medical) after placement.

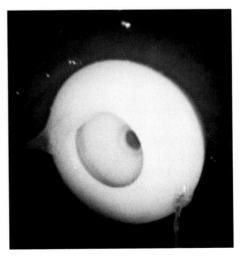

**Figure 11-9** Internal bumper of a PEG tube (Bard) after placement.

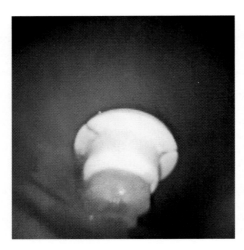

**Figure 11-10** Internal bumper of a PEG tube (Biosearch) as seen endoscopically after placement in a cat.

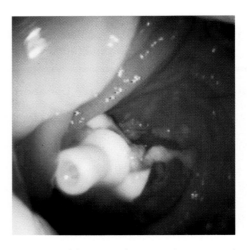

**Figure 11-12** Internal bumper of a PEG tube (Ross Laboratories) as seen endoscopically after placement.

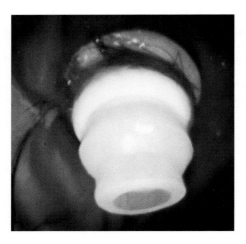

**Figure 11-11** Internal bumper of a PEG tube 6 weeks after it was placed in the cat in Figure 11-10.

comes into contact with the abdominal wall and displaces bowel, spleen, or liver from the insertion site (Figure 11-13). A site on the fundus of the stomach is selected by having an assistant apply sharp intermittent pressure with one finger just behind the last rib. The indentation of the gastric mucosa should be well visualized through the endoscope (see Figure 11-13). The site should be as dorsal as possible to minimize the risk of subsequent leakage of gastric contents through the gastrostomy site. Transillumination of light from the endoscope through the body wall may also help select the site for tube placement.

Once the final site is selected, the skin is prepared with surgical scrub. As a final check the gloved finger of the assistant is used to indent the gastric mucosa as before, and the mucosa should remain well visualized by the endoscopist. A 1-cm skin incision is made

at the chosen site. Through this incision a 14-gauge 2-inch over-the-needle catheter (supplied with many PEG tube kits) is placed percutaneously into the stomach with a sharp forceful thrust (see Figure 11-13, B). This should be directed toward the left shoulder, and the catheter piercing the stomach wall should be easily visualized through the endoscope. An endoscopic snare is placed around the catheter (Figures 11-14 and 11-15). The stylet is removed, and the looped end of the long suture (provided with the PEG tube kit) is placed through the catheter into the gastric lumen. The snare (preplaced around the catheter) is loosened and slid down to grasp the suture. If an endoscopic snare is unavailable, the suture can be grasped with endoscopic retrieval forceps (see Figure 11-13, D).

Once the suture is secured, the endoscope and suture are slowly retracted through the mouth. At this point the suture extends through the abdominal wall, stomach, and esophagus, with the looped end exiting through the mouth. The looped end of the suture is then secured to the wire loop attached to the tapered end of the PEG tube. This is done by placing the looped suture 1 to 2 inches through the wire loop of the tube. The opposite end of the tube (the end with the internal bumper attached) is brought up and through the inside of the looped suture. The end of the tube is pulled away from the suture, thus causing the two loops to interlock (Figure 11-16).

The tapered end of the tube is lubricated with sterile lubricant and is pulled into the mouth as the end of the suture through the body wall is pulled by the assistant. The assistant continues to pull the tube through the esophagus and stomach. When the tube comes into contact with the catheter, it is brought through the body wall with slow steady traction from the assistant. Placing the opposite hand on the body wall as the tapered

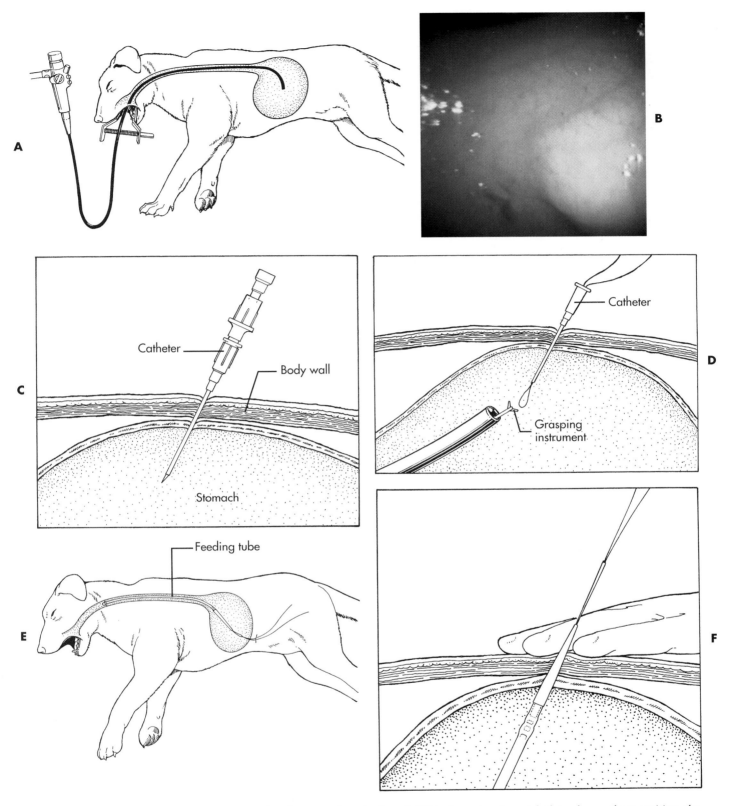

**Figure 11-13** Gastric insufflation and PEG tube placement site selection. **A,** With the patient in a right lateral recumbent position, the endoscope is advanced to the gastric body, and the stomach is fully insufflated so that the gastric wall abuts the body wall. **B,** Endoscopic view of depressed gastric mucosa. The endoscopist's assistant pressed on the skin during selection of the PEG insertion site. **C,** The spleen, bowel, or liver should not be between the stomach and the body wall. The light from the endoscope can be seen as it transilluminates the body wall. An over-the-needle catheter, supplied with most PEG kits, is placed percutaneously into the stomach. **D,** An over-the-needle catheter, supplied with the PEG kit, is placed percutaneously into the stomach. An endoscopic snare or other grasping instrument is used to capture the suture as it is advanced through the catheter by the assistant. A short grasping instrument is pictured here. **E,** Once the PEG tube is attached to the suture material, the assistant pulls the tube through the mouth and stomach. **F,** With firm counterpressure applied to the abdominal wall, the tip of the feeding tube is pulled through the stomach wall and then the body wall until the bumper sits against the gastric mucosal wall.

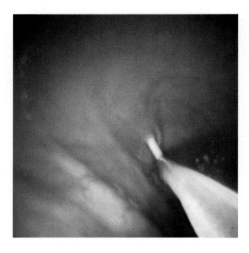

**Figure 11-14** Endoscopic snare grasping a 2-inch catheter after percutaneous puncture into stomach.

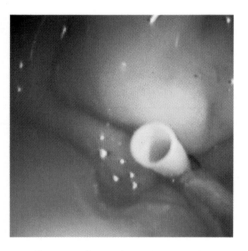

**Figure 11-15** Close-up of an endoscopic snare grasping a 2-inch catheter after the stylet has been removed.

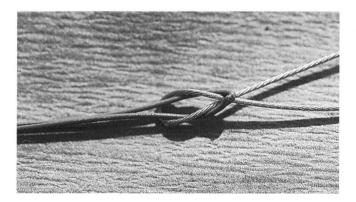

**Figure 11-16** Loop of suture interlocking with wire loop preattached to a PEG tube. This allows the tube to be pulled through the abdominal wall.

end of the tube exits can help in bringing the tube through (see Figure 11-13, *F*). Steady traction is continued as the tube is brought through the body wall. As the end of the tube with the internal bumper enters the esophagus, it is followed with the endoscope and visualized until it comes into contact with the gastric mucosa. *Care must be exercised to prevent pressure from being placed on the mucosa and to avoid having an excessive amount of tube protrude into the gastric lumen.* Pressure from the bulb or internal bumper could result in is-

chemic necrosis of the mucosa. Excessive tube extending into the gastric lumen could result in leakage around the tube or migration into the pylorus and subsequent outflow obstruction. Ideally the internal bumper should be just barely touching the gastric mucosa with minimal pressure (see Figures 11-8 through 11-12 and 11-32, *A*). The rounded internal bumper of customized feeding tubes is less likely to cause significant injury to the gastric mucosa than are the rectangular segments cut from and used with the homemade tubes.

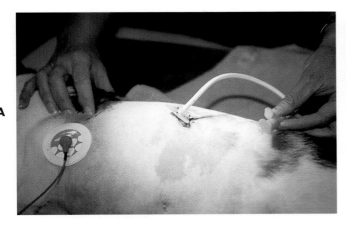
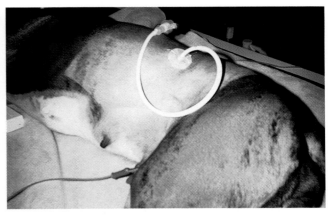

**Figure 11-17** Final placement of a PEG tube. **A,** Cat. **B,** boxer dog. Note the external retention disk that is just touching the skin. In **A,** the assistant is grasping the yellow feeding adapter at the end of the tube.

At this point an external retention disk is slid over the tapered end of the tube until it contacts the skin (Figure 11-17; see also 11-7, *B*). Some kits have an additional locking piece that is placed above the retention disk. Care must be taken to avoid excess pressure on the skin in order to prevent ischemic necrosis. If desired, the disk may be sutured to the skin. The tube is then cut at an appropriate length (usually about 12 inches), and a feeding adapter is placed in the end of the tube (see Figure 11-17). A final evaluation of the stomach is made with the endoscope to ensure that the internal bumper is properly placed. Air is evacuated from the stomach, the endoscope is withdrawn, and the animal is recovered from anesthesia.

The procedure for placing PEG tubes using the push method is identical to that for the pull method except that instead of a loop of suture, a guide wire (0.037-inch diameter) is placed in the stomach and brought out of the mouth. Kits that require placement using the push method have a tube with a hole in the tapered end that slides over the guide wire. The tube is pushed over the guide wire and subsequently out the body wall. The tapered end is then grasped by the assistant, who pulls the remainder of the tube out as described in the pull method.

### Maintenance

Once the PEG tube is in place, the tube site is protected by placing several ($\frac{1}{2}$ to 1 inch high) 3 by 3-inch gauze squares over the site (Figure 11-18 *A* and *B*). This is done by cutting half of the stack of gauze squares along one side up to the middle and then inserting the tube in this slot. A similar cut is made in the remaining gauze squares, with the cut slot 180 degrees opposite. Taping the two stacks together allows them to be secured with the tube exiting through the center. This also ensures that the tube exits the skin perpendicular to the body wall. A device supplied with the Corpak kit (distributed by Mila)

secures the tube and ensures that the tube exits the skin perpendicular to the body wall (Figure 11-18, *C*).

A piece of orthopedic stockinette (4 inches long for cats and small dogs and up to 6 inches long for large dogs) is used to create a "sweater" to protect the tube. Holes are cut for the animal's front legs, and a small hole is cut for the tube to keep the stockinette in place (Figure 11-19). The free end of the tube is secured to the stockinette with a safety pin attached to a small piece of tape near the end. Clients are instructed to change the bottom few gauze squares and flush around the tube exit site with dilute chlorhexidine solution (1:10) once daily for 7 to 10 days and as needed thereafter.

### Feeding

Feeding can begin as early as 3 hours after PEG tube placement but is usually instituted 12 to 24 hours later. Depending on the underlying disease, feeding can begin with maintenance requirements (divided into three to four feedings). In patients with prolonged anorexia the starting volume is approximately one fourth of maintenance requirements, with the volume then gradually increased. After feeding, approximately 10 mL of water should be flushed through the tube to prevent clogging. The details of feeding requirements and methods have been well described (Wheeler, McGuire, 1989; Abood, Buffington, 1992).

### Tube Removal

Once a PEG tube is in place, it should not be removed for 10 to 14 days so that the gastrostomy tract has sufficient time to mature with adequate fibrosis. Premature removal can result in the leakage of gastric contents into the abdominal cavity. Tubes can be removed in one of three ways:

1. The tube is cut off at skin level and allowed to pass in the feces.

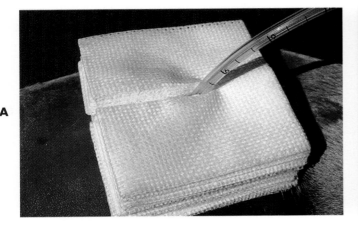

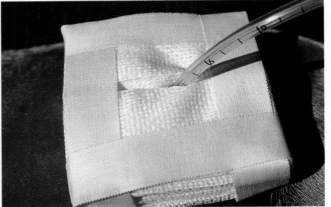

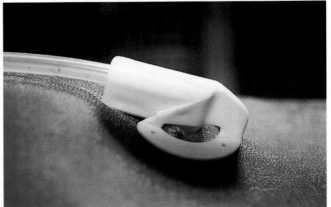

**Figure 11-18 A** and **B,** Stack of gauze squares used to protect tube site and ensure that the tube exits the skin perpendicular to the body wall. **C,** Device supplied with the Corpak kit (distributed by Mila) used to secure the tube and ensure that it exits the skin perpendicular to the body wall.

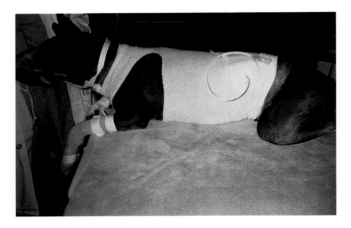

**Figure 11-19** Boxer following PEG tube placement. Note that a piece of 6-inch orthopedic stockinette has been used as a wrap to protect the tube site.

2. The tube is grasped and with positive traction is pulled through the abdominal wall.
3. The tube is cut off at skin level, and the remaining portion is removed endoscopically.

The choice of removal method generally depends on the style of the internal bumper and the personal preference of the clinician. Recommendations on removal method should be obtained from the manufacturer of the PEG tube kit that has been used.

I recommend allowing the cut portion of the tube to pass in the feces only in large dogs because of the potential for small intestinal obstruction in cats and small- to medium-sized dogs. Some PEG tube kits are specifically designed to be removed by positive traction (e.g., manufactured by Corpak; Kendall, Sherwood, Davis, and Geck; and Applied Medical Technologies). The endoscopic retrieval technique is simple and rapid. If an endoscope snare is available, it is used to encircle the end of the PEG tube for retrieval. Otherwise a grasping forceps can be used to capture a piece of 20-gauge orthopedic wire placed in a special loop around the cut portion of the tube before it is pushed into the stomach (Figures 11-20 through 11-22).

The gastrostomy tract closes in 24 hours (Figures 11-23 and 11-24). The stoma site may require superficial cleaning by the client for a few days, but it does not need to be sutured or bandaged.

## Replacement Tubes

If a PEG tube has been removed but ongoing gastrostomy tube feeding is needed, several types of replacement devices are available that do not require endoscopic placement, assuming the gastrostomy tract is still patent (i.e.,

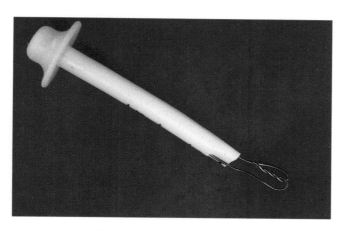

**Figure 11-20** Orthopedic wire (20-gauge) has been looped around the cut end of PEG tube and twisted to secure it. This wire facilitates endoscopic retrieval of the tube.

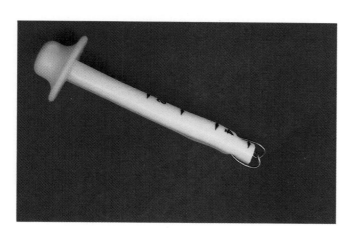

**Figure 11-21** The twisted end of the wire shown in Figure 11-20 is pushed into the lumen of the PEG tube before the tube is pushed into the stomach. This will allow easier removal with endoscopic retrieval forceps.

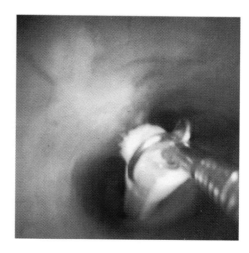

**Figure 11-22** Endoscopic forceps grasping the wire loop (placed as shown in Figures 11-20 and 11-21) during retrieval of the inner bumper.

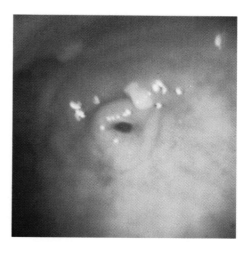

**Figure 11-23** Gastrostomy tract immediately after tube removal.

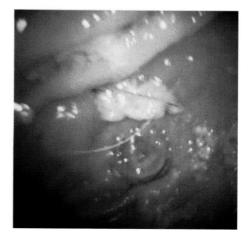

**Figure 11-24** Gastrostomy tract immediately after tube removal.

the PEG tube was removed less than 12 hours earlier). These replacement devices include balloon-type catheters (Figures 11-25 and 11-26), mushroom-type catheters, and skin-level devices with antireflux valves, termed *feeding buttons*. Feeding buttons are especially useful in patients with long-term or permanent gastrostomy feeding needs. I have successfully used low-profile feeding buttons for several years in dogs with esophageal diseases. These devices are constructed with a bulb- or mushroom-shaped tip that can be straightened with a metal stylet. This allows the feeding button to be placed through a patent gastrostomy tract with minimal sedation. When the stylet is removed, the tip regains its original bulb or mushroom shape and keeps the tube in the stomach. The proximal end of the feeding button is flush with the skin (low profile), making inadvertent removal more difficult. A feeding

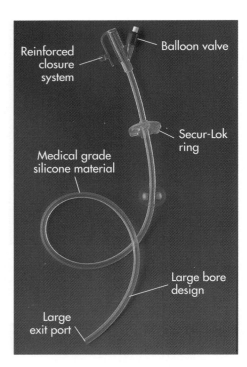

Reinforced closure system
Balloon valve
Secur-Lok ring
Medical grade silicone material
Large bore design
Large exit port

**Figure 11-25** Gastrostomy replacement tube (Ballard Medical) designed to go through an existing-gastrostomy tract. The distal balloon helps keep the tube in the stomach.

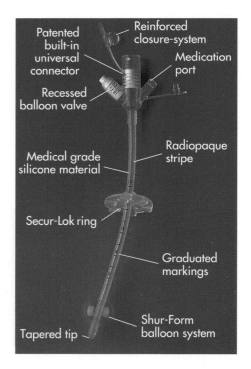

Patented built-in universal connector
Reinforced closure-system
Medication port
Recessed balloon valve
Medical grade silicone material
Radiopaque stripe
Secur-Lok ring
Graduated markings
Tapered tip
Shur-Form balloon system

**Figure 11-26** Gastrostomy replacement tube (Ballard Medical) designed to go through an existing gastrostomy tract. The distal balloon helps keep the tube in the stomach.

**Figure 11-27** One-Step Button kit (Surgitek). This kit allows placement of a low-profile feeding button as the initial procedure.

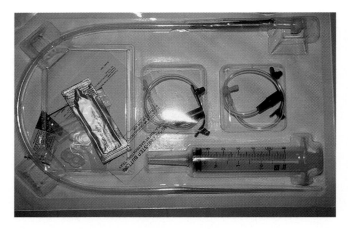

**Figure 11-28** One-Step Button kit (Surgitek). This allows placement of a low profile feeding button as the initial procedure for PEG placement.

adapter allows the introduction of food, and an antireflux valve in the bulb prevents reflux of food during feeding.

It is possible for the gastrostomy tract to be damaged during placement of a low-profile feeding button. This may result in direct access to the peritoneal cavity through the tube. Therefore, after the feeding button is in place, a radiopaque iodinated contrast medium should be injected through the tube. Then radiographs should be obtained to confirm that the contrast agent is in the stomach. Another potential complication is leakage of gastric contents around the tube and subsequent irritation of the skin. This can be managed by using a larger diameter tube.

Placement of a feeding button as the initial procedure has been described (Ferguson et al, 1993) and is also shown in Figures 11-27 through 11-30. This tube is placed in a manner identical to that described for PEG tubes. Once the feeding tube is in place, the end of a section of the tube as it leaves the stomach is peeled away, leaving a low profile button with an antireflux valve.

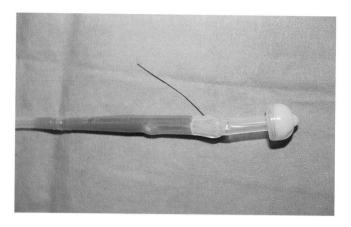

**Figure 11-29** Distal end of the One-Step Button, which converts into a low-profile feeding button. After the thread is pulled, the remainder of the tube is peeled away, leaving the feeding button flush with the skin. The bulb at the end helps keep it in the stomach.

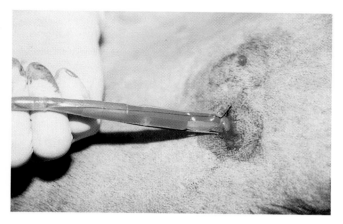

**Figure 11-30** One-Step Button as it exits the body wall of a dog, before the remainder of tube is peeled away.

These tubes are no more difficult to place than conventional PEG tubes.

## COMPLICATIONS OF PEG TUBE PLACEMENT

Major complications of PEG tube placement are uncommon and can usually be avoided with proper technique. Potential complications of PEG and PEJ tubes and suggested methods for avoiding them are presented in Table 11-3. Figure 11-31 shows both a normal-appearing stoma site at the time of tube removal and a stoma site with cutaneous ulceration and infection. The appearance of the gastric mucosal surface immediately after feeding tube removal is shown in Figures 11-23, 11-24, and 11-32.

## TECHNIQUE FOR JEJUNOSTOMY TUBE PLACEMENT

PEJ tubes can be placed through an existing PEG tube, or a nasojejunostomy tube can be placed with endoscopic guidance. A commercial PEJ tube designed for use in humans is shown in Figure 11-33.

### Placement of a PEJ Tube through an Existing PEG Tube

When a PEJ tube is placed through a PEG tube, jejunal feeding can be simultaneous with gastric decompression (through the PEG tube). A specialized PEJ tube (available in various kits for use in humans) is advanced into the stomach through the existing PEG tube. These tubes have a small plastic ball at the end that can be grasped with special endoscopic forceps passed through an endoscope introduced orally into the stomach. Once the plastic ball is grasped, the endoscope and tube are advanced as a unit into the duodenum. The tube is then released, and the endoscope is withdrawn, leaving the tube in the duodenum. On withdrawal of the endoscope, care must be taken to prevent retrograde migration of the jejunal feeding tube because of friction between the scope and feeding tube. Fluoroscopic imaging aids in this process. The tube is then advanced to the desired level in the jejunum. A stylet or guide wire in the tube makes tube advancement easier. An adapter is used to secure the PEJ tube to the PEG tube. Figure 11-34 shows the radiographic appearance of a PEJ tube in a cat.

A new method of placing a PEJ tube through a PEG tube has been described. A pediatric bronchoscope (3.5-mm-diameter insertion tube) is advanced through the PEG tube into the stomach and subsequently into the duodenum. A guide wire with a soft tip (0.035-inch diameter) is inserted through the channel of the bronchoscope into the duodenum and subsequently advanced into the jejunum. Fluoroscopic imaging aids in this process. The bronchoscope is slowly removed, with the guide wire left in place. The PEJ tube is then advanced over the guide wire into the jejunum.

### Placement of a Nasojejunostomy Tube

For placement of a nasojejunostomy tube, the endoscope is first inserted into the duodenum. A guide wire with a soft tip (0.035- or 0.037-inch diameter) is passed through the channel of the endoscope and advanced into the jejunum (Figure 11-35). The endoscope is removed, with the guide wire left in place. Fluoroscopic imaging helps prevent wire slippage. A 5- to 12-French feeding tube ("transfer tube") is used to "backload" the guide wire through the nose. This is accomplished by passing the transfer tube through the ventral nasal meatus until the distal tip can be seen exiting through the nasopharynx. The tip is grasped with forceps and brought out through

**Table 11-3** Complications of Percutaneous Endoscopic Gastrostomy Tube Placement

| Complication | Suggestions to avoid complication |
| --- | --- |
| Splenic laceration | Insufflate stomach adequately |
| Pneumoperitoneum* | Insufflate stomach adequately |
|  | Be certain that inner bumper is touching gastric mucosa |
| Gastric bleeding | Make a single, clean puncture with catheter |
|  | Rule out coagulopathy |
|  | Visualize and avoid large gastric vessels |
| Ischemic necrosis of gastric wall | Be certain that inner bumper is just touching gastric mucosa without excess pressure |
| Pyloric outflow occlusion | Avoid excessive tube length in stomach |
|  | Be certain that inner bumper is touching gastric mucosa |
| Delayed gastric emptying | Avoid excessive tube length in stomach |
|  | Administer metoclopramide or cisapride |
|  | Use small frequent feedings |
| Leakage of gastric contents at tube site | Be certain that inner bumper is touching gastric mucosa |
|  | Place tube in as dorsal location as possible |
| Animal biting tube | Use secure comfortable wrap |
|  | Use Elizabethan collar if necessary |
| Vomiting following feeding | Use small frequent feedings |
|  | Administer metoclopramide or cisapride prior to feeding |
| Skin ulceration at tube site | Do not place external retention disk tight against skin |
|  | Ensure proper cleaning by client |
| Infection at tube site | Use antibiotics as needed |
|  | Ensure proper cleaning of site by client |
| Clogging of tube | Flush tube with water after each feeding |
|  | Use blunt stylet from endotracheal tube to unclog tube |
|  | Flush cola through tube to help unclog it |

*This complication is usually of no clinical significance.

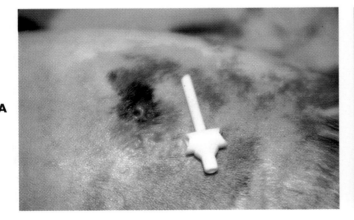 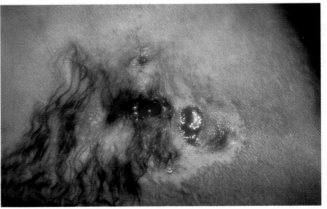

**Figure 11-31 A,** Normal-appearing stoma site at the time of PEG tube removal. The portion of the tube that was in the stomach is resting just to the right of the stoma. **B,** Stoma site with cutaneous ulceration and infection at the time of PEG tube removal. This complication probably occurred because the external retention disk exerted too much pressure against the skin.

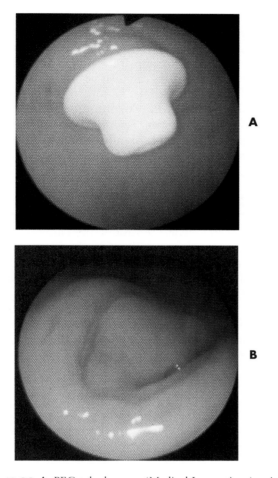

**Figure 11-32** **A,** PEG tube bumper (Medical Innovations) as it is positioned against the gastric wall. The feeding tube was placed 3 months earlier because of anorexia in this patient, a 6-year-old poodle with neoplasia. The tube was removed 3 weeks after the dog's appetite had returned to normal. **B,** Gastric wall immediately after tube removal. Note the absence of significant inflammation or erosive injury around the tube site. The tube was very well tolerated by the patient, and the owner had no problems performing tube feedings.

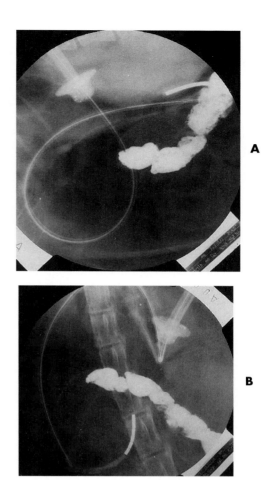

**Figure 11-34** PEJ tube placed through a PEG tube in a cat. **A,** Lateral radiograph. **B,** Ventrodorsal radiograph. The end of the tube is at the junction of the distal duodenum and proximal jejunum. This cat could not tolerate PEG tube feedings because of severe gastroesophageal reflux. Note the barium in the colon from an upper gastrointestinal contrast study performed two days previously.

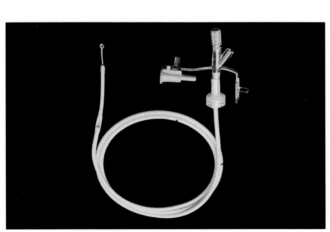

**Figure 11-33** Commercial PEJ tube designed for use in humans (Corpak). The plastic ball at the distal end allows the tube to be grasped with endoscopic forceps and dragged into the duodenum.

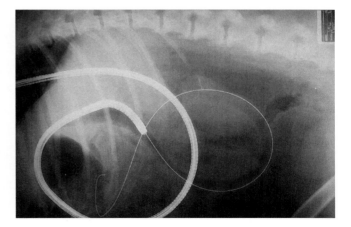

**Figure 11-35** Lateral radiograph demonstrating the placement of a nasojejunostomy tube in a rottweiler. The endoscope is in the proximal duodenum. The guide wire is placed through the channel of the endoscope and into the intestine. The tip of the guide wire is in the proximal jejunum.

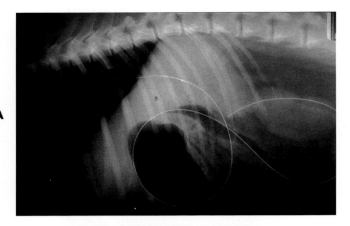

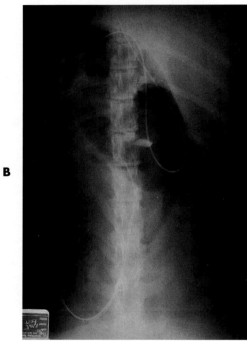

**Figure 11-36** Nasojejunostomy tube in place with the tip of the tube in the proximal jejunum of the same dog. as in Figure 11-35. **A,** Lateral radiograph. **B,** Ventrodorsal radiograph. A small amount of radiopaque iodinated radiographic contrast material was placed in the tube to better demonstrate its position.

the mouth. The proximal end of the guide wire is then placed several centimeters into the distal tip of the transfer tube. The entire transfer tube and guide wire are brought out of the nasal cavity as a unit. At this point the guide wire is entering the nasal cavity, with the other end in the jejunum. A water-soluble lubricant is applied to the guide wire, a vegetable spray–water suspension is used to flush out the nasojejunostomy tube lumen, and a water-soluble lubricant is applied to the outside surface of the nasojejunostomy tube. The nasojejunostomy tube is then advanced over the guide wire into jejunum to the desired level (Figure 11-36). The guide wire is kept taut to facilitate passage. Appropriate tube position is confirmed with

fluoroscopy or plain radiography. The guide wire is then removed, and the tube is secured in a manner identical to that for a nasogastric tube. If the tube is not radiopaque, a small amount of radiopaque iodinated contrast medium can be instilled, and fluoroscopic imaging or radiographs can be used to confirm tube position (see Figure 11-36). Feeding can begin when anesthetic recovery is complete. Radiographs should be obtained periodically to check for enterogastric migration of the tube.

## CONCLUSION

PEG, PEJ, and nasojejunostomy tubes are safe and cost-effective devices for providing short- or long-term nutritional support to patients who cannot or will not eat. Some of the newer kits designed for use in humans have made PEG and PEJ tube placement easier, with techniques that are relatively simple to learn. Client acceptance and patient tolerance are usually excellent, and minimal complications have occurred. Additional clinical studies are needed to better define patient selection and outcome.

### REFERENCES

Abood SK, Buffington CAT: Enteral feeding of dogs and cats: 51 cases (1989–1991), *J Am Vet Med Assoc* 201:619, 1992.

Armstrong PJ, Hardie EM: Percutaneous endoscopic gastrostomy: a retrospective study of 54 clinical cases in dogs and cats, *J Vet Intern Med* 4:202, 1990.

Baskin WN, Johanson JF: An improved approach to delivery of enteral nutrition in the intensive care unit, *Gastrointest Endosc* 42:161, 1995.

Bright RM, Burrows CF: Percutaneous endoscopic tube gastrostomy in dogs, *Am J Vet Res* 49:629, 1988.

Bright RM, DeNovo RC, Jones JB: Use of a low-profile gastrostomy device for administering nutrients in two dogs, *J Am Vet Med Assoc* 207:1184, 1995.

Bright RM, et al: Percutaneous tube gastrostomy for enteral alimentation in small animals, *Compend Contin Educ Pract Vet* 13:15, 1991.

Chaurasia OP, Chang KJ: A novel technique for percutaneous endoscopic gastrojejunostomy tube placement, *Gastrointest Endosc* 42:165, 1995.

DeBowes LJ, Coyne B, Layton CE: Comparison of French-Pezzar and Malecot catheters for percutaneously placed gastrostomy tubes in cats, *J Am Vet Med Assoc* 202:1963, 1993.

Ferguson DR, et al: Placement of a feeding button ("One-Step Button") as the initial procedure, *Am J Gastroenterol* 88:501, 1993.

Flanders JA: Gastrostomy and jejunostomy tubes for enteral nutrition in the cat, *Fel Pract* 22:6, 1994.

Mathews KA, Binnington AG: Percutaneous incisionless placement of a gastrostomy tube utilizing a gastroscope: preliminary observations, *J Am Anim Hosp Assoc* 22:601, 1986.

Mauterer JV: Endoscopic and nonendoscopic percutaneous gastrostomy tube placement. In Bonagura JD, editor: *Kirk's current veterinary therapy,* ed 12, Philadelphia, 1995, WB Saunders.

Orton EC: Enteral hyperalimentation administered via needle catheter-jejunostomy as an adjunct to cranial abdominal surgery in dogs and cats, *J Am Vet Med Assoc* 188:1406, 1986.

Wheeler SL, McGuire BH: Enteral nutritional support. In Kirk RW, Bonagura JD, editors: *Current veterinary therapy,* ed 10, Philadelphia, 1989, WB Saunders.

**Chapter 12**

# Endoscopy of the Upper Respiratory Tract of the Dog and Cat

**Philip A. Padrid and Brendan C. McKiernan**

## RHINOSCOPY

Rhinoscopy is the endoscopic visualization of the nasal cavity. It can be performed with a wide variety of instruments and often yields information that is difficult to obtain using other methods. The examination can be divided into two procedures based on anatomic site. *Anterior rhinoscopy* evaluates the nasal cavity using an approach through the external nares. *Posterior rhinoscopy* is used to evaluate the choanae and nasopharynx by inserting the endoscopic instrument through the oral cavity, maneuvering around the free edge of the soft palate, and looking backward (rostral) towards the choanae. Although anterior and posterior rhinoscopy can be performed separately, they are routinely combined to ensure that the nasal cavity and nasopharynx are completely examined.

### Indications

Animals with nasal, sinus, or nasopharyngeal disease may present with one or a combination of clinical signs, including sneezing, reverse sneezing, nasal discharge, epistaxis, stertor (snoring or snorting sounds), stridor

(inspiratory noise and wheezing), and facial swelling. Rhinoscopy is indicated as part of a complete diagnostic work-up in these patients. Typically, these clinical signs are chronic. In some cases, however, the clinical signs are acute and severe, and rhinoscopy may be the diagnostic and therapeutic procedure of choice.

Rhinoscopy is also indicated when a specific diagnosis is suspected and a biopsy or culture specimen is needed to confirm the location and extent of disease (e.g., nasal neoplasia before treatment is initiated.) At other times, rhinoscopy may be required for treatment, as in the removal of a foreign body or the instillation of drugs in the nasal cavity or sinuses of a dog with aspergillosis. Rhinoscopy may also be performed when the clinician and client want to exclude readily treatable disease such as a nasal polyp in a sneezing cat.

### Instrumentation

The instruments needed to perform rhinoscopy may include a simple otoscope, a dental mirror, and rigid and/or flexible endoscopes. Successful rhinoscopy requires instruments of the proper size for the patient being evaluated (Table 12-1).

357

**Table 12-1** Value of Equipment Used for Rhinoscopy in Dogs and Cats*

| Type | Anterior rhinoscopy | Posterior rhinoscopy | Approximate cost | Biopsy capability |
|---|---|---|---|---|
| Otoscope | + / + + | NA | Low | Yes |
| Dental mirror | NA | + / + + | Low | No |
| Rigid endoscope | + + + | NA/ + | Moderate | Yes |
| Flexible endoscope | + + +/ + + + | + + + + | High | Yes |

* Value is determined as follows: + , poor; + + , fair; + + + , good; + + + + , excellent. *NA* indicates that the instrument is not applicable for the procedure.

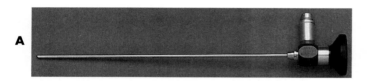

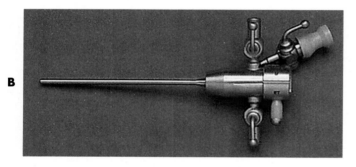

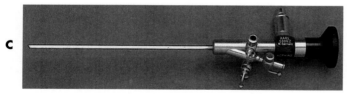

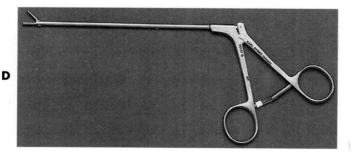

**Figure 12-1** Rigid endoscope and ancillary equipment suitable for use in canine and feline rhinoscopy. **A,** Telescope. **B,** Outer sheath with cannulae for simultaneous flushing and suction and the introduction of biopsy instruments. **C,** Telescope inserted into sheath. **D,** Biopsy forceps.

A simple otoscope is often sufficient to visualize the anterior portion of an animal's nasal cavity using the procedure described later in this chapter. The posterior nasopharynx in medium- and large-sized animals can be evaluated with a dental mirror although the view obtained is often quite limited.

Rigid endoscopes, including small arthroscopes and pediatric cystoscopes, are very useful for performing anterior rhinoscopy, especially if scopes with different viewing angles (typically 5 to 70 degrees) are available. The rigid scope used is typically 2 to 3 mm in diameter, with a sheath size ranging from 11- to 14-French. Rigid scope sets often have a flushing and/or biopsy channel (Figure 12-1).

Although small flexible endoscopes (2.5 to 5 mm in diameter) are expensive, they are the preferred instruments because they can be used for both anterior and posterior rhinoscopy. However, biopsy procedures may be limited or prohibited because of the small channel size in some flexible scopes (Figure 12-2).

## Patient Preparation and Restraint

General anesthesia is required for small animal rhinoscopy because of the persistence of a strong sneeze reflex in these patients. Rhinoscopy normally should be preceded by a full skull radiographic examination and followed by a thorough dental examination using a periodontal probe to measure sulcus depth on all maxillary teeth. Using these three diagnostic evaluations in combination and in sequence maximizes the likelihood that specific lesions will be detected in the nose, sinuses, and nasopharynx and minimizes the chance that one diagnostic test will interfere with the next (e.g., bleeding secondary to rhinoscopy resulting in an increased density on skull radiographs).

Before rhinoscopy is performed, a routine preanesthetic laboratory evaluation should be performed as in-

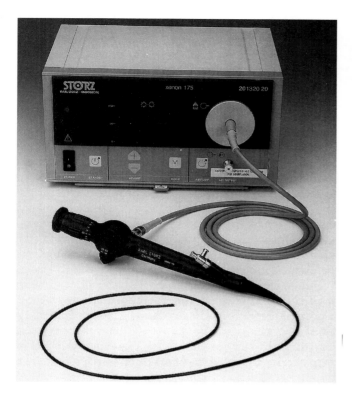

Figure 12-2 Flexible endoscope suitable for canine and feline rhinoscopy. A light source and connecting cable are also shown. The outer diameter (3.5 mm) of the flexible instrument is equivalent to the outer diameter of a rigid scope with accompanying sheath (see Figure 12-1). The increased maneuverability afforded by the flexible instrument must be weighed against its small-diameter (1.2-mm) single inner channel.

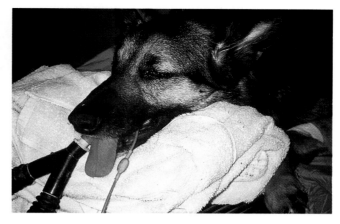

Figure 12-3 For both anterior and posterior rhinoscopy, the patient is ideally placed in a sternal recumbent position with muzzle resting horizontally on a padded support.

dicated by the patient's clinical signs and other known medical problems. Laboratory test typically include a complete blood count, a serum chemistry panel, and urinalysis. Animals with a history of nasal bleeding may require coagulation studies (e.g., prothrombin time, partial thromboplastin time, platelet count, mucosal bleeding time), serology for ehrlichiosis if this disorder is considered a possibility, and a systemic blood pressure determination to rule out systemic causes for the bleeding. Food should be withheld for 12 hours before rhinoscopy to minimize the risk of aspiration associated with general anesthesia.

Inhalation anesthesia is most commonly employed for rhinoscopy. A *cuffed endotracheal tube* is *mandatory* for the safe administration of gas anesthesia and the avoidance of fluid aspiration (e.g., blood, secretions, lavage fluid) during the procedure. Securing the tube to the mandible allows easier access to the nasopharynx. If significant hemorrhage occurs after biopsy, it is usually best to remove the endotracheal tube as late as possible during the anesthetic recovery phase. Extubation should be performed with the cuff still inflated so that any blood

clots that have accumulated in the proximal trachea are removed along with the cuffed tube.

For rhinoscopy the patient should be placed in a sternal recumbent position with the muzzle resting horizontally on a support to facilitate access to the nasal cavity through the external nares and access to the nasopharynx via the oral cavity (Figure 12-3). Two large mouth gags should be used to hold the mouth open and to prevent the patient from inadvertently biting the endoscope during the procedure. When the nasopharynx is being examined, a deep plane of anesthesia is required to prevent the strong gag reflex present in dogs and cats. Finally, viewing will be better if the examination is performed in a darkened room. This often allows the light from the tip of the endoscope to be seen through the maxilla, which can assist in localizing lesions within the nose and sinuses.

The mucosa of the nasal cavity may be viewed through an air or a fluid interface. Nasal secretions and bleeding secondary to mucosal trauma can obscure the endoscopist's view during the procedure. Thus a constant flow of fluid (e.g., saline) through a flexible endoscope or through the sheath that houses a rigid endoscope is sometimes necessary to flush secretions and blood away from the endoscope tip. However, fluid instilled in this manner tends to blanch capillaries, making the mucosa appear much paler than the typical pink color seen through an air interface. If air is instilled (our preference), intermittent flushing and careful suctioning are required to clear secretions and blood from the field of view.

Before the rhinoscopic procedure is started, the oral cavity should be evaluated visually and by palpation for mucosal and anatomic changes. Abnormalities that may be encountered include mucosal hyperemia, excess secretions, deformation of the hard palate (tumor), elongation and ventral depression of the soft palate (mass in the nasopharynx), draining tracts or foreign bodies, obvious dental or gingival disease (especially of the maxillary teeth), and tonsillar enlargement.

Rhinoscopy may be divided into two procedures: *anterior (nasal) rhinoscopy* and *posterior (nasopharyngeal) rhinoscopy*. We start with posterior rhinoscopy and then proceed with anterior visualization of the nasal cavities.

## Posterior Rhinoscopy

Posterior rhinoscopy is used to detect nasopharyngeal disease and/or confirm the caudal extent of the disease. Depending on the equipment used, the view of the nasopharynx and posterior aspects of the nasal cavity can vary greatly. A dental mirror and a spay hook (to pull the free edge of the soft palate forward) provide a cursory view of the nasopharynx in many medium- to large-sized animals. A better view of this region can usually be obtained by maneuvering a small flexible endoscope around the edge of the palate in one of two ways (Figure 12-4). In one maneuver, the tip of the endoscope is retroflexed 180 degrees outside the animal's mouth; the scope is subsequently advanced just past the free margin of the soft palate and then "hooked" and retracted against the soft palate. Alternatively, the scope tip is advanced to the free margin of the soft palate and is then retroflexed. As stated previously, because the nasopharyngeal mucosa is highly sensitive and the maneuvering space is small, the patient must be under a deep enough plane of anesthesia to facilitate examination without causing forceful sneezing or gagging.

Retroversion over the soft palate provides an inverted view of the nasopharynx and choanae (Figure 12-5). In this position the left nasal sinus is on the right side in the field of view, and the right nasal sinus is on the left. The nasopharyngeal border of the soft palate is in the upper area of the field of view. The view is enhanced by moving the endoscope aborally 1 to 2 cm, (thereby causing the endoscope tip to move closer to the choanae) or by rotating the insertion tube slightly to the left or right as needed to provide a clear view. As stated previously, if biopsy specimens are to be obtained, the tip of the biopsy instrument should be advanced to a point just inside the endoscope tip *before* the bending section of the scope is deflected to 180 degrees. This prevents damage from forcing the tip of the biopsy instrument against the channel inside an already deflected endoscope bending section.

The view obtained in animals with long noses is limited by the distance from the edge of the palate to the choanae (the view is like looking down a long tunnel). In some large animals, it is possible to allow the flexible endoscope to "unfold" and be inserted forward into the nasopharynx, providing a detailed close-up view of the choanae. Although limited maneuvering is possible when a flexible scope has been retroflexed in this man-

ner, biopsy specimens can be obtained through the scope. Alternatively, a flexible or rigid endoscope may be inserted straight over the soft palate using an approach similar to that for inserting a pharyngoscopy tube.

Healthy nasopharyngeal mucosa is pink and smooth. Irritated tissue often displays hypermia, mucosal friability (bleeding with only minimal pressure), excess secretions, and lymphoid follicular hyperplasia. Hyperplastic lymphoid tissue is typically seen in chronic reverse sneezing and is associated with long-standing antigenic stimulation of the nasopharyngeal mucosa (see Plate 12-1). Anatomic landmarks that can be identified include the eustachian tube orifices, soft palate, juncture of the hard and soft palates (identified by viewing the area while simultaneously pushing up on the palate from within the mouth), vomer bone and its continuation anteriorly as the nasal septum, pituitary gland area/projection, posterior choanae, and caudal aspects of the left and right nasal chonchae. Benign abnormalities that may be encountered include nasopharyngeal stenosis (in cats, a transverse web of tissue across the nasopharynx) and polyps. Malignant tumors are also commonly found in the posterior nasopharynx. Less often, foreign bodies or nasal mites may be visualized. (Examples of these conditions are shown in the color plates at the end of this chapter.)

Mild to moderate hemorrhage is to be expected after nasal biopsy specimens are obtained. Usually the hemorrhage subsides within several minutes. If hemorrhage is severe, the external nares and posterior nasal pharynx can be packed with sponges soaked in dilute epinephrine (1:100,000). Use of a cuffed endotracheal tube ensures that no blood is aspirated. Very rarely, severe epistaxis and blood loss may necessitate a blood transfusion. If hemorrhage is severe and persistent, the unilateral carotid artery can be permanently ligated in the neck.

## Anterior Rhinoscopy

Entry into the anterior nasal cavity is often difficult unless the endoscopist understands the direction of the pathway created by the large alar cartilage dividing the nares. Because of this cartilage the rhinoscope must be inserted medially and then straightened out to allow for insertion deeper into the nasal cavity. Once past the alar cartilage, the scope is placed so that the nasal septum (recognized by its nearly flat surface) is oriented vertically. In this position the chonchae can be recognized as three primary scrolls of bone rising laterally, and the major air passageways (meatuses) are also seen. Anterior rhinoscopy involves the assessment of the nasal mucosa, the three primary meatus, and the chonchae.

Nasal mucosa is normally pink and smooth (see Plate 12-13). A fine network of submucosal capillaries is seen (unless these vessels are obscured by mucosal edema or secretions). Although hemorrhage is often encountered

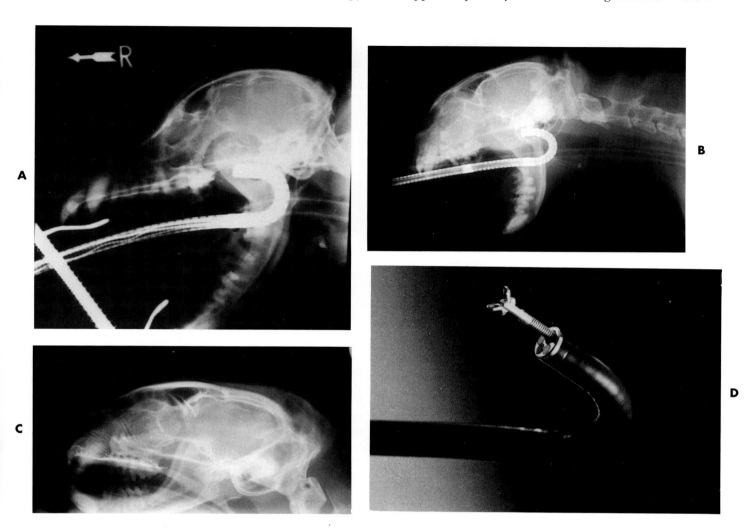

**Figure 12-4 A,** Lateral skull radiograph of a dog, demonstrating correct placement of a flexible endoscope for posterior rhinoscopy. (Note the configuration of the scope in the retroflexed position.) Examination of the choanae is facilitated by the use of a scope with a tip deflection capability of 180 degrees or more. A closer view of the choanae can be obtained if the insertion tube is grasped outside the animal's mouth and retracted. This moves the tube away from the patient. **B,** Lateral skull radiograph of a cat, demonstrating scope positioning for pharyngoscopy using a 5.0-mm-diameter bronchoscope. **C,** Lateral skull radiograph of a 10-year-old cat presented with a 2-week history of gradually worsening snorting. No coughing, sneezing, or nasal discharge was present. A soft tissue opacity is seen in the nasopharynx (the region just above soft palate and cranial to the bullae). Nasopharyngoscopy with biopsy was critical to obtaining the correct diagnosis. The histologic diagnosis was cryptococcosis. The animal responded well to itraconazole. (Courtesy Todd R. Tams.) **D,** Posterior nasal sinus lesions can be biopsied through the scope under direct visualization. A biopsy forceps instrument should be placed in the tip area of the scope *before* the bending section of the endoscope is deflected. This facilitates passage of the biopsy instrument through the accessory channel and guards against damage to the channel from forcing the tip of the biopsy instrument against the bending section (see text).

during small animal rhinoscopy, the ease with which bleeding occurs (e.g., the degree of mucosal fragility) may be one indicator of mucosal inflammation. Other nasal mucosal abnormalities may include hyperemia and surface irregularities such as erosions and ulcers.

Each airway passage should be evaluated during rhinoscopy. The endoscopist should note whether the normal amount of air space is present (i.e., the distance between each meatus). Increased meatal size (or cavitated appearance) is a sign of turbinate destruction. The normally narrow and convoluted nature of the air passageways limits the depth of rhinoscopic penetration. Our impression is that some degree of destruction must be present if the nasal cavity can be completely traversed

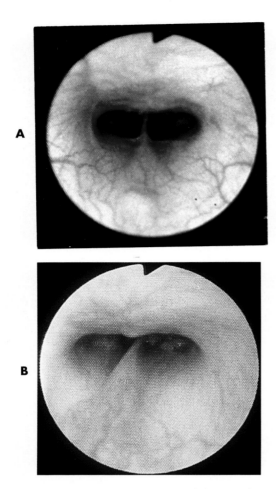

**A**

**B**

**Figure 12-5 A,** Normal posterior view of the nasopharynx of a dog (corresponds to scope position in Figure 12-4, *A*). **B,** Normal posterior view of the nasopharynx of a cat.

and the nasopharynx entered in all but the largest of dogs, unless a very small scope (2 to 3 mm) is used. Similarly, visualization of the nasofrontal duct and/or entry into the frontal sinus is impossible unless considerable turbinate destruction has occurred.

Destructive rhinitis is most commonly encountered in patients with chronic rhinitis (inflammation). Specific examples include chronic bacterial infection (secondary to a viral infection, dental disease, or foreign body) and chronic fungal infection in the dog (aspergillosis). With *Aspergillus* infection, fungal plaques may be seen as whitish mucoid to fluffy masses on the mucosal surface of the nose and/or the frontal or maxillary sinus (see Plate 12-15).

When secretions or tissue fill the channel, the nasal meatus appears smaller or completely obstructed. The endoscopist should note the presence and type of secretions and whether they are seen in one or both sides. The location of secretions should be correlated with the find-

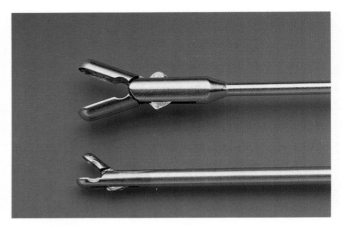

**Figure 12-6** Clamshell-type biopsy instruments used for obtaining biopsy samples from the anterior nasal passages. (Smaller biopsy instruments designed for passage through the sheath of a rigid endoscope are shown in Figure 12-1.)

ings of skull radiographs and the complete periodontal examination. Accumulated secretions may obscure an underlying foreign body or tumor. Secretions should be suctioned gently to minimize bleeding that could interfere with the procedure. Severe mucosal edema may narrow the apparent size of the meatus. Tissue present in the meatus is most often associated with neoplasia (e.g., adenocarcinoma, fibrosarcoma, lymphosarcoma) or fungal granulomas (e.g., feline cryptococcosis and sporothricosis, canine rhinosporidiosis).

## Ancillary Tools and Procedures

Endoscopic biopsy is indicated whenever nasal mucosal abnormalities are visualized and especially when tissue growth is present. Multiple biopsy specimens should be obtained to ensure adequate tissue for histologic analysis. Biopsy samples obtained with forceps instruments passed through a flexible endoscope or the sheath system of a rigid scope typically are quite small (i.e., <2mm. To keep the samples from being lost during processing, the endoscopist or an assistant should place the specimens on small (e.g., 1 × 1 cm) pieces of premoistened filter or lens paper before fixation in formalin. Larger clamshell-type instruments can be passed outside the sheath during anterior rhinoscopy or can be passed blindly into the nasal cavity (Figure 12-6). These instruments procure bigger tissue samples. Touch imprints for cytologic evaluation may be made from the biopsy samples. Biopsy specimens may be obtained under direct visual guidance during rhinoscopy (preferred) or blindly after the lesion has been located with the scope.

Chronic inflammatory conditions (especially canine nasal aspergillosis) are associated with bone destruction, and inadvertent penetration of structures with the biopsy forceps becomes a potential risk in these cases. *Care must be taken not to insert the biopsy forceps past the medial canthus of the eye* to avoid possible penetration of the globe (through the medial wall of the orbit) or brain (through the cribriform plate or posterior aspect of the frontal sinus). It is best to measure the biopsy instrument outside the nose up to the level of the medial canthus so that the *maximum* length of insertion is determined before the biopsy procedure is performed.

Foreign bodies frequently become lodged in the nasopharynx or caudal nasal cavity, presumably after an animal attempts to "spit out" a piece of foreign material from the oropharynx and it is thrown forward over the soft palate. Secretions may obscure the foreign material and should be carefully suctioned to obtain a clear view of the area. Forceps retrieval of foreign material in the nasal cavity is usually possible. Plant material, when present, often becomes soft and may fragment when grasped with a forceps. In many cases, even though a foreign body is not removed, simply dislodging the object allows it to be flushed or sneezed out later. Retroflushing the nasal cavity may facilitate the removal of secretions and/or small foreign bodies located in the nasal cavities or nasopharynx. This is accomplished using a soft rubber catheter (10- to 14-French Brunswick feeding tube) and a 60-ml catheter tip syringe. The cuff on the endotracheal tube must be inflated, and the animal's nose should be held down to facilitate the clearance of debris from the oropharynx. The catheter is inserted into the anterior nasal cavity, and the nostrils are held closed. Next 60 ml of saline is forcefully flushed into first one and then the other nostril. The fluid recovered from the oral cavity should be observed for tissue (save it for biopsy) and foreign bodies.

After the rhinoscopic procedure is completed, a thorough dental examination should be performed with a periodontal probe. Using the probe, the periodontal sulci (mesial, distal, lingual, and buccal) of all teeth are examined. The normal depth of a dental sulcus is 3 to 4 mm in dogs and 1 to 2 mm in cats. The presence of deep pockets (on maxillary teeth), especially when correlated with other clinical, radiographic, and endoscopic findings, is helpful in establishing the diagnosis of rhinitis secondary to dental disease. Regardless of the findings of previous radiographic and rhinoscopic procedures, strict adherence to this protocol ensures that subtle or coexisting lesions are diagnosed.

## LARYNGOSCOPY

Laryngoscopy is the visual examination of laryngeal anatomy and movement. This evaluation is indicated specifically for problems relating to laryngeal dysfunc-tion, including exercise intolerance, respiratory distress, increased inspiratory effort, prolonged inspiratory time, cyanosis, voice change, loss of bark/purr, coughing after eating or drinking, and inspiratory noise (stridor). As a general rule, laryngoscopy should be performed before a bronchoscopic examination.

### Instrumentation

The larynx can be examined with a wide variety of equipment. Any combination of instruments is adequate if it generates sufficient lighting on the larynx itself and also holds the epiglottis (and the dorsal pharyngeal wall in some animals) out of the viewing field. Adequate visualization can be obtained with a simple overhead examination light, a penlight, and a laryngoscope, or an actual endoscope may be used. The blade of the standard laryngoscope or a common wooden tongue depressor works well to depress the epiglottis and improve the view of the ventral portion of the larynx. The advantages of using an endoscope include visualization of details and the ability to extend the examination to adjacent areas (e.g., the nasopharynx and trachea) if indicated.

### Patient Preparation

Laryngoscopy is most easily performed when the patient is lightly anesthetized. Therefore, food should be withdrawn for 6 to 12 hours to minimize the risk of aspiration during the examination. Preanesthesia laboratory tests should be performed as indicated by the patient's age and health status.

### Patient Restraint and Positioning

Laryngoscopy is performed under light anesthesia or heavy sedation. The patient's plane of anesthesia should be deep enough to allow the oral cavity to be held open but light enough to retain normal laryngeal function. An animal that has been properly anesthetized for laryngoscopy still displays a strong gag reflex subsequent to pharyngeal or laryngeal stimulation and also has a good withdrawal reflex to deep pain. A level of anesthesia that allows easy intubation is too deep for proper assessment of normal laryngeal motion.

Injectable anesthetics are most typically used for laryngoscopy. Atropine or glycopyrrolate should be used as a premedication to decrease secretions and to prevent bradyarrhythmias that might be induced by vagal stimulation. Topical 1% lidocaine may occasionally be needed to decrease reflex responses (e.g., laryngospasm, swallowing, gagging) that may be encountered during the procedure. Laryngoscopy should be performed with the patient in a sternal recumbent position. A mouth gag may be used to facilitate oral examination and to ensure good visualization of the larynx.

## Procedure

A thorough laryngoscopic evaluation includes a complete *anatomic examination* and an assessment of *normal laryngeal function and motion*. In the period immediately after general anesthesia is induced, the patient may be too deeply anesthetized for proper evaluation of normal laryngeal motion (abduction). During this period, the endoscopist should perform a thorough anatomic evaluation.

As the anesthetic level lightens, laryngeal function and motion may be assessed. Care should be taken to *gently* depress the epiglottis from the visual field, because forceful maneuvers of the epiglottis can artifactually distort the appearance and movement of laryngeal structures.

Abnormalities in laryngeal function can be more readily detected if doxapram, 1.1 mg/kg (0.5 mg/lb), is given intravenously. Soon after administration, this medication increases the rate and depth of respiration, and the increased ventilation persists for a few minutes. Side effects are minimal and include salivation, muscular tremors, and (uncommonly) vomition.

Awake cats and dogs respond differently to doxapram. Dogs may have an inspiratory effort that holds the arytenoid cartilages in an abducted position. In contrast, the feline arytenoid cartilages cycle through full open and closed positions on inspiration and expiration respectively.

### Evaluation of Laryngeal Structure

Normal structures that should be evaluated during laryngoscopy include the cricoid, thyroid, and arytenoid (also the corniculate and cuneiform processes) cartilages, vestibular folds, vocal folds (cords), laryngeal saccules (lateral ventricles), epiglottis, and aryepiglottic folds (Figure 12-7). Normal mucosa should be pink in color, and significant amounts of secretions should not be present in the posterior oropharynx. Mucosal hyperemia and edema, excessive secretions, redundant pharyngeal mucosa, and laryngeal structural abnormalities are commonly encountered abnormalities. Structural abnormalities include everted saccules, laryngeal collapse or asymmetric motion (either above or within the glottic opening), and laryngeal webbing or granuloma formation (both typically secondary to previous surgery or trauma and resulting in stenosis of the glottic lumen). Less commonly a pharyngeal or laryngeal rannula, tumor, or foreign body may be found. (Laryngeal abnormalities are depicted in Plates 12-19 through 12-24.) The presence of secretions or blood should be noted, and the examiner should attempt to determine the anatomic source of the abnormal fluid accumulation. The examiner should remain aware that secretions (including blood) found in the region of the larynx may have originated in the trachea, lower airways, or lung parenchyma.

### Evaluation of Laryngeal Motion

For the examiner to appreciate both normal and abnormal laryngeal motion and function, the animal must be in a very light plane of anesthesia. A deep plane of anes-

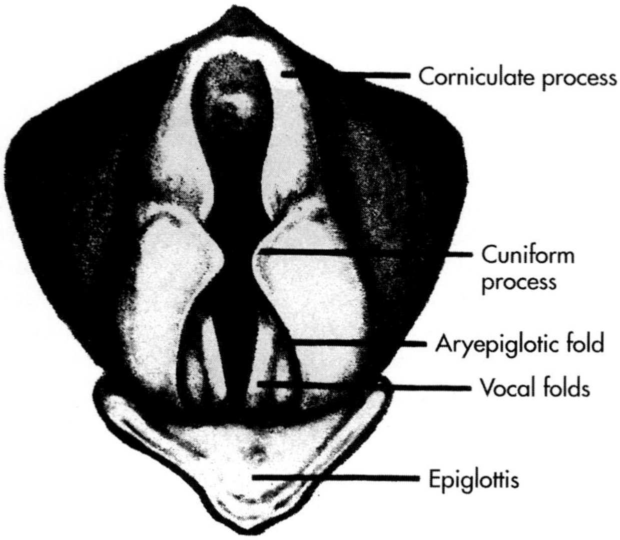

**Figure 12-7** Normal laryngeal anatomy (From Kagan K: Larynx. In Bojrab MJ, editor: *Current techniques in small animal surgery,* ed 2, Philadelphia, 1983, Lea & Febiger.)

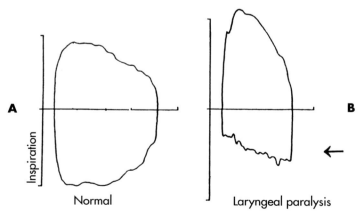

**Figure 12-8** A tidal breathing flow-volume loop (TBFVL) from a working-breed dog presented for decreased exercise ability during hunting. **A,** Note the loop shape in a normal dog. **B,** The loop shape on inspiration (*arrow*) is flattened. (From Amis TC et al: Upper airway obstruction in canine laryngeal paralysis, *Am J Vet Res* 47:1008, 1986).

thesia will inhibit motion of the arytenoid cartilages. Laryngeal motion related to vocalization (e.g., whining) or swallowing should not be confused with laryngeal abduction. Normally the size of the glottic lumen is increased on inspiration by an active abduction of the arytenoid cartilages. Failure of one or both arytenoid cartilages to abduct (increasing the size of the glottic lumen) is defined as *laryngeal paralysis* (unilateral or bilateral). Paradoxic motion (the opposite side is pulled across the midline during inspiration) involving the vocal cord or entire arytenoid cartilage on the affected side may be seen and is not a primary disorder.

## Ancillary Tools and Procedures

Radiographic evaluation of the larynx does not add significant diagnostic or prognostic information and is not indicated in the complete evaluation of laryngeal disorders. Tidal breathing flow-volume loops (TBFVL) have been used to document the presence of upper airway obstruction (Figure 12-8). However, an abnormal TBFVL still requires laryngoscopy to confirm the presence and extent of structural and functional laryngeal disorders. A laryngeal electromyogram or biopsy procedure may be used to delineate a specific etiology, but these tests are properly performed after the initial laryngoscopic evaluation has been made.

## Complications

A properly performed laryngoscopic examination is a low-risk procedure. However, the clinician should be aware that emergencies may occur during and immediately after laryngoscopy. In a small number of patients, stimulation of the larynx may provoke a very strong vagal response that may result in profound bradyarrhythmias. This complication is largely prevented by administering anticholinergic medication before anesthesia is induced. Laryngeal mucosal hyperemia and edema are commonly encountered in a variety of laryngeal disorders. The manipulation that occurs during laryngoscopy may cause additional mucosal irritation, edema, and, potentially, further narrowing of the airway (a complication that is more common in cats). In addition, some patients with laryngeal disease and upper airway obstruction may have great difficulty maintaining a patent airway during the immediate postanesthetic recovery phase. Therefore endotracheal and tracheostomy tubes and instruments should be available (in suspected cases). If a surgically correctable disorder of the larynx is suspected (e.g., laryngeal paralysis), the laryngoscopic examination should be scheduled so that surgical correction can immediately follow the examination, thereby avoiding a second anesthetic procedure.

## Differences Between Feline and Canine Laryngoscopy

The larynxes of dogs and cats have significant gross differences in anatomy. Specifically, the corniculate and cuneiform processes of the arytenoid cartilages are well developed and are much more prominent in dogs than in cats. Furthermore, structures that comprise the feline laryngeal vault become edematous after manipulations that cause no edema in canine patients. This edematous response may be dramatic and can result in serious airway obstruction (see Plate 12-24). The feline larynx may respond to light touch with spasm, further occluding the upper airway. For these reasons it is critical to place a few drops of *1% lidocaine* on the surface of the feline laryngeal structures before laryngoscopy is performed. It is also important for the operator to be very gentle when manipulating this area.

### SUGGESTED ADDITIONAL READINGS

Bjorling DE: Laryngeal paralysis. In Bonagura JD, editor: *Current veterinary therapy XII,* Philadelphia, 1995, WB Saunders.

Burk RL, Ackerman N: The skull. In Burk RL, Ackerman N, editors: *Small animal radiology and ultrasonography.* Philadelphia, 1996, WB Saunders.

Ford RB: Endoscopy of the upper respiratory tract of the dog and cat. In Tams TR, editor: *Small animal endoscopy,* St Louis, 1990, Mosby.

Hendricks JC: Recognition and treatment of congenital respiratory tract defects in brachycephalics. In Bonagura JD, editor: *Current veterinary therapy XII,* Philadelphia, 1995, WB Saunders.

## COLOR PLATES   PAGES 366-376

## POSTERIOR RHINOSCOPY

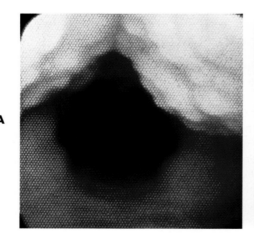 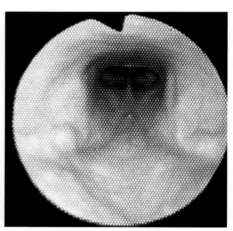

**Plate 12-1** A 9-year-old Siamese cat with a 1-year history of chronic mucoid nasal discharge and sneezing. **A,** The dorsal wall of the posterior nasopharynx is covered with pinpoint white plaques comprised of hyperplastic lymphoid tissue. No additional rhinoscopic abnormalities were found. The histologic diagnosis was follicular lymphoid nasopharyngitis. **B,** Normal posterior nasopharynx for comparison.

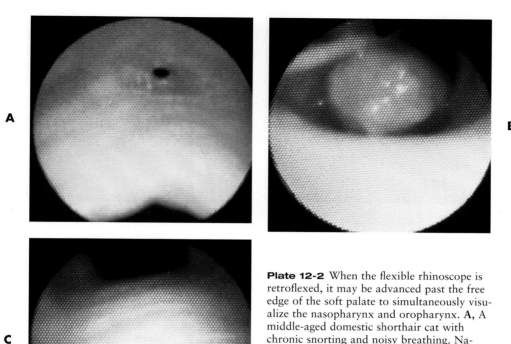

**Plate 12-2** When the flexible rhinoscope is retroflexed, it may be advanced past the free edge of the soft palate to simultaneously visualize the nasopharynx and oropharynx. **A,** A middle-aged domestic shorthair cat with chronic snorting and noisy breathing. Nasopharyngeal stenosis or web is seen dorsal to the edge of the soft palate (upper center in field of view). **B,** A young Burmese cat with snorting and noisy breathing. A round, red polyp is easily visualized in the dorsal nasopharynx. **C,** Edge of normal soft palate and entrance to nasopharynx and oropharynx for comparison.

## FOREIGN BODIES AND PARASITES

Chronic nasal discharge and sneeze occasionally result from foreign bodies or parasites. Endoscopy is a very valuable tool for diagnosing and in many situations managing these cases. Posterior rhinoscopy and pharyngoscopy should be considered early in dogs and cats with unexplained sneezing, snorting, or gagging.

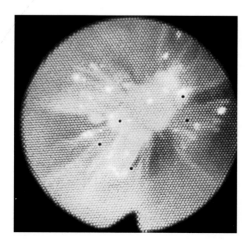

**Plate 12-3** Cockleburr in the posterior choanae of a young cat. Removal led to the resolution of all clinical signs.

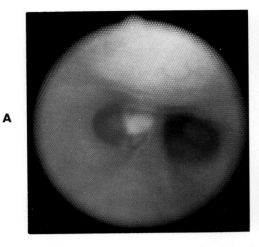 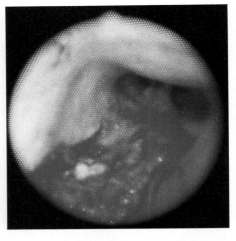

**Plate 12-4** Peanut foreign body in the internal nares of a miniature poodle presented with the acute onset of dyspnea after the owner observed the dog inhale a peanut. Bronchoscopy initially revealed no abnormal findings. **A,** The bronchoscope was subsequently retroflexed above the soft palate to examine the internal nares. A peanut lodged in this area was removed with foreign body grasping forceps. **B,** Nasopharynx after removal of the peanut. Hemorrhage resulted from minor trauma of the mucosa from contact with the foreign body grasper and peanut during retrieval. (Courtesy Keith P. Richter.)

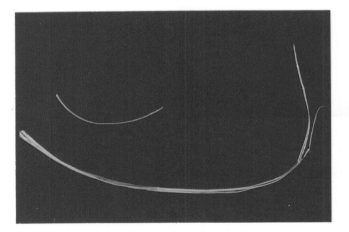

**Plate 12-5** A 4-cm blade of johnsongrass removed via endoscopy from the nasopharynx of a Labrador retriever presented with the acute onset of coughing and gagging. Several episodes of retching produced saliva with small grass fragments. Examination of the oral cavity revealed marked swelling of the caudal soft palate. Retroflex examination of the nasopharynx identified a grass blade extending into the internal nares as well as marked mucosal hyperemia (endoscopic photograph not available). The sharp base of the grass blade was embedded in the soft palate and therefore could not pass into the pharynx. A subsequent examination of the trachea and bronchi was normal. (Courtesy Todd R. Tams.)

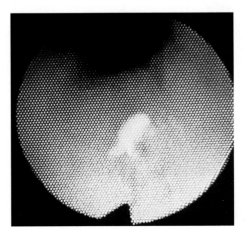

**Plate 12-6** Nasal mite in the posterior nasopharynx of a dog with chronic sneezing.

## NEOPLASIA

Neoplasia may cause chronic sneezing and nasal discharge. If the lesion and resulting mucoid or bloody discharge occlude both choanae, the animal may lose its sense of smell. In cats especially this may lead to inappetence and weight loss.

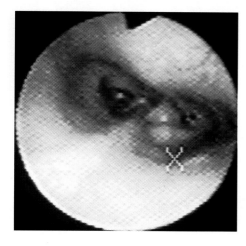

**Plate 12-7** Lymphosarcoma in the left posterior choanae of a cat. Note the relatively normal appearance of surrounding mucosa in the absence of abnormal mucus or discharge.

A 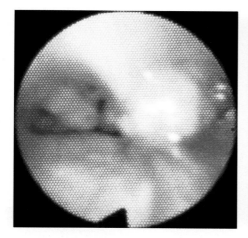 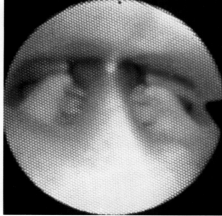 B

**Plate 12-8 A,** Undifferentiated carcinoma in the right posterior choanae of an 8-year-old domestic shorthair cat with chronic sneezing and nasal discharge. Note the bloody fluid surrounding the mass and totally occluding the choanal opening. **B,** Normal appearance of posterior choanae.

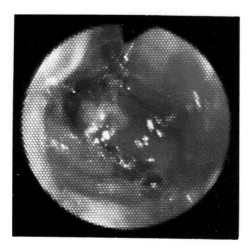

**Plate 12-9** Nasal tumor (center of the field) extending into the caudal nasal cavity of a dog presented because of sonorous breathing. The histologic diagnosis was adenocarcinoma. (Courtesy Richard B. Ford.)

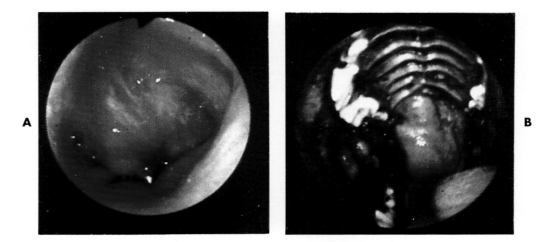

**Plate 12-10 A,** Nasopharyngeal neoplasm extending from the hard palate into the nasopharynx of a 6-month-old rottweiler presented with stertor and halitosis. The histologic diagnosis was fibrosarcoma. **B,** Photoendoscopy of the hard palate. The neoplasm extends from the palate into the lumen of the oral cavity. (Courtesy Richard B. Ford.)

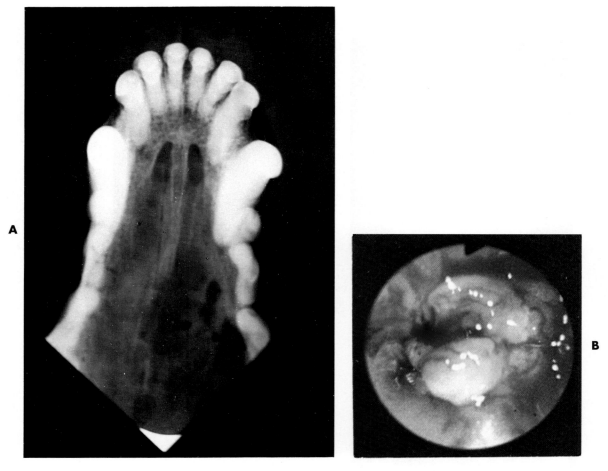

**Plate 12-11 A,** Nasal radiograph of a 12-year-old poodle with a 3-month history of progressively worsening nasal discharge, including epistaxis, stertor, sneezing, and recent swelling of the caudal aspect of the nose. Diffuse densities are seen in both nasal sinuses, and turbinate detail has been lost. **B,** Endoscopic view of the nasopharynx. A soft tissue mass is occluding the caudal nasal sinus. The histologic diagnosis was adenocarcinoma. (Courtesy Todd R. Tams.)

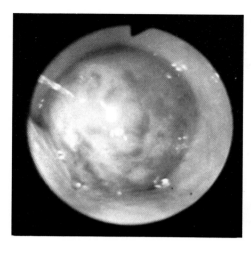

**Plate 12-12** Large nasal tumor extending into and occluding the caudal nasal sinus of a 2-year-old Labrador retriever presented for sneezing and stertor. No nasal discharge or epistaxis was present. The histologic diagnosis was rhabdomyosarcoma. (Courtesy Todd R. Tams.)

## ANTERIOR RHINOSCOPY

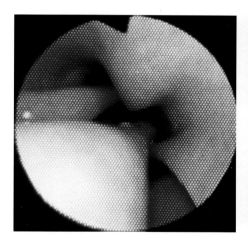 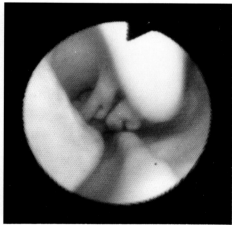

**Plate 12-13** Normal appearance of anterior nasal mucosa. Note the pink firm smooth tissue and the absence of mucus or other discharge.

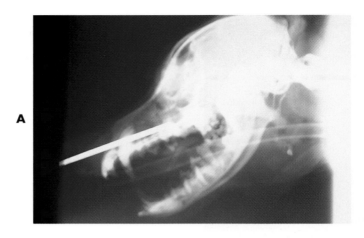

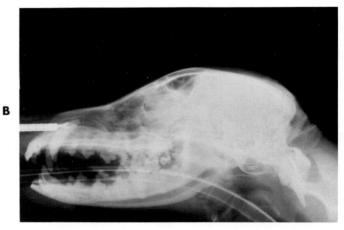

**Plate 12-14  A,** Lateral skull radiograph of a 20-kg (44-lb) dog, demonstrating the correct placement of a 2.7-mm-diameter rigid endoscope within a sheath for anterior rhinoscopy. **B,** Lateral skull radiograph of a 17-kg (37-lb) dog, demonstrating the correct placement of a bronchoscope (5-mm outer diameter) for rhinoscopic examination. Note that the insertion depth is maximal. Biopsy forceps have been passed through the instrument channel and are in position to procure a biopsy specimen.

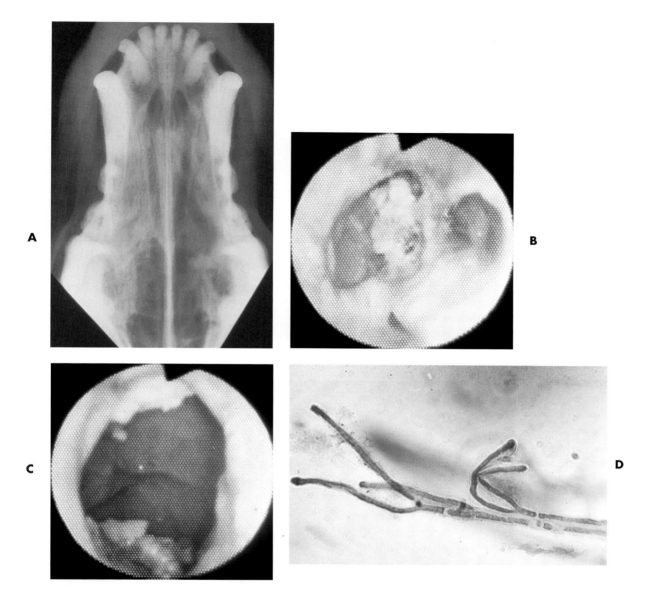

**Plate 12-15** Good-quality high-contrast radiographs of the nasopharyngeal region are important for determining the potential value of rhinoscopy in an animal with chronic nasal discharge, sneezing, and/or gross nasofacial deformity. In this case a 7-year-old boxer with adrenal-dependent hyperadrenocorticism was presented to the University of Chicago veterinary referral center with chronic nasal discharge and explosive bloody sneezing **A,** Open-mouth radiograph demonstrates patchy areas of increased density bilaterally and increased lucency on the left. The normal fine reticular pattern of the nasal turbinates is lost bilaterally. **B,** Destruction of the nasal choanae and the appearance of a "fungal ball" typical of nasal aspergillosis. **C,** Further exploration of the left nasal cavity demonstrated severe destruction of the normal nasal architecture and the creation of a "tunnel effect." **D,** Nasal flushing demonstrated the hyphae of *Aspergillus* species.

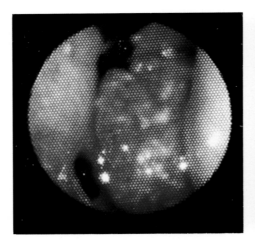

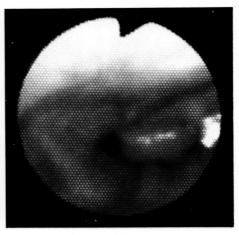

**Plate 12-16** Rhinosporidiosis growth (*Rhinosporidium seeberi*) in the nasal cavity of a dog. The lesion typically occurs as a pink nasal polyp that is pedunculated or sessile and usually less than 3 cm in diameter. White specks (sporangia) may be seen on the surface.

**Plate 12-17** Discrete, benign nasal polyp in the rostral aspect of the nasal cavity in a dog with paroxysmal sneezing.

A

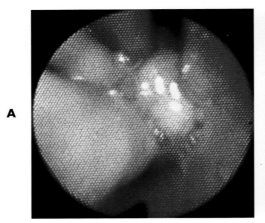

B

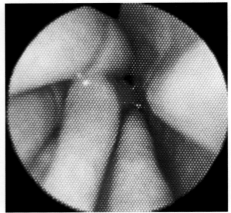

**Plate 12-18** A 5-year-old mixed-breed dog was presented to the University of Illinois veterinary medicine teaching hospital with a 4-month history of chronic unilateral nasal discharge and intermittent sneezing. The dog's clinical signs resolved partially with antibiotic therapy. **A,** The left nasal cavity is filled with a 2-cm mass that is coated with yellow, purulent, filmy material. The surrounding nasal mucosa is grossly hyperemic and friable, and it bled very easily when touched. Rhinoscopically guided biopsy resulted in a diagnosis of adenocarcinoma. **B,** For comparison, normal right nasal cavity demonstrating intact pink mucosa.

## LARYNGEAL DISORDERS

Tracheobronchoscopy should always be preceded by a thorough evaluation of the posterior pharynx and laryngeal area. Regardless of cause, disorders of the vocal folds or surrounding structures result in variable bark changes, noisy breathing (especially during inspiration), and exercise intolerance.

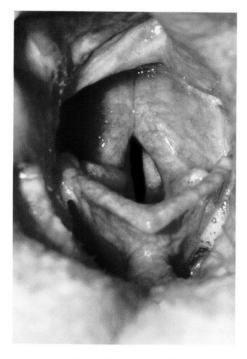

**Plate 12-19** Partial laryngeal collapse in a 12-year-old Labrador retriever with a 6-month history of noisy breathing. Only partial bilateral abduction of the arytenoid cartilages occurs during maximal inspiration. The left vocal fold is visible in the lumen of the normally clear laryngeal opening. Note also hyperemia, excessive secretions, and edema distributed throughout the laryngeal vault.

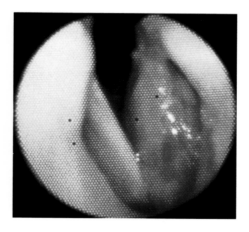

**Plate 12-20** Vocal fold granuloma in a 6-year-old boxer. The dog's owners had noticed a gradual change in the quality of the animal's bark.

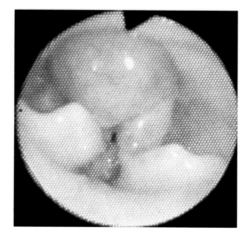

**Plate 12-21** Thyroid carcinoma causing significant airway obstruction and exercise limitation in an 8-year-old terrier.

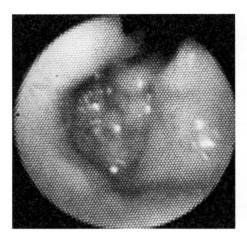

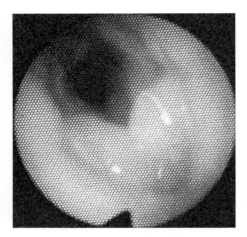

**Plate 12-22** Laryngeal granuloma in a dog presented for noisy breathing 4 months after a "de-barking" surgical procedure.

**Plate 12-23** Saccular edema and eversion in a cat with inspiratory distress following extubation.

A

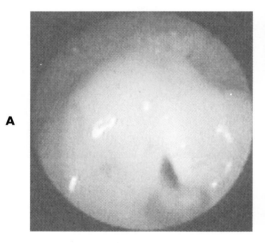

B

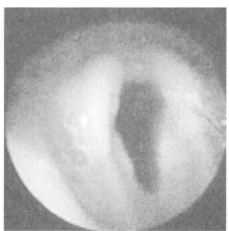

**Plate 12-24 A,** Severe laryngeal edema and obstruction that developed within 5 minutes of a traumatic attempt at intubation in a 4-year-old domestic shorthair cat. **B,** Normal feline larynx for comparison.

# Chapter 13

# Tracheobronchoscopy of the Dog and Cat

Philip A. Padrid and Brendan C. McKiernan

The first reported endoscopic procedure of the lower respiratory tract may have occurred in 1897 when Dr. Gustav Killian, using light from the Black Forest as a guide, passed a hollow tube down the trachea of a woodcutter to remove a pork bone from the unfortunate man's right mainstem bronchus. In 1904 Dr. Chevalier Jackson developed a rigid bronchoscope, and the medical specialty of bronchoscopy subsequently became firmly established. However, it was not until 1968 that the flexible fiberoptic bronchoscope was introduced into the clinical practice of human medicine.

In the past 10 years, respiratory endoscopy has become an important diagnostic technique in the practice of high-quality veterinary medicine. Before bronchoscopes were used, the evaluation of veterinary patients with clinical signs referable to the respiratory system was limited to chest auscultation, thoracic radiography, and transtracheal washing. Bronchoscopy has greatly expanded the veterinarian's understanding of respiratory disease in dogs and cats and has facilitated the diagnosis and treatment of many respiratory disorders. Bronchoscopic evaluation of the pulmonary tree can reveal the nature, vascularity, extent, and distribution of many pathologic changes in airway wall structure and function. Areas of focal infection can be microbiologically sampled without contamination of "healthy" sites, a complication that can occur during unguided transtracheal washing or a bron-

chopulmonary wash through an endotracheal tube. Exfoliated cells from primary or metastatic neoplastic lesions can be identified within lung tissue using the technique of bronchoalveolar lavage, which has made it possible to stage and treat cancer more effectively. Left atrial compression of a mainstem bronchus can be identified (see Plate 13-14), thereby confirming cardiomegaly as a cause of cough and ruling out primary respiratory disease. The general experience of most clinicians who have incorporated bronchoscopy into the practice of veterinary medicine and surgery can be summarized in one line: *How did we ever get along without it?*

## INDICATIONS

The numerous indications for tracheobronchoscopy in dogs and cats are summarized in Box 13-1. The two most frequent reasons to perform bronchoscopy in veterinary patients are (1) acute or chronic cough that is unanticipated or unresponsive to standard medical therapy and (2) suspicious radiographic infiltrates. Less commonly appreciated reasons to perform respiratory endoscopy include the advanced evaluation of abnormal breathing patterns and the grading of chronic bronchitis or tracheal collapse. Bronchoscopy can also be invaluable in distinguishing cardiac from respiratory causes of cough and for staging metastatic lung cancer. Tracheo-bronchoscopy should also be considered in veterinary patients with noisy breathing or stridor for which laryngoscopy fails to confirm the cause.

Ancillary procedures performed under bronchoscopic visualization include biopsy, microbiologic sampling and bronchoalveolar lavage. Tracheobronchial biopsy is primarily performed to obtain a histologic diagnosis for abnormal endobronchial growths or parenchymal infiltrates. Microbiologic sampling of potentially infected areas within the respiratory tree is greatly assisted by bronchoscopic guidance because the sampling brush can be directed into specific areas of interest. This technique offers the best chance of retrieving diagnostic samples and minimizes the risk of cross contamination of less involved sites, as can occur when nonspecific washing techniques are used. Bronchoalveolar lavage is a technique that can be used to assess the morphology and distribution of cells that line individual lung segments, and

the retrieved samples can be processed to include total and differential counts of the cells obtained.

Bronchoscopy itself has no specific contraindications. However, the procedure should not be performed in patients that are not candidates for general anesthesia.

## INSTRUMENTATION

Before 1968 tracheobronchoscopy was performed exclusively with rigid instruments. With the introduction of flexible bronchoscopes the veterinarian is now able to visualize and manipulate a much larger area of the respiratory tree. Nevertheless, rigid bronchoscopy is still indicated in the following situations:

1. When very small patients (cats, toy-breed dogs) require examination
2. When the area of interest is the trachea and carina
3. When photographic quality needs to be enhanced

In most cases, however, veterinary practitioners will have the greatest success performing tracheobronchoscopy using a flexible bronchoscope.

Bronchoscopes used to evaluate adult human patients are 4.8 to 5.2 mm in outer diameter, have a 2.0-mm inner channel diameter, and are between 55 and 60 cm in length. These scopes are appropriate for complete evaluation of the respiratory tree in medium- to large-sized dogs. As previously noted, cats and small (toy) dogs are more safely evaluated with smaller diameter rigid instruments. Alternatively, bronchoscopes designed for use in children may be used in small patients. Flexible pediatric instruments are generally 3.5 to 3.7 mm in outer diameter, have a 1.2-mm inner channel diameter, and are 40 to 60 cm in length. Although these instruments are much safer for use in smaller patients, their narrow inner channel does not permit passage of commonly used ancillary tools, including biopsy and culture forceps, that require an inner channel diameter of 2 mm or greater. Specific dimensions of instruments designed for bronchoscopy are summarized in Table 13-1.

**Box 13-1   Indications for Tracheobronchoscopy**

Acute cough for which an inhaled foreign body is the suspected cause
Chronic cough that has an unknown cause or does not respond to standard therapy
Unexplained lung infiltrate
Unexplained abnormal breathing pattern
Confirmation and staging of tracheal collapse
Staging of chronic bronchitis, including the presence and degree of airway collapse
Distinction of cardiac disease from respiratory disease as a cause of cough by demonstration of left mainstem bronchial collapse
Stridor not explained by laryngoscopic findings
Diagnosis and staging of primary or metastatic pulmonary neoplasia
Removal of mucoid obstruction in atelectatic lung lobes

**Table 13-1   Dimensions of Flexible and Rigid Instruments for Use in Tracheobronchoscopy in Dogs and Cats**

| Bronchoscope | Outer diameter (mm) | Working length (cm) | Inner channel (mm) | Up deflection (degrees) | Down deflection (degrees) |
|---|---|---|---|---|---|
| Flexible | 5 | 55 or 85 | 2 | 180 | 80 |
| Flexible | 3.7 | 54 | 1.2 | 180 | 80 |
| Flexible | 2.5 | 100 | 1.2 | 170 | 90 |
| Rigid | 2.7 | 53 | None | None | None |
| Rigid | 1.7 | 34 | None | None | None |

In general, animals should be intubated with an appropriate-sized tube to permit easy passage of the bronchoscope with sufficient area for easy gas exchange around the scope. An exception to this rule is the bronchoscopic evaluation of very large and giant-breed dogs. In these, animals the standard adult bronchoscope is not long enough to reach past the carina if the scope is first passed through an endotracheal tube. Therefore, bronchoscopy may need to be performed without an endotracheal tube so that the bronchoscope can be advanced farther into the airways. Alternatively, these animals may be evaluated using a pediatric *gastroscope* with an outer diameter of 7.8 to 9 mm, an inner channel diameter of 2 to 2.8 mm, and a length of 100 to 150 cm.

## PATIENT PREPARATION

Tracheobronchoscopy requires the induction and maintenance of general anesthesia. Beyond the risks associated with general anesthesia, no significant concerns are usually related to the procedure. Thus the work-up prior to tracheobronchoscopy should include the tests that are routinely performed in patients undergoing anesthesia, including a complete physical examination, a complete blood count, serum chemistries, and urinalysis. In addition, patient-specific tests may include chest radiographs, a heartworm test, fecal flotation, and a cardiac ultrasound examination to rule out primary heart disease as the cause of clinical signs. In some universities, additional pulmonary function tests may be available and appropriate, including measurement/analysis of total lung resistance, dynamic compliance, and tidal breathing flow-volume loops.

Special *precautions* are required for endoscopy in patients with upper airway obstruction from such causes as posterior pharyngeal polyp, elongated and thickened soft palate, laryngeal paralysis or paresis, and tracheal mass or collapse. These patients tend to wake up with a vague increased awareness of the obstruction, and consequently adopt a very aggressive inspiratory breathing strategy. This leads to further upper airway collapse and a vicious cycle that may necessitate tracheostomy. These patients must be kept at a very light plane of anesthesia, and they should be monitored aggressively until they are fully awake. If an endotracheal tube is placed, it should not be removed until the awakening patient is forcefully attempting to cough it out.

### Oxygen

Patients should always be given 100% oxygen for 10 to 15 minutes before tracheobronchoscopy and again for 10 to 15 minutes after the procedure. This prevents the hypoxemia that routinely develops in animals that are not oxygenated before respiratory endoscopy. Oxygen may be delivered through an endotracheal tube or by a tight-fitting face mask.

### Previously Prescribed Medications

The decision to continue or discontinue medications prescribed before endoscopy depends on the situation. For example, if infection is suspected and the endoscopist anticipates taking airway secretions for culture, it may be wise to stop antibiotics for 3 days before endoscopy. However, the withholding of antibiotics may not be indicated if the infection is severe and/or withdrawal of antibiotics may lead to a deterioration in a patient's clinical status. Thus the endoscopist must evaluate each clinical situation in concert with the primary veterinarian to determine if and what drugs should be withheld and for how long.

### Bronchodilators

Bronchodilators are only indicated for cats with a clinical history or signs consistent with asthma. These cats should be given terbutaline, 0.011 mg/kg (0.005 mg/lb) intramuscularly, 15 minutes before tracheobronchoscopy is performed.

### Topical Lidocaine

Lidocaine (1% without epinephrine) should be applied to the larynx of all cats. This may be accomplished using a 1-ml syringe and a 26-gauge needle to gently "spray" the larynx before an endotracheal tube or bronchoscope is inserted. Lidocaine should also be applied to the trachea of all dogs and cats undergoing tracheobronchoscopy. This can be accomplished by "spraying" lidocaine (≤0.5ml) through the vocal folds using endoscopic or laryngoscopic visualization. The endoscopist should then wait 5 minutes before proceeding with endoscopy. This valuable procedure minimizes tracheal sensitivity and the cough reflex; it also decreases the level of general anesthesia required for the procedure.

### Specific Anesthetic Recommendations

A number of different and sophisticated protocols have been developed and advocated for anesthetizing patients with respiratory compromise. These protocols are generally sound and safe, and it is well worth the time needed to become proficient in their use. Alternatively, in our experience (and for most practitioners) the best method of anesthetizing a patient for respiratory endoscopy is the method that is most commonly and safely used by the practitioner who is responsible for administering the anesthesia. Common sense and good judgment should determine the techniques used in this and all anesthetic cases. We do recommend the use of rapidly cleared gas anesthetics because of the quick recovery time involved.

Experienced bronchoscopists may complete a thorough endoscopic evaluation and sampling of the respiratory tract in 10 minutes. In these uncomplicated cases it is not usually necessary to intubate the patient, and a short-acting injectable anesthetic is adequate. The primary advantage to this approach is the increased airflow that is available to the patient because an endotracheal tube is not in place and does not further decrease airway diameter. However, when a prolonged procedure is anticipated, it is wise to place an endotracheal tube prior to insertion of the bronchoscope. The advantage of this approach is that the endoscopist has a protected airway if the health of the patient deteriorates during the procedure. This approach requires a T-piece type adapter so that the endoscopist can connect the endotracheal tube to the gas anesthetic/oxygen source and simultaneously pass the endoscope into the respiratory tract (Figure 13-1). Practitioners need to remember that a standard bronchoscope with a 5-mm outer diameter requires at least a 7-French endotracheal tube so that adequate airflow can be maintained within the tube and around the bronchoscope.

For the reasons previously discussed, smaller dogs and cats should be evaluated with a pediatric (3.5-mm outer diameter) bronchoscope, with or without prior endotracheal intubation (4.5-French or greater). If intubation is not planned, supplemental oxygen can be administered through the biopsy channel of the endoscope or through a tube passed alongside the scope into the trachea.

## PATIENT RESTRAINT AND POSITIONING

Tracheobronchoscopy of dogs and cats is always performed using general anesthesia. The position of the patient is determined by the preference and previous expe-

rience of the endoscopist. We place dogs and cats in a sternal recumbent position and support the ventral neck with a rolled towel. The mouth is kept open by insertion of a metal speculum (Figure 13-2).

## PROCEDURE

### When Infection is Not a Significant Concern

The endoscopist should learn to travel the tracheobronchial tree in the same direction, from one specific lobe to the next, in the identical order in each patient. This makes it easier to remember the anatomic location from moment to moment. The bronchoscope should always be passed in a nontraumatic fashion through the rimma glottis (between the vocal folds) with complete visualization. If the endoscope is passed through an endotracheal tube, a small amount of lubricating jelly (K-Y or equivalent) should be placed on the outside of the instrument. This makes it easy to slide the instrument within the endotracheal tube and minimizes trauma to the bronchoscope.

The trachea is first evaluated for color, vascularity, rigidity, size, and position and movement of the dorsal membrane. The bronchoscope is advanced toward the carina while the tip is maintained directly within the lumen of the trachea. If the bronchoscopist loses sight of the carina, the endoscope should not be advanced until the carina is again located. Once the tip of the bronchoscope approaches the carina, we begin to examine each lobar bronchi in the following order: right cranial, right

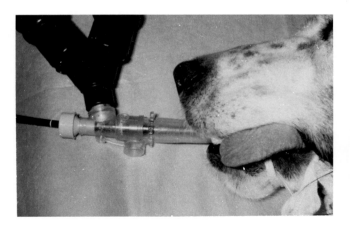

**Figure 13-1** T-piece adapter for endotracheal tube. This adapter allows the flexible bronchoscope to be inserted through the endotracheal tube without disrupting the simultaneous administration of anesthetic gas and oxygen.

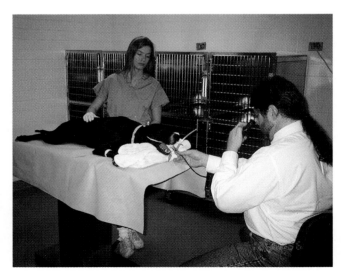

**Figure 13-2** Proper position of endoscopist and patient for bronchoscopy. Note that the dog is in a sternal recumbent position and square to the table to prevent distortion of normal anatomic relationships. The bronchoscopist is seated to avoid fatigue.

middle, accessory, right caudal, left cranial subsegment, left caudal subsegment, left caudal lobe (Figure 13-3).

The segmental and smaller branches of many lobar bronchi have a similar appearance to the new bronchoscopist. If the bronchoscopist is not sure of the exact position of the bronchoscope tip, the scope should be withdrawn to the carina and positioned so that the tracheal membrane is dorsal. The bronchoscope can then be repositioned into the area of interest. This maneuver should be repeated as many times as necessary to confirm the position of the instrument within the respiratory tree. Few situations in respiratory medicine are more frustrating than visualizing a discrete bronchial lesion during bronchoscopy, withdrawing the bronchoscope for the placement of ancillary tools such as biopsy forceps, and then not being able to find the lesion again. This situation can be prevented if the bronchoscopist is always aware of the anatomic position of the scope within the pulmonary tree.

## When Infection is a Concern

The infected area should be visited first if secretions are going to be obtained for culture and/or cytologic examination. This approach decreases the chance of sample contamination by colonizing bacteria from noninfected areas. Otherwise the infected area should be the last area visited by the bronchoscope to minimize the chance of carrying infectious material to other areas of the bronchial tree.

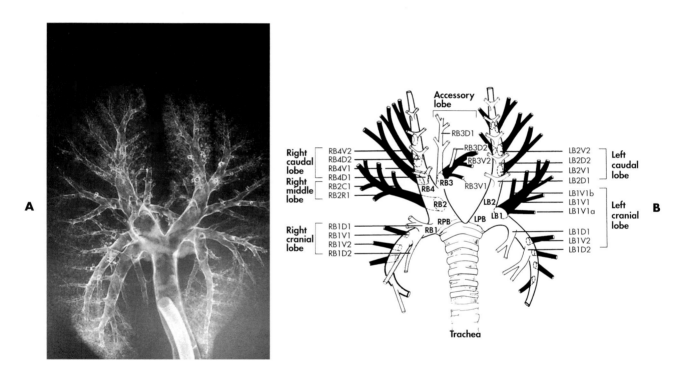

**Figure 13-3** Tracheobronchial anatomy. The respiratory tree is a series of connected, branching tubes that serve to conduct air into and out of the respiratory exchange units (alveoli). Because the multiple airway branches arborize into thousands of small respiratory bronchioles, the task of learning tracheobronchial anatomy may seem overwhelming. In practice, however, the bronchoscopist need only learn the names and appearances of the seven major lung segments. In almost all cases, disease or pathology localized to a particular lung segment with radiography can be confirmed and explored bronchoscopically if the endoscopist learns the appearance of the entrance to these seven lung lobes. Because the trachea is long, wide, and straight, it is an easy area to navigate with an endoscope. However, once the mainstem bronchi are entered, even the experienced bronchoscopist can become confused about the particular branch or airway segment. If uncertainty exists regarding the placement of the bronchoscope, the endoscopist should retract the instrument to the carina so that the tracheal membrane is dorsal and then begin again, noticing the specific segment and subsegment entered. **A,** Tantalum bronchogram demonstrating the vast arborization of the canine respiratory tree. (The canine and feline respiratory trees are basically identical.) **B,** Diagram of the canine respiratory tree, showing the seven principle lung lobes (lobar bronchi) and primary branches within each lung lobe. (From Amis TC, McKiernan BC: Systematic identification of endobronchial anatomy during bronchoscopy in the dog, *Am J Vet Res* 47: 2649, 1986.)

## Normal Appearance

The normal canine airway generally does not contain mucus or free fluids of any kind (see Plate 13-1). The mucosa is pink and glistening. A fine network of submucosal vessels is easily seen unless the mucosa is edematous or covered with mucus. The tracheal rings are also easily identified. The dorsal tracheal membrane is tight, does not protrude into the lumen of the trachea, and may extend past the carina and blend into either or both of the mainstem bronchi. The smaller intrathoracic airways tend to widen and narrow very slightly on inspiration and expiration respectively, and the timing and degree of these shape changes should be noted.

Normal airway mucosa in cats has a yellowish tinge (see Plate 13-2). Importantly, it is common to find small amounts of mucus in otherwise healthy feline airways. (This mucus would be considered a sign of inflammation in canine airways.)

## Abnormal Appearance

Mucosal inflammation from any cause tends to result in various degrees of hyperemia, edema, and mucus secretion. The presence of hyperemia alone can be due to cough from any cause, and the finding of increased mucosal reddening does not indicate any specific disease process. Tracheal collapse that results in cough typically causes general hyperemia. During a normal cough the tracheal lumen may narrow transiently by as much as 75%, and this finding should not be interpreted as a sign of tracheal collapse. However, during normal expiration the tracheal lumen should be unaffected. Dogs with tracheal collapse often have a weakened or flaccid dorsal tracheal membrane that intrudes into the tracheal lumen during passive inspiration. This flaccid membrane may occlude part or all of the lumen of the trachea (see Plate 13-3). With segmental collapse, mucosal erosion may be seen in the areas where the dorsal membrane comes into contact with the ventral floor of the trachea (see Plate 13-4).

More chronic inflammatory processes, including parasitic infection with *Filaroidea* nematodes or chronic bronchitis, may cause the formation of nonneoplastic polyps or nodules (see Plate 13-5). These tissues are usually friable and therefore bleed easily if touched by the tip of the bronchoscope or an ancillary instrument. Chronic inflamed airways may contain large amounts of thick tenacious mucus, which in rare cases may result in mucus plugs. In severe cases, scarring and mucus may lead to total obliteration of an airway. This is seen more commonly in cats with asthma. Airway collapse is another common finding in chronic inflammatory airway disease. Inflammatory lesions are depicted in Plates 13-6 through 13-12.

Pulmonary fungal infections or neoplasia that cause enlarged hilar lymph nodes may be suspected broncho-scopically because of the resulting distortion of normal anatomy (see Plate 13-13). An enlarged left atrium from congestive heart failure may also cause a characteristic distortion of normal airway architecture as it compresses only the left mainstem bronchus without affecting other airway segments (see Plate 13-14).

Tracheobronchial foreign bodies are found and removed more often than they are reported in the veterinary literature. This is especially true in warmer climates where plant material, including foxtail grass, is frequently inhaled by hunting dogs. In the majority of cases this plant material is quickly coughed up and expelled without apparent complications. Occasionally, however, foxtails or blades of other grasses become trapped within the respiratory tree and cause acute, explosive coughing. Entrapped plant material should be suspected in any dog that has an acute, explosive cough and has recently been in a field or woody environment (see Plate 13-15). In addition to plant material, we have discovered and removed unusual objects, including rocks and sewing pins, from the airways of both dogs and cats.

## ANCILLARY TOOLS AND PROCEDURES

### Culture

Most dogs and cats with chronic signs of cough, gag, or expiratory difficulty that are otherwise systemically well do not have clinically significant respiratory bacterial infections. Nevertheless, bacteria may be found in material obtained from the tracheobronchial tree of these patients. This apparent paradox is easily explained by the finding that the tracheobronchial tree of many species, including the dog and cat, is not routinely sterile. As in almost all situations in clinical medicine, culture results should be interpreted in light of the patient's clinical history, physical signs, and other diagnostic test results.

When infectious bacterial airway disease is suspected, airway secretions should be cultured for aerobic bacteria and *Mycoplasma organisms* (cats only). When a patient's radiographic signs and travel history are consistent with a fungal infection, cultures should be obtained. The exception to this suggestion is possible infection with *Coccidioides immitis*. In cultures, *C. immitis* develops mycelia, which are highly infectious and therefore represent a public health hazard.

The *guarded microbiology brush* (Microvasive, Milford, Mass.) is an alternative to the transtracheal wash for retrieving airway material for culture. The brush is designed to be passed through the biopsy port (2-mm diameter) of a previously positioned adult (5-mm outer diameter) bronchoscope (Figure 13-4). The inside brush is extruded, gently passed into the region of suspected infection, and resheathed. It is then withdrawn from the

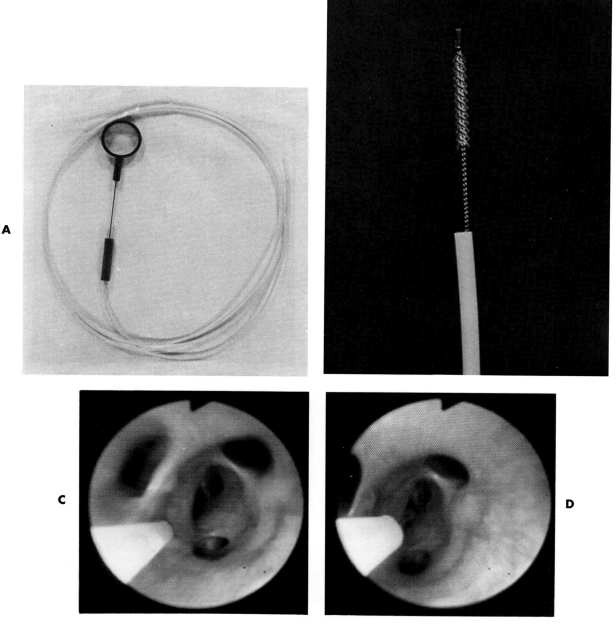

**Figure 13-4** Double lumen sheathed microbiology brush. **A,** The brush is retracted into the sheath to ensure that sterility is maintained. **B,** The tip of the brush is extended from the sheath. The 140-cm-long sheathed brush is first passed through the biopsy port of the bronchoscope. Under bronchoscopic guidance the brush and the sheath are passed into the airway. The brush is extruded from the sheath and passed into the area of interest within the airway to collect samples for microbiologic analysis. Under bronchoscopic visualization the brush is resheathed before it is withdrawn into the distal end of the scope. Once the apparatus has been removed from the bronchoscope, the end of the brush is extruded from the sheath so that the tip, along with the airway sample, can be clipped off into a sterile clot tube for further processing. **C,** Endoscopic appearance of tubing extended from the scope. **D,** The brush is extended into the airways under direct visualization. After a brushing sample is obtained, the brush is withdrawn into the sheath before the sheath is retracted into the working channel of the scope. (Courtesy Todd R. Tams.)

bronchoscope and processed by cutting off the end of the brush into a sterile red top tube containing 0.25 to 0.5 ml of sterile water to prevent the brush from drying out.

Secretions obtained using a guarded microbiology brush may be cultured routinely or in a quantitative fashion. Quantitative bacterial cultures have been used to distinguish colonization from infection in human patients with bacterial pneumonia. In these cases, bacterial growth at a concentration of less than $10^4$ colony-forming unit (CFU)/ml is believed to represent nonpathologic colonization, and antibiotic therapy is not recommended. Healthy cats and dogs may harbor an aerobic bacterial population within their mainstem bronchi at a concentration of as high as $10^3$ CFU/ml. In practice, quantitative cultures are prohibitively expensive. Nevertheless, the clinical significance of a positive culture result can be inferred from the finding that growth was obtained on a primary culture plate (more than $10^4$ CFU/ml indicates infection) or only after the airway material was subcultured in enrichment broth such as thioglycolate (fewer than $10^3$ CFU/ml indicates commensal growth).

## Cytology

Cytologic evaluation of respiratory secretions obtained from dogs and cats with signs of tracheobronchial dis-

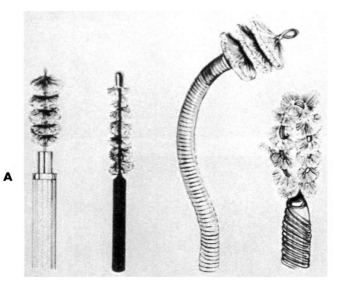
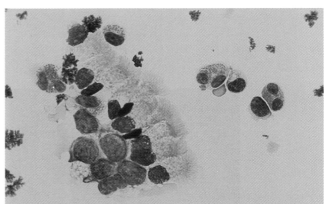

**Figure 13-5** Tracheal, bronchial, and pulmonary cytology. The diagnosis of neoplastic and infectious diseases of the respiratory tract may be significantly aided by the cytologic evaluation of cells collected during bronchoscopy. Occasionally, respiratory cytology may also be helpful in the differential diagnosis of noninfectious nonneoplastic pulmonary inflammatory disorders, including chronic bronchitis, feline asthma, and pulmonary infiltrates with eosinophilia (PIE syndrome). Common methods used to collect airway and parenchymal cells include bronchial brushings, bronchial wash, and bronchoalveolar lavage (BAL). Various brushes are available to collect cells from the respiratory mucosa; however, these instruments have been designed for human patients with focal endobronchial lesions. Because the majority of bronchopulmonary disorders seen in veterinary practice do not involve such lesions, these brushes are not appropriate for the routine collection of airway specimens for cytology. Bronchial washings are advantageous compared to transtracheal washings because the former technique is performed under bronchoscopic guidance and the fluid can be instilled into specific lung segments. However, the analysis of cells obtained by the method of bronchial wash is limited to a subjective appraisal of the number and kind of cells present. BAL is a more recently developed technique in which the bronchoscope is guided into an affected lung segment until the size of the scope is as large as the entered airway. At this point the instrument is said to be in a "wedged" position. With this technique, large amounts of fluid may be instilled and gently aspirated without fear of flooding the lung, because the majority of instilled fluid can be retrieved while the endoscope is in a wedged position. Both differential and total cell counts can be determined for the cells collected by BAL, and these counts can greatly aid the endoscopist in determining the respiratory cause of clinical signs. **A,** Bronchial brushes available for use when a focal lesion is suspected or visualized by radiography or during bronchoscopy. **B,** Cytologic specimen collected using a bronchial brush. The majority of cells are mucosal epithelial cells.

ease is most helpful for confirming the presence of suspected infectious organisms or exfoliated neoplastic cells. It is less helpful for diagnosing the cause of noninfectious inflammation of the lower airway. This is especially true in cats because eosinophils (cells that might reflect inflammation in other body fluids) are normal inhabitants of the feline lower airway (Figure 13-5). In addition, total cell counts are not routinely determined from airway fluids.

Cytology brushes designed for use in humans with respiratory disease are made to sample endobronchial cells, or cells that line the airway wall. This is appropriate in humans, for whom endobronchial masses are relatively common. Because endobronchial lesions are very rare in dogs and cats, cytology brushing is not the method of choice to retrieve samples for cytologic analysis.

In general, large numbers of nonseptic neutrophils support the finding of bronchitis *or* asthma, and overwhelming populations of eosinophils (greater than 75%) are consistent with the diagnosis of allergic asthma.

## Bronchoalveolar Lavage

A major limitation in the cytologic interpretation of tracheobronchial secretions is the lack of uniformity in the collection, processing, and reporting of the samples. Unlike analysis of other body fluids such as whole blood,

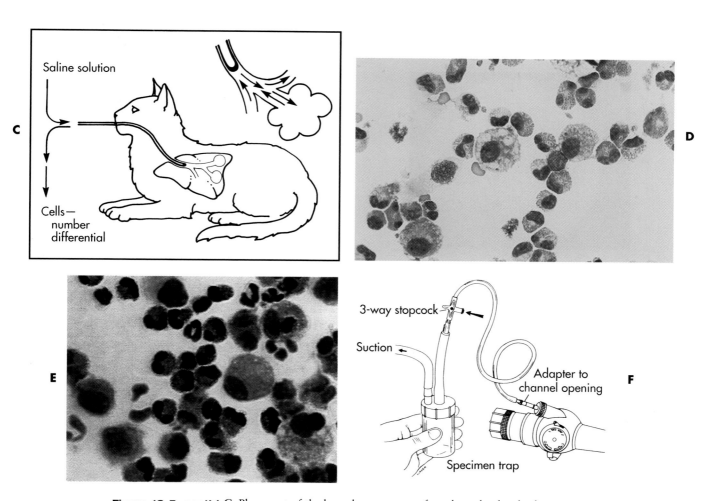

**Figure 13-5, cont'd** C, Placement of the bronchoscope to perform bronchoalveolar lavage. Note that the majority of aspirated fluid is withdrawn back through the bronchoscope because the instrument is wedged into position, thus minimizing the amount of fluid that may be lost around the bronchoscope. D, Cytologic specimen collected using the BAL technique. Alveolar macrophages are the predominant cell type recovered from healthy dogs and cats. E, Large number of eosinophils in a BAL sample from a healthy cat. F, Sterile suction trap, which can be placed in series between the suction catheter (not shown) and the bronchoscope. The aspirated fluid can be cultured or prepared for cytologic evaluation.

urine, and spinal or joint fluid, total and differential cell counts from tracheobronchial washings are not routinely determined. This is partially due to the various methods used to collect and analyze the samples and the subsequent lack of uniformity in the results that are obtained. The technique of bronchoalveolar lavage was developed to better standardize the collection, analysis, and reporting of bronchial and alveolar lining cells and secretions.

To ensure maximal return of fluid, bronchoalveolar lavage should be performed through a flexible broncho-scope that has been "wedged" into a segmental or sub-segmental branch of a lung lobe (see Figure 13-5). Using this technique, relatively large volumes of fluid (2 ml/kg [0.9 ml/lb] of body weight) may be repeatedly instilled and recovered. Because of the potential loss of large volumes of fluid within the lung, only clinicians experienced in this technique should perform bronchoalveolar lavage

in cats. The administration of 100% oxygen for at least 10 minutes before and after bronchoalveolar lavage is necessary to prevent the development of hypoxemia.

## Biopsy

Endobronchial biopsy is more commonly performed and more rewarding diagnostically in human medicine because of the more frequent occurrence of endobronchial cancer associated with cigarette smoke. For veterinarians, endobronchial biopsy is occasionally helpful in diagnosing neoplastic lesions and identifying nonneoplastic polyps. This technique can also increase the index of suspicion for chronic bronchial inflammation.

The biopsy cup is less than 2 mm in width and can retrieve tissue from the bronchial tree that is usually only 1 to 1.5 mm in size. Full-thickness samples are not retrieved using this method. Furthermore the specimen

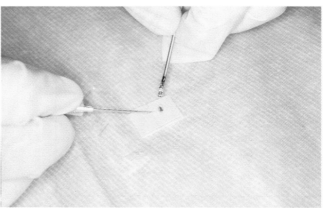

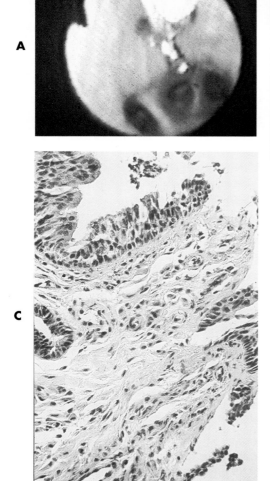

**Figure 13-6** Endobronchial biopsy. **A,** Biopsy cup (at the tip of a biopsy instrument designed for endobronchial biopsy) within the lumen of the right mainstem bronchus of a dog with chronic bronchitis. The cup appears relatively large because of the magnification effect that occurs during bronchoscopic visualization. **B,** After the biopsy instrument is withdrawn from the airway, the sample is retrieved and placed on a piece of a wooden tongue depressor. Note the actual size of the biopsy cup relative to the hands of the operator. **C,** Processed tissue obtained by endobronchial biopsy of the airways of the dog in *A.* The epithelium is fragmented due to "crush artifact." However, the epithelium can still be appreciated to be increased in size, and the submucosa is infiltrated with neutrophils. A single enlarged submucosal gland is seen at the 9 o'clock position.

that is obtained is frequently "crushed," and the presence of "crush artifact" makes histologic interpretation of the sample difficult. The bronchoscopist may also be initially fooled into thinking that a larger piece of tissue can be obtained because the appearance of the biopsy instrument tip is magnified when viewed through the endoscope (Figure 13-6).

*Transbronchial biopsy* may be performed using standard flexible biopsy forceps or by introducing a Stifcor needle (Microvasive Inc.). Using the former approach, the flexible bronchoscope is introduced into the affected lung segment, and the closed biopsy forceps is delivered into the lung periphery, past the operator's field of vision. When resistance is met or the appropriate area reached (if fluoroscopy is used), the forceps instrument is retracted 1 to 2 mm and its jaws are opened. At this point the lungs of the anesthetized patient are expanded, and the biopsy instrument is advanced until resistance is again met. The patient's lungs are allowed to deflate, the jaws of the biopsy forceps are closed, and peribronchial alveolar tissue is obtained. At this point the bronchoscopist usually feels a characteristic tug of parenchyma. While the forceps is removed, the flexible bronchoscope is maintained in the biopsied lung segment to monitor for bleeding or to confine bleeding to the isolated bronchial segment.

We have used the transbronchial biopsy technique successfully without encountering significant complications. In human medicine, however, the technique has been associated with persistent bleeding and pneumothorax, potential complications that should be of concern to anyone attempting the procedure. It is emphasized that although transbronchial biopsy is a promising technique, it requires specialized equipment and sophisticated operator training.

Closed-chest techniques are available to acquire lung parenchyma for histologic analysis. However, we emphasize that open-lung biopsy probably provides a greater chance of obtaining quality diagnostic samples most likely as safe as closed-chest techniques.

## SUGGESTED ADDITIONAL READINGS

Amis TC, McKiernan BC: Systematic identification of endobronchial anatomy during bronchoscopy in the dog, *Am J Vet Res* 2649, 1986.

Beaumont PR: Intratracheal neoplasia in two cats, *J Small Anim Pract*, 23:29, 1982.

Breary MJ, Cooper JE, Sullivan M, editors: *Color atlas of small animal endoscopy,* St Louis, 1991, Mosby.

Creighton SR, Wilkens RJ: Transtracheal aspiration biopsy technique and cytologic evaluation, *J Am Anim Hosp Assoc* 10:219, 1974.

Hawkins EC, DeNicola DB: Collection of bronchoalveolar lavage fluid in cats using an endotracheal tube, *Am J Vet Res* 5:855, 1989.

Hernandez BL, Hernandez IMS, Garido VdMV: Safety of the transbronchial biopsy in outpatients, *Chest* 99:562, 1991.

McKiernan BC, Smith AR, Kissil M: Bacteria isolated from the lower trachea of clinically healthy dogs, *J Am Anim Hosp Assoc* 20:139, 1984.

Moise NS et al: Clinical radiographic and bronchial cytologic features of cats with bronchial disease: 65 cases (1980–1986), *J Am Vet Med Assoc* 194:1467, 1989.

Padrid PA et al: Canine chronic bronchitis. A pathophysiologic evaluation of 18 cases, *J Vet Intern Med* 4:172, 1990.

Padrid PA, Amis TC: Chronic tracheobronchial disease in the dog, *Vet Clin North Am Small Anim Pract* 22:1203, 1992.

Wang K-P, Mehta AC, editors: *Flexible bronchoscopy,* Cambridge, Mass, 1995, Blackwell.

Wheeldon EB, Pirie HM: Measurement of bronchial wall components in young dogs, adult normal dogs, and adult dogs with chronic bronchitis, *Am Rev Respir Dis* 110:609, 1974.

Wimberly N, Faling LJ, Bartlett JG: A fiberoptice bronchoscopy technique to obtain uncontaminated lower airway secretions for bacterial culture, *Am Rev Respir Dis* 119:337, 1979.

## COLOR PLATES    PAGES 387-396

### NORMAL CANINE AND FELINE TRACHEA AND BRONCHI
**Plate 13-1,** p. 388, Canine trachea and bronchi
**Plate 13-2,** p. 388, Feline trachea and bronchi

### PRIMARY TRACHEAL COLLAPSE
**Plate 13-3,** p. 389, Tracheal collapse in a Welsh corgi
**Plate 13-4,** p. 389, Segmental tracheal collapse with mucosal erosion

### PARASITIC TRACHEOBRONCHITIS
**Plate 13-5,** p. 390, Parasitic nodules (Filaroides osleri)

### CHRONIC BRONCHITIS AND ASTHMA
**Plate 13-6,** p. 391, Nodule formation caused by chronic bronchitis in a dog
**Plate 13-7,** p. 391, Hyperemia and occlusive nodules in a dog
**Plate 13-8,** p. 391, Scarring and mucus formation in a dog
**Plate 13-9,** p. 392, Bleeding at the carina after bronchoscopy in a dog
**Plate 13-10,** p. 392, Open airway in a dog with tracheal collapse and chronic bronchitis
**Plate 13-11,** p. 392, Dorsoventral radiograph of a cat with asthma
**Plate 13-12,** p. 393, Mucus cast from the right caudal lobe of a cat with asthma

### ENLARGED TRACHEOBRONCHIAL LYMPH NODES
**Plate 13-13,** p. 393, Blastomycosis in a dog

### LEFT ATRIAL COMPRESSION OF LEFT MAINSTEM BRONCHUS
**Plate 13-14,** p. 394, Left mainstem bronchus collapse caused by left atrial enlargement in a dog

### TRACHEOBRONCHIAL FOREIGN BODIES
**Plate 13-15,** p. 395, Foxtail foreign body in bronchus of a dog
**Plate 13-16,** p. 396, Cat with rock lodged in trachea

## NORMAL CANINE AND FELINE TRACHEA AND BRONCHI

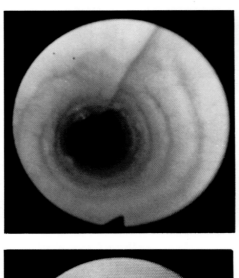

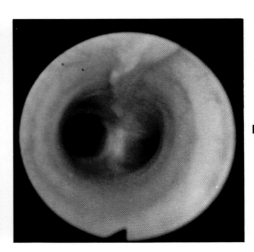

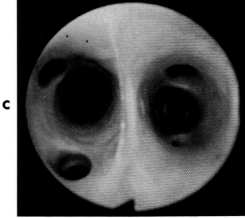

**Plate 13-1 A,** Bronchoscopic appearance of the normal canine trachea with a bronchoscope positioned at mid-trachea. The dorsal tracheal membrane appears as a distinct thin strip of muscle (12 o'clock position). **B,** Carina, which appears as a sharp wedge dividing the trachea into the right and left principal bronchi. The dorsal tracheal membrane is visualized at the 12 o'clock position in this field of view. The right principal bronchus (seen at the left) appears as an almost direct extension of the trachea. The left principal bronchus forms a more acute angle with the trachea. **C,** Normal canine lobar and segmental bronchi. Note the rounded structure of the individual airway segments, their pink color, and the absence of mucus or free fluids. (**B** and **C** courtesy Todd R. Tams.)

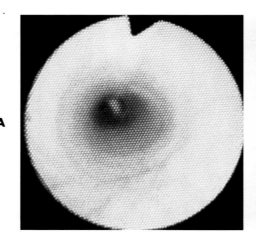

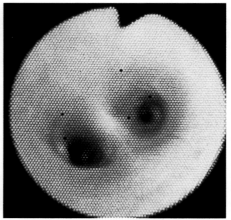

**Plate 13-2 A,** Lumen of a feline trachea and carina with a bronchoscope positioned at the level of the mid-trachea. Feline airway mucosa has a distinctly yellow tinge compared to canine and human airways. **B,** Same airway at the level of the carina. Slight hyperemia at the entrance to both the right and left mainstem bronchi is due to irritation from the tip of the bronchoscope. Compare with the appearance of canine carina (see Plate 13-1, *B*).

# PRIMARY TRACHEAL COLLAPSE

Deviation of the dorsal tracheal membrane into the lumen of the trachea may occur as a primary condition (primary tracheal collapse) or in association with chronic bronchitis. The collapse point may be focal or may involve the entire length of the trachea. Coughing greatly exacerbates the condition and can lead to complete airway obstruction, syncope, and respiratory arrest.

**A**                    **B**

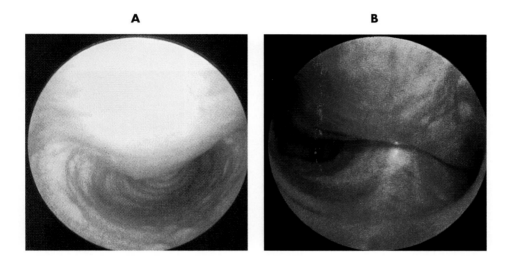

**Plate 13-3 A,** Generalized tracheal collapse in a Welsh corgi with a chronic honking cough. The tip of the bronchoscope is at the level of the mid-trachea. More than 50% of the tracheal lumen is occluded during normal breathing. **B,** As seen with a bronchoscope at the level of the carina, the tracheal membrane has occluded two thirds of the entrance to the right mainstem bronchus.

**A**                    **B**

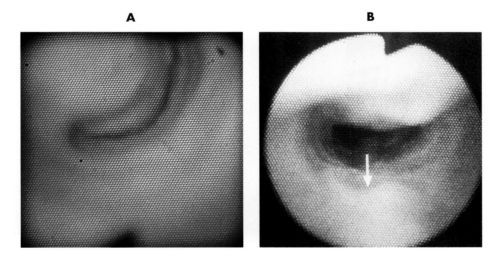

**Plate 13-4** Segmental tracheal collapse with mucosal erosion. **A,** Tracheal collapse causing cough may result in communication between the dorsal and ventral mucosa. **B,** This may lead to mucosal erosion (*arrow*), which can cause continued cough and a destructive cycle of cough-mucosal damage-cough. Mucosal erosion cannot be appreciated radiographically but is easily seen with a bronchoscope.

## PARASITIC TRACHEOBRONCHITIS

Common tracheobronchial parasites include *Filaroides (Oslerus) osleri* in dogs and *Aelurostrongylus abstrusus* in cats. The lungworm *F. osleri* produces small granulomas in the tracheal and bronchial mucosa adjacent to the carina. Coughing is the major clinical symptom, and wheezing and dyspnea may occur if a large number of nodules are present. Radiographs may reveal soft tissue densities (granulomas) in the caudal trachea. Characteristic nodules are readily visible on bronchoscopic examination, and mature worms may be observed within the nodules. The diagnosis is confirmed by identifying larvae in bronchial washings or in a fresh fecal sample after larvae are coughed up and swallowed.

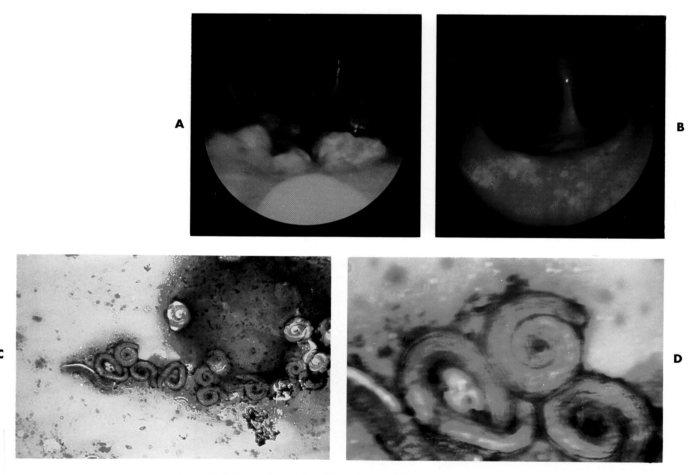

**Plate 13-5** Parasitic nodules. More chronic inflammatory processes, including parasitic infection with *Filaroides* species, may cause the formation of nonneoplastic polyps or nodules. **A,** *Filaroides (oslerus) osleri* nodules in the distal trachea of a greyhound with chronic cough, wheezing, and weight loss. **B,** The same greyhound's trachea after therapy (1 year from the time the original endoscopic photograph was made). Tracheal hyperemia is seen, but no nodules remain. **C,** *F. osleri* larvae from a tracheal wash sample (low-power magnification). **D,** *F. osleri* larvae (high-power magnification). (A and B courtesy Flora E.F. Lindsay; C and D courtesy Anne E. Wagner.)

# CHRONIC BRONCHITIS AND ASTHMA

Chronic noninfectious inflammatory diseases in dogs and cats are most commonly due to chronic bronchitis (both species) or asthma (cats)

**A** 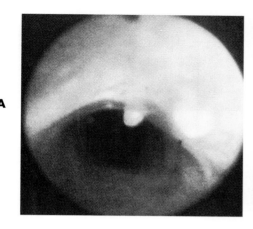 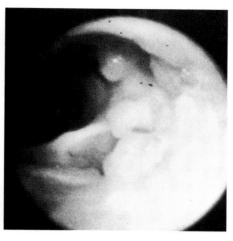 **B**

**Plate 13-6 A,** Single nodule caused by chronic bronchitis in a 12-year-old mixed-breed dog. **B,** Advanced nodular formation in the same dog.

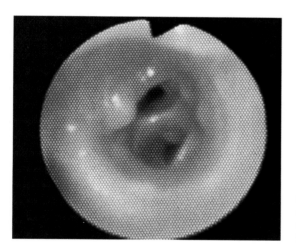

**Plate 13-7** Hyperemia and nodules occluding almost 90% of the airway lumen in a 9-year-old Labrador retriever with a cough for 2 years.

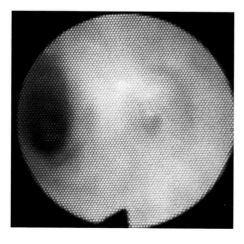

**Plate 13-8** Scarring and mucus formation causing complete obliteration of the airway of a 10-year-old Welsh corgi with a chronic cough.

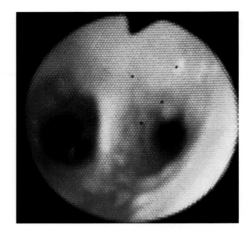

**Plate 13-9** Bleeding at the carina after bronchoscopy in a 14-year-old chocolate Labrador retriever with chronic cough. Nodules are present at the entrance to both mainstem bronchi.

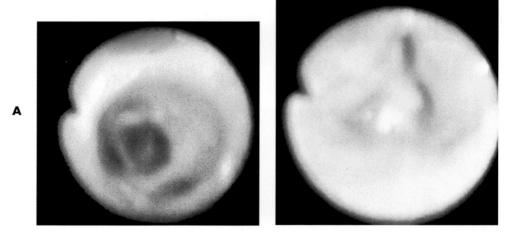

A

B

**Plate 13-10** A, Open airway at inspiration in an 11-year-old poodle with tracheal collapse and chronic bronchitis. B, Airway in the same dog, now collapsed during passive inspiration.

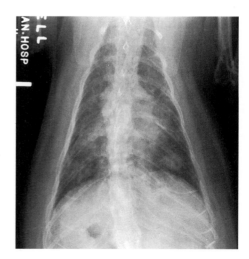

**Plate 13-11** Dorsoventral radiograph of a cat with asthma. Note the areas of apparent consolidation due to the accumulation of thick, tenacious mucus that is occluding major airways. (This radiographic appearance is never seen in dogs with bronchitis and can be easily mistaken for pneumonic lesions.)

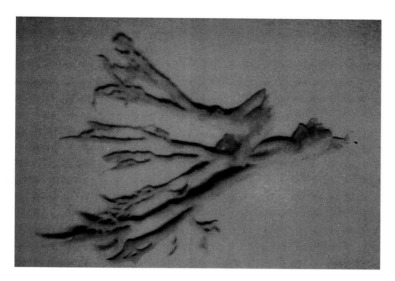

**Plate 13-12** Mucus cast removed at necropsy from the right caudal lobe of a cat with asthma.

## ENLARGED TRACHEOBRONCHIAL LYMPH NODES

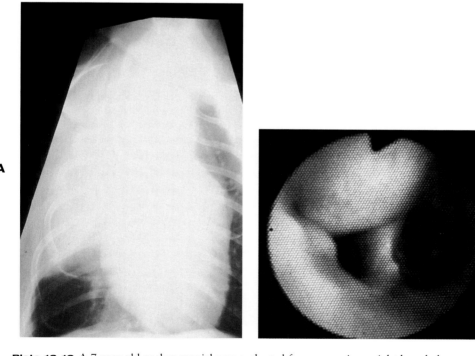

**A**

**B**

**Plate 13-13** A 7-year-old cocker spaniel was evaluated for progressive weight loss, lethargy, and cough persisting for 1 to 2 months. **A,** Dorsoventral thoracic radiograph revealed complete consolidation of the right cranial and middle lung lobes. **B,** Bronchoscopy revealed massive lymphadenopathy resulting in obstruction of the entrance to the right principal and right cranial bronchus. Bronchoalveolar lavage samples revealed thick-walled yeast cells typical of *Blastomyces dermatitidis*. Biopsy confirmed the diagnosis of blastomycosis.

## LEFT ATRIAL COMPRESSION OF LEFT MAINSTEM BRONCHUS

Congestive heart failure can result in enlargement of the left atrium, which may push up into the ventral floor of the respiratory tree at the level of the left mainstem bronchus. As a result, the ventral and dorsal mucosa come into contact with every heartbeat. This situation can result in chronic cough.

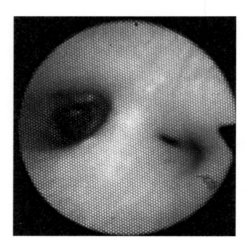

**Plate 13-14** A 12-year-old retriever cross was evaluated for chronic cough. Chest radiographs demonstrated normal lung parenchyma and left atrial enlargement. Through the bronchoscope the left mainstem bronchus was seen to collapse from the ventral floor up in time with the heartbeat. The right mainstem and segmental bronchi, as well as the left-sided bronchi past the collapse point, were all normal. Diuretic therapy resulted in left atrial shrinkage and resolution of the cough.

## TRACHEOBRONCHIAL FOREIGN BODIES

A chronic cough that does not respond to treatment with antibiotics, cough suppressants, and other medications is usually the most common presenting sign of a tracheobronchial foreign body. Inhaled foreign bodies are often small enough to pass beyond the carina into the lobar bronchi. Grass awns, nails, bone fragments, and a variety of other types of foreign material have been retrieved from the airways. Survey thoracic radiographs may be unremarkable if the foreign material is not radiodense. In most airway foreign body cases a mucopurulent exudate is found originating from the bronchus in which the foreign body is located. Biopsy forceps or foreign body graspers can be passed through or around the scope to retrieve the foreign material. In most cases, clinical signs resolve shortly after the foreign body is removed.

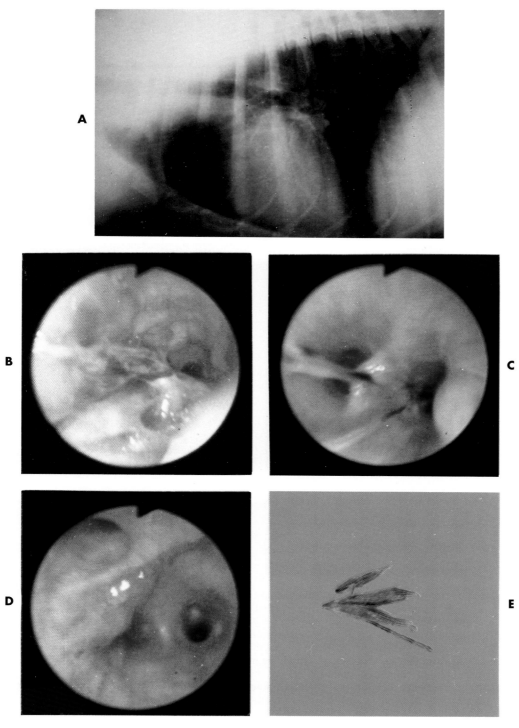

**Plate 13-15** A 2-year-old golden retriever was presented with a 2-month history of nonproductive cough. Radiographs showed mild interstitial and peribronchial densities that suggested mild chronic bronchitis. A complete blood count was unremarkable. A corticosteroid and a cough suppressant controlled the clinical signs, but the cough recurred as soon as the drugs were discontinued. **A,** Lateral thoracic radiograph showing mild interstitial densities. **B,** Endoscopic view of the bronchus, with mucopurulent exudate covering what appears to be a foreign body (7 to 9 o'clock position in the field of view). **C,** After the mucus was cleared away, two projections from a foxtail (*Hordeum jubatum,* a common weed in California) were identified. The foxtail was retrieved with a biopsy forceps. Note the generalized airway hyperemia. **D,** Swelling around the bronchus where the foxtail was lodged. **E,** Foxtail (length, 2.5 cm) removed from the bronchus. The cough stopped immediately after the foreign body was retrieved (Courtesy Todd R. Tams.)

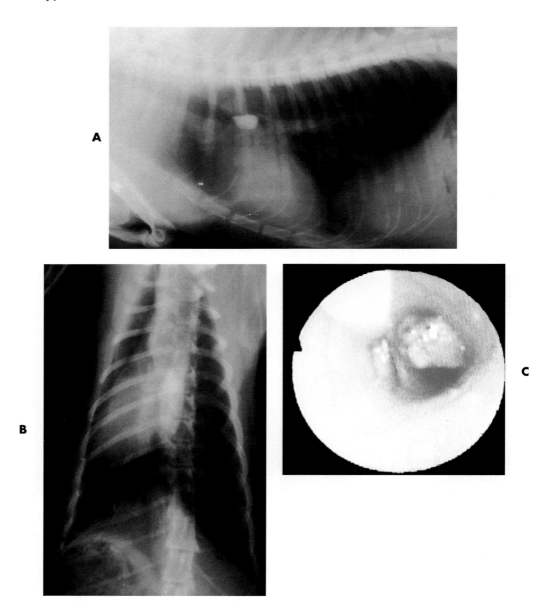

**Plate 13-16** A 2-year-old domestic long-haired cat was presented to the emergency clinic at the University of California at Davis Veterinary Medicine Teaching Hospital because of the acute on-set of respiratory distress. On admission the cat was coughing; however, no other respiratory signs were apparent. During physical examination the cat acutely began gasping, became cyanotic, and suffered respiratory arrest. **A,** Lateral thoracic radiograph revealing a radiopaque foreign body over the base of the heart, within the intrathoracic trachea. **B,** Dorsoventral thoracic radiograph suggesting mediastinal and cardiac shift toward the left hemithorax. The large amount of air in the stomach is a common finding in animals suffering from acute and significant respiratory impairment. **C,** Rock found within the tracheal lumen. When the rock moved cranially, the cat coughed but was otherwise stable. When the rock rolled caudally, it obstructed a mainstem bronchi, leading to acute respiratory distress. The bronchoscopist was not able to use normal forceps to remove the rock. The foreign body was finally retrieved using a Foley catheter that was advanced alongside the bronchoscope until the balloon tip was caudal to the rock. The catheter balloon was blown up and brought out of the trachea with the bronchoscope and the rock. The cat survived the procedure and was released the following morning. The mediastinal shift was attributed to an obstructed right mainstem bronchus at the time the radiograph was taken.

# Chapter 14

# Laparoscopy: Instrumentation and Technique

**Michael L. Magne and Todd R. Tams**

Laparoscopy is an operative procedure designed for the visual inspection and biopsy of the peritoneal cavity and its organs. For many years laparoscopy has been a valuable diagnostic and therapeutic tool in human clinical medicine. Only in the last 25 years, however, has this operative procedure been widely used for research and clinical diagnostic and therapeutic purposes in various animal species.

The first canine laparoscopy procedures were performed in the early 1900s using essentially the same technique employed today. Initially veterinary laparoscopy was most widely used for reproductive function studies in food animal, equine, nonhuman primate, and various zoo or exotic species. The first *clinical* application of laparoscopy in dogs was in ovarian function studies performed in the early 1960s, and the first laparoscopic liver biopsy procedure in a dog was reported in 1972 (Lettow).

With the development of flexible fiberoptics and advanced illumination systems, laparoscopy has become a sophisticated technique that has many applications in companion-animal clinical medicine. Although we have most commonly employed laparoscopy to procure hepatic and renal tissue samples, we have also used the technique to obtain biopsy samples from pancreatic, adrenal, prostatic, and ovarian tissues.

## ROLE OF LAPAROSCOPY IN HUMAN SURGERY

Laparoscopic surgical techniques in humans have both improved and expanded in the past decade. In Lyons, France, Mouret and colleagues performed the first successful laparoscopic cholecystectomy in 1987. After a year of intensive work in animals, the technique was refined. In the United States the first laparoscopic cholecystectomy on a human patient was performed in 1988. By 1989 medical centers in several countries were offering laparoscopic cholecystectomy as an alternative to the much more invasive, traditional open-abdomen technique. The advantages of laparoscopic cholecystectomy over open cholecystectomy include much shorter hospitalization (1 to 2 days versus 5 to 7 days), fast recuperation, and very small incision size. Another early development in laparoscopy improved accuracy in the diagnosis of acute appendicitis. As the less invasive "keyhole" surgical techniques have gained favor and public demand for them has increased, many surgeons have undergone extensive training in laparoscopic surgery.

The developments in human surgery have led to an explosion in the field of laparoscopy, and the great demand for video, laser, and laparoscopy instrumentation has not uncommonly resulted in 3- to 9-month backlogs in equipment orders. The strong interest in laparoscopy has helped fuel the development of new applications and instruments for this surgical technique. Procedures now commonly performed laparoscopically in humans include appendectomy, herniorrhaphy, pelvic and paraaortic lymphadenectomy, splenectomy, nephrectomy, and subtotal colectomy. Laparoscopy is also used in the staging of pancreatic and gastric neoplasm, the surgical treatment of gastroesophageal reflux disease, and a variety of gynecologic procedures.

## INSTRUMENTATION

### Basic Equipment

The basic equipment for laparoscopy includes the laparoscope (telescope) and corresponding trocar-cannula

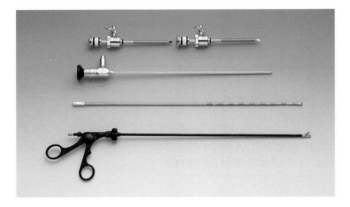

**Figure 14-1** Instrumentation for laparoscopy (*top to bottom*): two trocar-cannula units (with trocars inside the cannulas), a 5-mm-diameter laparoscope (telescope), a palpation probe, and a punch biopsy instrument. The size of the cannula corresponds to the size of the telescope being used.

unit (Figure 14-1), a light source, the Veress (insufflation) needle, and a gas insufflator.

The size of the trocar-cannula unit corresponds to the diameter of the laparoscope being used. Trocar tips are either conical or pyramidal. A pyramidal tip is preferred because it facilitates easier abdominal wall penetration. The cannula, or sleeve, consists of a channel (to accommodate the laparoscope) with a trumpet valve that prevents insufflated gas from being lost when the trocar is removed or the laparoscope is inserted (Figure 14-2). Most cannulas also have a Luer-lock adaptor that allows continued insufflation or fluid aspiration while the laparoscope is being used.

Laparoscopes applicable for use in dogs or cats range from 1.7 to 10 mm in diameter (Figure 14-3). Because the 10-mm laparoscope requires a 2-cm incision for insertion, it is only used in animals weighing more than 10 kg (22 lb). The smallest laparoscope (1.7 mm) is used with a 2.2-mm cannula that can be inserted through an incision no longer than the diameter of a 14-gauge needle; this scope is useful in even the smallest animals. A significant disadvantage of smaller laparoscopes is their limited field of vision. Furthermore, because smaller laparoscopes contain fewer light bundles, a more powerful light source is required for good image quality. A 5- to 7-mm-diameter laparoscope is versatile and can be used in dogs and cats of almost any size. Therefore, if only one laparoscope is to be purchased, we recommend a unit in this size range.

For veterinarians interested in performing a variety of rigid endoscopic procedures (e.g., cystoscopy in female dogs, rhinoscopy, avian endoscopy, otoscopy), we recommend purchase of 2.7-mm oblique-viewing and 5-mm forward-viewing scopes (Figure 14-4). The 2.7-mm scope is very versatile; in small patients (e.g., small dogs and cats, iguanas, birds), laparoscopy can easily be

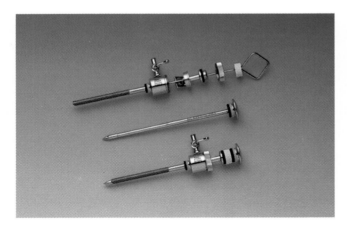

**Figure 14-2** Trocar-cannula unit. *Top,* Disassembled cannula with cleaning pin in place, holding the valve open. *Middle,* Trocar with a pyramidal tip. *Bottom,* Cannula with trocar inserted.

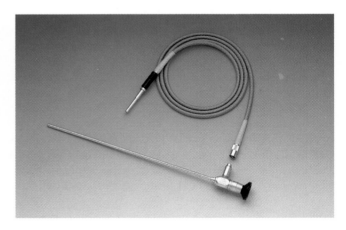

**Figure 14-3** Laparoscope (telescope) and fiberoptic light cable. This 5-mm-diameter scope (Karl Storz Co., Goleta, Calif.) is an ideal size for performing laparoscopy in both dogs and cats.

performed with this scope, especially if a video camera is used to enhance the image. The 5-mm scope is an excellent instrument for performing laparoscopy in dogs and cats of any size.

Laparoscopes with various directions of vision (Figure 14-5) are also available. A 0- or 180-degree direction of vision provides the operator with a "normal" field of view and in our experience has proved most useful for laparoscopy. Oblique-angle and retrograde-view laparoscopes are also available and are preferred by some endoscopists.

Operating laparoscopes have an offset eyepiece and contain a channel for the introduction of accessory instruments (Figure 14-6). These scopes were designed to allow organ biopsy or manipulation without the insertion of a secondary (accessory) cannula. However, the insertion cannula for operating laparoscopes is large (11 to 12 mm in diameter), which limits the use of these instruments in smaller animals. Double-puncture insertion of a laparoscope and an accessory cannula allows a versatility in biopsy procurement and organ manipulation that is not possible with a single-puncture operating laparoscope.

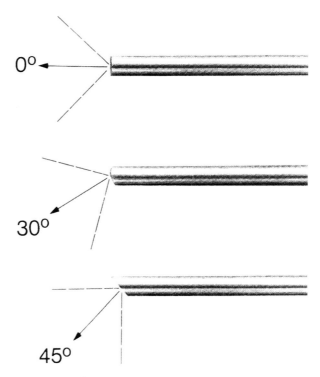

**Figure 14-5** Telescope angles of view. The most commonly used are the 0-degree and 30-degree angled telescopes (Courtesy Karl Storz Veterinary Endoscopy-America, Inc.).

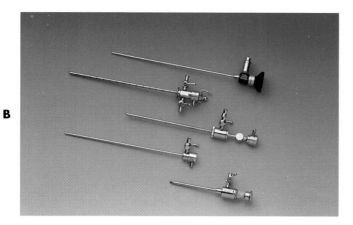

**Figure 14-4** Multifunction telescopes. **A,** A 5-mm, 0-degree (forward-viewing) laparoscope/thoracoscope (*top*); a 2.7-mm, 30-degree (oblique-viewing) scope (Karl Storz Co.) (*bottom*) for use in the following procedures: laparoscopy in cats and small dog, rhinoscopy, cystoscopy in small- to medium-size female dogs, otoscopy, arthroscopy, and avian endoscopy. **B,** Multipurpose rigid telescope (2.7 mm in diameter, 30-degree oblique-angle view) with various sheaths (*top to bottom*): telescope, operating sheath that accommodates 5-French instruments, arthroscopy sheath (many uses), examination and protection sheath, and laparoscopy/thoracoscopy trocar and cannula (Karl Storz Co.).

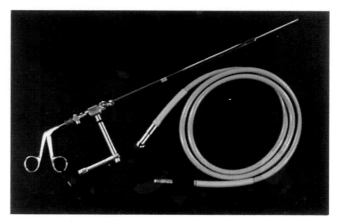

**Figure 14-6** Operating laparoscope with offset eyepiece and fiberoptic light cable. Note the attached channel for the insertion of accessory instruments. A biopsy forceps instrument is shown in the channel.

Various light sources are available. Some are only suitable for diagnostic purposes, whereas others are also applicable for photographic and video recording. A light source containing a 150-W lamp is sufficient for routine diagnostic laparoscopy (Figure 14-7), but photographic documentation requires either a 300-W lamp or a flash generator. A flexible fiberoptic cable is required to transmit light from the light source to the laparoscope (see

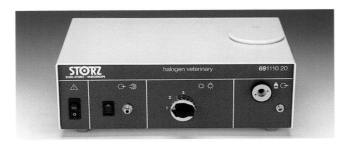

**Figure 14-7** Halogen veterinary light source, 150 W. This versatile light source can be used for a number of endoscopic procedures. It has an insufflation pump for use in flexible gastrointestinal endoscopy. Note, however, that a laparoflator is necessary for laparoscopy.

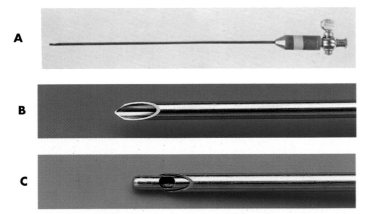

**Figure 14-8 A,** Veress needle used in establishing the pneumoperitoneum. Note the Luer-lock at the far right of this photograph. The Veress needle consists of two detachable parts: a sharp outer trocar and a blunt inner stylet. Tubing is used to connect the gas insufflation unit with the Veress needle. **B,** Close-up of a Veress needle with its inner needle retracted and its sharp outer trocar exposed. Abdominal wall puncture is accomplished with the Veress unit in this configuration. **C,** As soon as the Veress needle is positioned within the abdominal cavity, the outer trocar is retracted and the blunt inner stylet, as shown here, is exposed. With this positioning, the abdominal organs are less likely to be damaged. Gas is insufflated through the small opening at the tip of the Veress needle.

Figure 14-3). Light-transmitting cables are produced in a variety of diameters, with larger cables providing more light transmission and greater internal illumination. A 4- to 5.5-mm cable is recommended for general use in dogs and cats.

The Veress needle (Figure 14-8) is a spring-loaded, blunt-tipped needle used to establish a pneumoperitoneum. A Veress needle 120 mm in length and equipped with an on-off Luer-lock adaptor is suitable for use in small animals.

Various types of automatic gas insufflators are available (Figure 14-9). These units are called either *laparoflators* or *endoflators*. A carbon dioxide tank ("E" tank) is attached to the laparoflator, and gas is channeled through the unit. Although an automatic insufflator adds to the expense of the total system, it provides a great deal of convenience and safety during a procedure because it allows measurement of both the total gas volume delivered and the intraabdominal pressure.

Automatic insufflation is another valuable feature of the laparoflator. The unit detects the pressure in the gas hose that is connected to the Veress needle (or insertion cannula after the Veress needle has been removed), and gas is insufflated if the abdominal pressure level is below the level that has been preset on the insufflation unit. We typically set a maximum abdominal pressure of 12 to 13 mm Hg in cats and 15 mm Hg in dogs. Once the preset pressure level has been reached, the laparoflator will not pump any more gas until the abdominal pressure level drops below the preset level. During laparoscopy some gas typically leaks out of the abdominal cavity. With the gas hose connected to one of the insertion cannulas, gas volume can be quickly replaced and consistently maintained during a procedure, without the operator having to be concerned about manual insufflation.

The use of a gas anesthesia machine with nitrous oxide as the insufflation gas has also been described. Insufflation can also be achieved with hand syringes, bulb pumps, gas tanks, and carbon dioxide dispensers, although these methods are either unsafe or inconvenient. We strongly recommend the routine use of a laparoflator in laparoscopic procedures. Gas insufflation makes laparoscopic procedures easier and more efficient.

## Selection of Gas for Insufflation

Air, nitrous oxide, and carbon dioxide have been successfully and safely used for insufflation. The ideal gas for pneumoperitoneum should be nontoxic, colorless, readily soluble in blood, easily ventilated through the lungs, nonflammable, and inexpensive. Carbon dioxide most closely fits these requirements. This gas is highly soluble in blood and readily expired by the lungs. Because of its high solubility coefficient, carbon dioxide is rapidly absorbed (nitrous oxide is 68% as rapidly absorbed into the blood) and then quickly eliminated after a procedure. Consequently, its use provides a high margin of safety. In animal experiments on gas embolism induction, carbon dioxide has been found to be less lethal than both room air and oxygen. A potential minor disadvantage of carbon dioxide is that it turns into carbonic acid on peritoneal surfaces and therefore can cause discomfort. In contrast, nitrous oxide is inert on peritoneal surfaces. Nitrous oxide has been shown to cause no pain in human patients receiving local anesthesia for diagnostic procedures. However, this gas must not be used in procedures involving a laser because of the potential for explosion resulting from the combination of particulate matter, an oxidizing gas, and the high temperatures created when laser energy hits smoke particles.

Gas embolism is a rare but potentially dangerous complication of pneumoperitoneum. Embolism results from the injection of gas into the circulation. At the start of the laparoscopic procedure, care should be taken to ensure that the Veress needle is correctly placed within free peritoneal cavity before insufflation is started (see the discussion of procedure). Initial insufflation should also be done slowly. These measures should decrease the likelihood of gas being injected into a venous channel. With proper technique and gas selection, the risk of complications related to pneumoperitoneum in small animals is quite low.

## Accessory Instruments for Biopsy Procedures

Organ biopsy procedures require several accessory instruments. We prefer either a grasping-type biopsy forceps or a Tru-Cut needle (Travenol Labs, McGaw, Ill.)

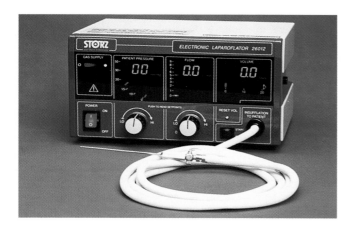

**Figure 14-9** Laparoflator (gas insufflation unit) and gas tubing with a Veress needle attached. Gauges that measure intraabdominal pressure, amount of gas insufflated, and amount of gas remaining in the external tank are located on the front of the unit.

(Figure 14-10) and routinely use both of these instruments to obtain tissue samples from liver, kidneys, pancreas, spleen, and adrenal glands, and intraabdominal masses. Palmer forceps (for manipulation and electrocoagulation) and scissors-type forceps are also available. Most accessory instruments are insulated and equipped for use with electrocoagulation units.

## Instrumentation for Complete Laparoscopy

Instruments and other equipment that may be needed to perform a complete laparoscopic procedure are listed in Box 14-1. One required item is a minor surgery pack that contains scalpel and blade (number 10 or 15), thumb forceps, needle holder, scissors, towel clamps, and hemostats. Absorbable suture material (2-0 to 3-0) is used to close the cutaneous and abdominal wall incision sites, and spinal needles (10 to 20 gauge, 10 cm in length) are necessary when performing splenoportography or cholangiography. Trays for equipment sterilization are also useful. Equipment may be sterilized using ethylene oxide (ETO) gas. An appropriate aeration period is required before use of instruments that have undergone ETO sterilization. Cold sterilization solutions such as 2% glutaraldehyde (Cidex) may also be used, but the equipment should then be rinsed with warm sterile saline before use. Laparoscopic equipment should not be autoclaved.

## LAPAROSCOPIC TECHNIQUE

### Preparation and Restraint

Animals should be fasted for 12 to 24 hours before laparoscopy, and water should be withheld the morning of the procedure. Ideally, the urinary bladder, stomach, and colon should be empty. We do not routinely catheterize the urinary bladder; a moderately full bladder does not seem to interfere with the procedure. However, when the urinary bladder is distended, there may be an increased risk of an inadvertent traumatic puncture of the bladder while inserting the trocar-cannula unit Veress needle into the abdominal cavity in very small animals.

Laparoscopy may be performed with the patient either under general anesthesia or sedation. In the past we often used a narcotic analgesic such as oxymorphone (0.1 mg/kg [0.045 mg/lb] intravenously [IV]) plus a local anesthetic (2% lidocaine) infiltrated at the site of trocar puncture. Oxymorphone provides adequate analgesia and sedation, and narcotic antagonists such as naloxone can be administered if problems are encountered. We have also administered a low dose of phenothiazine tranquilizer (acepromazine, 0.25 mg to a total dose of 2 mg IV) in conjunction with oxymorphone to deepen seda-

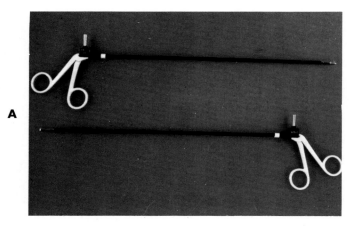

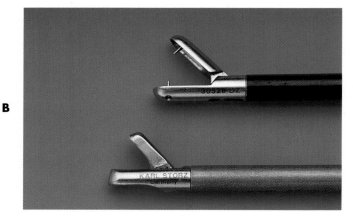

**Figure 14-10 A,** Biopsy forceps for use with an accessory cannula. **B,** Close-up of the jaws of biopsy forceps instruments: double-spoon grasping-type forceps (*top*) and cutting-type forceps (*bottom*).

---

**Box 14-1    Instrumentation for General Laparoscopy**

**SUPPLIES FOR LOCAL ANESTHESIA, SKIN INCISION, AND CLOSURE**
Syringes for anesthetic solutions
Lidocaine or carbocaine
Towel pack and fenestrated drape
Towel clamps
Scalpel blades (no. 10, no. 15)
Thumb forceps
Gauze sponges
Bowl and sterile saline
2 Curved mosquito forceps
2 Straight mosquito forceps
Needle holder
Suture scissors
2-0 or 3-0 catgut
2-0 or 3-0 nylon

**LAPAROSCOPE INTRUMENTATION**
Veres needle
Laparoscope (telescope)
Fiberoptic light cable
Gas insufflation tubing
Laparoscope cannula (sleeve) with trocar
Second puncture cannula with trocar
Tactile (palpatating-measuring) probe
Set of assorted rubber sealing caps
Tru-Cut biopsy needle
Biopsy forceps

---

tion and have encountered no apparent ill effects with this combination. Ketamine (5 to 10 mg/kg [2.3 to 4.6 mg/lb] IV), diazepam (0.1 mg/kg [0.045 mg/lb] IV), and a local anesthetic may also be used together. Currently, however, laparoscopic procedures are more commonly performed using general gas anesthesia, with isoflurane the preferred agent. In severely depressed patients, a local anesthetic agent may be sufficient, used either alone or in conjunction with a combination of diazepam and butorphanol. Oxymorphone or butorphanol provides analgesia, which is often beneficial to the patient during recovery. Barbiturates should not be used in patients with hepatic insufficiency, and ketamine is contraindicated in patients with renal insufficiency.

## Procedure

For laparoscopy, the selection of a midline, right, or left lateral abdominal approach depends on several factors. The right lateral approach is used for diffuse or multifocal hepatopathies, right-sided liver masses, and biopsy of the pancreas, right kidney, or adrenal gland. This approach allows visualization of the caudate, right lateral, right medial, and quadrate lobes of the liver, as well as the gallbladder, common bile duct, descending duodenum, right limb of the pancreas, pylorus, diaphragm, right kidney, and small intestine.

A left lateral abdominal approach is employed for the evaluation of left-sided liver masses and for splenoportography, visualization and biopsy of the spleen, and measurement of splenic pulp pressure. Obviously, visualization and biopsy of the left kidney or adrenal gland can also be achieved with this approach. Although some authors have recommended a ventral midline approach, falciform fat in the anterior ventral abdomen may obscure visualization. We have not found this approach to be particularly useful.

For laparoscopy the animal is placed on the table in either a left or right lateral recumbent position. A table that can be tilted is recommended because shifting the abdominal viscera can enhance visualization in some patients. When laparoscopy is performed using sedation and local anesthesia, the animal's legs are secured to the table to prevent movement during the procedure. Surgical sterility is maintained throughout the procedure. The lateral abdominal region is clipped from approximately the 10th intercostal space caudally to the flank and from the dorsal to ventral midlines. This area is then surgically scrubbed, disinfected, and draped. Before the final surgical scrub, if a local anesthetic is to be used, it is injected both subcutaneously and intramuscularly in the anticipated area of trocar puncture.

The first step is the establishment of a pneumoperitoneum to produce a gas layer that separates the abdominal wall from the underlying viscera. The internal blunt tip of the Veress needle is retracted; this exposes the sharp outer stylet point, which is used to facilitate abdominal wall penetration (see Figure 14-8). Before the Veress needle is inserted, the underlying area should be palpated to avoid puncture of masses or organs. Once the needle has penetrated the abdominal wall, the spring is released, allowing the blunt tip to protrude. The needle is swept gently in a circular pattern against the inner abdominal wall to free any adhesions or omentum that might interfere with insufflation.

The gas hose from the insufflator is then attached to the Luer-lock of the Veress needle, and a moderate pneumoperitoneum is established using a flow rate of approximately 1 L/min to a final intraabdominal pressure of approximately 12 to 13 mm Hg in cats and 13 to 15 mm Hg in dogs. Naturally the required insufflation volume increases with increasing body size. With experience the operator can assess the pneumoperitoneum by ballottement and the degree of abdominal distension. Respirations and capillary perfusion should be closely monitored because overdistension of the abdomen can lead to cardiopulmonary compromise and even death.

Once the appropriate pneumoperitoneum has been established, the Veress needle is withdrawn and, depending on trocar size, a 1- to 2-cm skin incision is made on the ventrolateral abdominal wall at a variable distance caudal to the ribs. A typical entry site is 3 to 4 cm caudal to the last rib and halfway between the ventral midline and the lumbar vertebral transverse processes. The exact position of the puncture site depends on the organ of interest and the size and body condition of the animal. The operator's personal preference and experience also play a role in determining the puncture site. In animals with microhepatica (e.g., cirrhosis) the puncture site should be closer to the ribs and more ventrally placed, whereas in animals with hepatomegaly a more caudal site is preferred. Because of fat deposition a "ventral shift" of abdominal organs occurs in obese animals; thus a more ventral site should be selected for abdominal puncture. Inexperienced operators commonly place the puncture site too close to the organ being examined, thereby hindering visualization.

Blunt separation of muscle layers is performed with a hemostat to minimize abdominal wall trauma at the time of trocar puncture. The *size* of the skin incision and blunt dissection should be kept to a *minimum* to avoid gas leakage around the cannula. The trocar-cannula unit is held with the base of the trocar seated against the heel of the hand and the fingers grasping the cannula (Figure 14-11). The Luer-lock should be closed to avoid insufflation loss. The trocar-cannula unit is inserted with a quick, steady twisting motion of the hand and wrist; an audible "pop" is usually heard on penetration of the abdominal wall. Ramming or stabbing motions should be avoided!

After the sleeve has fully penetrated the abdominal wall, the trocar is immediately withdrawn to avoid trauma to underlying organs. Once the trocar is removed from the sleeve, the operator can easily insert the sleeve farther, using gentle forward force and slight left-right axial rotation. With complete removal of the trocar the trumpet valve of the sleeve closes automatically to prevent further escape of gas. The gas insufflation hose is then attached to the Luer-lock of the cannula so that pneumoperitoneum can be maintained during the procedure. If necessary, the Leuer-lock can be used to withdraw ascitic fluid from the abdomen. Alternatively a special aspiration instrument can be advanced into the abdominal cavity through the accessory cannula, and fluid can be aspirated under laparoscopic guidance (Figure 14-12).

Before the laparoscope is inserted, it should be warmed to prevent fogging of the distal lens. When a cold optics instrument enters the abdominal cavity, where the temperature is higher and humidity is 100%, vapor tends to condense on its glass surfaces (Figure 14-13, *A*). Warming can be easily and most economically accomplished by inserting the laparoscope tip into sterile saline (Figure 14-13, *B*) or water that is slightly warmer than body temperature or by holding the tip of the laparoscope in the palm for several minutes just before the scope is inserted through the cannula. Busy human endoscopy units use a commercial endoscope

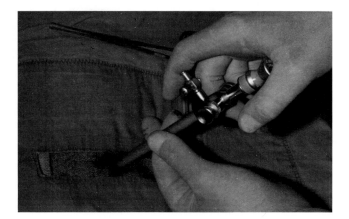

**Figure 14-11** Proper technique for holding the trocar-cannula unit during abdominal puncture after a pneumoperitoneum has been established. The trocar handle is positioned directly against the hand so that it stays in place during the advance across the body wall to the abdominal cavity.

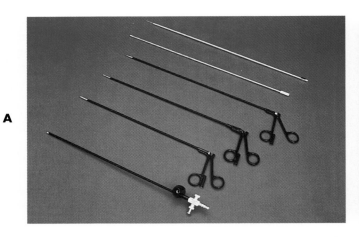

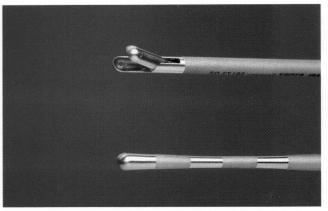

**Figure 14-12 A,** Assorted laparoscopic hand instruments (*top to bottom*): injection/aspiration needle, palpation probe, scissors; grasping forceps, biopsy forceps, and suction cannula (Karl Storz Co., Goleta, Calif.). **B,** Close-up of laparoscopic hand instrument tips: double-spoon biopsy forceps (*top*) and palpation probe (*bottom*).

**Figure 14-13** Prevention of fogging. **A,** Schematic of human abdominal cavity, depicting the mechanism of fogging on the tip of the telescope. **B,** Scope warming in sterile saline. **C,** Commercial endoscope warmer. **D,** Use of a sterile antifogging solution. (From Hulka JF, Reich H: *Textbook of laparoscopy,* Philadelphia, 1998, WB Saunders.)

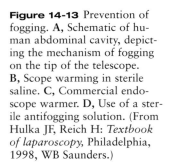

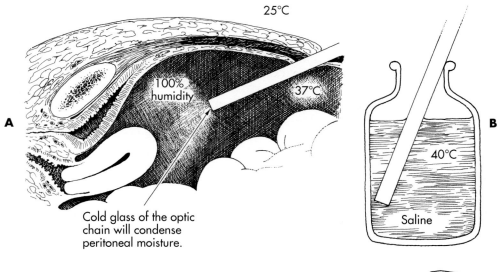

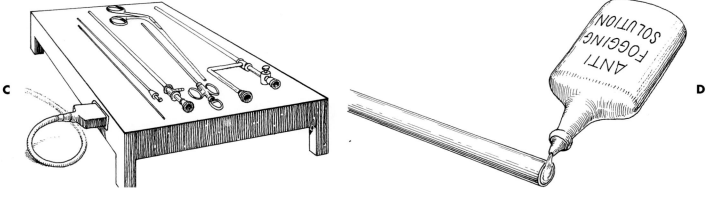

warmer (Figure 14-13, *C*). An antifogging solution (Figure 14-13, *D*) can also be applied to proximal and distal lenses. However, an ordinary detergent (e.g., hexachlorophene emulsion [pHisoHex]) has the same effect, causing droplets of condensed steam to spread rapidly and almost invisibly over the surface of the cold lens. For photographic purposes, warming techniques are preferred over the use of antifogging solutions because the extra coating of solution and condensed water can distort the lens surface enough to blur photographs. Based on our experience, a laparoscope can be warmed sufficiently by inserting the tip in a warm solution or holding it in the palm of the hand.

During the course of the procedure the distal lens of the laparoscope occasionally becomes fogged or contaminated with abdominal fluid or blood. When this occurs, touching the laparoscope tip gently against abdominal organs (e.g., liver, kidney) usually clears the distal lens. Sometimes, however, the laparoscope must be withdrawn and the distal lens cleaned with a gauze sponge moistened with saline or sterile water. A sterile bowl should be prepared for each laparoscopic procedure so that sterile water or saline is readily available for cleansing either telescope lens (see Box 14-1). As the scope is reinserted into the abdominal cavity, blood or fluid that has made its way into the instrument cannula may become attached to the lens, further obstructing the view. In such instances, wiping the tip of the scope against an abdominal organ frequently clears the lens. Alternatively it may occasionally be necessary to flush a small amount of sterile fluid through the instrument cannula.

The operator should begin viewing as soon as the laparoscope is moved into the cannula (Figure 14-14). Proper placement of the cannula within the abdominal cavity should be confirmed. Rarely the cannula may be placed inadvertently within muscle layers or adipose tissue. If this occurs, the cannula must be reinserted before the procedure can be continued. Before proceeding, the operator should determine the presence of intraabdominal adhesions and the adequacy of the pneumoperitoneum. Viscera immediately underlying the puncture site are inspected to identify any traumatic injury or hemorrhage caused by trocar insertion. The entire abdomen should then be systematically examined to detect any abnormalities. A blunt probe may be used to manipulate organs or retract omentum to improve visualization (see Figure 14-12).

Tissue specimens can be obtained by passing a biopsy needle (e.g., a Tru-Cut needle) through a small skin incision at a site close to the organ to be sampled (Figure 14-15). The laparoscope is retracted so that the biopsy needle can be visualized as it enters the abdominal cavity and is directed to the biopsy site. Caution must be exercised to prevent inadvertent puncture of underlying structures. Grasping biopsy forceps may also be used to obtain tissue samples (see Figure 14-10). The instrument is inserted through an accessory cannula (second puncture) (Figure 14-16) or through the channel of an operating laparoscope. Because of the length of grasping biopsy forceps, we have found this instrument to be particularly useful in larger dogs, especially those with microhepatica.

Biopsy sites are observed for several minutes after the biopsy procedure to check for excessive bleeding. Excessive postbiopsy hemorrhage is rare. If excessive bleeding occurs, it can usually be controlled by applying direct pressure with the laparoscope tip or by inserting a blunt probe through the accessory cannula. If direct pressure fails to control hemorrhage, topical hemostatic agents such as absorbable gelatin sponge (e.g., Gelfoam) can be directly applied or electrocoagulation can be performed at the biopsy site.

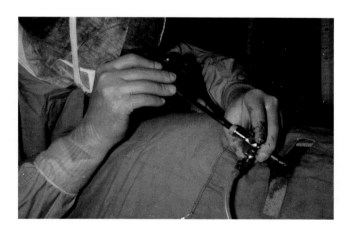

**Figure 14-14** The trocar has been removed from the cannula, and the telescope has been advanced through the cannula for visualization of the abdominal organs. One of the operator's hands maintains the cannula at a consistent depth while the other hand controls advance and retraction of the telescope. The operator must be careful not to pull the cannula too far back through the abdominal wall to the exterior; doing so may result in loss of pneumoperitoneum. The hose for carbon dioxide insufflation is fastened to the cannula, and the fiberoptic light cable is attached to telescope (close to the operator's right hand).

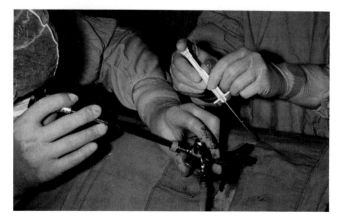

**Figure 14-15** Positioning of the Tru-Cut biopsy needle during organ biopsy.

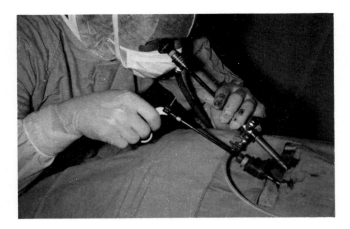

**Figure 14-16** Use of accessory cannula and biopsy forceps for organ biopsy. A single operator can handle both instruments easily.

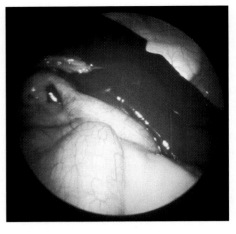

**Figure 14-18** The duodenum in a dog is visualized in the foreground of this photograph, the gallbladder and cystic duct are seen in the middle, and the normal liver and oval window of the diaphragm (light area) are visible in the background.

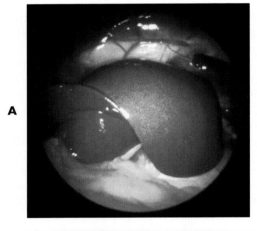

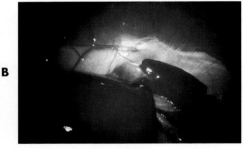

A

B

**Figure 14-17 A,** Normal canine liver viewed from a right lateral approach. Organ color, texture, and shape can be clearly evaluated during laparoscopy. The diaphragm is in the background. **B,** Oval window (white area) of the diaphragm and parts of several liver lobes. Note the excellent detail of the blood vessels coursing along the diaphragm. Rigid scopes provide magnification that enhances visualization significantly. A small section of the gallbladder and the cystic duct can be seen at the 5 o'clock position in the field of view.

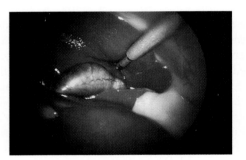

**Figure 14-19** Liver and gallbladder in a cat with lymphocytic, plasmacytic cholangiohepatitis. An accessory cannula and palpation probe (*upper right*) are being used to lift a liver lobe away to facilitate visualization of the gallbladder.

Sample photographs illustrating laparoscopic views are presented in Figures 14-17 through 14-25. A distinct advantage of laparoscopy is the clarity of the views and the fact that biopsies can be obtained under direct visualization. Ancillary procedures that may be performed during laparoscopy include cholecystocholangiography, splenoportography, and splenic pulp pressure measurements (see Chapter 15). When the laparoscopic examination is completed, the pneumoperitoneum is completely evacuated through the cannula, and the abdominal wall and skin incisions are closed with synthetic suture material.

## CONTRAINDICATIONS

Laparoscopy is contraindicated in several situations. Cardiopulmonary decompensation precludes the use of this procedure until clinical control of the underlying

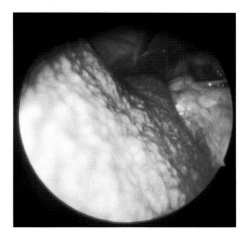

**Figure 14-20** Marked diffuse granularity of the liver in a 4-year-old Maltese with chronic active hepatitis. This is an unusual appearance. The dog was clinically normal; however, screening laboratory tests done before a dental procedure suggested that the animal had a liver disorder, and both preprandial and postprandial serum bile acid levels were significantly elevated. Liver biopsies were obtained laparoscopically. Compare the appearance of this liver to that of the normal liver shown in Figure 14-17.

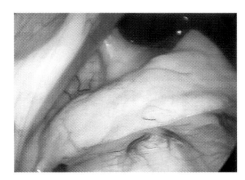

**Figure 14-21** Normal canine pancreas (left lobe). The duodenum is seen below the pancreas, and a small section of the liver is visible at the 12 to 1 o'clock position.

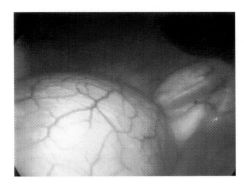

**Figure 14-22** The right kidney is seen in the foreground, and the adrenal gland is the light-colored ovoid structure visualized to the right in the field of view.

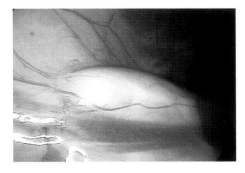

**Figure 14-23** Normal canine adrenal gland. The posterior vena cava is below the adrenal gland. A palpation probe (not in view) was advanced through a second cannula and used to deflect the right kidney caudally (by engaging the cranial pole of the kidney) so that the adrenal gland could be more clearly visualized. The cranial pole of the right kidney is located just beyond the field of view at the 9 o'clock position.

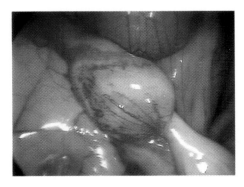

**Figure 14-24** Right canine ovary.

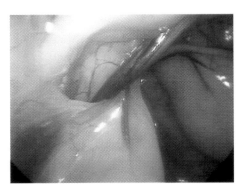

**Figure 14-25** Inguinal ring, spermatic cord, and vessels in an intact male dog.

disorder has been achieved. For obvious reasons, laparoscopy and organ biopsy should not be performed in animals with coagulopathies, and we routinely evaluate coagulation function before laparoscopy. Because visceral puncture may occur during laparoscopy in animals with extensive intraabdominal adhesions from previous surgery or disease, exploratory laparotomy is recommended in these patients. Profound ascites can complicate laparoscopy and increase the likelihood of visceral puncture. Consequently, ascites should be reduced by medical management or abdominocentesis before laparoscopy is performed. Bacterial peritonitis and abdominal herniation (diaphragmatic or inguinal) are obvious contraindications to laparoscopy.

## COMPLICATIONS

A number of complications have been associated with laparoscopy. In our experience, complications are rare and can be minimized by caution and rigorous attention to proper technique. During establishment of the pneumoperitoneum, a hollow organ (e.g., stomach, urinary bladder, intestine) can be punctured, resulting in gas distension of the organ. Gas embolization has been reported after a Veress needle was inadvertently placed within a major vessel, spleen, or vascular tumor. More commonly, subcutaneous or body wall emphysema can occur if the Veress needle is not introduced completely into the abdomen. The use of carbon dioxide or nitrous oxide as insufflation gases minimizes these risks because both gases rapidly diffuse through tissue. As previously mentioned, excessive pneumoperitoneum can result in cardiopulmonary compromise, and deaths have been reported from this complication.

Improper technique in inserting the trocar-cannula carries the greatest risk of immediate, severe complications. Significant trauma to the abdominal wall or viscera can occur. Problems can be avoided by proper patient preparation (i.e., empty the bladder and colon), use of appropriately sized equipment, proper abdominal wall dissection, and establishment of an adequate pneumoperitoneum. Reviewing prelaparoscopic abdominal radiographs and performing thorough palpation before laparoscopy minimize risks by identifying masses or adhesions.

Organ biopsy can also lead to complications. The most commonly reported problem is biopsy needle puncture of structures underlying the target organ. Diaphragmatic puncture can result in severe pneumothorax because of the positive intraabdominal pressure. Thus the use of grasping-type biopsy forceps rather than needle instruments is recommended in cats, very small dogs, and animals with microhepatica. Inadvertent puncture of major vessels has been reported as a fatal complication in humans. Excessive hemorrhage from the biopsy site can occur, especially in patients with advanced liver disease or coagulopathies. Other reported complications include bile and bacterial peritonitis; however, neither of these problems has occurred in our experience.

A case review of 100 laparoscopies on canine patients found a very low rate of complications directly related to the procedure. Two dogs developed disseminated intravascular coagulopathy after the procedure. One of these animals had severe, acute, fulminant hepatitis, and the other showed histologic changes of end-stage cirrhosis. After laparoscopy another dog with cirrhosis developed apparent hepatorenal syndrome, characterized by progressive, nonresponsive, anuric renal failure. After renal biopsy one animal developed profuse, subcapsular hemorrhage, but the bleeding resolved without specific treatment. An unusual complication was the procurement of a full-thickness gastric wall biopsy sample during a procedure to obtain needle biopsy specimens of the liver in a dog. This complication was at least partially attributable to clinician inexperience. Interestingly, no clinical problems resulted from the gastric puncture. A minor complication in some animals with ascites is the leakage of ascitic fluid from the puncture site into the ventral subcutaneous tissues, resulting in ventral edema. This problem generally resolves with appropriate therapy.

## REFERENCES

Boyer TD: Laparoscopy. In Sleisenger MH, Fordtran JS, editors: *Gastrointestinal disease*, ed 3, Philadelphia, 1983, WB Saunders.

Harrison RM, Wildt DE, editors: *Animal laparoscopy*, Baltimore, 1980, Williams & Wilkins.

Hulka JF, Reich H: Light: optics and television. In Hulka JF, Reich H, editors: *Textbook of laparoscopy*, ed 3, Philadelphia, 1998, WB Saunders.

Hulka JF, Reich H: Gas and pneumoperitoneum. In Hulka JF, Reich H, editors: *Textbook of laparoscopy*, ed 3, Philadelphia, 1998, WB Saunders.

Johnson GF, Twedt DC: Endoscopy and laparoscopy in the diagnosis and management of neoplasia in small animals, *Vet Clin North Am* 7:77, 1977.

Lettow E: Laparoscopic examinations in liver diseases in dogs, *Vet Med Rev* 2:159, 1972.

Nichols SL, Tompkins BM, Henderson PA: Probable carbon dioxide embolism during laparoscopy: a case report, *Wis Med J* 80:27, 1981.

Patterson JM: Laparoscopy in small animal medicine. In Kirk RW, editor: *Current veterinary therapy VII*, Philadelphia, 1981, WB Saunders.

Sherlock P: Gastrointestinal endoscopy. In Wyngaarden JB, Smith LH, editors: *Cecil's textbook of medicine*, ed 17, Philadelphia, 1985, WB Saunders.

Svenberg T: Pathophysiology of pneumoperitoneum. In Ballantyne GH, Leahy PF, Modlin IM, editors: *Laparoscopic surgery*, Philadelphia, 1994, WB Saunders.

Wildt DE, Kinney GM, Seager SWJ: Laparoscopy for direct observation of internal organs of the domestic cat and dog, *Am J Vet Res* 38:1429, 1977.

# Chapter 15

# Laparoscopy of the Liver and Pancreas

**David C. Twedt**

L aparoscopy consists of the transabdominal placement of a rigid endoscope after the establishment of a pneumoperitoneum. Based on the location of the endoscope insertion, certain organs are visualized and various manipulations can be performed. The reader is advised to review Chapter 14 for a complete description of the basic techniques involved in laparoscopy.

Although laparoscopy has been used in small animals for several decades, it has only more recently become an important diagnostic tool in veterinary hospitals for the routine evaluation of the liver and pancreas in small animals. Liver biopsy is now the major indication for the use of laparoscopy at my institution. The information presented in this chapter is based on the results of observations made in a review of the first 360 consecutive laparoscopic procedures performed at Colorado State University. In this series the major indication for laparoscopy was evaluation of the liver, and liver biopsy was performed in 282 of the cases. The information regarding indications, techniques, and complications in this chapter is the result of the experience at Colorado State University with these and subsequent cases.

The preference for laparoscopy in evaluating the liver and to a lesser extent the pancreas lies in the fact that a great amount of information can be obtained quickly using a relatively noninvasive procedure that costs considerably less than other diagnostic procedures. It is recog- nized that most disorders of the liver and pancreas are nonsurgical and that a definitive diagnosis is often made only after tissue biopsy specimens are obtained. These samples are procured via exploratory laparotomy, by laparoscopy, or through percutaneous needle biopsy often performed under ultrasound guidance. Compared with exploratory laparotomy, laparoscopy has the advantages of lower morbidity and mortality rates (because the technique causes minimal trauma), an uncommon need for general anesthesia, and a greatly reduced procedure time. Surgery does, however, allow the entire abdominal cavity to be evaluated and a number of specific surgical procedures to be performed. Unlike percutaneous needle biopsy, laparoscopy provides visualization of the liver or pancreas and allows precise direction of the biopsy instrument to the area that is to be evaluated. Thus the operator's visual impressions become important in correlating the histologic diagnosis with the clinical diagnosis. For example, nodular hyperplasia, a common condition in older dogs, is often missed on ultrasound examination or needle biopsy. Furthermore, the larger liver biopsy samples necessary for hepatic copper determination or other types of tissue analysis can be obtained with laparoscopy but not always with percutaneous needle biopsy methods. Compared with laparoscopy, the percutaneous ultrasound-directed liver biopsy technique has a lower retrieval rate and a greater risk of inadvertent organ perforation.

## INDICATIONS AND CONTRAINDICATIONS

### Indications for Liver Evaluation

Laparoscopy is indicated to obtain liver biopsy specimens in animals known or suspected of having liver disease. The many specific indications for evaluating the liver and a comprehensive discussion of these indications are beyond the scope of this chapter. Among others, these indications for laparoscopy include findings such as unexplained abnormal liver-specific biochemistries, abnormal liver function tests, and abnormal liver size; the evaluation of therapeutic response in patients with liver disease; and the procurement of liver tissue to screen for suspected copper hepatotoxicities. Less absolute indications include evaluation of the extrahepatic biliary system; concurrent evaluation of other organs such as the spleen or kidneys; and performance of specific ancillary laparoscopic procedures such as splenoportography, splenic pulp pressure measurements, and gastrostomy or jejunostomy tube placement.

Laparoscopy for evaluation of the liver should not be considered a major diagnostic procedure with the same risks as exploratory abdominal surgery. Instead, laparoscopy should be regarded as an additional relatively low-risk diagnostic modality that should be considered in the work-up of the patients with suspected liver disease.

### Indications for Pancreatic Evaluation

Laparoscopy has been used to evaluate the pancreas in a small number of cases. Because of the limited experience with this procedure, a complete list of indications has not been generated. However, a recent abstract on laparoscopic pancreatic biopsies in normal dogs reported no postbiopsy complications (Harrington DP, Jones BD, 1996). The diagnosis of pancreatitis and its differentiation from extrahepatic liver disease are often difficult, in that pancreatitis frequently causes secondary hepatic inflammation, which occasionally extends around the common bile duct, causing partial or complete obstruction of bile flow. In selected cases, laparoscopy has been an aid in differentiating primary pancreatic disease from primary liver disease. It appears that laparoscopic evaluation and biopsy of the pancreas are of most benefit in diagnosing chronic recurring pancreatitis and may offer little information in patients that have obvious acute inflammatory pancreatitis without secondary biliary tract involvement. Cats with cholangitis or cholangiohepatitis commonly have concurrent chronic fibrosing pancreatitis. Simultaneous biopsy of both the liver and pancreas during laparoscopy aids in establishing the extent of involvement in this syndrome.

### Contraindications

Laparoscopic evaluation of the liver and pancreas appears to have relatively few contraindications. If there is any evidence that the patient has a surgically treatable disease, laparoscopy obviously should not be performed. In some patients, however, a definitive tissue diagnosis may be useful in planning the specific surgical technique. When a *complete* examination of the abdominal cavity is required, exploratory laparotomy is the appropriate procedure. Conditions such as obvious hepatic masses and extrahepatic biliary disorders generally require surgical intervention. Hepatic ultrasonography has proved useful in localizing focal hepatic masses and demonstrating extrahepatic biliary obstructions. This modality is commonly used before the decision is made to perform exploratory laparotomy or laparoscopy. Laparoscopy does not replace complete exploratory laparotomy. When choosing laparoscopy, the operator must know the organ or area of the abdominal cavity to evaluate for the procedure to be successful.

Laparoscopy should never be undertaken in an animal that has a coagulation disorder, septic peritonitis, or multiple abdominal adhesions. Before the procedure is performed, the patient's status should always be carefully evaluated. If the animal is in a critical state or is unable to adequately tolerate sedation or the stress of the procedure, laparoscopy should not be done. Other potential contraindications to laparoscopy include diaphragmatic hernia and abdominal effusion.

## INSTRUMENTATION

The equipment discussed in the preceding chapter constitutes the basic instrumentation required for evaluation of the liver and pancreas. We prefer to use a diagnostic telescope 5 to 7 mm in diameter. This endoscope has a forward-viewing 0-degree field of view and is the best suited for evaluation of the liver in dogs and cats. Telescopes with an angled field of view are more difficult to operate and are not required to adequately evaluate the liver. Operating telescopes containing a biopsy channel within the scope are larger in size, can be cumbersome, and are not required to perform various laparoscopic manipulations.

Liver and pancreatic biopsies and various manipulations are performed using the two-puncture technique. With this technique a second 5-mm or larger pyramidal trocar with trocar cannula must be placed through the abdominal wall to pass instruments for biopsy or manipulation of the liver and pancreas. Instruments commonly passed through the second puncture cannula include a calibrated palpation probe and biopsy forceps. To biopsy the liver, we prefer double-spoon forceps with grasping teeth (see Figure 14-10, *A*). Tissue sample size with these forceps is adequate for additional diagnostic testing. We prefer to use punch biopsy forceps for pancreatic biopsies because of the cutting action of the forceps (see Figure 14-10, *B*). Less tissue tearing occurs with these forceps; however, smaller samples are obtained. The palpation probe, a straight rod with centimeter calibrations, is used for various manipulations, such as lifting up liver lobes, sweeping omentum away from the liver or pancreas, and palpating the gallbladder. Biopsy forceps cause minimal tissue trauma and minimal bleeding.

Also available are special biopsy needles that can be passed through the second puncture cannula. In lieu of the second puncture technique, standard liver biopsy needles, such as the 6-inch Tru-Cut disposable biopsy needle (Baxter Healthcare Corporation, Deerfield, Ill.), can be passed directly through the abdominal wall adjacent to the laparoscope and directed to the area to be biopsied. Needle aspiration samples for cytology are obtained in a similar manner for the evaluation of the liver and pancreas. A 6-inch needle or longer is required to enter the gallbladder to aspirate bile or to inject radiographic contrast agents; we generally use 18- to 20-gauge spinal needles with stylets. This size is suitable for all but large, deep-chested dogs or dogs with very small livers; in these animals, longer needles are required to reach the area to be sampled.

## PATIENT PREPARATION

Patient preparation for laparoscopy of the liver and pancreas is generally minimal. Food should be withheld for at least 12 hours before the procedure to ensure that the stomach is empty. In addition, the urinary bladder and colon should be evacuated. Catheterization of the urinary bladder is usually not necessary unless the bladder is significantly distended and difficult to express manually. The blood's clotting ability should always be evaluated before laparoscopy and liver biopsy. This is especially true in animals with suspected liver disease because most of the plasma coagulation factors are produced by the liver and they may be depleted with advanced liver disease. Only factor VIII, whose most likely primary source is the vascular endothelium rather than hepatocytes, is an exception. The one-stage prothrombin time, activated partial thromboplastin time, and total platelet count are the preferred tests for evaluating hemostasis. The minimum coagulation tests to detect evidence of gross bleeding disorders are a total platelet count and an activated clotting time.

Decreases in total platelet numbers may be only a relative contraindication for laparoscopy and liver biopsy. The clinical observation of associated thrombocytopenia with normal clotting factors and its failure to be associated with bleeding after liver biopsies has been reported in humans undergoing laparoscopy and liver biopsy. We have taken liver biopsy samples from a number of dogs, with the only hemostatic abnormality being platelet numbers as low as 60,000/mm$^3$. In these animals, no bleeding complications occurred after liver biopsy. This does not mean, however, that the operator should have a total disregard for decreased platelet numbers. Animals that are predisposed to von Willebrand's disease (e.g., Doberman pinschers) should ideally be screened with a von Willebrand factor assay or should at least have a bleeding time evaluated before the procedure. Bleeding associated with this disorder can be a significant complication; thus it is wise to have a source of fresh blood available for potential problem cases.

Ascites can also complicate laparoscopy. When the abdominal fluid is a clear transudate, it is often possible to transilluminate the fluid and see the liver. However, even the slightest amount of bleeding clouds this fluid and hinders visualization of the abdominal organs. The abdominal organs and omentum usually float in the fluid, making the evaluation difficult. When ascites is present, it is wise to remove most or possibly all of the fluid before laparoscopy. This is best accomplished by placing an abdominal drain and slowly removing the fluid over several hours before the laparoscopic procedure.

## PATIENT RESTRAINT

Laparoscopy may be performed using either sedation and local anesthesia or general anesthesia. The patient should be thoroughly evaluated, and the appropriate sedation or anesthetic regimen should be selected for each case. In dogs, a combination of narcotic analgesia (oxymorphone, 0.05 mg/kg [0.023 mg/lb] intravenously [IV]) and tranquilization (acepromazine, 0.05 mg/kg IV) with a local anesthetic (2% lidocaine) infiltrated into the abdominal wall at the site of the trocar and biopsy puncture is usually effective. Even though these drugs require hepatic metabolism for their removal, this protocol is attractive because the drugs are given in low doses and the narcotic portion of the combination can be reversed with naloxone if problems arise.

Laparoscopy in cats is generally performed using ketamine (0.5 to 1 mg/kg [0.023 to 0.45 mg/lb] IV). In some cases, additional tranquilization with acepromazine (0.05 mg/kg IV) or diazepam (0.5 to 1 mg IV) may be required. Ketamine is excreted by the kidneys and does not require hepatic metabolism. Local anesthesia at the trocar entry site is required, with the use of 2% mepivacaine (rather than lidocaine) preferred in cats.

In most patients, general anesthesia is not required for laparoscopy. If the previously described sedation is inadequate, the animal can be given an inhaled anesthetic by mask. When general anesthesia is necessary, inhaled isoflurane is preferred and is considered the safest agent to use in animals with liver disease. Isoflurane undergoes almost no hepatic metabolism, whereas other gas anesthetics, such as halothane and methoxyflurane, require hepatic breakdown and also have the potential to cause an idiosyncratic hepatotoxicity reaction. Barbiturates are considered unacceptable agents for laparoscopy because of the large dose that is required for adequate restraint of the patient and the fact that most barbiturates undergo hepatic metabolism.

## PATIENT POSITIONING

The site of laparoscope entry for evaluation of the liver depends on a number of factors. A right lateral mid-abdominal approach is generally considered the entry site of choice. With the patient in a left lateral recumbent position the usual entry point is located on the right lateral abdominal wall equidistant between the costal arch and the proximal aspect of the iliac crest and intersected with the midpoint of the ventral abdominal midline and the ventral aspect of the lumbar muscles. A right-side approach is chosen because a significantly greater area of liver can be visualized than with a ventral or left lateral approach. The right lateral, right medial, and caudate lobes of the liver, as well as the gallbladder and extrahepatic biliary tract, can be visualized from the right side. In larger animals and those with very small livers the entry site should be shifted closer to the costal arch to adequately reach the liver with the laparoscope. In very small animals or animals with very large livers the entry site is shifted caudally to give more working space between the laparoscope and the liver.

The left lateral mid-abdominal approach is generally used only when lesions in the left lateral or medial lobes of the liver are suspected or when visualization of the spleen is required. The point of entry on the left side is similar to that described for the right-side approach. Care should be taken when using the left-side approach because the spleen can be easily traumatized during entry with the trocar. Laparoscopically directed splenic punctures for splenic biopsy, splenoportography, splenic pulp pressure measurements, or gastrostomy feeding tube placement are performed using this approach.

Some authors have recommended the ventral midline approach for evaluation of the liver. The entry site is located near the umbilicus, with the patient in a ventral recumbent position. This approach often has the disadvantage of limited visualization of the liver and the anterior abdominal structures, which may be obscured by the falciform fat found in the anterior ventral abdominal wall. This is a major problem when examining an obese patient. A ventral midline approach is best for evaluating posterior abdominal structures such as the ovaries and uterus.

Evaluation of the pancreas requires a right lateral abdominal wall entry. Using this entry, the examiner can almost always visualize the right lobe of the pancreas lying adjacent to the duodenum. With manipulation using the palpation probe, a portion of the left lobe of the pancreas can sometimes be seen through this entry site.

Once the site of entry is determined, the animal is placed in the appropriate position on a surgical table. The animal's legs should be secured to prevent movement during the procedure. A surgical table that can be tilted is ideal. Slightly elevating the front end of the body (5 to 10 degrees) often shifts the abdominal viscera and omentum caudally, thus improving the view of the liver. Obscured views commonly occur in animals with ascites, very small livers, or obesity. A sterile surgical preparation is done before the procedure.

## LAPAROSCOPIC PROCEDURE

### Evaluation and Biopsy of the Liver

The liver is generally evaluated through the right lateral mid-abdominal approach. Following the described entry guidelines and after moving the laparoscope into the abdomen, the operator should see the diaphragmatic aspect of the liver. A complete examination of the liver and adjacent structures is then undertaken in an orderly sequence. With experience an operator can inspect the abdomen in only a few minutes. It is advisable to use the second puncture technique so that a palpating probe or biopsy forceps can be passed. During the initial examination the appropriate location for the second trocar-cannula insertion should be determined. The second trocar-cannula is then introduced into the abdomen under laparoscopic direction. The palpating probe can be used to move the omentum about, palpate the gallbladder, and elevate the liver lobes to examine the undersurface.

The normal liver should extend caudally to the level of the costal arch and should have a smooth surface with sharp borders. The liver should be of a uniform deep red color (see Plate 15-1). As the laparoscope is moved close to the liver, the operator is able to detect the portal areas and a uniform sinusoidal configuration. (This is possible because of the magnification capabilities of most laparoscopes as they are moved close to the tissue being examined.) Gentle palpation of the liver with either the laparoscope or the palpation probe causes temporary blanching and depression of the organ's surface. The liver should not tear or bleed excessively when palpated.

Pathologic changes of the liver are often detected grossly. Abnormal liver changes include hepatic lipidosis, in which the liver appears pale mustard in color and is friable on manipulation (see Plate 15-3). The portal triads are usually prominent in livers with extensive hepatic lipidosis. A glycogen-laden liver or steroid hepatopathy of dogs looks similar to a fatty liver, but the organ tends to be more pink in color. Passive hepatic congestion results in a large, dark, black-red liver with rounded borders, and prominent distended hepatic sinusoids are seen on close inspection of the surface. Livers with chronic passive congestion have been described as "nutmeg" in appearance. Metastatic or multifocal neoplasia usually has a characteristic appearance. The tumor nodules are raised from the hepatic surface, are usually discolored, and often have cavitations or depressions in their center. In contrast, nodular hyperplasia, a common condition in older dogs, may be mistaken for neoplasia. Nodular hyperplasia is seen as variably sized, frequently multiple, raised nodules with a yellow fatty appearance and depressions over their surface. A needle biopsy specimen obtained through a nodule may only show vacuolar changes and fail to demonstrate to the pathologist that it is the cross section of a hyperplastic nodule. Laparoscopy offers the added dimension of a gross description to aid in the histologic interpretation of nodular hyperplasia. Animals with biliary tract disease, such as cats with cholangitis or cholangiohepatitis, have prominent green-black portal triads. With extrahepatic biliary obstructions the entire liver becomes green-black from the excessive bilirubin accumulation, and the gallbladder and extrahepatic bile ducts are distended and turgid on palpation.

Cirrhosis often has a characteristic appearance. In fact, the gross impression of cirrhosis is often more accurate in making a diagnosis than are the histopathology findings. This is because small biopsy samples sometimes do not represent all the changes in the liver. The surface may have an irregular "cobblestone" texture, or it may contain various-size regenerative nodules extending from the surface of the liver and resembling a cluster of grapes. Cirrhotic livers are generally small in size and firm on palpation as a result of an increase in fibrosis. The liver capsule may be thickened, giving the surface a whitish appearance. Ascites may be present, or acquired collateral shunting of the portal circulation may be indicated by the presence of multiple venous plexuses around the pararenal area. Acquired collateral portal shunts are best observed in the area of the left kidney.

## Liver Biopsy Techniques

After the visual examination of the liver and adjacent visceral structures has been completed, a directed liver biopsy is performed and photographs are taken to document gross findings and to correlate these findings with the histologic evaluation. The distinct advantage of laparoscopy over percutaneous needle biopsy techniques is the capability for visual selection of the areas to be sampled. Areas of increased vascularity, necrosis, or dis-

tended bile ducts should be avoided. With patchy or multifocal changes, it is best to obtain biopsy samples not only from the area that is considered abnormal but also from the areas that appear normal. Often a suspected abnormal area may actually be normal. Consequently, several biopsy specimens representative of all areas should be obtained. Tissue samples may be collected for histologic evaluation, copper analysis, or culture.

Several laparoscopically directed liver biopsy methods may be used. In larger dogs with normal to large livers, a biopsy needle such as the Tru-Cut disposable biopsy needle (an 18-gauge and 6-inch needle) may be adequate. The needle must be sufficiently long to span the abdominal wall plus the established pneumoperitoneum and still reach the liver. The point of entry of the biopsy needle should be close to the costal arch and as near as possible to the area to be sampled. The laparoscope is generally withdrawn slightly to give a wider view of the anterior abdomen and to facilitate visualization of the biopsy needle as it enters the abdominal cavity. The needle is then directed to the biopsy site. The operator should be aware of the adjacent structures in the biopsy area to avoid inadvertent puncture of the diaphragm, gastrointestinal tract, large blood vessels, or gallbladder. It is advisable to direct the needle in a plane parallel to the long axis of the liver lobe rather than pass it through the lobe at right angles, which could result in inadvertent perforation of the underlying structures (see Plate 15-15). With a biopsy needle, the samples can be obtained from deep within the liver; in contrast, biopsy forceps only retrieve tissue from the organ's surface. The disadvantage of needle biopsies is the small size of the tissue samples.

An alternate method for liver biopsy involves the use of biopsy forceps passed through a second trocar cannula placed adjacent to the laparoscope (Figure 14-16). The right-handed operator should make the second puncture to the right and usually slightly cranial to the laparoscope. A distance of at least 5 cm between the two cannulas is required to have enough space to manipulate both instruments. The biopsy forceps technique has a number of advantages. Biopsy forceps are longer than most standard biopsy needles and are capable of reaching the livers of even large, deep-chested dogs. Biopsy forceps are also considered much safer for taking samples from small livers in that the risk of perforation or trauma to adjacent organs is minimal (see Figure 14-10 and Plate 15-8). The crushing action of the biopsy forceps also generally results in minimal bleeding. When a patient is suspected of having diffuse disease based on visual inspection, the biopsy specimens are usually obtained from the edge of one of the representative liver lobes (see Plate 15-17). Focal lesions on the surface of the liver are biopsied in a pinching manner over the area to be sampled. The biopsy forceps technique involves grasping the area to be sampled and applying forceps pressure. Double-spoon–type biopsy forceps generally do not cut the liver sample completely free unless the instrument is exceptionally sharp and the liver has minimal fibrosis. In most cases the sample must be pulled away from the liver with slow steady tension. This cutting, crushing, and tearing technique does not significantly damage the liver or biopsy sample; it also does not cause increased bleeding.

Bleeding from liver biopsies is minimal and amounts to no more than 5 to 10 ml of blood. Generally, a little more bleeding can be expected with needle biopsies than with the biopsy forceps method (see Plates 15-15 and 15-18). Once the biopsy sample has been obtained, the area should be scrutinized until adequate clotting is detected. This takes usually no more than 3 minutes to occur. If more than the expected amount of bleeding should result, the biopsy site may be occluded by placing the blunt palpation probe, the biopsy forceps, or even the tip of the laparoscope over the area. If bleeding persists despite the application of direct pressure, hemostatic agents such as an absorbable gelatin sponge (e.g., gelfoam) or 1:1000 epinephrine can be applied topically under laparoscopic direction. Many biopsy forceps are also equipped for electrocoagulation at the tip of the instrument. If available, coagulation at the biopsy site could be used. Rarely, if ever are hemostatic or coagulation agents needed.

## Evaluation and Biopsy of the Pancreas

The pancreas is evaluated by a right lateral mid-abdominal approach. Commonly the omentum may cover the surface of the pancreas. Such cases require a second puncture and the use of a palpation probe or biopsy forceps to sweep the omentum away. The right lateral wing of the pancreas is found adjacent to the duodenum; its length should be followed, beginning from the right distal end, and then traced as far to the left side as possible. Generally only the proximal portion of the left pancreatic lobe is visualized with this approach before the rest of the organ becomes lost among the surrounding deeper structures. In some cases the entire pancreas can be visualized with a ventral abdominal approach. The normal pancreas should be a pale cream color and should be coarsely lobulated, which gives the surface a regular nodular appearance with irregularly crenated margins (see Plates 15-13 and 15-16). In some instances the common bile duct may be observed as it passes adjacent to the pancreas before entering the duodenum.

Clinical experience with pancreatic biopsy is limited, but a considerable number of these procedures have been performed in normal dogs with no serious complications. In our series of 360 consecutive laparoscopies, six pancreatic biopsies were performed in clinical cases.

All six patients were suspected to have pancreatitis, and tissue samples were obtained using double-spoon biopsy forceps with grasping teeth. (We are currently using the cutting punch biopsy forceps for pancreatic biopsy.) Pancreatic biopsies should be taken from the margin of the distal portion of the right pancreatic wing. Note that samples should not be obtained near the duct system, which is located in the center of the gland. The tissue is grasped, and a small sample is taken from the pancreas (similar to the technique described for liver biopsies). The animals we evaluated displayed no clinical evidence of postbiopsy pancreatitis, and we recognized no increase in the severity of ongoing pancreatitis in the affected dogs. The latter instance must be recognized as a potential complication, however.

Pathologic changes observed in our cases included both acute and chronic pancreatitis. Chronic pancreatitis is characterized by markedly irregular, nodular pancreatic architecture. There may also be evidence of parapancreatic fat nodules that represent calcification, fibrosis, or necrotic tissue. In patients with acute pancreatitis, severe parapancreatic inflammation often obscures visualization of the pancreas itself. Local hyperemia, adhesions, tissue edema, and parapancreatic fat necrosis are characteristic. Because of the inflammatory changes the pancreas commonly cannot be visualized. The diagnosis of acute pancreatitis is sometimes made based only on visual inspection of the adjacent tissue and biopsies showing necrotic and inflammatory parapancreatic tissue. We advise always obtaining biopsies of the *liver* when evaluating the pancreas because concurrent liver disease is often present. In general, laparoscopy is not indicated for the patient with obvious acute pancreatitis and peritonitis and is contraindicated if the patient has evidence of a bacterial peritonitis. Great care must be exercised when evaluating the patient with suspected pancreatitis because of the potential for adhesions and the danger of perforation after trocar placement. Laparoscopic evaluation may be beneficial in the patient with suspected pancreatic adenocarcinoma, but it should not be used to confirm a suspected case of islet cell tumor. Islet cell tumors are small and often difficult to find. If present, these tumors usually require surgical excision.

We often use laparoscopy to confirm the presence of acute pancreatitis or to laparoscopically place a jejunostomy feeding tube in a patient with continued vomiting and a nutritional imbalance. Laparoscopy may also prove to be beneficial in the placement of peritoneal lavage tubes in selected patients.

## ANCILLARY PROCEDURES

Additional diagnostic and therapeutic procedures can be performed in conjunction with laparoscopy. As with all invasive procedures, the diagnostic benefit must be weighed against the risk in each case. Ancillary diagnostic procedures include gallbladder puncture to collect bile or perform cholecystocholangiography and splenic puncture to perform splenoportography or obtain splenic pulp pressure measurements. Therapeutic procedures include laparoscopic placement of gastrostomy feeding tubes and temporary decompression of bile duct obstructions prior to surgical intervention.

## Biliary Evaluation

A right-side approach is used to evaluate the gallbladder, extrahepatic ducts, and common bile duct. A second puncture technique and the use of a palpating probe are required to adequately visualize the biliary system. The right lateral lobe of the liver must be elevated to observe the hilus of the liver, the gallbladder, and the remainder of the biliary system. When palpated, the normal gallbladder should be soft and fluctuant, and the ductal system should not be distended.

Obstructive biliary tract disease is often associated with a hard, firm gallbladder, and the liver usually appears dark green-black in color as a result of bile pigment accumulation. Marked bile staining is often present around the hilus of the liver in animals with significant cholestatic disease. The common bile duct should be evaluated and followed as it courses to the duodenum.

After the extrahepatic biliary system and adjacent structures have been completely evaluated, bile can be aspirated from the gallbladder. For bile aspiration a needle is inserted through the abdominal wall in close approximation to the gallbladder. Normally a 20-gauge, 10-cm spinal needle is satisfactory for this procedure. In larger animals a longer needle is required. Under direct visualization the needle tip is inserted into the gallbladder (see Plate 15-19). Bile is aspirated into a syringe and then submitted for cytologic examination and bacterial culture and sensitivity studies. The bile should be cultured for both aerobic and anaerobic organisms.

A contrast study (cholecystocholangiography) can be performed under laparoscopic direction in the patient suspected of having an extrahepatic bile duct obstruction. The needle is inserted into the gallbladder as described previously, and as much bile as possible is aspirated. In some cases only a small amount can be removed because of the usually viscous consistency of the bile in extrahepatic biliary tract disease. After the bile has been aspirated, a sterile radiopaque iodine contrast agent designed for IV use is injected into the gallbladder. A volume of 5 to 10 ml is usually adequate to properly distend the biliary system and delineate any abnormalities. The volume of contrast material placed into the gallbladder should, however, not be so great that the gallbladder becomes overly distended. Overdistension may result in leakage of the contrast agent. If the biliary tract is patent, contrast material should easily pass into the duodenum; this passage must be demonstrated by fluoroscopy or with routine static radiographs. The contrast agent generally remains in the biliary system long enough to perform radiographic studies. If possible, the gallbladder should be decompressed by removing the contrast material to prevent excessive pressure and leakage. This is especially important in the patient with obstructive biliary tract disease. Leakage of a small amount of contrast agent is common and generally does not cause any significant problems. Great concern is warranted, however, if the bile is septic.

In the series of 360 laparoscopies evaluated, five dogs underwent gallbladder puncture and bile collection and were then followed with a contrast study. Three of the dogs were found to have complete bile duct obstructions that subsequently were surgically corrected.

## Splenic Pulp Pressure Measurement

Splenic pulp pressure measurements can be obtained during laparoscopy when suspected portal hypertension secondary to liver disease is to be documented. In most cases this procedure is used only for research or academic purposes because the information gained offers limited clinically useful information except in selected cases. Barbiturates and phenothiazine tranquilizers should not be used for patient restraint because resultant splenic engorgement could alter splenic pulp pressures.

For this procedure, the animal must be approached from a left mid-abdominal site. Care must be taken when entering at this level because the spleen is often lying under or close to the entry site and can easily be traumatized. The liver should first be adequately evaluated and biopsied. Portal hypertension from liver disease commonly results in acquired portal systemic shunting of blood. Collateral vessels usually develop in the left renal area and form an anastomosis with the posterior vena cava. The presence of these abnormal vessels should be noted: they signify portal hypertension.

An 18- to 20-gauge 10-cm spinal needle is inserted through the ventrolateral abdominal wall near the area of the spleen. The needle is then directed in such a manner that it traverses the spleen parallel with the long axis (see Plate 15-24). Under direct visualization the needle is inserted 1 to 3 cm into the center of the splenic parenchyma. Once the needle is seated firmly within the spleen, the laparoscope is removed and insufflated gas is evacuated before pressure recordings are made. Splenic pulp pressures are usually reported in centimeters of water and are taken using a simple manometer. The zero point of the manometer should be level with the right atrium of the heart. Normal splenic pulp pressures in dogs range from 10 to 15 cm of water. Dogs with acquired portal hypertension, usually the result of chronic liver disease, have splenic pulp pressures ranging from 20 to 40 cm of water.

After pressure recordings, the needle is removed and the spleen is observed for evidence of bleeding. A small hematoma usually develops at the area of the needle insertion, but excessive bleeding is uncommon. If prolonged bleeding occurs, the measures described for controlling liver biopsy hemorrhage are used. In our series, splenic pulp pressure measurements were performed in 31 animals without complications.

## Splenoportography

Splenoportography is used to demonstrate portal blood flow and can be accomplished under laparoscopic control. This procedure is usually performed on the radiology table. The technique described for splenic pulp pressure measurements is similar to the method for splenoportography. When the two procedures are performed together, portal pressure measurements should be taken before contrast studies are obtained.

Once the needle has been placed firmly in the body of the spleen and splenic pulp pressure measurements have been taken, an IV iodine contrast agent is injected. A dose of 0.25 to 0.5 ml/kg (0.55 to 1.1 ml/lb) body weight of the contrast agent is injected by hand at a rate of approximately 1 to 2 ml per second. A radiograph is obtained immediately after completion of the contrast agent infusion. When possible, however, a series of radiographs should be made during the last half of the injection and for 5 to 10 seconds after the injection. This series will delineate portal blood flow patterns. In our 360 laparoscopy cases, 30 animals underwent splenoportography to document the presence of congenital or acquired portal collateral circulation abnormalities. Each procedure was considered diagnostic and was completed without complications.

## Percutaneous Laparoscopic Gastrostomy Tube Placement

Percutaneous laparoscopic gastrostomy (PLG) tube placement is useful when a patient is undergoing laparoscopy and requires enteral nutrition, with tube feeding through the stomach. The technique can be performed in cats with hepatic lipidosis that require tube feeding for management of their disease, while obtaining a liver biopsy. The technique is contraindicated in the patient that is vomiting or has gastric disease and/or outflow obstruction.

Proper placement of the PLG tube in the greater curvature of the stomach requires a left lateral approach with the patient in a right lateral recumbent position. Because the liver and pancreas are best evaluated with a

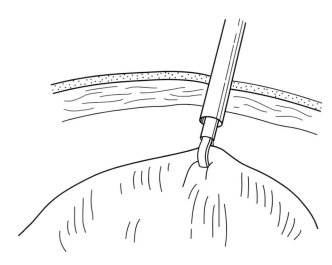

**Figure 15-1** Placement of a percutaneous laparoscopic gastrostomy tube. The forceps instrument is grasping the stomach.

right lateral approach, tube placement should be planned before the procedure. The abdomen is insufflated routinely, and the scope trocar-cannula is introduced through the left caudoventral body wall. Then a routine examination is performed. The working trocar-cannula (5 mm or larger if possible) is introduced under direct visualization in the craniodorsal wall just caudal to the last rib. Site selection for the PLG tube can be made by externally indenting the abdominal wall digitally while assessing the location with the laparoscope.

After the working cannula has been introduced, ancillary procedures such as liver biopsy should be performed prior to PLG tube placement.

For PLG tube placement an avascular area of the lateral stomach wall is grasped in the area of the junction of the fundus and gastric body. Slight insufflation of the gastric lumen via an orally introduced stomach tube sometimes aids in the visualization and localization of gastric anatomy. Insufflation should be done only after all other diagnostic tests are performed because a gas-distended stomach can hamper visualization. The area of the stomach for tube placement is firmly grasped with racheting-type tissue graspers (Figure 15-1). The stomach is withdrawn until it comes into contact with the cannula sleeve; then both the cannula and graspers are withdrawn in unison until the stomach wall is slightly protruding (or exteriorized) through the abdominal puncture. If a small-diameter cannula is used, the abdominal wall opening will probably have to be carefully widened while the exteriorized stomach is held securely with the graspers. The stomach is then secured with absorbable stay sutures (Figure 15-2). A purse string of synthetic absorbable suture is placed in the stomach wall for the tube placement, and a small 1-cm incision is then cut into the lumen of the stomach at the center of the area where the purse-string

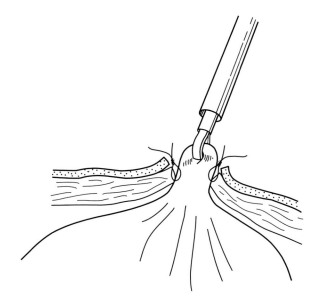

**Figure 15-2** The stomach has been pulled outside the body through the trocar-cannula opening. The stomach has been stabilized with stay sutures prior to placement of the percutaneous laparoscopic gastrostomy tube.

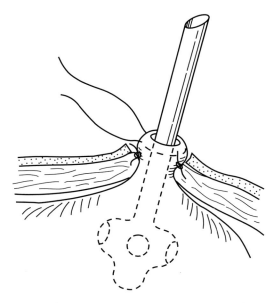

**Figure 15-3** The percutaneous laparoscopic gastrostomy tube is placed into the stomach lumen through a purse-string suture.

suture has been placed. While the full wall of the stomach is grasped with hemostats or tissue-grasping forceps, the lubricated feeding tube is passed into the gastric lumen (Figure 15-3). We routinely use an 18- to 22-French Pezzer mushroom-tip catheter (Bard Urological Division, Covington, Ga.). The catheter mushroom must be stretched onto a stylet to flatten the tip in order to advance the catheter into the stomach lumen. The feeding tube is opposed to the stomach and body wall. The purse-string suture is closed around the tube, and the suture is then used to close the muscle wall and skin. This final technique is identical to the surgical placement of a gastrostomy tube. An exterior gasket or bumper is slid down to the skin, with care taken to avoid excessive compression, and the bumper is secured with suture, tape, or glue. Under laparoscopic visualization the tube is flushed with a small amount of sterile water to check for leakage. The tube should be kept in place for at least 1 week before removal in order to allow sufficient time for a permanent adhesion to form.

## COMPLICATIONS

The complication rate for laparoscopy in the evaluation of the liver and pancreas is low (Box 15-1). In our institution, laparoscopy procedures were performed by a number of residents and faculty members with variable skills. The overall major complication rate for the series was 3.3%. The complications were due in part to oper-

---

> **Box 15-1**    Complications of Laparoscopy in the Evaluation of the Liver and Pancreas
>
> **MAJOR COMPLICATIONS**
> Bleeding
> Air embolism
> Organ perforation
> Infection
> Gallbladder perforation
> Diaphragmatic puncture (pneumothorax)
> Anesthetic complications
>
> **MINOR COMPLICATIONS**
> Instrumentation problems
> Subcutaneous emphysema
> Leakage of ascites
> Overdistension of pneumoperitoneum

ator inexperience and failure to identify appropriate indications for the procedure. Problems associated with instrumentation technique comprised the most common minor complaints and were attributed to operator inexperience. Potential major complications include air embolism, cardiopulmonary arrest, pneumothorax, damage to internal organs, bleeding, and infection.

Several complications occurred in the laparoscopic evaluation of dogs with either hepatic or pancreatic disease in our series. Two fatalities were associated directly with the procedure: one was the result of laceration of the posterior vena cava in a cat from the biopsy needle, and the other was an anesthetic death in a dog with end-stage liver disease. Three other deaths that occurred within 36 hours of the procedure were felt to be partially associated with the procedure. These three animals had advanced liver disease at the time of laparoscopy, and the procedure was thought to have contributed to their clinical decompensation.

Other complications included one instance of pneumothorax caused by a biopsy needle puncturing the diaphragm and one instance of excessive bleeding that occurred during needle biopsy of the liver and required a blood transfusion. The animal that needed the transfusion was a Doberman pinscher with chronic active hepatitis and concurrent von Willebrand's disease.

Minor complications in our series included subcutaneous emphysema and subcutaneous leakage of ascitic fluid around the puncture site. The latter problem can be prevented if the operator uses a tight three-layer closure in the abdominal wall.

## REFERENCES

Harrington DP et al: Laparoscopic biopsy of the normal canine pancreas. JVIM 10(3): 156, 1996.

Harrison RM, Wildt DE, editors: *Animal laparoscopy*, Baltimore, 1980, Williams & Wilkins.

Jones BD: Laparoscopy, *Vet Clin North Am Small Anim Pract* 20:1243, 1990.

Jones BD, Hitt M, Hurst T: Hepatic biopsy, *Vet Clin North Am* 15:39, 1985.

Lettow E. Laparoscopic examinations in liver diseases in dogs, *Vet Med Rev* 2:159, 1972.

Patterson JM. Laparoscopy in small animal medicine. In Kirk RW, editor: *Current veterinary therapy VII*, Philadelphia, 1981, WB Saunders.

Rothuizen J: Laparoscopy in small animal medicine, *Vet Q* 7:225, 1985.

Twedt DC: Laparoscopy in small animals. In *Proceedings of the Fifth Annual American College Veterinary Internal Medicine Forum*, 1987.

Wildt DE, Kinney GM, Seager SWJ: Laparoscopy for direct observation of internal organs of the domestic cat and dog, *Am J Vet Res* 38:1429, 1977.

## COLOR PLATES   PAGES 419-426

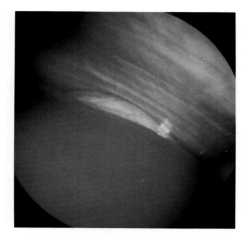

**Plate 15-1** Normal surface of the right lateral lobe of the liver (lower aspect of the field of view), with the peritoneal reflection of the diaphragm (upper aspect of the field) and a small portion of the gallbladder (narrow structure in the center of the field).

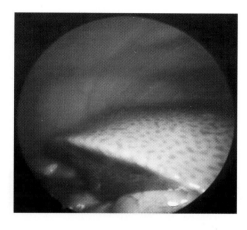

**Plate 15-2** Liver of a cat with cholangiohepatitis. Note the prominent portal areas, which give the liver a mottled appearance. The peritoneal reflection of the diaphragm is in the background.

**A**

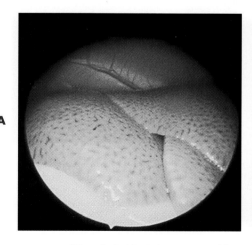

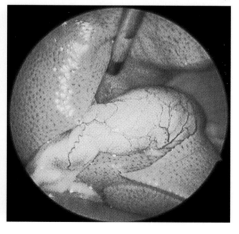

**B**

**Plate 15-3** Hepatic lipidosis in a 5-year-old cat with a history of anorexia, weight loss, and jaundice. **A,** Note the pale yellow appearance of the liver. The liver parenchyma was friable. The diaphragm can be seen in the background. **B,** A palpation probe is being used to lift the right liver lobes for clear visualization of the gallbladder. The gallbladder is normal in size, and the cystic duct can be seen exiting it (7 o'clock position in the field of view).

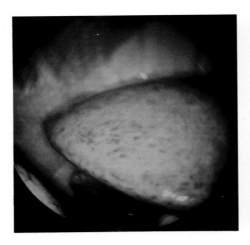

**Plate 15-4** Swollen discolored liver lobe of a dog with diffuse hepatic lymphosarcoma. The diaphragm can be seen in the background.

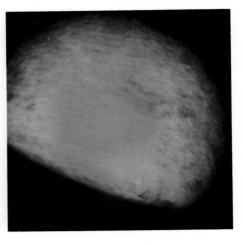

**Plate 15-5** Close-up of the liver shown in Plate 15-4 (hepatic lymphosarcoma). The swollen and rounded border is characteristic of infiltrative disease.

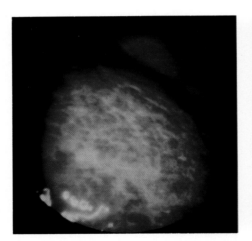

**Plate 15-6** Irregular cobblestone surface of the liver in a Bedlington terrier with chronic active hepatitis and early cirrhosis. The pale areas over the surface represent fibrosis.

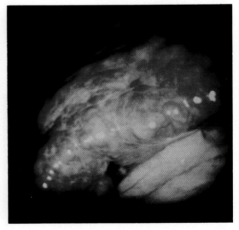

**Plate 15-7** Liver of a Doberman pinscher with cirrhosis. Marked hyperplastic nodules, fibrosis, and necrosis of the liver are present. This dog had ascites and clinical signs related to hepatic encephalopathy.

**A**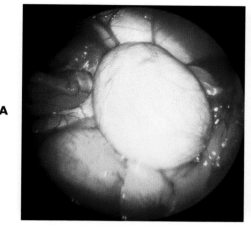
**B**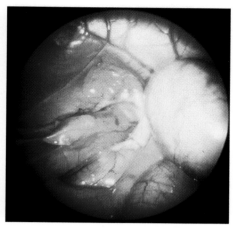

**Plate 15-8** Microhepatica in a 3-year-old cocker spaniel with a 3-week history of intermittent vomiting and anorexia. Liver enzyme levels were only mildly elevated, but both resting and postprandial bile acid values were markedly increased. **A,** As the laparoscope is advanced to the abdominal cavity, the gallbladder is clearly in view (center of the field). The gallbladder is so prominently seen because all of the liver lobes are very small. Biopsies confirmed a diagnosis of micronodular cirrhosis. Hepatic copper levels were significantly elevated (5600 ppm [normal: less than 400 ppm]). **B,** Several small liver lobes can be seen to the left of the gallbladder. The caudal vena cava is seen between two of the lobes (8 o'clock position). The oval window of the diaphragm is in the background (light area at the top of the field). The dog lived 15 months after the diagnosis of severe liver disease was made. NOTE: Laparoscopy is an ideal method for safely and quickly obtaining liver biopsies in animals with a small liver. (Courtesy Todd R. Tams.)

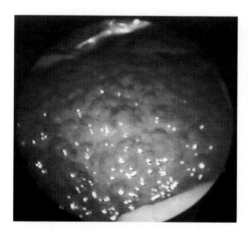

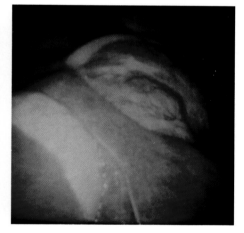

**Plate 15-9** Nodular liver of a 12-year-old dog with hepatocutaneous syndrome. The nodules are hyperplastic, and the liver has a cirrhotic appearance.

**Plate 15-10** Hepatic adenoma, just adjacent to a normal gallbladder (pale structure in left foreground), in the right lateral lobe of a dog's liver. This tumor was successfully removed surgically.

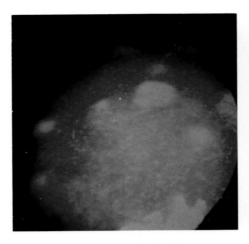

**Plate 15-11** Numerous raised, white metastatic tumor nodules in the liver. These nodules represent spread from a mammary gland adenocarcinoma.

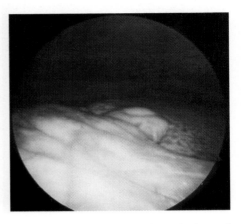

**Plate 15-12** Metastatic nodule in the liver of a dog. The primary tumor was a pancreatic adenocarcinoma. Note the crater depression over the surface of the tumor. This is often characteristic of neoplasia. In front of the metastatic nodule are adhesions of omentum around the pancreatic tumor.

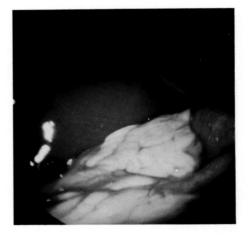

**Plate 15-13** Normal right lateral lobe of the pancreas (lower right foreground) adjacent to the right medial lobe of the liver (upper aspect in field of view).

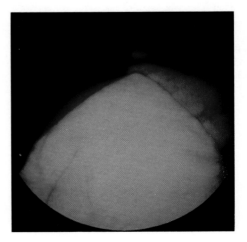

**Plate 15-14** Close-up of a normal right lobe of the pancreas. The proximal duodenum is located just to the right of the pancreas.

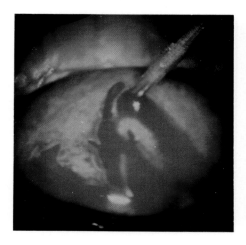

**Plate 15-15** A Tru-Cut biopsy needle in the liver, with a small amount of bleeding at the biopsy site. Note that the needle is directed along the long axis of the liver lobe.

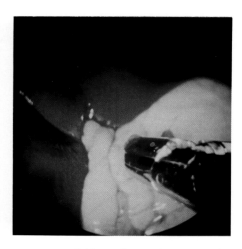

**Plate 15-16** A biopsy forceps instrument that has been passed through a second puncture and is grasping a portion of a normal pancreas. The pancreas is adjacent to a grossly normal liver (upper and left aspect in the field of view).

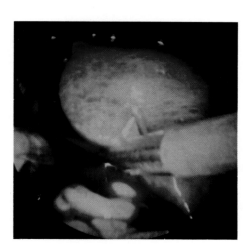

**Plate 15-17** Biopsy forceps instrument grasping an edge of a liver lobe. The sample is pinched and then pulled away from the liver. A small amount of blood has pooled below the liver lobe.

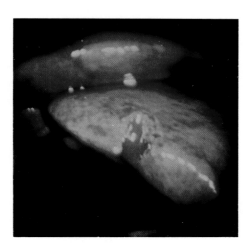

**Plate 15-18** The liver in Plate 15-17 after forceps biopsy. Note that minimal bleeding or tissue trauma occurs when this technique is used.

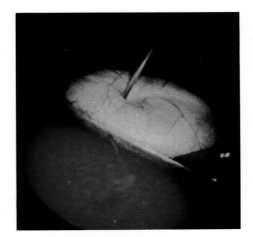

**Plate 15-19** A 20-gauge spinal needle placed in the gallbladder of a normal dog. The gallbladder is located between the right lateral and medial liver lobes.

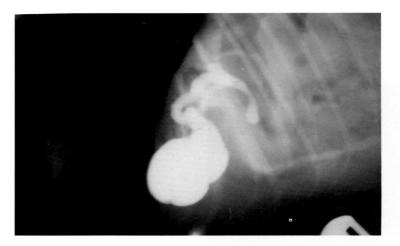

**Plate 15-20** Radiograph of a normal cholecystocholangiography study that was performed under laparoscopic direction. The contrast material is entering the duodenum, indicating a patent biliary system.

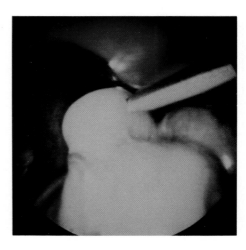

**Plate 15-21** A 20-gauge spinal needle placed in the distended common bile duct of a dog. A biliary stone in the duodenal papilla has resulted in complete bile duct obstruction. The common bile duct can be seen as it enters the duodenum, which is ventral (5 to 6 o'clock position). A lobe of the liver is seen in the left aspect of the field. The liver is black-green in color because of the chronic bile duct obstruction.

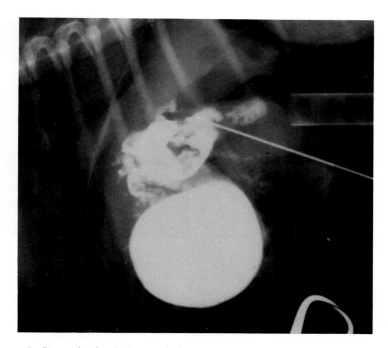

**Plate 15-22** Radiograph of a cholecystocholangiography study performed on the patient represented by Plate 15-21. No contrast material is entering the duodenum, and the gallbladder is distended because of the complete bile duct obstruction.

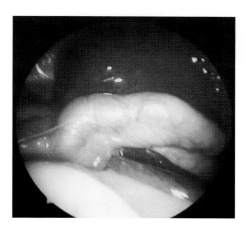

**Plate 15-23** Liver and distended bile ducts in a cat with choleliths in the common bile duct.

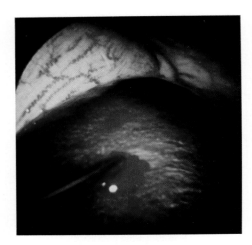

**Plate 15-24** An 18-gauge spinal needle is seated in the spleen (grossly normal) to perform splenic pulp pressures and splenoportography. Under laparoscopic direction the needle is placed parallel to the long axis of the spleen.

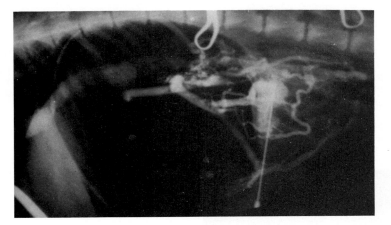

**Plate 15-25** Splenoportography performed under laparoscopic direction in a dog with cirrhosis and portal hypertension. The portal circulation consists of multiple venous plexuses draining into the posterior vena cava. No portal circulation is observed entering the liver.

# Chapter 16

# Laparoscopy of the Urinary Tract

## Gregory Grauer

Kidney inspection and biopsy are the major indications for laparoscopic examination of the urinary tract. In many cases, kidney biopsy specimens are obtained using ultrasound guidance. However, with the aid of laparoscopy, these biopsy specimens may be safely procured under direct visualization without the disadvantages of laparotomy and usually without general anesthesia. Laparoscopy is especially well suited for serial kidney biopsies, which are often needed to follow the progression of renal disease or to assess response to therapy. Direct visualization of the kidney allows the operator to obtain multiple biopsy specimens for light, immunofluorescent, and electron microscopy while avoiding previous biopsy sites. Laparoscopy can also be used to inspect the serosal surface of the urinary bladder and in many cases the distal portion of the ureters.

## INDICATIONS

Laparoscopy should be considered any time that a kidney biopsy is required. Laparoscopic direction of renal biopsy has several advantages over the keyhole renal biopsy technique. Visualization of the kidney before biopsy results in the procurement of a higher percentage of diagnostic tissue, especially when focal renal disease is present. Furthermore, inspection of the kidney can often provide immediate valuable information. In contrast, digital palpation with the keyhole biopsy technique may miss renal tumors, infarcts, and petechiae, as well as an irregular renal surface. Visualization of the kidney after biopsy also allows the operator to determine the amount of hemorrhage and, if necessary, to apply pressure to the biopsy site with the laparoscope. In addition, several other abdominal organs (e.g., liver, spleen, pancreas, large and small bowel, omentum) can be visualized and biopsied or aspirated. Sedation and local anesthesia requirements for laparoscopy are similar to those for the keyhole renal biopsy technique.

Biopsy artifact may be created with the keyhole biopsy technique because the kidney often has to be displaced a considerable distance from its normal location to facilitate proper exposure. This can result in the congestion of peritubular and glomerular capillaries and resultant extravasation of erythrocytes into the tubular lumina and Bowman's space. These artifacts are not observed in kidney biopsies obtained via laparoscopy. Another artifact may be caused by the compression of tissue by the biopsy needle, which has been reported with the use of Franklin-modified and Vim-Silverman biopsy needles, but it is usually not a problem with true-cut type biopsy needles (Sherwood Medical, St. Louis, Mo.).

Compared with laparotomy, laparoscopy takes less time, usually does not require anesthesia, and is less invasive. Delayed incision healing and ascites fluid leakage can complicate recovery from a ventral midline laparotomy incision in hypoproteinemic patients. These problems are rarely encountered with the small midparalumbar incision used for laparoscopy.

The major disadvantage of laparoscopy compared with laparotomy is limited visualization of abdominal organs. Although parts of the peritoneal cavity can be seen well, a thorough laparoscopic exploration is not possible because the entry site of the scope limits the number of organs that can be inspected. For example, a right midparalumbar entry allows inspection of the right half of the liver, the gallbladder, the right kidney and right adrenal gland, and part of the omentum, pancreas, and large and small bowel, but it does not allow visualization of the left kidney, the spleen, and most of the stomach. Thus, if both kidneys need to be inspected, laparotomy should be performed.

## PATIENT PREPARATION AND RESTRAINT

Laparoscopy and renal biopsy should not be performed before basic laboratory tests and coagulation studies have been obtained. In many cases, prelaparoscopic studies also include quantitation of urine protein excretion, evaluation of renal excretory function, ultrasonography, and intravenous (IV) urography.

Food should be withheld for at least 8 hours before the procedure. A combination of oxymorphone and acepromazine or butorphanol, acepromazine, and glycopyrrolate given IV provide adequate sedation in most dogs. Excessive abdominal insufflation is poorly tolerated by sedated patients and should be avoided. In cats, inhalation anesthesia is often preferred to sedation. A light plane of general anesthesia with isoflurane is also well tolerated by most patients. Adequate support with IV fluids should be provided. If the urinary bladder is large, it should be expressed or emptied by catheterization to avoid bladder perforation by the trocar when the cannula is introduced into the abdomen.

## PROCEDURE

### Kidney Evaluation and Biopsy

A biopsy sample from the right kidney (see Plates 16-1 and 16-3) is routinely obtained unless plain radiography, ultrasonography, or IV urography indicates unilateral left renal involvement. The biopsy sample can be procured from either kidney via laparoscopy. However, the right kidney is more stable in that the caudate lobe of the liver provides resistance to movement during the biopsy procedure. For biopsy of the right kidney, the patient is placed in a left lateral recumbent position. The right midparalumbar region caudal to the last rib is then clipped, prepared as for aseptic surgery, and draped. Lidocaine is used for local anesthesia of the abdominal wall in nonanesthetized patients.

After pneumoperitoneum is established with a Veress needle and compressed carbon dioxide, the laparoscope cannula containing a trocar is introduced into the abdomen through a 1-cm skin incision. The incision should

be approximately 5 cm caudal to the last rib and 3 to 5 cm ventral to the border of the lumbar muscles. The trocar and cannula should be pointed in a cranial-dorsal direction and should enter the abdomen at a shallow angle. A crisp, short thrust with a slight twisting motion facilitates entry of the pyramidal trocar point into the abdomen. The right kidney usually lies 5 to 8 cm in a cranial-dorsal direction from the point of entry. The kidney is pale gray and has a readily apparent capsular vasculature (see Plates 16-1 and 16-3). As the tip of the scope is moved in a cranial-dorsal direction, the kidney is seen to the right of the dorsal body wall and to the left of the liver and diaphragm. If ascites is present, tilting the table so that the patient's head is slightly elevated usually improves visualization of the kidney.

For renal biopsy procedures a 6-inch Tru-Cut biopsy needle is introduced into the abdomen approximately 3 cm above or below the cannula. The biopsy needle is then "walked" down the laparoscope until it is in the field of view. A biopsy sample can be more easily obtained from the cranial pole of the kidney, which is usually larger than the caudal pole. The biopsy needle is directed away from the hilum of the kidney and at a shallow angle to the kidney capsule. Then an assistant holds the laparoscope, freeing the operator's hands for the biopsy procedure. The operator should observe the kidney both as the biopsy specimen is procured and also afterward for hemorrhage (see Plate 16-4). If hemorrhage is arterial or does not abate within 2 to 3 minutes, pressure should be applied over the biopsy site using the tip of the laparoscope. Once the bleeding has stopped, a sterile isotonic saline "rinse" to dislodge the blood clot rarely results in further hemorrhage and may help prevent future adhesions. A needle attached to a syringe and introduced through a separate abdominal puncture can be used to apply the rinse.

### Bladder and Ureter Evaluation

In addition to inspecting the kidney and performing a biopsy, the operator can also use the laparoscope to examine the serosal surface of the urinary bladder (see Plate 16-7) and commonly the distal one third to one half of the ureters (see Plate 16-6). Although it is possible to diagnose an ectopic ureter, a hydroureter, a urachal remnant, a bladder wall tumor, or bladder wall trauma via laparoscopy (see Chapter 18), conditions affecting the bladder and ureter are usually best diagnosed with ultrasonography, cystoscopy, or contrast radiography. Laparoscopy is, however, useful for obtaining biopsy specimens from a bladder wall tumor that does not extend to the mucosal surface and for aspirating urine from a hydroureter for culture.

The urinary bladder and nondependent ureter can be visualized using the same abdominal entry site as for kidney evaluation and then directing the laparoscope caudally. If the primary purpose of laparoscopy is evaluation of the bladder, the patient should be placed in a dorsal recumbent position and the entry site for the laparoscope should be the ventral midline midway between the umbilicus and xiphoid. The trocar and cannula unit should be directed cranially and toward the ventral diaphragm as the unit is advanced through the abdominal wall. The bladder should be emptied before abdominal placement of the cannula. Once the laparoscope is in place, sterile saline is instilled via a urethral catheter to facilitate bladder identification. The bladder is gray with tortuous serosal vessels (see Plate 16-8). Slight lowering of the patient's head or abdominal manipulation by an assistant often increases the visible surface area of the bladder.

The nondependent ureter is best visualized with the nonobese patient in a lateral recumbent position. The distal portion of the ureter can usually be found ventral to the lumbar muscles and dorsal to the large and small bowels in the caudal abdomen. The ureter descends toward the trigone of the bladder, loops cranially around the ductus deferens in the male, and then enters the bladder in a cranial direction.

## Peritoneal Cavity Evaluation and Completion of Procedure

Any time laparoscopy is performed, the operator should assess the gross appearance of as much of the peritoneal cavity and its contents as possible. This is best done by a systematic clockwise and then counterclockwise half rotation of the scope around the entry site. The examination should be performed before biopsy specimens are procured.

Before the cannula is removed from the abdomen, the gas used for abdominal insufflation should be removed. Sutures should be placed in the subcutaneous tissues and skin to close the laparoscopy site. Renal biopsy patients should usually be observed in the hospital for 12 to 24 hours before discharge.

### SUGGESTED ADDITIONAL READINGS

Bartges JW, Osborne CA: Canine and feline renal biopsy. In Osborne CA, Finco DR, editors: *Canine and feline nephrology and urology,* Baltimore, 1995, Williams & Wilkins.

Grauer GF, Twedt DC, Mero KN: Evaluation of laparoscopy for obtaining renal biopsy specimens from dogs and cats, *J Am Vet Med Assoc* 183:677, 1983.

Wildt DE: Laparoscopy in the dog and cat. In Harrison RE, Wildt DE, editors: *Animal laparoscopy,* Baltimore, 1980, William & Wilkins.

## COLOR PLATES   PAGES 430–432

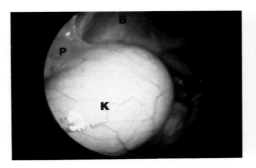

**Plate 16-1** Laparoscopic view of the right kidney *(K)* in a dog. The laparoscope has entered the right midparalumbar region and is directed cranially and dorsally. The kidney is pale gray with readily apparent capsular vasculature. The dorsal body wall *(B)*, a reflection of the peritoneum *(P)*, and the caudate lobe of the liver can also be seen.

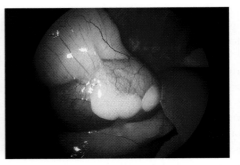

**Plate 16-2** Normal kidney with a large amount of perirenal fat. The liver is to the right in the field of view. An advantage of laparoscopy is that kidney biopsy specimens can be obtained under direct visualization.

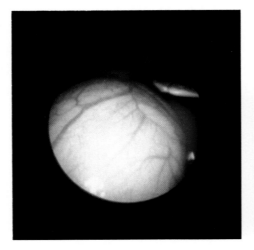

**Plate 16-3** Close-up of the right kidney shown in Plate 16-1. The tip of a Tru-Cut biopsy needle is in the field of view. The biopsy needle should be directed at a shallow angle to the capsule and away from the hilum of the kidney.

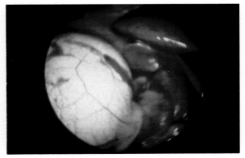

**Plate 16-4** Typical amount of hemorrhage from the kidney after Tru-Cut needle biopsy. If hemorrhage is severe, pressure may be applied to the biopsy site with the tip of the laparoscope. Liver lobes are observed anterior and to the right of the kidney.

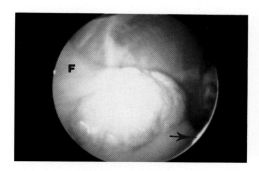

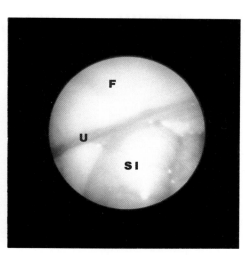

**Plate 16-5** Laparoscopic appearance of a canine kidney with chronic end-stage renal disease. The peritoneal reflection contains a large amount of fat *(F)*. The tip of the laparoscope has been pulled back into the cannula and the rim of the cannula is reflecting light *(arrow)*.

**Plate 16-6** Laparoscopic view of the distal portion of the right ureter *(U)* in a dog. The laparoscope has entered the right midparalumbar region and is directed caudally and dorsally. The kidney is to the right and the urinary bladder is to the left. Sublumbar fat *(F)* is seen dorsal to the ureter, and a loop of small intestine *(SI)* is seen ventrally.

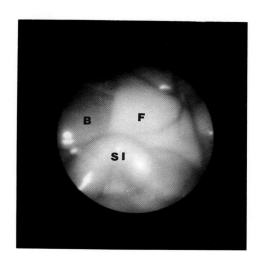

**Plate 16-7** Laparoscopic view of the canine urinary bladder *(B)*. The laparoscope has entered the right midparalumbar region and is directed caudally and ventrally. The serosal surface of the bladder is gray. Sublumbar fat *(F)* and a loop of small intestine *(SI)* can also be seen.

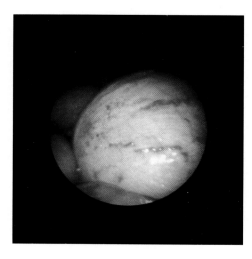

**Plate 16-8** Close-up of the urinary bladder shown in Plate 16-7. The dog is in a left lateral recumbent position, and the scope has entered the right midparalumbar region. An assistant has reached under the dog and elevated the bladder to facilitate inspection. The tortuous serosal vessels of the bladder are apparent.

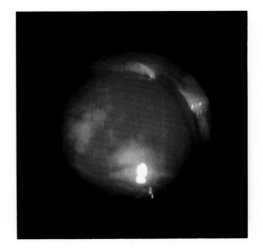

**Plate 16-9** Close-up of a canine urinary bladder with moderate intramural hemorrhage secondary to blunt abdominal trauma.

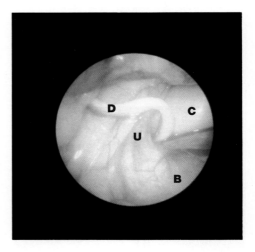

**Plate 16-10** Close-up of the right ureter *(U)* in a male dog as the ureter joins the urinary bladder *(B)*. The dog is in a left lateral recumbent position, and the scope has entered the abdominal cavity approximately 5 cm ventral to the wing of the ilium on the right side. The colon *(C)* and ductus deferens *(D)* can also be seen.

# Chapter 17

# Endoscopy in Birds and Reptiles

**Michael Taylor**

Fine-diameter rigid endoscopes have been used for diagnostic purposes in birds and reptiles since the late 1970s. During the 1980s veterinarians in zoologic and private practice began employing endoscopy more routinely. These practitioners quickly recognized the value of a minimally traumatic procedure that allowed excellent visualization of internal structures even in very small patients. However, enhanced diagnostic sampling procedures were slower to develop. The knowledge base for avian medicine has expanded tremendously over the past 15 years. Reptile medicine is now experiencing many of the same exciting changes.

## AVIAN ENDOSCOPY

Rigid endoscopes were first employed in birds to visualize gonads for the purpose of sex identification in species for which external characteristics did not clearly differentiate male from female. As private and public captive breeding programs began to flourish, the need for reliable sex identification services motivated the early clinical applications of endoscopic technology (Harrison GJ, 1978; McDonald SE, 1982; Jones DM et al, 1984). The superior resolution and light transmission characteristics of even the earliest rod-lens endoscopes made these instruments far superior to other optical systems for avian applications.

A number of pioneering avian veterinarians soon realized that endoscopy offered far more than sex identification in that the unique anatomy of the avian respiratory system allowed relatively easy access to many

organ systems. Soon the diagnostic uses of endoscopy were extended beyond organ visualization (Satterfield W, 1981; Kollias GV, 1984). Secondary hand instruments could be guided into the viewing field to collect biopsy specimens or retrieve materials. Endoscopic collection of hepatic and renal tissue samples allowed precise targeting of lesions with minimal patient trauma. In 1987, Lumeij provided the first comprehensive overview of endoscopic access points in the bird with the pigeon used as a model. He was also the first to suggest the use of some method whereby hand instruments could be manipulated in concert with the endoscope. In 1992, I developed a new endoscope and sheath system for use in birds (14.5-French sheath-065 CC and 2.7-mm endoscope-018 BS; Karl Storz Veterinary Endoscopy–America, Goleta, Calif.) (Figure 17-1). The sheath design allowed a variety of hand instruments to be guided to the tip of the endoscope through an instrument channel, thereby increasing operator ease and preventing iatrogenic trauma. Then I described an anatomic approach to better understand the most applicable access points for avian endoscopy in a comprehensive review published in 1994. For the first time, endophotographic techniques and line illustrations were combined to document and teach the common avian endoscopic approaches and anatomy.

### Avian Anatomy and Endoscopy

The unique anatomy of the avian respiratory system facilitates endoscopic examination. The air sacs of the bird are self-pneumatizing and extensive. These air sacs pro-

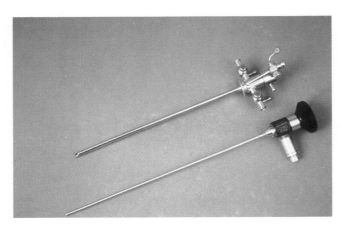

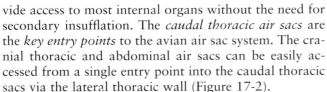

**Figure 17-1** Avian sheath system with a 2.7-mm telescope (Karl Storz Veterinary Endoscopy–America, Inc.). The telescope is inserted and locked into the sheath. The two side ports are used for the infusion of air and/or water. The top instrument port allows the introduction of semirigid and flexible instruments.

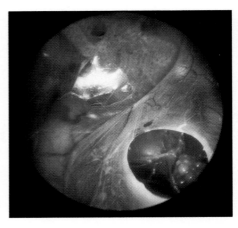

**Figure 17-2** Left caudal thoracic air sac in a red-tailed hawk *(Buteo jamaicencis)*. Note the puncture made through the confluent walls of the left caudal thoracic and abdominal air sacs. The confluent membranes of the caudal thoracic and cranial thoracic air sacs are also visible (9 to 11 o'clock position).

vide access to most internal organs without the need for secondary insufflation. The *caudal thoracic air sacs* are the *key entry points* to the avian air sac system. The cranial thoracic and abdominal air sacs can be easily accessed from a single entry point into the caudal thoracic sacs via the lateral thoracic wall (Figure 17-2).

The traditional left lateral surgical approaches used by poultry caponizers and later by many field ornithologists took advantage of air sac anatomy to reach the gonads by directly entering the abdominal air sac or by entering the caudal thoracic air sac first and then passing into the abdominal air sac through a small incision made in their contiguous wall. The first descriptions of the lateral endoscopic approach in birds were derived from these early techniques (Harrison GJ, 1978; Satterfield W, 1981; Kolias GV, 1984; McDonald SE, 1984). For endoscopy the patient is placed in a true lateral recumbent position with wings extended dorsally. The upper leg is extended and held caudally. The point of insertion is located by approximation, using palpation. This insertion point is in the triangle cranial to the muscle mass of the femur, ventral to the synsacrum, and caudal to the last rib. The body wall may be penetrated by a trocar and cannula or by blunt separation. In psittaciformes the entry site is usually between the seventh and eighth ribs (Harrison GJ, 1986), not behind the last rib as had been frequently stated. With this approach the tip of the endoscope enters the cranial to middle portion of the caudal thoracic air sac in most species.

The approach to the caudal thoracic air sacs that I developed is based on precise landmarks that are reproducible in a wide variety of species. The entry site is located by finding the point where the semimembranous muscle *(musculus flexor cruris medialis)* crosses the last rib (Figure 17-3, *A* and *B*). The ventral fascia of the semimembranous muscle is bluntly separated from the underlying body wall, and the muscle is reflected dorsally. I recommend blunt entry through the thin body wall just caudal to the last rib and beneath the reflected semimembranous muscle (Figure 17-3, *C*). Except in birds with moderately to markedly increased fat reserves, these landmarks are located easily, and the entry site has been reproducible in members of a wide variety of orders, including psittaciformes, passeriformes, columbiformes, gruiformes, anseriformes, falconiformes, and strigiformes. A major advantage of placing the bird's upper leg forward is that the thin, lateral body wall can be more easily approached without interference from femoral musculature. This becomes particularly important in birds with heavily muscled upper thighs (e.g., many psittaciformes).

With this approach the endoscope enters the caudal thoracic air sac at or near its caudal border. Once the scope is in the left caudal thoracic air sac, the operator can look cranially and view the lateral septal surface of the lung with its large ostium (Figure 17-4, *A*). The transparent membrane formed by the confluent walls of the caudal thoracic and the abdominal air sacs can be seen at about the 2 to 3 o'clock position. Passing through this membrane would place the endoscope within the abdominal air sac (Figure 17-4, *B*). At the 4 to 6 o'clock position is the ventrolateral border of the proventriculus and ventriculus. At the 7 to 8 o'clock position the lateral edge of the left lobe of the liver may be seen draped on the ventriculus. From the 9 to 10 o'clock position is another transparent membrane composed of the walls of the confluent caudal and cranial thoracic air sacs. Passing through this membrane would place the tip

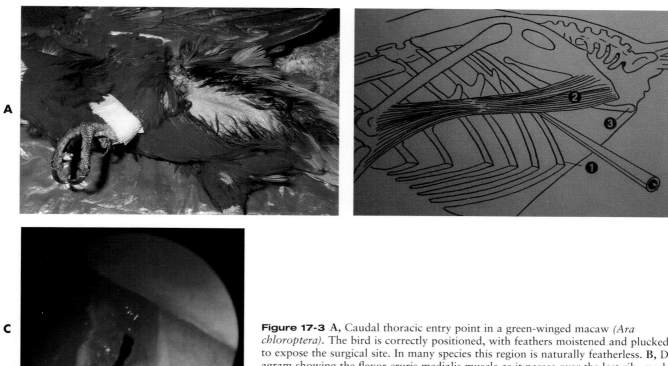

**Figure 17-3 A,** Caudal thoracic entry point in a green-winged macaw *(Ara chloroptera).* The bird is correctly positioned, with feathers moistened and plucked to expose the surgical site. In many species this region is naturally featherless. **B,** Diagram showing the flexor cruris medialis muscle as it passes over the last rib, marking the insertion point. (From Taylor M: Endoscopic examination and biopsy techniques. In Ritchie BW, Harrison GJ, Harrison LR, editors: *Avian medicine: principles and application,* Lake Worth, Fla., 1994, Wingers.) **C,** Close-up of the blunt puncture made through the thin body wall. The flexor cruris medialis muscle can be seen coursing diagonally across the top of the photograph.

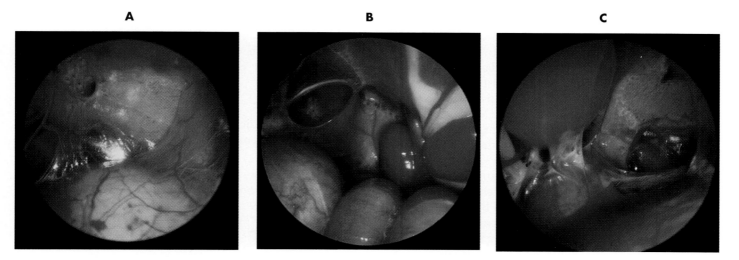

**Figure 17-4 A,** Left caudal thoracic air sac in an orange-winged amazon *(Amazona amazonica).* This view, seen after the operator moves the scope into the air sac and looks cranially, illustrates the internal anatomy. Notice the prominent ostium of the lung, visible at the 11 o'clock position. **B,** Left abdominal air sac as seen after the endoscope tip has passed through the confluent walls of the caudal thoracic and abdominal air sacs. The proventriculus, loops of intestine, and kidney are prominent in this photograph. **C,** Left cranial thoracic air sac after the endoscope has passed through the confluent walls of this air sac and the cranial thoracic air sac (9 to 10 o'clock position in **A**). The heart beating in the pericardial sac is the most prominent landmark.

of the endoscope in the cranial thoracic air sac (Figure 17-4, C).

The caudal thoracic air sacs in some diving birds are much larger than those in other species. This size difference is assumed to represent an anatomic adaption to the increased air requirements when diving birds swim underwater.

## Indications for Endoscopic Examination

Endoscopic examination is indicated whenever visual inspection of an organ or site may yield additional diagnostic information. Diagnostic endoscopy is usually preceded by certain laboratory tests (e.g., complete blood count, biochemistry profile) and/or radiographic studies. The patient's history, the findings of the physical examination, and the results of laboratory and radiologic studies are frequently inconclusive or may suggest that endoscopic examination of a specific site may prove valuable (Box 17-1). Although conventional radiographic studies are useful, I have found that the direct visualization provided by endoscopic follow-up of suspicious findings frequently yields much additional diagnostic information.

## Biopsy

Like the pathologist, the endoscopist needs to be familiar with the normal and pathologic appearances of the tissues to be examined. The operator should attempt to describe lesions accurately in terms of their location, color, size, shape, and consistency. Photographic or video documentation can be a tremendous aid in this process. However, assessing the appearance of tissue is but the first step in the diagnostic utilization of endoscopy. Improved instrumentation has made it possible to routinely collect specimens of suspicious- or abnormal-appearing tissue and debris for histologic, cytologic, and microbiologic examination. The Storz avian system allows a variety of flexible instruments to be introduced into the sheath, passed alongside the endoscope, and guided to a specific site with relative ease. Iatrogenic tissue trauma is markedly reduced because instruments are directed to the visual field through the integral sheath, avoiding possible injuries during the blind manipulation required to place a second, rigid instrument.

Precise target biopsy of specific organs is a natural extension of endoscopic examination. Compared to open surgical procedures, endoscopically guided biopsy is a far less traumatic method for obtaining diagnostic specimens in small avian patients. Carefully selected biopsy samples from affected organs may be critical in establishing a diagnosis, thereby allowing more precise therapeutic decisions to be made. Clinical signs may be absent or unclear. Birds endeavor to hide outward signs of disease for as long as possible; furthermore, when they do show signs of illness, they express them in a limited number of ways. Based on the biopsy specimens, a lesion may be staged as acute or chronic. Using endoscopic and biopsy findings, the clinician can often give clients prognostic information.

## Indications for Biopsy

The indications for biopsy are similar to those for the visual inspection of tissues, and therefore endoscopy (see Box 17-1). Abnormal radiographic findings, biochemical parameters outside the reference range, chronic respiratory disease, and polyuria and polydipsia are some of the most common reasons for *organ biopsy*. The operator should be prepared to collect biopsy specimens during even the most routine examination. Not uncommonly, unexpected lesions are found during endoscopy for sex identification. Specimens from obvious lesions are easily collected from the border zone between abnormal and normal tissue. Sometimes gross lesions may not be recognized, particularly in patients with renal disease. If the history, physical examination, or biochemical findings suggest that a patient has renal or hepatic abnormalities, I biopsy the *kidney* or *liver* respectively even if the organ appears normal. Based on my experience and that of others, tissues frequently appear grossly normal even though significant histologic lesions are present.

## Contraindications to Biopsy

The major contraindications for biopsy are related to the blood's clotting system. Biopsy specimen collection should be delayed in avian patients with evidence of hemostatic abnormalities. Clotting problems usually become evident at the time of preendoscopic blood collection. Most birds exhibit clot formation in 5 to 10

---

**Box 17-1   Indications for Endoscopic Examination**

Acute or chronic dyspnea, sneezing
Ingluvitis, crop burns, or trauma
Abnormal radiographic findings, such as organomegaly or abnormal air sacs, lungs, or gastrointestinal organs
Abnormal biochemical studies, such as elevated uric acid levels (kidney) or elevated bile acid levels (liver)
Persistent leukocytosis that is unexplained or does not respond to treatment
Acute or chronic systemic disease
Suspected infertility
Polyuria and/or polydipsia
Follow-up examination to check on lesion resolution

minutes. Vitamin K deficiency is the coagulation disorder most commonly recognized in my hospital. This deficiency can be corrected by the administration of vitamin $K_1$ (AquaMephyton) at a rate of 1 to 2 mg/kg. The blood film should be examined for the presence of an adequate number of thrombocytes.

Ascites is a relative contraindication to biopsy. If a lateral approach to the caudal thoracic air sac is used, the bulging ventral hepatic peritoneal cavity may be torn, releasing ascitic fluid into the air sac and therefore into the lung. Thus a poststernal ventral midline approach to the ventral hepatic peritoneal cavities is safer when the presence of fluid is strongly suspected.

## Biopsy Instrumentation and Technique

The biopsy cup shape and diameter must be appropriate to the size of the patient and organ to be biopsied. If the forceps instrument is too large, excessive organ trauma and hemorrhage may occur. Biopsy cups generally come in two shapes: round or elliptical. Round cups do not penetrate as deeply into tissue as elliptical cups of the same diameter. Forceps with round cups may be indicated for biopsy of organs such as the kidney and testes. However, for general use in birds weighing 200 to 2000 g, I recommend an elliptical cup with a 5- to 7-French (1.7- to 2.3-mm) diameter.

Inexperience with the instrumentation and approaches to the organ are the two most common causes of iatrogenic biopsy complications. A knowledge of regional anatomic relationships is essential to good endoscopic technique.

Biopsy of the left kidney and spleen can be achieved by entering the left abdominal air sac from the standard (left) caudal thoracic air sac. With the same approach, specimens can be obtained from the left liver lobe, left septal surface of the lung, and several air sacs. Right caudal thoracic air sac approaches allow access to the right liver lobe, right septal surface of the lung, air sacs, and by entering the right abdominal air sac, the right kidney and the pancreas.

When approaching the liver to perform a biopsy, the operator should remember that this organ lies within the ventral and dorsal hepatic peritoneal cavities. Using a standard lateral approach to the caudal thoracic air sacs, the endoscopist needs to incise the left or right ventral hepatic peritoneal cavity and overlying air sac wall in order to be able to grasp the edge of liver parenchyma with the forceps. This is a useful approach in the patient with generalized hepatic disease. In a patient with focal disease (e.g., granulomas, neoplasia) the lesion should be specifically targeted, with the operator being careful not to open the forceps jaws too widely when pushing the cups into the liver. This should reduce crush artifact and ensure that the abnormal tissue is included in the biopsy specimen.

In most species the caudal thoracic air sac is the one most frequently involved in air sac pathology. Lesions may be more prominent on one side than another, or they may involve the cranial thoracic air sac more extensively. Radiographs are essential in selecting the preferred entry site. Cup biopsy forceps may be used to grasp a small piece of air sac from the border of an air sac puncture site (e.g., caudal thoracic-abdominal air sac puncture) or to harvest focal lesions directly from the surface of the air sac. Exudate may also be collected with a cup or grasping forceps for microbiologic, cytologic, and antigen-capture examination. The latter study is particularly useful when chlamydial airsacculitis is suspected.

I prefer to perform a diagnostic evaluation first, using only the telescope. If lesions worthy of sampling are discovered, the scope is withdrawn and the sheath with its blunt obturator is introduced with the same standard approach. With the sheath held stationary, the obturator is removed and the telescope is reintroduced and locked into place. The system can then be guided visually into position, and an appropriate biopsy forceps can be inserted into the sheath's instrument port. The sheath should be held somewhat away from the expected site of biopsy as the forceps is slowly passed down the instrument channel until it appears in the viewing field. Only then should the unit be moved into position for collection of the specimen. Practice and the use of good technique will reduce the risk of iatrogenic trauma to negligible levels (Figure 17-5). Additional hand instruments available for use with the avian system include semirigid scissors (Karl Storz Veterinary Endoscopy–America, Inc.), a flexible 22-gauge needle with Teflon guide, and several grasping forceps. The scissors are particularly useful for incising air sac and peritoneal membranes. Examples of biopsy techniques are depicted in Figures 17-6 through 17-9.

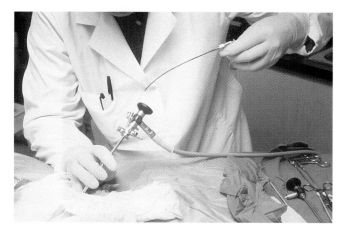

**Figure 17-5** Avian system in use. Note how the operator stabilizes the sheath with one hand while inserting the hand instrument with the other hand.

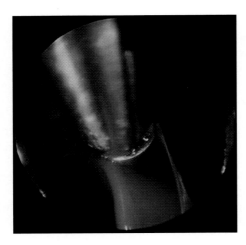

**Figure 17-6** View through the telescope as the 5-French elliptical cup biopsy forceps is guided into place along the lateral border of the liver. The overlying air sac and ventral hepatic peritoneal membrane have been incised to allow access to the liver. For manipulation purposes the forceps instrument has been extended to the limit of the best visual field of the endoscope, but this is not the recommended distance for sample collection (see Fig. 17-8).

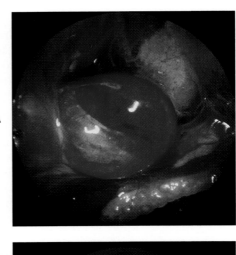

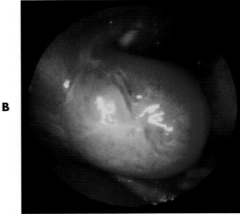

**Figure 17-7 A,** 7-French renal biopsy of the cranial division of the kidney in an amazon parrot 2 minutes after sample collection, showing clot formation and a lack of hemorrhage. Note the large size of the biopsy site. A 5-French forceps instrument is more suitable for a patient of this size. **B,** Same biopsy site 6 weeks later, demonstrating healing even with a large biopsy site.

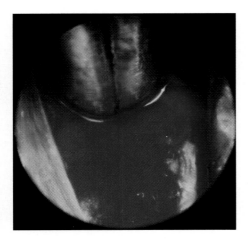

**Figure 17-8** 5-French biopsy forceps guided into the correct position for sample collection. In most circumstances it is best to adjust the position of the forceps to just within the visual field while holding the sheath away from the target organ. Then the entire sheath system may be moved into position to collect the specimen.

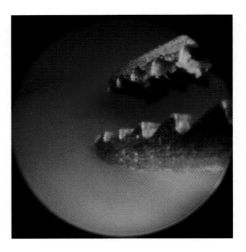

**Figure 17-9** Grasping forceps, which is useful for dissection, capturing foreign objects, and harvesting caseous debris. These 3-French (1-mm-diameter) forceps have fine teeth. Note how the inherent magnification of the endoscope makes the teeth appear coarse.

## Preparation of Small Biopsy Specimens

Small specimens are obtained with the forceps types recommended for avian endoscopic biopsy procedures. These tissue samples must be handled with care so that they are not lost or damaged. Various techniques have been recommended to enable the histotechnologist to locate and properly embed small specimens for processing. Wrapping tiny pieces of tissue in filter paper or very fine cloth before immersion in the fixative is one method. My current preference is to place specimens into a small stoppered blood collection container without anticoagulant (e.g., a red-top 3-ml tube). This simple, effective system allows the technician to visualize the sample(s) clearly. No more than three specimens should be placed in each clearly labelled container. Compared with larger specimens, small tissue samples require far less time for fixation (probably no more than 2 hours in formalin). Buffered 10% formalin specifically intended for tissue fixation should be used. Failure to use the correct formalin can result in precipitates and artifact. If the specimens cannot be processed immediately, sample quality should be ensured by storing the specimens in a solution similar to the first processing solution used by the endoscopist's laboratory (e.g., 97% methyl alcohol). Specific storage recommendations should be obtained from that laboratory.

## REPTILIAN ENDOSCOPY

Rigid endoscopy for the evaluation of reptiles was described by Bush in 1980. This technology has since been applied in a number of reptile orders (Wood JR, 1983; Schildger BJ, 1987; Cooper JE, Schildger BJ, 1991). In 1992 Schildger described the use of a small-diameter pediatric cystoscope with an integral sheath in reptiles. This system allowed the insertion of 3-French (1-mm) hand instruments through the channel in the sheath. Targeted biopsy samples could be collected under direct visualization. Insufflation was also possible using a laparoflator connected to one of the infusion ports on the sheath. Reptile medicine is currently in a rapid growth phase reminiscent of the one avian medicine experienced in the early 1980s.

A number of endoscopic applications for reptiles are likely to arise out of work already completed in avian endoscopy. The focal, directed illumination and magnification achieved with modern rod lens endoscopes such as the Storz 018 BS are highly applicable to work in a variety of reptile species. I have used the previously described avian sheath and 2.7-mm endoscope system with 5-French instruments to examine and collect specimens from chelonians (turtles and tortoises) and the green iguana. Insufflation is achieved in a manner similar to

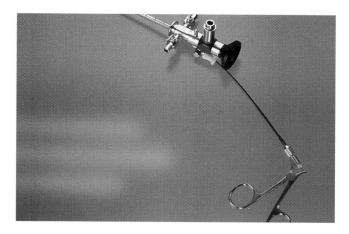

**Figure 17-10** Flexible biopsy forceps inserted into the instrument port of the avian sheath. Note the white rubber sealing bonnet in place on the instrument port opening.

that described by Schildger. Carbon dioxide from a manual or electronic laparoflator is infused through one of the lateral stopcocks of the sheath at a pressure of 10 mm Hg. Fine regulation of intracoelomic pressure can be achieved by selectively venting the valve of the opposite stopcock (Fig. 17-10). A white rubber sealing bonnet (Karl Storz Veterinary Endoscopy–America, Inc) placed over the instrument port prevents excessive air leakage during instrument placement. Biopsy specimens may be routinely collected from the liver, kidney, and spleen by introducing a flexible cup biopsy forceps through the rubber fitting and into the instrument channel. As in the bird, the forceps tip may be guided precisely to the site of collection in the reptile. In some species it may be necessary to incise the peritoneum over the kidney with semirigid scissors.

In chelonians an entry incision is made in the left prefemoral region, which is first surgically prepared using standard techniques of skin cleansing. The incision site is equidistant from the horizontal margins of the carapace and plastron and approximately midway between the femur and the cranial portion of the carapace margin; this is similar to a surgical approach described previously for laparotomy (Brannian RE, 1984). A fine mosquito forceps is then introduced through the body wall in a craniomedial direction. The jaws of the forceps are opened to gently spread the muscle layers. In lizards such as the green iguana *(Iguana iguana)* an incision is made in the region analogous to the mammalian "paralumbar fossa" caudal to the last rib. The fine musculature of the lizard's body wall may be spread using a mosquito forceps, as in the chelonians. Insufflation with an inert gas such as carbon dioxide is not always necessary in chelonians but is essential to allow adequate visualization in lizards. From the insertion point and looking cranially, the operator can view the liver, spleen, stomach, lung, and heart. No diaphragm is present. With increased intracoelomic pressure the lungs may not inflate well. In such cases, intermittent positive pressure ventilation at two to three breaths per minute is recommended.

## CONCLUSION

Rigid endoscopy in birds and reptiles has never offered more potential to the exotic animal practitioner. Improved instrumentation designed to meet the needs of the avian or reptile clinicians has made clinical sampling easier and increased diagnostic return. Improved imaging technologies, especially video cameras for use in endoscopy, have dramatically altered the way endoscopic techniques can be demonstrated and taught. It is now possible to participate in intensive two-day courses on avian and reptilian endoscopy. The new technologies are also making it possible for colleagues to consult on cases in a manner not possible before. The potential for new endosurgical procedures is great.

## REFERENCES

Brannian RE: A soft tissue laparotomy technique in turtles, *J Am Vet Med Assoc* 185:1416, 1984.

Bush M: Laparoscopy in birds and reptiles. In Harrison RM, Wildt DE, editors: *Animal laparoscopy*, Baltimore, 1980, Williams & Wilkins.

Cooper JE, Schildger BJ: Endoscopy in exotic species. In Brearly MJ, Cooper JE, Sullivan M, editors: *Color atlas of small animal endoscopy*, St Louis, 1991, Mosby.

Harrison GJ: Endoscopic examination of avian gonadal tissue, *Vet Med Small Anim Clin* 73:479, 1978.

Harrison GJ: Endoscopy. In Harrison GJ, Harrison LR, editors: *Clinical avian medicine and surgery*, Philadelphia, 1986, WB Saunders.

Jones DM et al: Sex determination of monomorphic birds by fibreoptic endoscopy, *Vet Rec* 115:596, 1984.

Kollias GV: Liver biopsy techniques in avian clinical practice, *Vet Clin North Am* 14:287, 1984.

Lumeij TJ: Endoscopy. In *A contribution to clinical investigative methods for birds with special reference to the racing pigeon (Columbia livia domestica)*, Utrecht, Netherlands, 1987.

McDonald SE: Surgical sexing of birds by laparoscopy, *Calif Vet* 5:16, 1982.

Satterfield W: Early diagnosis of avian tuberculosis by laparoscopy and liver biopsy. In Cooper JE, Greenwood AG, editors: *Recent advances in the study of raptor diseases*, Keighley, U.K., 1981, Chiron.

Schildger BJ: Endoscopic sex determination in reptiles. In *Proceedings of the 1st international conference on zoological and avian medicine*, Oahu, Hi, AAV/AAZV, 1987.

Schildger BJ, Wicker R: Endoscopie bei Reptilien und Amphibian—Indikationen, Methoden, Befunde, *Praktische Tierzart* 6:516, 1992.

Taylor M: Diagnostic application of a new endoscopic system for birds. In *Proceedings of the European Conference on avian medicine and surgery*, Utrecht, Netherlands, 1993.

Taylor M: Endoscopic examination and biopsy techniques. In: Ritchie BW, Harrison GJ, Harrison LR, editors: *Avian medicine: principles and application*, Lake Worth, Fla., 1994, Wingers.

Wood JR et al: Laparoscopy of the green sea turtle, *Chelonia mydas, Br J Herp* 6:323, 1983.

## COLOR PLATES   PAGES 441-445

**Plate 17-1,** p. 441, Hypovitaminosis in a yellow-naped amazon

**Plate 17-2,** p. 441, Palatine abscess in an african gray parrot

**Plate 17-3,** p. 441, Normal tracheal mucosa in an amazon parrot

**Plate 17-4,** p. 441, Normal cranial and middle divisions of the kidney in a cockatoo

**Plate 17-5,** p. 442, Normal ventral hepatic peritoneal cavities in a pigeon

**Plate 17-6,** p. 442, Normal juvenile ovary in a blue and gold macaw

**Plate 17-7,** p. 442, Normal juvenile testicle in a blue and gold macaw

**Plate 17-8,** p. 442, Normal mature testicles in an amazon parrot

**Plate 17-9,** p. 443, Normal mature ovary in amazon parrot

**Plate 17-10,** p. 443, Normal spleen in an amazon parrot

**Plate 17-11,** p. 443, Normal pancreas in green-winged macaw

**Plate 17-12,** p. 443, Chronic granulomatous airsacculitis in a blue and gold macaw

**Plate 17-13,** p. 444, Severe mycotic airsacculitis in a scarlet macaw

**Plate 17-14,** p. 444, Pneumoconiosis in a yellow-naped amazon

**Plate 17-15,** p. 444, Bile duct carcinomas in a yellow-headed amazon

**Plate 17-16,** p. 444, Hepatic amyloidosis in a trumpeter swan

**Plate 17-17,** p. 445, Subserosal granuloma in a blue-headed pionus

**Plate 17-18,** p. 445, Mature ovary in a green iguana

**Plate 17-19,** p. 445, Mature testicle in a green iguana

**Plate 17-20,** p. 445, Hepatic lipidosis in a snapping turtle

**Plate 17-21,** p. 445, Hepatic lipidosis with inflammation in a green iguana

## BIRDS AND REPTILES

The following photographs depict case examples from birds (Plates 17-1 through 17-17) and reptiles (Plates 17-18 through 17-21). These photographs highlight the clinical utility of endoscopy in these species.

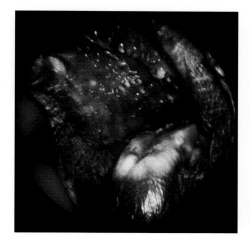

**Plate 17-1** Severe chronic hypovitaminosis in a yellow-naped amazon *(Amazona ochracephala)*. The white plaques on the tongue are caused by squamous metaplasia of the epithelium of the lingual salivary glands.

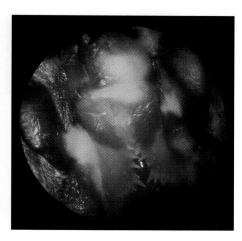

**Plate 17-2** Palatine abscess in an african gray parrot *(Psittacus erithacus)*. Endoscopy of the oral cavity is a powerful, yet frequently overlooked tool for the diagnosis of oral and upper respiratory diseases. The patient must be suitably anesthetized to prevent inadvertent trauma to the operator or equipment.

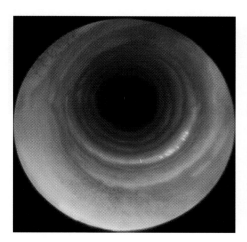

**Plate 17-3** Normal tracheal mucosa in an amazon parrot *(Amazona* sp.). Examination of the tracheal lumen to the level of the syrinx is frequently possible in medium-sized birds.

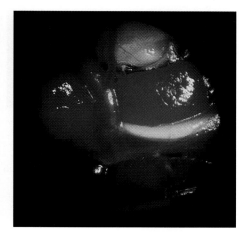

**Plate 17-4** Normal cranial and middle divisions of the kidney in a cockatoo *(Cacatua* sp.). The ureter (filled with urates) is clearly visible as it tracks caudally from beneath the iliac artery and vein. Note the deeply melanistic testicle that is present in some avian species.

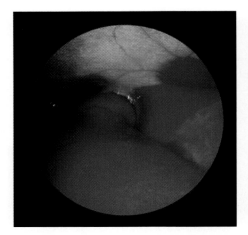

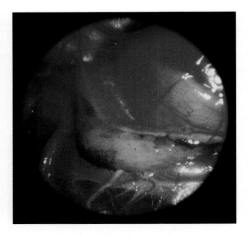

**Plate 17-5** Normal ventral hepatic peritoneal cavities (VHPCs) in a pigeon *(Columbia livia).* A ventral midline approach just caudal to the sternal border places the endoscope within the VHPC. The right lobe of the liver is larger than the left lobe. Pigeons frequently lack a prominent ventral mesentery separating the left and right VHPCs.

**Plate 17-6** Normal juvenile ovary in a blue and gold macaw *(Ara ararauna).* The juvenile ovary is shaped like a comma and lacks visible primary follicles. Partial or complete melanism of the gonad varies by and within species. In most species only the left ovary develops. The dorsal ligament of the oviduct is prominent and can be seen traversing the cranial division of the kidney.

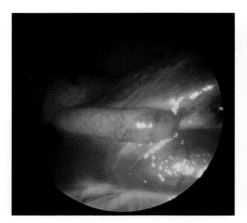

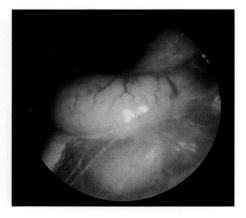

**Plate 17-7** Normal juvenile testicle in a blue and gold macaw *(Ara ararauna).* The testicles are paired and cylindrically shaped in this bird, which is about the same age as the one in Plate 17-16. The right testicle can usually be seen through the dorsal mesentery. No structure comparable to the dorsal ligament of the oviduct is present.

**Plate 17-8** Normal mature testicles in an amazon parrot *(Amazona* sp.). The right testicle is visible through the dorsal mesentery

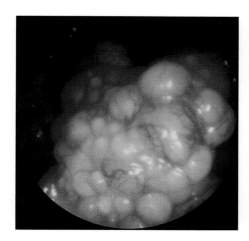

**Plate 17-9** Normal mature ovary in an amazon parrot (*Amazona* sp.). Primary follicles are prominent and resemble a cluster of grapes.

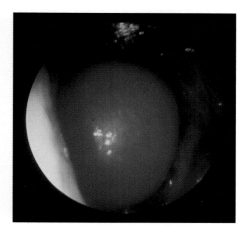

**Plate 17-10** Normal spleen in an amazon parrot (*Amazona* sp.). The spleen is located using a left caudal thoracic air sac approach to the abdominal air sac and following the border of the proventriculus dorsally.

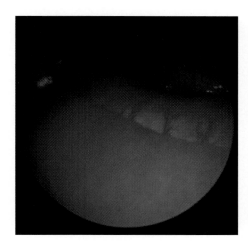

**Plate 17-11** Normal pancreas in a green-winged macaw *(Ara chloroptera)*. The pancreas is best viewed via a right caudal thoracic air sac approach to the right abdominal air sac. The descending and ascending duodenum are the most ventral loops of intestine. The pancreas is situated between the duodenal loops.

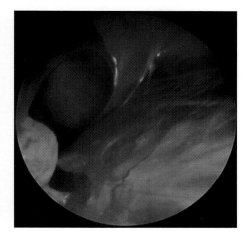

**Plate 17-12** Chronic granulomatous airsacculitis in a blue and gold macaw *(Ara ararauna)*. The air sac is markedly thickened and opaque. New blood vessels course over the surface, and yellow caseous debris has accumulated focally.

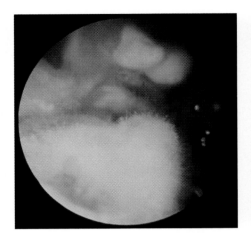

**Plate 17-13** Severe mycotic airsacculitis in a scarlet macaw *(Ara macao)*. Endoscopic examination of the right abdominal air sac revealed this aggressive growth of fungal mats with fruiting bodies and branching septate hyphae. *Aspergillus niger* was cultured.

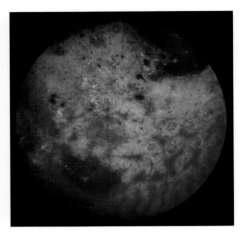

**Plate 17-14** Pneumoconiosis in a yellow-naped amazon *(Amazona ochracephala)*. Particulate debris has accumulated in the fixed macrophages of the lung and is grossly visible on the septal surface. This was an incidental finding in a pet amazon that lived in an industrial shop.

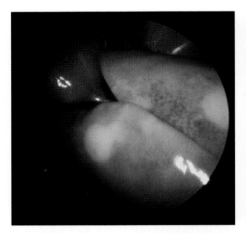

**Plate 17-15** Bile duct carcinomas in a yellow-headed amazon *(Amazona ochracephala)*. The two prominent, focal pale areas in the hepatic parenchyma represent bile duct neoplasia. The cause of this neoplasm remains unknown; however, bile duct neoplasia commonly occurs in amazon parrots with papillomatous disease.

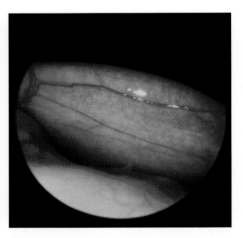

**Plate 17-16** Hepatic amyloidosis in a trumpeter swan *(Cygnus buccinator)*. The accumulation of large amounts of amyloid in the liver, spleen, and kidney of anseriformes is frequently reported. Here the liver is pale tan and moderately swollen because of the amyloid.

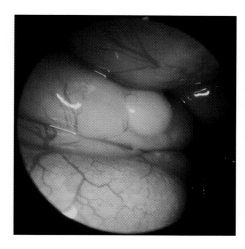

**Plate 17-17** Subserosal granuloma in a blue-headed pionus *(Pionus menstratus)*. Granulomas of the intestinal wall are most frequently associated with *Mycobacterium avium-intracellulare* infection. Endoscopy may be one of the best early screening tools for this chronic infection *if* the operator is willing to examine tissues closely and collect appropriate samples for culture or acid-fast staining.

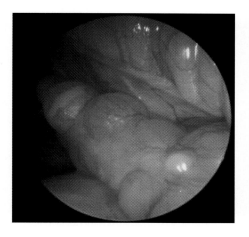

**Plate 17-18** Mature ovary in a green iguana *(Iguana iguana)*. The reptile ovary is very similar in appearance to the avian ovary. The iguana develops both a right and left ovary.

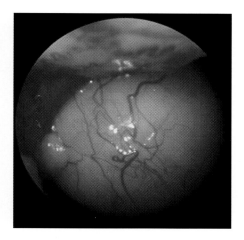

**Plate 17-19** Mature testicle in a green iguana *(Iguana iguana)*. The moderate enlargement of this testicle is a sign that this male lizard is entering a period of seasonal hormonal activity.

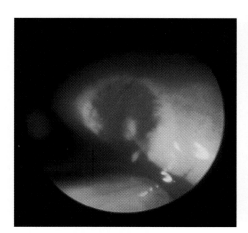

**Plate 17-20** Hepatic lipidosis in a snapping turtle *(Chelydra serpentis)*. The pale yellow color of the liver parenchyma in this captive turtle reflects the accumulation of fat. A biopsy site is visible.

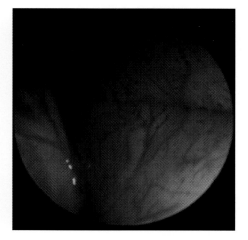

**Plate 17-21** Hepatic lipidosis with inflammation in a green iguana *(Iguana iguana)*. The liver is pale yellow-brown with prominent vasculature. Histologic evaluation revealed increased lipids as well as inflammatory cells suggestive of septicemia.

# Chapter 18

# Cystoscopy

**David F. Senior**

Recent advances in endourology may improve patient management, eliminate the need for open surgery of the urinary tract, and provide a more accurate diagnosis in several clinical circumstances. During cystoscopy the bladder mucosa can be examined when the wall of this organ is distended. The magnified cystoscopic appearance is much more revealing than the appearance at open surgery when the bladder has been incised and is contracted. Clients often request nonsurgical treatment options, and cystoscopic procedures can be used in place of open surgery for many indications (Table 18-1). The bladder and urethra of female dogs and cats can be examined using a rigid cystoscope similar or identical to the instruments used in human endourology.

Several flexible fiberscope models are suitable for performing cystoscopy in male dogs, and a very small fiberscope can be passed through the urethra of male cats. However, the size of the male urethra severely limits the diameter of the endoscope that can be passed through the urethra and into the bladder. In both male cats and male dogs the bladder can be examined using a small endoscope passed through a centesis needle. This procedure can be performed with a needle arthroscope, or equipment can be purchased as a dedicated unit designed specifically for this purpose.

**Table 18-1** Indications and Procedures for Cystoscopy

| Indications | Procedures |
| --- | --- |
| Hematuria | Locate bleeding site; cauterize |
| Recurrent urinary tract infection | Identify and eliminate predisposing causes (e.g., polyps) |
| Lower urinary tract inflammation | Fragment and remove uroliths; resect polyps and tumors |
| Urolithiasis | Perform lithotripsy; determine composition from fragments |
| Urinary incontinence | Ectopic ureters; locate and catheterize |
| | Urethral incompetence; inject Teflon or collagen |
| Bladder tumors | Biopsy; resect |
| Urethral obstruction | Determine the cause; remove uroliths; resect polyps and tumors |
| Suspected trauma | Localize and define injuries |
| Renal disease | Catheterize the ureters |
| | Obtain differential glomerular filtration rate |
| | Sample ureteral urine for urinalysis and culture |
| | Perform retrograde pyelography |

## EQUIPMENT

### Rigid Endoscopy

A rigid cystoscope consists of an outer sheath through which all instruments are passed (Figure 18-1); an obturator designed to make the leading end of the cystoscope smooth and rounded so that the scope can be passed through the urethra without causing traumatic injury (Figure 18-2); a bridge that adapts the telescope to the sheath (Figure 18-3); and a telescope (Figure 18-4). The bridge also has openings for the channels through which biopsy and operating instruments can be passed. Special bridges (see Figure 18-2) with deflecting mechanisms allow flexible instruments (e.g., catheters, biopsy forceps, electrocautery electrodes, laser fibers) to be redirected at the tip of the sheath. This allows specific direction or angling of the instruments to perform specific tasks.

Rigid cystoscope sheaths for use in humans have two usual lengths: 22 cm (adult) and 16 cm (pediatric). In addition, sheaths of several unique lengths (both short and very long) are available for veterinary use. Many of these sheaths (as well as other cystoscopy equipment) are manufactured by Karl Storz Veterinary Endoscopy–America, Inc., Goleta, Calif. For female dogs weighing 2 to 5 lb, female cats, and male cats with a perineal urethrostomy, a

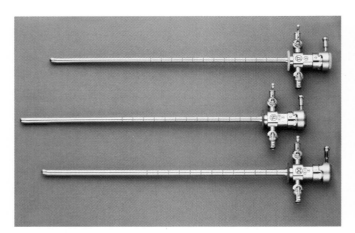

**Figure 18-1** Cystoscope sheaths with obturator locked in place (17-, 19-, and 20-French outer diameter).

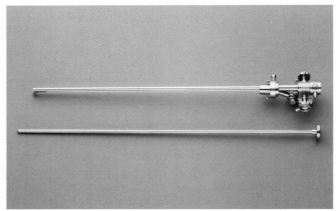

**Figure 18-2** *Top,* Albarran deflecting bridge, which is passed into the lumen of the cystoscope sheath and locked in place. When the wheellike devices are rotated, a short section at the distal tip of the bridge hinges away from the axis of the instrument. This action deflects flexible instruments (e.g., catheters, biopsy instruments) away from the axis of the central instrument channel. *Bottom,* Obturator.

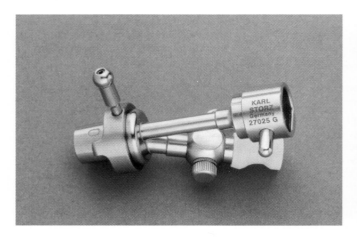

**Figure 18-3** Standard cystoscope bridge. One end of this device (left end in this photograph) locks into the back of the cystoscope sheath. In turn, the telescope locks into the back of the bridge (right end in this photograph). The rubber cap sits on the entry to the instrument channel.

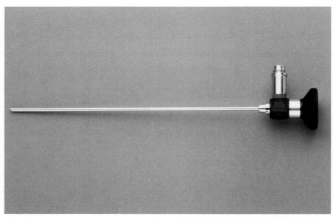

**Figure 18-4** Telescope with a 2.7-mm diameter and a 30-degree oblique angle of view.

10-French-diameter, 14.3-cm-long rigid cystoscope sheath is suitable. For female dogs weighing 7.7 to 15 kg (17 to 33 lb), a 14.5-French-diameter, 16-cm-long rigid cystoscope sheath is appropriate. For female dogs weighing 11.8 to 25 kg (26 to 55 lb), 17- to 22-French-diameter, 22-cm long cystoscope sheaths are suitable. A 22-French-diameter, 29-cm extended-length cystoscope sheath with a matching extra-length telescope is also available. The extra length is necessary for examining the cranial pole of the bladder in very large female dogs. In male dogs, rigid cystoscopes introduced through a perineal urethrotomy incision have been used experimentally, but clinical application of the technique has not been reported.

The diameter of the operating channels varies with the size of the cystoscope sheaths. When planning procedures, the endoscopist must be cognizant of operating channel size because small channels preclude the passage of some instruments. Although instruments come in many sizes, the larger ones generally are easier to work with, are more effective and, in the case of biopsy forceps, procure more diagnostic tissue samples.

Wide-angle telescopes are available with lenses that provide a 0-degree viewing direction (viewing angle of 180 degrees) and a 30-degree viewing direction (viewing angle of 180 degrees) (Karl Storz Veterinary Endoscopy–America, Inc.). These rigid cystoscopes enable visualization of the entire bladder and urethra and are suitable for most operative procedures.

## Flexible Endoscopy

In male dogs weighing more than 7.7 kg (17 lb), a 2.5- to 2.9-mm-diameter, 100-cm-long specialty flexible fiberoptic endoscope (Karl Storz Veterinary Endoscopy–America, Inc.) can be passed into the bladder via the urethra. This endoscope has an operating channel for the passage of fine instruments, but the capability of such instruments is limited because the narrow lumen of the male canine urethra restricts the scope diameter that can be used. Although a flexible endoscope can be easily moved in and out of the bladder and its tip can be pointed in various directions, the end of the scope cannot be as readily advanced in any particular direction in the same way as a rigid endoscope. However, with experience an operator can gain a sense of orientation and can manipulate the scope effectively.

A 1.2-mm-diameter flexible cystourethroscope (Mitsubishi, New York, N.Y.) can be passed via the urethra into the bladder of male cats. This instrument allows direct visualization and the infusion of irrigating solution, but it has no operating channel for passing instruments such as biopsy forceps. Because deflection of the distal tip of the scope cannot be controlled, examination of different sites is achieved by manipulating the bladder and urethra around the endoscope. Bladder biopsy procedures can be performed through a cystocentesis channel under endoscopic guidance.

## Prepubic Percutaneous Endoscopy

Prepubic percutaneous cystoscopy can be performed in small dogs and cats of both sexes using a specially designed needle endoscope introduced through a retractable needle (Karl Storz Veterinary Endoscopy–America, Inc.) or using an endoscopic trocar and cannula. In either instance the visual field is readily cleared and kept clear by in-and-out flushes of irrigation solution through a urethral catheter during the entire procedure. Instruments for biopsy and cautery can be directed into the bladder via a second needle passed through the abdominal wall.

A wide variety of procedures can be performed during cystoscopy. Rigid, flexible, and percutaneous endoscopy all allow direct visualization, biopsy, and photography. Light sources used for other endoscopic equipment are adaptable to most cystoscopes.

## PREPARATION OF EQUIPMENT AND OPERATING ENVIRONMENT

Although all equipment for cystoscopy should be sterilized and organized on a sterile drape, full asepsis does not have to be maintained in the operating theater. Sterile gloves should be worn, but the use of surgical masks is not usually warranted. It is impossible to pass instruments into the urethra and maintain a sterile environment because of the normal urethral flora. However, constantly flushing the endoscope with irrigating solution can keep the bladder clean and clear of infectious agents. Serious infection is unlikely even after the rare instances in which the bladder or urethra is ruptured during cystoscopy.

## PATIENT POSITIONING AND PREPARATION

Cystoscopy is performed using general anesthesia. For rigid cystoscopy, dogs and cats can be placed in a lateral or dorsal recumbent position. For flexible and prepubic cystoscopy the lateral recumbent position is most commonly used, and the prepuce or lateral abdomen can be prepared. In female dogs, introduction of the cystoscope and examination are easiest when the patient is positioned so that its hindquarters extend slightly beyond the end of the examination table. This allows the operator to angle the scope toward all areas of the bladder.

Perivulval hair should be clipped, and the perineum should be prepared with a surgical scrub. If vaginal discharge is excessive or purulent, an antiseptic douche may be used before the endoscope is introduced. In male dogs the prepuce can be rinsed before cystoscopy. Finally, the patient is surgically draped with the vulva or prepuce exposed.

## VISUALIZING THE URETHRA BEFORE INSTRUMENT PASSAGE

For the introduction of devices into the bladder via the urethra, the urethral os must be observed directly with the aid of a speculum and light source. In female dogs the urethral os can be visualized using a 3-inch Killian nasal speculum with a built-in light source or, alternatively, using the same speculum and a head lamp. Whatever light source is used, visualization of the urethral os is facilitated by simultaneously providing caudoventral traction to the tip of the vulva. In male cats the penis can be extruded from the prepuce by placing stay sutures at the reflection of the penile and preputial mucosa. Gentle traction can be applied to the stay sutures by hanging mosquito forceps clamped to the stay sutures over the edge of the operating table.

## INTRODUCTION OF THE RIGID CYSTOSCOPE

All devices should be liberally coated with sterile lubricant before they are passed through the urethra. The cystoscope can be fully assembled with telescope, bridge, and irrigation lines attached and then introduced through the urethra into the bladder under direct visualization. Maintaining a constant flow of irrigation fluid from the front of the cystoscope facilitates this procedure. The irrigation fluid tends to balloon first the vestibule and vagina and then the urethra in front of the advancing cystoscope sheath. Sometimes initial orientation and visualization of the urethral os can be difficult to achieve because the mucosa of the vestibule maintains direct contact with the telescope lens. This problem can be overcome by gently constricting the outer vestibule around the cystoscope sheath to prevent the infused fluid from leaking out of the vulva. The vulva and vagina will expand with the infusion fluid, the mucosa will separate away from the front of the telescope, and the anatomic orientation of the urethral os will become apparent.

Alternatively, the cystoscope sheath with obturator in place can be guided into the urethral os under direct visualization and then advanced blindly through the urethra into the bladder. The smooth, rounded end of the obturator allows the endoscope sheath to pass more easily through the urethra. Once the cystoscope sheath has moved into the bladder, the obturator can be withdrawn

and the bridge and telescope can be locked in place to complete the assembly. Irrigation lines, drainage lines, and the light cable can be connected, and examination of the bladder can begin.

Passage of the fully assembled endoscope is preferable to blind passage because it allows direct visualization of the urethra as the sheath is advanced. Under direct visualization, special angles that need to be adopted to ease passage of the sheath through the urethra can be appreciated. Also, trauma can be avoided if urethral lesions and strictures are seen before passage of the sheath is attempted.

## IRRIGATION SOLUTIONS

The irrigation solution should be warmed to prevent the patient from becoming hypothermic. To prevent overdistension, the bladder bag containing the irrigation solution should be raised no higher than 80 cm above the level of the bladder. For rigid cystoscopy the bladder is flushed as soon as the endoscope is introduced into the bladder. However, for flexible endoscopy the small diameter of the operating channel reduces the speed at which irrigation fluid can be flushed in and out of the bladder. The development of a clear field of view can be hastened by irrigating the bladder several times via a urinary catheter before the endoscope is introduced.

Any physiologic salt solution is a satisfactory irrigant for routine examination. For *electrocautery,* a nonelectrolyte solution such as 1.5% glycine is preferable; the osmolality of this solution prevents osmolar damage of tissue samples taken for histologic examination. For *electrohydraulic shock-wave lithotripsy (EHL),* 0.01% saline allows better spark generation and hence more powerful transmission of shock waves, although the procedure can also be performed successfully with normal saline as the irrigant.

## BALLOON DILATION OF THE URETHRA

Sometimes it is advantageous to pass a cystoscope sheath with a relatively larger diameter than a patient's urethra (e.g., when large biopsy or operating instruments are required). In female dogs the introduction of relatively large sheaths can be eased and urethral trauma can be minimized by prior urethral dilation with a balloon dilator (Cook Urological, Spencer, Ind.). The uninflated dilator is passed through the urethra. Once the balloon is positioned so that it extends beyond both the proximal and distal ends of the urethra, the balloon cuff is inflated to high pressure. The pressure is maintained for 1 to 2 minutes during which the urethral smooth muscle gradually stretches. The cuff is then deflated, and the dilator is removed. After the urethra has been dilated, the cystoscope sheath can be introduced into the bladder fully assembled or with the obturator in place.

## EXAMINATION OF THE LOWER URINARY TRACT

Initially the bladder must be rinsed several times with irrigation fluid to allow clear visualization and photography. Rinsing is particularly necessary when inflammation with abundant cellular debris and hemorrhage is present. As mentioned previously, when a flexible endoscope is used for cystoscopy in male dogs, the bladder is best rinsed via a urinary catheter before passage of the endoscope. However, with rigid endoscopes, fluid can be rapidly infused into the bladder using gravity flow from a bag through an infusion line connected to the endoscope sheath. Subsequent drainage can be achieved by opening the drainage valve or more rapidly by disconnecting the bridge from the sheath and expressing fluid from the bladder using direct compression through the abdominal wall. Even more rapid cleansing of the bladder can be achieved by successive ingress and egress of fluid using an Ellik evacuator (Karl Storz Endoscopy–America, Inc., Culver City, Calif.).

In cats a dorsal longitudinal ridge of tissue is usually present along the length of the urethra. The normal urethra has a pale pink appearance, and submucosal vessels can be observed if the scope is pressed sideways against the urethral wall.

The mucosal surface of the bladder should be observed both when the bladder is partially contracted and again when it is distended. Small lesions may become flattened and less obvious once the bladder wall is stretched. Overdistension of the bladder induces artifactual submucosal petechial hemorrhages. Bladder rupture is also a possibility, particularly if the bladder wall is weakened by the presence of an infiltrative neoplasm. During placement of the cystoscope a small quantity of air is always introduced into the bladder. When the patient is in a dorsal recumbent position, the air bubble remains at the ventral (uppermost) region of the bladder. The entire bladder wall should be examined systematically by successively advancing and retracting the cystoscope followed by partial rotation. In this way even small lesions are not missed. Useful landmarks include the cranial pole of the bladder, the trigone and neck of the bladder, the air bubble (which always remains uppermost in the bladder), and the ureteral orifices. In cats the ureteral openings may appear to be in the proximal urethra if the bladder is not distended. Once the bladder is distended, these openings adopt a more expected position in the trigone area. Urine can be observed intermittently flowing out of the ureteral orifices. The bladder

neck and urethra are best examined by slowly advancing or withdrawing the cystoscope with the irrigation fluid running.

The ureteral orifices should always be identified. If difficulty is encountered in identifying either or both ureteral orifices, another technique usually proves beneficial. First the scope is withdrawn to the urethra. As the scope is readvanced just beyond the trigone area, it is rotated just slightly to provide a different angle view. Because the ureters attach on the dorsal wall of the bladder, it may occasionally be necessary to rotate the scope a full 180 degrees so that the angle of illumination is directed more toward the dorsal wall. Then slow sweeping motions and slight rotation generally lead to successful visualization of the ureteral orifices. Changing the degree of bladder distension may also be helpful. In a fully distended bladder the ureteral orifices tend to be more slit-like, whereas with moderate distension the orifices often protrude a little more, which makes them easier to see. Occasionally, identification of a ureteral orifice is first confirmed when a small spurt of urine is seen flowing from it. With increased operator experience, ureteral orifices can usually be identified rapidly.

When the bladder is contracted, the mucosa develops irregular folds and appears more pink (see Plate 18-6). When distended, the normal bladder has a flat, pale, blanched appearance, and the submucosal vascular pattern becomes apparent (see Plate 18-7). Abnormalities such as uroliths (see Plate 18-12), inflammatory polyps (see Plate 18-13), neoplasms (see Plates 18-14 to 18-16), and ectopic ureters (see Plates 18-17 to 18-20) are easily seen. All structures should be examined before biopsy or other procedures are initiated because bleeding causes the irrigation fluid to become cloudy, obscuring anatomic and pathologic details.

## CYSTOSCOPIC PROCEDURES

Operating instruments that can be passed through cystoscopes include forceps for grasping and biopsy (Karl Storz Veterinary Endoscopy–America, Inc.); wire baskets for recovering large pieces of resected tissue and uroliths (Mill-Rose Laboratories, Mentor, Ohio); laser fibers and electrocautery electrodes for tissue resection; laser fibers and electrohydraulic shock-wave electrodes for lithotripsy; and needles for giving submucosal injections.

Several procedures that can be performed via cystoscopy are direct visual examination and biopsy of lesions in the bladder and urethra; resection of superficial polyps and tumors by electrocautery or laser; identification and location of ectopic ureters (see Plates 18-17 to 18-20); catheterization of ectopic ureters as an aid to subsequent surgical correction; ureteral catheterization for differential renal function studies, urine collection for urinalysis, retrograde pyelography, and retrograde establishment of a nephrostomy tract; EHL (see Plate 18-21); and periurethral injection of substances to control urinary incontinence resulting from urethral incompetence. In diffuse bladder disease, representative biopsy specimens of the bladder mucosa can be obtained by blindly passing biopsy forceps through the urethra to the bladder.

Cystoscopic evaluation can define the location and extent of urethral disease to determine the feasibility of subsequent prepubic urethrostomy. Biopsy can be performed to differentiate carcinoma and granulomatous urethritis. Direct visualization of the bladders in cats with lower urinary tract disease has allowed classification of a subsection of patients with a feline disease that has some of the same characteristics as human interstitial cystitis. In cats, useful clinical information may be obtained by observing the mucosal vasculature after distending the bladder fluid at 5 cm $H_2O$ pressure and then again at 80 cm $H_2O$ pressure. Affected cats exhibit submucosal hemorrhages, called *glomerulations,* when the bladder is distended to 80 cm $H_2O$ pressure (see Plate 18-22).

Polyps are readily excised by transection of the stalk using electrocautery or a laser fiber. The electrocautery should be set at cutting/coagulation. For laser resection a neodymium:yttrium-aluminum-garnet (Nd:YAG) laser with a contact fiber set at 35 W is effective.

Transection of the stalk of a polyp at its base can be facilitated by placing simultaneous traction on the polyp with grasping forceps. This procedure requires a double-channel bridge to carry both instruments simultaneously. In addition, a second operator makes manipulation easier. Delicate resection procedures are made more difficult by the tissue motion caused by normal respiration. Under these circumstances the operative field can be stabilized by suppressing respiration with neuromuscular blocking agents and controlled ventilation.

Laser resection causes the production of gas bubbles that can interfere with the operative field. The uppermost lesions are best resected first, when the operative field is still clear. Alternatively, the patient can be repositioned so that the operative field rotates away from the uppermost position. In addition, direct external pressure on the abdominal wall by an assistant can reposition the bladder so that lesions are better located for resection.

The removal of tissue and stone fragments from the bladder lumen after resection or fragmentation is facilitated by the rapid flushing of irrigation fluid in and out through the cystoscope sheath using an Ellik evacuator. Solid material that passes out of the cystoscope sheath during the egress phase is trapped because it gravitates into the evacuator bulb and tends not to be flushed back into the bladder with each subsequent ingress phase.

If tissue fragments and polyps resected from the bladder wall are too large to pass through the cystoscope sheath, they can be snared in a wire basket and withdrawn through the urethra along with the whole cystoscope assembly. This procedure is facilitated by the liberal application of lubricant to the cystoscope sheath before the extraction of each fragment. Balloon dilation of the urethra to a very large diameter using a 8 or 10-mm (24 to 30 French) esophageal balloon dilator (Cook Urological) can facilitate the removal of very large pieces of tissue or uroliths.

Ureteral catheterization usually cannot be achieved by the direct passage of a catheter into the ureteral os. Catheterization is facilitated by the successive advancement of a flexible J-tipped guide wire (Cook Incorporated, Bloomington, Ind.) and the surrounding ureteral catheter (Bard Urological Division, C.D. Bard Inc., Murray Hill, N.J.). Collection of ureteral urine allows urinalysis, cultures to test for pyelonephritis, and cytologic examination of cells when tumors of the upper urinary tract are suspected. With the infusion of a radiographic contrast agent, retrograde pyelography can be performed to closely examine the architecture of the renal collection system.

Cystoscopy can be a fundamental procedure in the diagnosis of hematuria. After the visual field in the bladder is clarified with irrigation fluid, all areas of the urethral and vesicular mucosa can be minutely examined. Because of the magnifying effects of the endoscopic image, it is possible to identify extremely small mucosal lesions that may be biopsied and cauterized. If the source of bleeding is located in the upper urinary tract, direct visualization of the ureteral openings allows identification of the affected side. The ureters should be examined for hematuria as soon as possible after anesthesia is induced. Prolonged anesthesia with reduced blood pressure can cause idiopathic renal bleeding to cease during the diagnostic procedure. Pharmacologic intervention to increase blood pressure can overcome this problem.

EHL is used to fragment large uroliths so that they can be flushed out through the cystoscope sheath. The EHL electrode is held against the urolith and activated for 1- to 2-second bursts. Larger fragments can then be further broken down into subunits until all pieces are small enough to pass through the cystoscope sheath. An Ellik evacuator facilitates the removal of these fragments via the cystoscope sheath. The EHL electrode must not be activated when it is held against the bladder wall because of the risk of perforation.

Incontinence caused by urethral incompetence has been treated with the periurethral injection of polytetrafluoroethylene (Teflon) paste (Polytef; Mentor, Norwell, Mass.) using special flexible needles and high-pressure syringe devices (Karl Storz). Teflon paste deposits should be placed just distal to the junction of the bladder and the urethra. In a single report of this procedure three injections placed equidistant circumferentially around the urethra until the urethral lumen was partially occluded improved urinary incontinence in female dogs (Arnold et al, 1989). Because Teflon can induce granuloma formation and can migrate to other tissues, collagen (Contigen; C.R. Bard Inc., Covington, Ga.) has been suggested as an alternative material for periurethral injection. However, this product is expensive.

## POSTOPERATIVE CARE

Cystoscopic procedures are intrinsically clean because of the constant flow of sterile irrigant through the instruments. However, even the most experienced operator with extremely gentle technique can cause small tears in the bladder and urethral mucosa (see Plate 18-23). Because these tears may predispose patients to postoperative infection, broad-spectrum antimicrobials are usually prescribed for 3 to 5 days after the procedure.

An indwelling catheter can be maintained for 48 to 72 hours after prepubic cystoscopy to allow complete sealing of the holes created by the centesis instruments. It is not known if this extended period of catheterization is necessary when patients can urinate normally (i.e., when they have no urethral outflow obstruction).

## CONTRAINDICATIONS AND COMPLICATIONS

Contraindications to cystoscopy in human patients are few, although acute inflammatory processes such as cystitis, prostatitis, or urethritis should be resolved before the procedure is performed. Urethral obstruction can preclude examination of the bladder with instruments passed through the urethra, but endoscopic examination of the obstruction site allows identification of the cause, which may include stricture, urolithiasis, granulomatous inflammation, or tumors. The last two possibilities must be differentiated by either cytologic evaluation or histologic examination of biopsy specimens.

In cats, rigid transurethral cystoscopy should not be performed within 6 weeks of a perineal urethrostomy procedure. In addition, prepubic cystoscopy is difficult or impossible to perform in cats that have contracted, thick-walled bladders with small lumens.

Iatrogenic rupture of the urethra during cystoscopy is usually due to the use of excessive force and operator inexperience. In certain circumstances, however, even gentle pressure can cause the rigid endoscope to pass through the wall of the urethra. Retroperitoneal fat and loose fibrous connective tissue are seen if the scope is outside the urethra. The scope should be withdrawn, the procedure should be discontinued, and broad-spectrum antimicrobials should be administered postoperatively. The necessity of positioning a stent across the ruptured urethra is not clear. In three cases of urethral rupture, stents were not placed and side effects were not noted.

If cystoscopy is performed with the Albarran deflecting bridge, the deflector should be rotated up inside the sheath whenever it is not in use. Movement of the sheath with the deflector extended, particularly in and out of the urethra, can cause mucosal injury.

## REFERENCES

Arnold S et al: Treatment of urinary incontinence in dogs by endoscopic injection of Teflon, *J Am Vet Med Assoc* 195:1369, 1989.

Brearley MJ, Cooper JE: The diagnosis of bladder disease in dogs by cystoscopy, *J Small Anim Pract* 28:75, 1987.

Chew DJ et al: Urethroscopy, cystoscopy, and biopsy of the feline lower urinary tract, *Vet Clin North Am* 26:441, 1996.

Cooper JE et al: Cystoscopic examination of male and female dogs, *Vet Rec* 115:571, 1984.

Hunter PT et al: Hawkins-Hunter retrograde transcutaneous nephrostomy: a new technique, *Urology* 22:583, 1983.

McCarthy TC: Cystoscopy and biopsy of the feline lower urinary tract, *Vet Clin North Am* 26:463, 1996.

McCarthy TC, McDermaid SL: Prepubic percutaneous cystoscopy in the dog and cat, *J Am Anim Hosp Assoc* 22:213, 1986.

Osborn S et al: Cystoscopic identification of glomerulations in cats with interstitial cystitis [Abstract], *J Vet Intern Med* 8:169, 1994.

Senior DF: Electrohydraulic shock-wave lithotripsy in experimental canine struvite bladder stone disease, *Vet Surg* 13:143, 1984.

Senior DF, Newman RC: Retrograde ureteral catheterization in female dogs, *J Am Anim Hosp Assoc* 22:831, 1986.

Senior DF, Sundstrom DA: Cystoscopy in female dogs, *Comp Contin Educ Pract Vet* 10:890, 1988.

Wan J et al: The treatment of urinary incontinence in children using glutaraldehyde cross-linked collagen, *J Urol* 148:127, 1992.

**COLOR PLATES   PAGES 454-459**

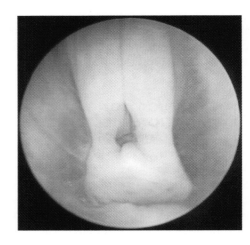

**Plate 18-1** Urethral os (center of the field of view) with moderate distension of the vestibule.

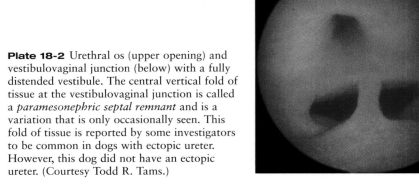

**Plate 18-2** Urethral os (upper opening) and vestibulovaginal junction (below) with a fully distended vestibule. The central vertical fold of tissue at the vestibulovaginal junction is called a *paramesonephric septal remnant* and is a variation that is only occasionally seen. This fold of tissue is reported by some investigators to be common in dogs with ectopic ureter. However, this dog did not have an ectopic ureter. (Courtesy Todd R. Tams.)

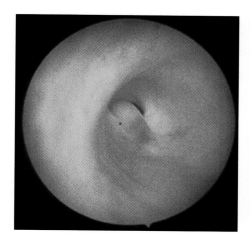

**Plate 18-3** Normal vagina with full distension.

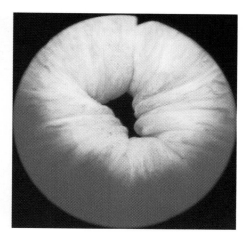

**Plate 18-4** Normal urethra.

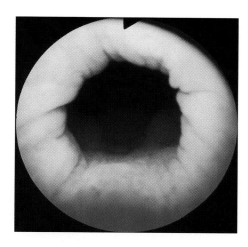

**Plate 18-5** Normal urethra at the junction of the urethra and the bladder. The ureteral papillae are visible in the trigone region of the bladder (center of the field and extending to the left and right).

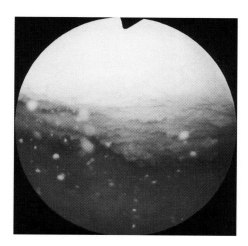

**Plate 18-6** Normal appearance of the bladder mucosa when the bladder is not fully distended. The mucosa has a wrinkled appearance, and submucosal vessels cannot be seen. The particles in the bladder fluid are sloughed cells and debris that are normally present on initial introduction of a cystoscope. This material is removed by successive in-out washes of irrigation fluid to allow better visibility.

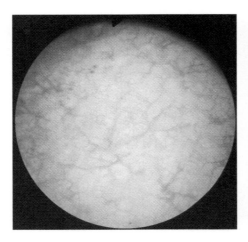

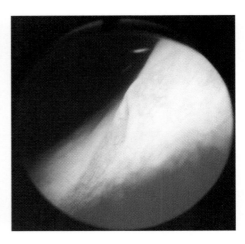

**Plate 18-7** Normal appearance of the bladder mucosa when the bladder is fully distended. Because the epithelium of the distended bladder is only one cell thick, the intricate submucosal vascular pattern becomes obvious.

**Plate 18-8** Normal appearance of the right ureter when the bladder is distended. (The patient is in a dorsal recumbent position.)

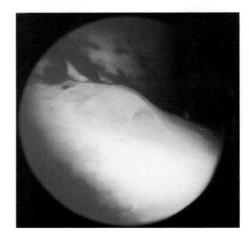

**Plate 18-9** Normal appearance of the left ureter when the bladder is not fully distended. The ureteral opening appears to be on a raised papilla. (The patient is in the dorsal recumbent position.)

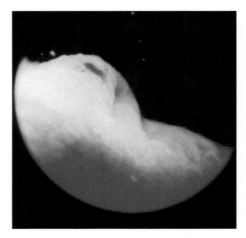

**Plate 18-10** Normal appearance of the left ureter when the bladder is not fully distended. The ureteral papilla is raised above the surface of the surrounding bladder. The hemorrhage on the rim of the ureteral opening is due to instrument-induced trauma. (The patient is in a dorsal recumbent position.)

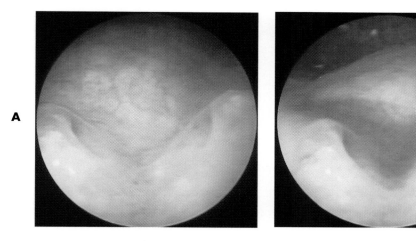

**Plate 18-11 A,** Ureteral papillae with the bladder partially distended. **B,** A spurt of urine has flowed into the bladder from the right ureter (left opening in the field of view).

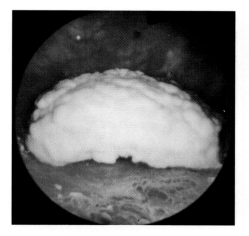

**Plate 18-12** Struvite urolith in the bladder of a dog. The mucosa appears hyperplastic.

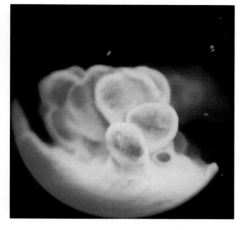

**Plate 18-13** Inflammatory polyp in the bladder of a dog.

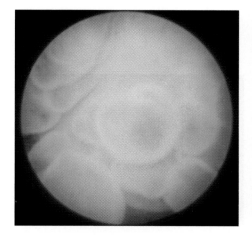

**Plate 18-14** Close-up of the surface of a transitional cell carcinoma in the bladder of a dog.

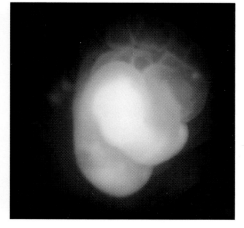

**Plate 18-15** Close-up of the necrotic tip of a transitional cell carcinoma in the bladder of a dog.

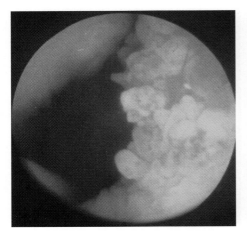

**Plate 18-16** Adenocarcinoma in the bladder of a dog.

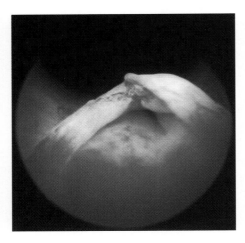

**Plate 18-17** Opening of an ectopic ureter in the proximal urethra of a young female dog.

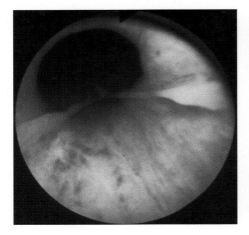

**Plate 18-18** Opening of an ectopic ureter in the proximal urethra of a young female dog.

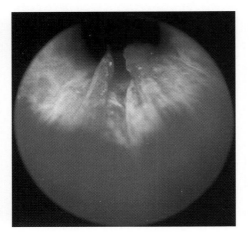

**Plate 18-19** Lateral ridges of redundant tissue that continue caudally from the opening of an ectopic ureter for the full length of the urethra in a dog.

**Plate 18-20** Lateral ridges of redundant tissue that continue caudally from the opening of an ectopic ureter for the full length of the urethra in a dog.

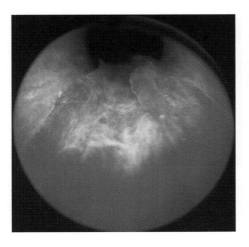

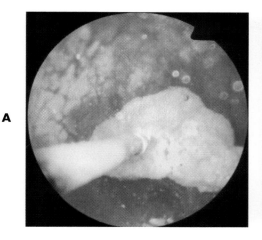
**A**

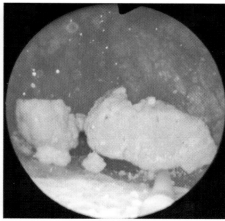
**B**

**Plate 18-21 A,** Electrohydraulic shock-wave lithotripsy of a struvite urolith in the bladder of the dog. The spark is visible at the distal tip of the electrode placed on the surface of the urolith. **B,** The same urolith immediately after brief activation (1 to 2 seconds) of the electrohydraulic shock-wave lithotripter on the surface. The urolith is fragmented.

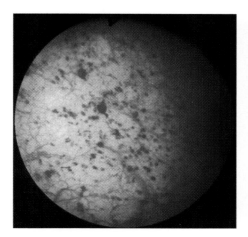

**Plate 18-22** Submucosal hemorrhages (glomerulations) in the bladder of a cat. The bladder has been distended to 80 cm $H_2O$ pressure. Glomerulations are associated with inflammatory conditions of the bladder and can be seen in many cats with idiopathic lower urinary tract inflammation.

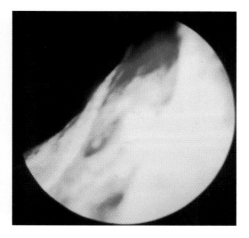

**Plate 18-23** Instrument-induced tear in the mucosa of the bladder in a dog. The mucosa is very fragile, and although trauma is easily induced, postoperative side effects related to such trauma are uncommon.

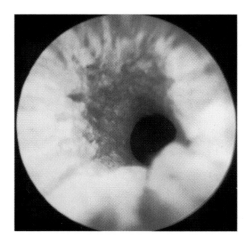

**Plate 18-24** Hyperemic mucosa of an inflamed urethra in a dog with bacterial cystitis.

# Chapter 19

# Arthroscopy

Robert A. Taylor

Arthroscopic examination of the canine stifle was first described more than two decades ago (Siemering GH, 1978). Since then, techniques for arthroscopic examination of the coxofemoral joint, scapulohumeral joint, cubital joint, and tarsus have been developed. Although most reports detail the use of arthroscopy for diagnosis, the technique has also been used to remove osteochondral fragments associated with osteochondrosis of the canine scapulohumeral joint.

In one comparative study of arthroscopy and arthrotomy in 24 dogs, arthroscopy not only provided adequate examination of the stifle but also was found to be less traumatic than conventional arthrotomy (Miller CW, Presnell KR, 1985). Similar work was conducted in ponies (Nixon AJ, 1984), and arthroscopic surgery is now widely used for diagnosis and therapeutic interventions in horses. Despite the early enthusiasm for arthroscopy and its proven clinical efficacy (Siemering GH, 1978; Kivumbi CW, Bennett D, 1981; Person MW, 1989), the technique still is not a commonly used diagnostic and surgical tool in small animal medicine. However, this situation is changing, and small animal surgeons are beginning to use arthroscopy more frequently (Van Ryssen B, Van Bree HJ, 1997; Van Bree HJ, Van Ryssen B, 1998.).

The advantages and disadvantages of arthroscopy in dogs are listed in Box 19-1. Arthroscopy requires expensive equipment and a procedure time that is frequently longer than with conventional arthrotomy. In addition, the learning curve to achieve excellence in arthroscopy is steep and often very frustrating. When the size difference between the canine stifle and the equine or human stifle is considered, it is easy to understand how difficult it can be to access the joints of the dog. However, with the smaller telescopes now available, all important canine joints can be accessed.

Arthroscopy offers unparalleled visualization of joint structures. Furthermore, it is a minimally invasive technique from which postoperative recovery is rapid. The arthroscopic findings can be documented in the patient's record with photographs and/or videotapes. In certain cases, such as elusive fragmentation of the medial coronoid process of the ulna, arthroscopy is preferable to conventional radiography and more cost effective than computed tomographic imaging.

---

**Box 19-1** Relative Advantages and Disadvantages of Arthroscopy Compared with Arthrotomy

**ADVANTAGES**
Unparalleled view (under magnification) of joint pathology
Diagnosis and therapeutic intervention
Reduced morbidity
Faster functional return
Cost savings

**DISADVANTAGES**
Expensive, fragile equipment
Exacting technique with a long, difficult learning curve

---

| Box 19-2 | Equipment Required for Diagnostic Arthroscopy |
| --- | --- |

**GENERAL SUPPLIES**
Surgical gloves and gowns
Surgical preparation solutions and sponges
Scalpels and blades (no. 11)
Intravenous tubing
Needles: 1½ inch long, 18 gauge
Sterile fluids: lactated Ringer's solution or saline

**EQUIPMENT AT EACH ARTHROSCOPY STATION**
Video camera
Light source
Video recorder
2.7-mm, 30-degree Storz arthroscope*
2.7-mm arthroscope sheath
2.7-mm blunt obturator
Light cable
Dyonics power source†
Dyonics hand piece†
3 Dyonics burrs†

*Storz Veterinary Endoscopy–America, Inc., Goleta, Calif.
†Dyonics-Smith Nephew, Andover, Mass.

Canine arthroscopy is currently used primarily for diagnostic purposes. However, as abilities are refined and more surgeons use the technique, therapeutic arthroscopic procedures are expected to become commonplace. The frequent occurrence of fragmentation of the medial coronoid process in the cubital joint and osteochondrosis of the scapulohumeral joint, tarsocrural joint, and cubital joint makes these joints prime candidates for operative intervention.

## EQUIPMENT

### Telescopes

Veterinary arthroscopy can be performed with a variety of surgical telescopes. A forward-viewing or 20-degree forward-viewing scope is best for most work in dogs. Although telescopes with a diameter of 1.9 or 2.4 mm (Karl Storz Veterinary Endoscopy–America, Inc. Goleta, Calif.) are easier to place in smaller joints, they have a limited field of view and their shorter length makes them less applicable to other uses.

In my opinion the best general-purpose telescope is the Storz 2.7-mm scope (Box 19-2 and Figure 19-1). Because of its larger field of view and longer length, this telescope is extremely useful for rigid endoscopy. The 2.7-mm scope is long enough (18 cm) to be used for ex-

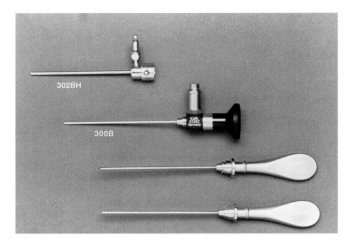

**Figure 19-1** Rigid 2.7-mm arthroscope, insertion sheath *(top)*, and trocars.

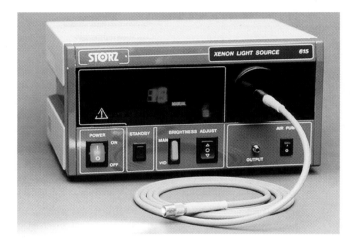

**Figure 19-2** Xenon fiberoptic light sources provide excellent intraarticular illumination.

amination of the bladder and urethra in female dogs weighing 2.5 to 20 kg (5.5 to 45 lb). The scope is also ideal for rhinoscopy, and it is frequently used in birds and many small exotic animal species.

Larger telescopes such as 4-mm instruments are commonly used in human and equine patients. Scopes of this size are too large for routine use in canine joints.

### Light Source

An adequate light source is mandatory because arthroscopy is performed in smaller joints and narrow-diameter telescopes are used for visualization. Most light sources can be used with other fiberoptic equipment such as flexible and rigid endoscopes. With this in mind it is probably wise to purchase the highest quality light source possible. A xenon light source is preferable (Figure 19-2), but any good-quality fiberoptic light source may be used.

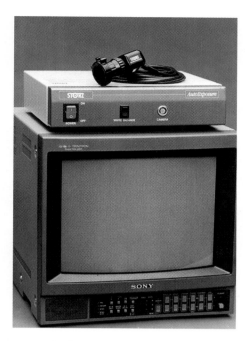

**Figure 19-3** Single-chip video camera and monitor used for diagnostic and therapeutic arthroscopy.

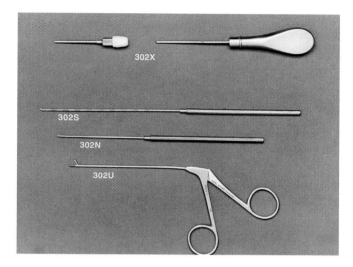

**Figure 19-4** A blunt probe (second from bottom) or hooked manipulator (third from bottom) is useful for probing and for retracting intraarticular structures.

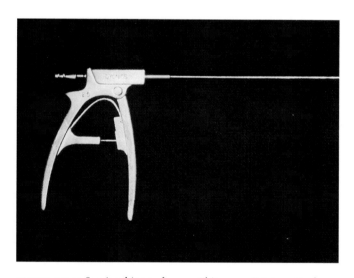

**Figure 19-5** Suction biopsy forceps "bite away" intraarticular structures; the small fragments are suctioned through the instrument.

## Video Camera and Monitor

Canine arthroscopy was first performed under direct visualization through the telescope. Contemporary methods dictate the use of a small video camera that is attached to the telescope (Figure 19-3). Use of a video camera increases operator agility, allows two or more people to work together, and provides an accurate record of the procedure. The camera used for video endoscopic documentation is able to withstand immersion in sterilizing solutions and sterilization with ethylene oxide gas. A single-chip video camera is quite suitable for canine arthroscopy and can be adapted for use with other fiberoptic equipment. (Video equipment is discussed in more detail in Chapters 1 and 2.)

## Instruments

A vast array of equipment is available for use in human and equine arthroscopy. The smaller instruments are quite amenable for use in small animal arthroscopy. For diagnostic arthroscopy the only required extra equipment is a *blunt probe* (Figure 19-4). Although the probe can be inserted through a simple stab incision, it is better to use an *insertion cannula* so that adequate joint capsule distension can be maintained and periarticular fluid extravasation is minimized. With progression from diagnostic to therapeutic procedures, more instrumentation is required.

*Suction biopsy forceps* are particularly useful for intraarticular work. The small tissue fragments "bitten off" by the forceps are suctioned through the instrument and out of the joint (Figure 19-5). Thus the forceps instrument does not have to be removed from the joint as each bite is taken. Because the instrument has a small diameter, tissue fragments may occlude its suction portal. In addition, the amount of suction must be regulated to prevent joint capsule collapse.

*Ferris Smith-type cup rongeurs* (Figure 19-6) can be useful for removing small osteochondral fragments, osteophytes, intraarticular debris, and bone and meniscal

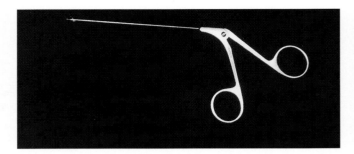

**Figure 19-6** Ferris Smith rongeur forceps are suitable for fragment retrieval and synovial biopsy procedures.

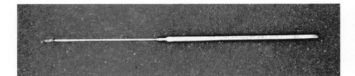

**Figure 19-7** Meniscal knives can be used to sever meniscal attachments.

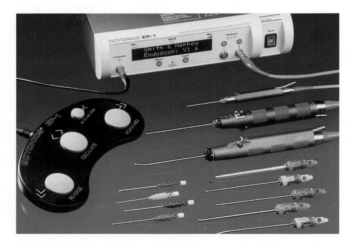

**Figure 19-8** The head of a power-driven shaver or cutter is shielded to protect intraarticular structures. Debris is suctioned through the instrument.

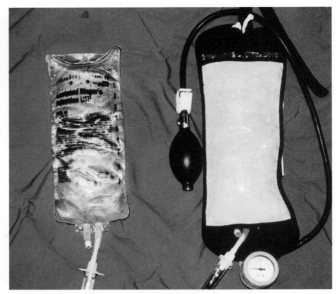

**Figure 19-9** A simple fluid infusion system suitable for joint infusion.

fragments. Small *meniscal knives* suitable for placement through an arthroscopy cannula can be helpful in removing torn pieces of meniscus (Figure 19-7).

Arthroscopic procedures can also be performed using power-driven instruments. The heads of these instruments are shielded so that intraarticular structures can be protected. A number of head attachments are available for intraarticular use. As intraarticular work is being done, debris is suctioned out of the field through the instrument. *Power-driven shavers* and *cutters* make precise work easier to accomplish (Figure 19-8). This equipment is expensive and requires the addition of another instrument portal into the already small operating space

of canine joints. In some cases, calcified pieces of the meniscus and osteophytes are difficult to remove with this equipment.

## Fluid Infusion Equipment

Sterile fluid ingress is necessary for diagnostic and therapeutic work within the joints. The fluid is used to clean telescope lenses, wash away debris, and maintain capsular distension. A simple fluid infusion system can be fashioned from conventional plastic fluid bags and a pressure infusion bag (Figure 19-9). Lactated Ringer's solution in a collapsible 1-L bag is ideal for infusion. The bag filled with this solution is placed in a pressure infusion bag that, using gravity alone, is capable of providing fluid flow to infusion pressures of up to 200 mm Hg.

A small amount of fluid may be introduced to distend the joint capsule before the telescope cannula is introduced. This fluid is typically injected through an 18- or 20-gauge needle or, alternatively, a Veress needle. Once the telescope is in the joint, the fluid line is attached to a port on the sheath. The fluid is then allowed to flow through the lumen of the sheath, around the telescope, and into the joint. The placement of a Veress needle at a separate location is important to allow fluid egress and debris removal.

## PRINCIPLES OF ARTHROSCOPY

Rigid surgical asepsis is mandatory because as few as 100 microorganisms can infect a joint. The extremity should be draped so that open arthrotomy, if indicated,

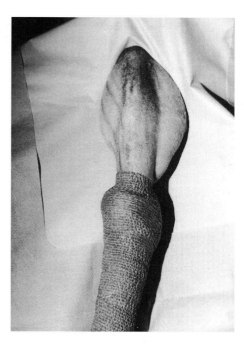

Figure 19-10 The patient has been positioned, and the extremity has been draped to provide rigid asepsis.

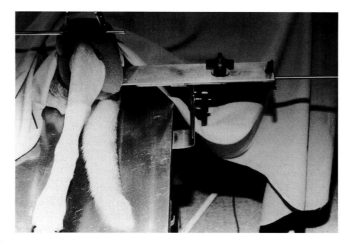

Figure 19-11 This custom-designed leg holder allows the operator to grasp the leg and apply medial or lateral stresses to the stifle. These maneuvers facilitate the visualization of intraarticular structures.

can be performed after the arthroscopic examination has been completed.

The joint or extremity should be positioned for maximum advantage. The extremity must be held firmly because movement may cause the telescope and instrument cannula to shift, making it difficult to access the joint (Figure 19-10). When possible, a fixed leg positioner should be used (Figure 19-11). No leg positioners are commercially available, but several have been described in the literature.

A no. 11 blade is used to make the initial skin incision, which should be just large enough to allow insertion of the telescope cannula and trocar. Next a blunt trocar is placed in the cannula, and the unit is slowly inserted into the joint. At this juncture it is helpful for the operator to manipulate the cannula and blunt trocar to verify placement. If the joint has been predistended with saline solution, some of this solution and some joint fluid will escape when the blunt trocar is removed from the cannula.

Once the telescope is in the joint, a thorough diagnostic examination is performed before treatment is attempted. It may be helpful to move the joint through its normal range of motion to allow inspection of all intraarticular structures. This maneuver is important in the stifle, but it is difficult to accomplish in the cubital joint because too much motion may cause the telescope to become dislodged from this joint.

Although fluid distension of the joint capsule is important, dogs are very susceptible to fluid extravasation. Infusion pressures greater than 550 mm Hg are generally

felt to be unnecessary and can result in fluid extravasation. This complication, which seems to occur more frequently in the shoulder joint, can be minimized by careful selection of equipment, proper portal location, conservative use of infusion fluids, prevention of excessive limb movement, and avoidance of excessive joint capsular distension prior to telescope insertion. Once fluid extravasation occurs, it can displace and collapse the joint capsule, distort tissue planes, and increase postarthroscopy morbidity. Severe fluid extravasation may cause the procedure to be abandoned.

When the telescope is used for diagnostic purposes and no other instruments are to be placed in the joint, *triangulation* is not important. However, when a therapeutic procedure is planned, the scope is positioned to allow adequate visualization, but careful thought must also be given to the proper location of the instrument cannula. A no. 11 blade is used to make the initial incision. The instrument cannula and blunt probe are then inserted. Having the telescope already in the joint allows the operator to ascertain the ideal location for the instruments. Using triangulation, the operator can position instruments to facilitate continuous and direct visual control throughout the procedure.

To use a video camera with the arthroscopic image displayed on the monitor screen, the operator needs to become familiar with the positions of the telescope (especially a forward-viewing scope) and the camera. The manipulation of instruments introduced into the joint is viewed on the video monitor. Extensive experience is necessary before most operators develop expertise in manipulating and coordinating instruments based on video images. In my opinion this is the most challenging part of learning arthroscopy. While no minimum number of procedures is required to achieve proficiency, there seems to be an almost linear relationship between the number of joints examined arthroscopically and operative expertise. The transition from diagnostic to therapeutic arthroscopy requires the performance of at least 50 surgical arthroscopic procedures.

## STIFLE ARTHROSCOPY

The dog is positioned in a dorsal recumbent position with the affected leg partially extended so that the stifle is flexed about 160 degrees. The leg is clipped and surgically prepared. A leg holder is helpful for preventing movement during the procedure and reduces the number of assistants required (see Figure 19-11). The leg holder is positioned proximal to the stifle in such a way that the knee is immobilized but the holder is out of the way to ensure maintenance of a sterile field. The holder should restrain the knee securely, allowing the operator to provide either valgus or varus stress to increase exposure of the menisci.

An 18-gauge, 1½-inch needle or a Veress needle (see Figure 14-8) is then introduced into the proximal joint space, and the joint capsule is distended with saline. For optimal visualization of the cranial cruciate ligament and medial meniscus, the arthroscope is introduced laterally (Figure 19-12). A no. 11 blade is used to create an insertion portal through the skin just lateral to the straight patellar tendon and distal to the lateral femoral condyle. (One disadvantage to this location is the poten-

tial for penetrating the large and sometimes vascular patellar fat pad.) Next the arthroscope sheath and blunt trocar are advanced into the joint. The blunt trocar is manipulated in the joint to orient the operator and ascertain the location. The trocar is removed, and the arthroscope and camera are placed in the arthroscopic sheath and positioned to provide proper orientation within the joint. The saline infusion set is attached to the arthroscope sheath, and the valve is opened to allow saline flow, which will clean debris from the lens. The previously placed Veress needle now serves as an egress port, and its patency and position are verified.

Once the telescope has entered the joint, it should first be directed proximal and dorsal to locate the trochlear groove of the femur and the articular surface of the patella (Figure 19-13). The groove is then followed distally to identify the intercondylar notch and the most proximal aspect of the cranial cruciate ligament (Figure 19-14). Both ligaments are visible as the telescope is deflected far-

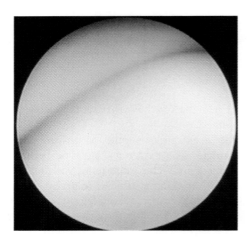

**Figure 19-13** Trochlear groove and articular surface of the patella.

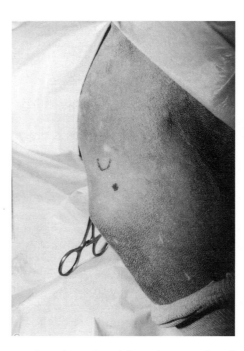

**Figure 19-12** Insertion point of the arthroscope into the stifle joint.

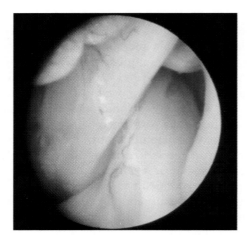

**Figure 19-14** Proximal aspect of the intercondylar notch and both cruciate ligaments.

ther distal. The cranial cruciate spirals distally to attach to the tibial plateau (Figure 19-15). The cranial edge of the medial meniscus and intermeniscal ligament should be visible. At this juncture the stifle joint is flexed to 160 degrees and stressed medially. By alternatively internally and externally rotating the tibia, the operator can see all of the medial meniscus (Figure 19-16). This maneuver can prove difficult in dogs with chronic degenerative joint disease or an intact meniscus. Synovial biopsies, if necessary, can be obtained with the Ferris Smith cup rongeurs.

If indicated, a partial meniscectomy can be performed, but an instrument portal must be added for the ancillary instrumentation. I prefer to enter the stifle from the lateral side and stay roughly parallel to the scope. When the posterior horn of the medial meniscus is torn or detached, medial rotation can increase exposure. A simple biopsy instrument, suction biopsy forceps, or

power instrument can be used to remove the meniscal fragments, which are then flushed out with the continuous saline flow or suctioned out through the instruments (Figure 19-17).

After the arthroscopic examination has been completed, the saline infusion is discontinued and the scope and sheath are removed along with any instrument cannulas. The joint is cycled through a range of motion and gently massaged to remove excess saline via the Veress needle. If necessary, the stab incisions are closed with small, simple, interrupted sutures or skin cement.

## CUBITAL JOINT ARTHROSCOPY

The cubital joint can be examined to evaluate the coronoid process and humeral condyle (Figure 19-18). This joint is very tight, and the intraarticular space is small, even in a large dog. After the affected leg has been prepared for surgery, it is draped proximal to the elbow to allow access to the medial aspect of the cubital joint. An assistant can grasp the leg and lever it over the edge of the operating table by abducting the distal extremity.

An 18-gauge needle is introduced into the joint space just between the caudal aspect of the medial humeral condyle and the medial collateral ligament. If necessary, a 21-gauge 1½-inch needle can be used to probe for the joint space. A no. 11 blade is used to create a stab incision caudal to the collateral ligament and immediately distal to the medial humeral condyle. The arthroscope sheath and blunt trocar are advanced into the joint. This placement allows good visualization of the coronoid process, the medial joint structures, the medial humeral condyle, and a portion of the anconeal process. Visualization of the intraarticular structures is enhanced by abduction of the distal extremity and by external rotation

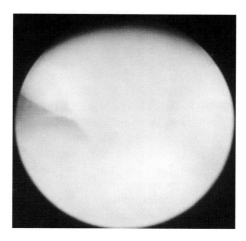

**Figure 19-15** Cranial cruciate ligament near its point of insertion on the tibia.

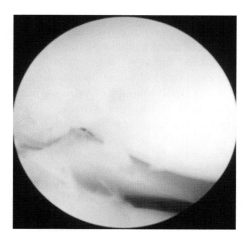

**Figure 19-16** Manipulation of the stifle joint, using alternating internal and external rotation of the tibia, allows the entire medial meniscus to be seen.

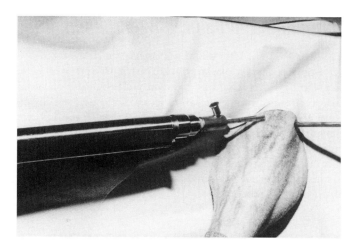

**Figure 19-17** Handheld power cutter inserted in an effort to remove the caudal portion of the medial menisci.

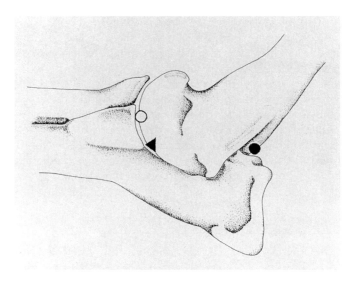

**Figure 19-18** Elbow with the key anatomic structures and insertion points marked. (▲, scope; ○, instrument; ●, egress cannula.)

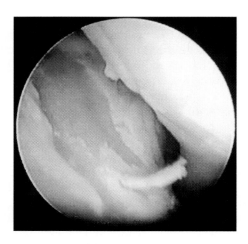

**Figure 19-19** Erosion of the humeral articular cartilage erosion caused by cubital joint incongruence.

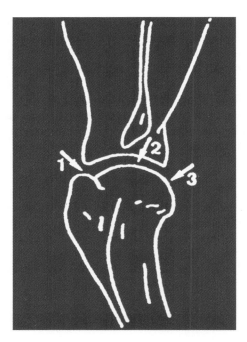

**Figure 19-20** Scapulohumeral joint, showing anatomic structures and the insertion point. (*1*, Egress cannula; *2*, scope; *3*, instrument.)

(Figure 19-19). After the diagnostic procedure has been completed, the arthroscope and sheath are removed. The infusion needle is held in position with the limb elevated to promote drainage of saline from the joint.

The needle is removed, and the skin incisions are treated as previously described. Arthroscopic removal of fragments of the coronoid process, while very challenging, is possible and hopefully will become commonplace as more expertise is gained and more surgeons begin performing arthroscopy.

## SCAPULOHUMERAL ARTHROSCOPY

The dog is positioned in a lateral recumbent position with the affected limb uppermost. It is advantageous to position the limb with a leg holder or large roll of cotton so that the joint can be slightly extended and the distal extremity can be abducted. When the leg is distracted, the acromion process aligns directly over the joint space. With the scapulohumeral joint held in 120 degrees of extension, an 18-gauge needle or a Veress needle is placed just lateral to the biceps tendon as it crosses the joint. The joint is then distended with a small quantity of sterile saline.

A no. 11 blade is used to make a skin incision for the arthroscopy cannula and blunt probe. The joint is flexed to nearly 90 degrees, and the incision is made caudal to the midpoint between the acromion and the greater tubercle of the humerus (Figure 19-20). A more caudal placement favors examination of the humeral head but may make cranial advancement of the scope more difficult. The saline infusion line is attached to the arthroscopy cannula, and saline flow is initiated to clear the lens. Only a small amount of saline is instilled until visual confirmation of location is made.

The scapulohumeral joint is inspected, beginning with the humeral head. The scope can be slightly withdrawn and advanced cranially to visualize the tendon of the biceps brachii. Distraction or levering of the joint against the rolled cotton can enhance visualization of the medial aspect of the glenoid surface and the medial glenohumeral ligament.

A separate instrument portal is needed for the arthroscopic removal of osteochondritic lesions of the humeral head. A stab incision is made cranial to the telescope cannula but lateral to the Veress needle. Ancillary instrumentation is passed through this portal. While it is easy to dislodge large fragments, it is difficult to remove fragments from the joint unless they are small enough to pass through the Veress needle or one of the cannulas. A suction biopsy forceps or power instrument can be used to create vascular access channels in the bed of the osteochondritic lesion. At the completion of the procedure the instrument and arthroscope cannulas are removed. Then the Veress needle is removed. The skin incisions can be closed with sutures or staples.

## REFERENCES

Kivumbi CW, Bennett D: Arthroscopy of the canine stifle joint, *Vet Rec* 109:241, 1981.

Miller CW, Presnell KR: Examination of the canine stifle: arthroscopy versus arthrotomy, *J Am Anim Hosp Assoc* 21:623, 1985.

Nixon AJ: Arthroscopic approaches and intra-articular anatomy of the equine elbow, *Vet Surg* 19:93, 1990.

Person MW: Arthroscopic treatment of osteochondritis dissecans in the canine shoulder, *Vet Surg* 18:175, 1989.

Siemering GH: Arthroscopy of dogs, *J Am Vet Med Assoc* 172:575, 1978.

Van Ryssen B, Van Bree HJ: Arthroscopic findings in 100 dogs with elbow lameness, *Vet Rec* 140:14, 1997.

Van Bree HJ, Van Ryssen B: Diagnostic and surgical artroscopy in osteochondrosis lesions, *Vet Clin North Am Small Anim Pract*, 18:1, 1998.

**ABNORMAL FINDINGS IDENTIFIED AT ARTHROSCOPY**
**Plate 19-1,** p. 470, Osteochondral fragment

**Plate 19-2,** p. 470, Power shaver for breaking down osteochondral fragment

**Plate 19-3,** p. 470, Partial tear of cranial cruciate ligament
**Plate 19-4,** p. 470, Small tear of medial meniscus

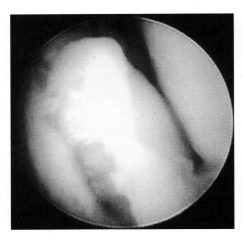

**Plate 19-1** Large osteochondral fragment associated with fragmentation of the medial coronoid process.

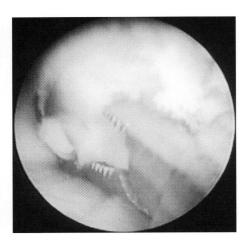

**Plate 19-2** Power shaver used to break an osteochondral fragment into smaller, more easily removed pieces.

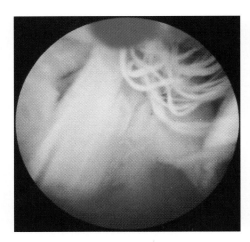

**Plate 19-3** Partial tear of the cranial cruciate ligament. (Courtesy Tim McCarthy.)

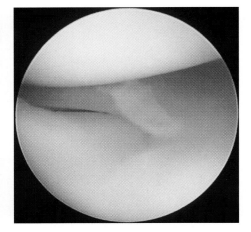

**Plate 19-4** Small midsubstance tear of the medial meniscus.

# Chapter 20

# Thoracoscopy

## Ronald S. Walton

Thoracoscopy is a minimally invasive operative procedure designed for visual inspection of the thoracic cavity and its organs. The technique of thoracoscopy was developed in 1910 by Jacobes, who attempted to break down adhesive tuberculosis lesions in human patients using a modified cystoscope. For the next 35 years operative thoracoscopy was widely used in human medicine. However, with the development of antibiotics such as streptomycin and the improvement of surgical and anesthesia techniques, thoracoscopy was supplanted by more invasive open thoracotomy techniques. Today, with expanded efforts to explore minimally invasive surgical techniques, thoracoscopy is receiving significant renewed attention in human medicine. The introduction of the miniature surgical video camera has in large part facilitated the development and performance of operative procedures using endoscopic instrumentation.

Only a few isolated reports of thoracoscopy have appeared in the veterinary literature. Although the use of thoracoscopy has been limited to a few veterinarians and referral centers, both universities and private practices are now showing considerable interest in adding thoracoscopy capabilities. In 1983 Bauer and Thomas published the first report on the use of thoracoscopy in clinical small animal practice. The development of more sophisticated and cost-effective instrumentation has made the performance of this procedure possible for many veterinary clinicians.

The basic techniques of thoracoscopy are in many ways easier to perform than standard laparoscopy. A sound knowledge of anatomy, appropriate preoperative staging, and a comfortable working knowledge of the equipment are prerequisites for performing the procedure. Descriptions of new uses and techniques for diagnostic and operative thoracoscopy regularly appear in the human literature. The application of these techniques is limited only by the skill and imagination of the clinician.

## INSTRUMENTATION

Thoracoscopy and laparoscopy (see Chapter 14) use the same basic instrumentation. This is convenient for the average veterinary practice because one basic instrument set can be used to examine both the thoracic and abdominal cavities. Traditionally, thoracoscopic instruments are shorter than these commonly used in laparoscopy. The decreased length of instruments and trocars makes them easier to use and reduces the risk of trauma to tissues in the limited confines of the thoracic cavity.

Laparoscopic instruments can easily be used for thoracoscopy in the veterinary patient. This markedly decreases the cost of instrumentation in a practice that is already set up to perform laparoscopy. A noted exception is the thoracic cannula trocar apparatus. The shorter barrel of the typical thoracic cannula decreases the likelihood of damage to underlying tissue. However, I have frequently used standard laparoscopic cannulas during thoracoscopic procedures and have encountered no problems. Thoracoscopy does not require the use of a laparoscopic insufflator.

**Box 20-1    Instrumentation for General Thoracoscopy**

**BASIC SUPPLIES**
Standard surgical set
Six towel packs and a fenestrated drape
Telescope and instrument tray
Standard suture materials
Thoracic drain and accessories
Three way stopcock
Extension tubing
Adapter coupling

**BASIC THORACOSCOPIC INSTRUMENTATION**
Telescope
Fiberoptic light cable
Light source
Three trocar-cannula units
Palpation probe
Scissors
Grasping forceps
Biopsy forceps
Tru-Cut biopsy instrument*

*Travenol Labs, McGaw, Ill.

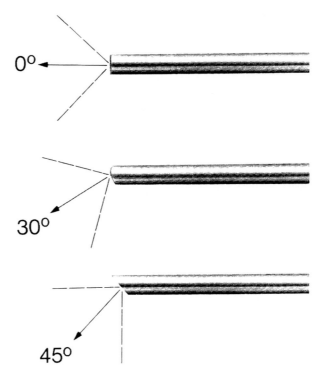

**Figure 20-1** Telescope with various angles of view. The most commonly used are the 0-degree and 30-degree angled telescopes. (Courtesy Karl Storz Veterinary Endoscopy–America, Inc., Goleta, Calif.)

The basic equipment for performing thoracoscopy includes a surgical telescope, a trocar-cannula unit, a light source, a basic set of endoscopic manipulation and surgical instruments, and a minor surgery pack. The components of the complete instrument set are listed in Box 20-1. A miniature video camera can be attached to the telescope to allow video-assisted thoracoscopic procedures. This camera provides a superior image that facilitates the performance of diagnostic and therapeutic procedures.

The telescope is the key to the instrument package. Telescopes available for general veterinary use are 1.2 to 10 mm in diameter. Some telescopes are even available as disposable units (US Surgical Corporation, Norwalk, Conn.). The 4-, 5-, and 10-mm scopes are appropriate for most general veterinary applications in dogs and cats. Exceptionally narrow scopes (1.2 mm in diameter) are available for the smallest patients. However, the limited field of vision and illumination of these very small scopes restrict their practical applications. The telescope that is most versatile for the widest range of animal patients is an instrument with a 4- to 5-mm diameter. This scope size allows examination of almost any dog or cat.

Telescopes with a variety of visual directions are available (Figure 20-1). Most clinicians prefer a forward-viewing 0-degree angle because it provides a more natural field of view. The 0-degree scope also gives a normal perspective to organ orientation. Oblique-angle and retrograde telescopes are preferred for a large number of applications. Many human and veterinary thoracoscopists favor the use of a forward-oblique 30-degree angled telescope because this scope provides a wider view of the thoracic cavity. Angled telescopes can, however, be difficult for an inexperienced operator to use. If just one telescope is to be purchased for both abdominal and thoracic procedures, I suggest a straight-forward 0-degree scope.

The operating thoracoscopes designed for humans can be used to perform diagnostic and therapeutic interventions using only one trocar placement. An operating scope has a 5- or 6-mm instrument channel that accommodates the passage of surgical or manipulative instruments (Figure 20-2). Surgical and biopsy procedures are very limited with this type of scope because to maneuver the instrument, the operator must also change the orientation of the field of view. The telescope diameter is quite large (10 to 12 mm) and is not satisfactory for routine work. When the "view only" telescope (most common type) is used, at least one additional trocar cannula site is required ("second puncture") for instrument insertion to perform any manipulative, biopsy, or surgical procedure.

The trocar-cannula unit is another key accessory to the thoracoscopy set. This instrument can provide a nearly airtight sealed portal through which the telescope

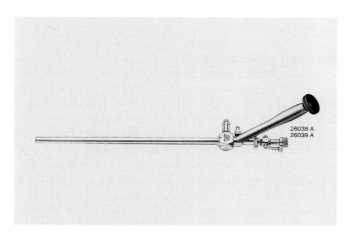

**Figure 20-2** Typical design of an operating telescope with a biopsy/instrument channel built into the telescope. Note that the eyepiece is offset from the instrument channel. (Courtesy Karl Storz Veterinary Endoscopy–America, Inc.)

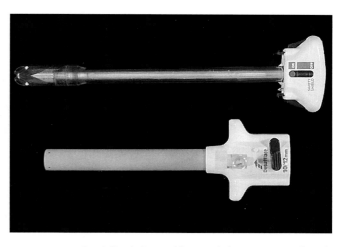

**Figure 20-4** Specialized disposable guarded trocar tip Endopath surgical trocar (Ethicon Endo-Surgery, Inc.) used to minimize the possibility of damage to underlying tissue and organs on insertion of the laparoscope. This cannula can also be easily used for thoracoscopic procedures.

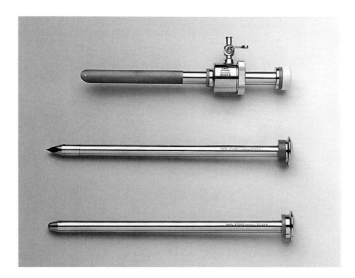

**Figure 20-3** Typical laparoscope trocar-cannula unit. The cannula unit *(top)* has a one-way valve. When the cannula is inserted, this valve provides a nearly airtight seal to the body cavity being examined. A sharp trocar *(middle)* and a blunt *(lower)* trocar are also shown. (Courtesy Karl Storz Veterinary Endoscopy–America, Inc.)

and surgical and manipulating instruments are inserted and biopsy specimens are withdrawn. Trocar-cannula units come in a variety of sizes corresponding to the diameters of the instruments or telescopes that can be used. Typically the standard laparoscopy cannula unit consists of a multifunctional valve apparatus and a variable-length cannula barrel with a removable sharp or blunt trocar (Figure 20-3). The trocar tips are typically pyramidal, conical, or blunt. Some disposable trocar cannula units designed for human laparoscopy even

have guarded trocar tips to minimize potential damage to underlying tissues and organs (Figure 20-4).

A typical trocar-cannula unit designed for thoracoscopy is shorter than the units used for laparoscopy, and its trocar has a blunt tip. The shorter length of the cannula increases maneuverability in the tight confines of the thoracic cavity. Some standard thoracoscopy cannulas do not have an airtight seal or a valve at the end. When these cannulas are used, mechanical ventilation is necessary because of the open communication between the thoracic cavity and the atmosphere. The primary advantage of the standard laparoscope cannula is that it allows the operator to regulate precisely the degree of induced pneumothorax and to remove air rapidly through the insufflation valve after the procedure has been completed.

A number of human units have flexible sleeve material on the cannula. Some of these units are reusable and have a threaded surface that helps keep them from migrating out once they have been placed (Figure 20-5). Newly designed disposable flexible units are very easy to place and are retained by stay sutures (Figure 20-6). The flexible material minimizes damage to underlying tissue and is also reported to lessen postoperative pain in human patients.

A standard laparoscopic light source is used for thoracoscopic procedures. Light sources typically range from 150 to 300 W. The greater the wattage, the more versatile the light source is for performing a wide range of procedures. Photographic documentation is greatly enhanced by a more powerful light source. The light source provides illumination to the telescope via a light cable. Light cables are available in a variety of diameters. As a general rule, the larger the cable, the greater the amount of light that is delivered to the scope and the greater the cavity is illuminated.

Video cameras have revolutionized endoscopic examination and surgery in both human and veterinary medicine. The use of a small surgical video camera attached to the telescope (see Fig. 2-5) makes the procedure considerably easier to perform and enables the operator and assistant to view a simultaneous, enlarged, clear image. Ready documentation for record keeping and review is obtained by attaching the camera to a video cassette recorder and/or video printer. Sterile camera bags are commercially available from many sources and are relatively inexpensive. Certain camera systems can also be gas sterilized directly. The manufacturer's recommendations should be reviewed before a camera system is subjected to chemical sterilants.

Numerous instruments are available for endoscopic exploration and surgery. The basic instrument set consists of a grasping forceps, scissors, a punch biopsy instrument, and a palpation probe. Tissue biopsy instruments are usually of the grasping or Tru-Cut–needle type (Travenol Labs). Forceps and scissors are often insulated for electrocautery. Adapters that fit most standard electrocautery units are available. Most major manufacturers even make electrocautery units designed exclusively for endoscopic use. Electrocautery provides easy coagulation of mild to moderate bleeding that may occur during a procedure. In human thoracoscopy, specialized stapling devices have eliminated much of the difficult, time-consuming, and tedious actions involved in suturing and cutting tissue (Figure 20-7). In addition, pretied ligatures (Endoloop; Ethicon Endo-Surgery, Inc., Cincinnati, Ohio) have greatly simplified knot tying during endoscopic procedures (Figure 20-8). Additional instruments can be added to the basic set as the operator gains

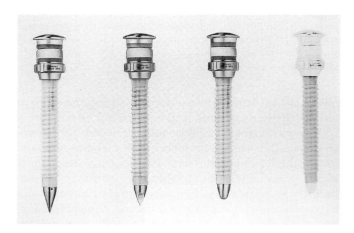

**Figure 20-5** Reusable flexible trocars with threaded cannula barrels and a variety of blunt and sharp trocar tips. (Karl Storz Veterinary Endoscopy–American, Inc.)

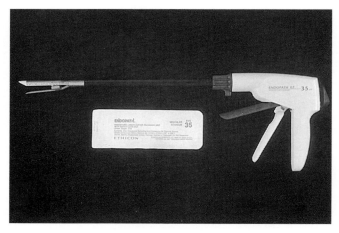

**Figure 20-7** Surgical stapling device. This unit places a set of six staggered staples and has a knife blade that cuts between the staple lines (Endopath EZ, 35-mm linear cutter, Ethicon Endo-Surgery Inc.)

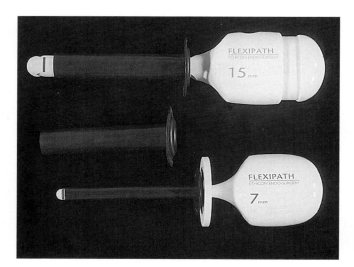

**Figure 20-6** Disposable flexible thoracic cannulas (7 to 15 mm in diameter). The trocars have smooth sides and holes placed at the flange for stay suture placement (Flexipath flexible surgical trocar, Ethicon Endo-Surgery Inc.)

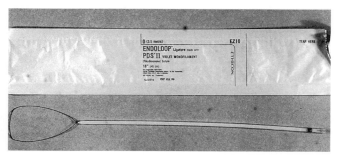

**Figure 20-8** Specially designed pretied suture material. The loop of the material is slipped over the lesion or structure of interest, and a plastic sleeve is used to slide the knot securely in place (Endoloop, Ethicon Endo-Surgery Inc.)

experience and begins to perform more complex surgical procedures. Most instrument manufacturers offer classes and "wet labs" on the use of advanced surgical stapling and suturing devices.

Because of concerns regarding the potential transmission of infectious disease, some of the instruments designed for use in human medical centers are disposable. These disposable instruments include trocars, telescopes, and ancillary operating instruments. The use of disposable instruments is not cost effective in veterinary medicine. The purchase of stainless-steel instrumentation represents an initially greater investment, but the instruments can be used for many years. Although many disposable human instruments can be resterilized, they are designed for use in a single patient and should not be expected to have a prolonged life span.

Instruments can be safely sterilized using ethylene oxide gas. Cold sterilization is also effective and safe for endoscopic instruments and can be easily performed using commercially available solutions such as 2% glutaraldehyde (Cidex). Cold sterilization solutions must be rinsed from instruments with warmed sterile saline or water to prevent tissue irritation when the equipment is used. Many newer telescopes are even autoclavable. Damage to endoscopic instrumentation can be prevented by obtaining specific guidelines from the equipment manufacturer *before* any sterilization method is used on these precision instruments.

## INDICATIONS

The indications for thoracoscopic exploration in humans include the following: general thoracoscopic exploration for pleural disease; management of malignant pleural effusion; staging of neoplasia; assessment of lesion resectability; implantation of defibrillator lead wires; pulmonic resection and biopsy; pericardectomy; esophageal surgery; sympathectomies; anterior mediastinal exploration; and the correction of vascular anomalies. New techniques and instrumentation continually expand the applications of thoracoscopy.

The primary indication for thoracoscopy in veterinary medicine is the evaluation and visual inspection of the thoracic cavity using a minimally invasive technique. Thoracoscopy is far less invasive than a typical open thoracotomy, and it has a much lower morbidity and mortality rate. The view obtained with thoracoscopy is often superior to that obtained via thoracotomy because any structure within the thorax can be accessed and evaluated with a magnified and well illuminated view. Thoracoscopy provides very consistent results in the diagnosis of intrathoracic pathology. For example, it provides definitive information when radiographic or ultrasonographic evaluations indicate hilar and mediastinal

masses, when fluid loculations cannot be differentiated from solid masses, and when a definitive diagnosis of malignant pleural effusions or pericardial disease is needed. In my hospital, thoracoscopy is used primarily for the staging of neoplastic disease and the preoperative evaluation of resectability. We have also used this technique to biopsy masses, lymph nodes, lung, and pericardial tissues. To date, our clinical surgical techniques have been limited to pericardectomies. However, extensive surgical procedures have been performed (on dogs) in research settings. These procedures have included complete lung lobectomies, intrathoracic intervertebral discectomies, diaphragmatic repair, and sympathectomies. The limitations of thoracoscopy are largely determined by the operator's level of experience. It is well known that most if not all new human techniques were developed in animal models.

## CONTRAINDICATIONS

Thoracoscopy is not indicated for every thoracic surgery case. Limitations in instrumentation, tactile discrimination, and vascular control, as well as the lack of three-dimensional vision, have impeded the use of thoracoscopy in human patients. Technologic advances have begun to bridge many of these gaps. Unfortunately the cost of such instrumentation precludes its use in the average veterinary patient.

Certain conditions, however, are absolute contraindications for thoracoscopy. The first is a clotted hemothorax. In this condition, visibility is negligible and the procedure can exacerbate a severe hemorrhage, which may then be difficult to control. The second is coagulopathy disorder. Chronic empyema can be a relative contraindication if severe adhesions limit trocar placement.

## THORACOSCOPY TECHNIQUE

### Preparation and Anesthesia

The patient must receive a thorough preanesthetic evaluation. This evaluation helps the clinician select the anesthetic regimen and determine the specific approach for the procedure. As for a standard thoracotomy, the patient is clipped and prepared in the region of interest. General anesthesia and endotracheal intubation are required. Gas inhalation anesthesia and mechanical ventilation are recommended but are not absolutely necessary. Some animal patients can be evaluated under heavy sedation, although this technique is not recommended. Patient movement that disrupts the sterile field can easily occur whenever a painful manipulation is performed in a sedated but not anesthetized patient. Movement during manipulation can endanger the patient.

The choice of induction agent and maintenance anesthetic depends on the patient's condition and the clinician's preferences. Some patients may require assisted ventilation. However, I have performed many procedures during which the patient spontaneously ventilated and have not experienced any problems. Regardless of the anesthetic regimen chosen, supplemental oxygen should always be delivered. A high fractional inspired oxygen concentration helps compensate for the ventilation perfusion mismatching that occurs during a partial pneumothorax. Adequate monitoring is essential to ensure patient safety. Patient monitoring can also include pulse oximetry, capnography, blood gas analysis, blood pressure measurement (direct or indirect), and a running electrocardiogram.

During many human surgical procedures *one* lung ventilation is performed to increase intrathoracic visibility. The technique involves selective bronchial intubation, which then allows the nonintubated lung to collapse. The dependent lung is ventilated, allowing the contralateral lung to collapse. Thus far this technique has primarily been used in a research setting on animals. If extensive thoracoscopic techniques are developed, the physiologic effects of one-lung ventilation techniques need to be studied in dogs and cats. Normal research dogs seem to tolerate one-lung ventilation without serious cardiopulmonary compromise; however, the dog has only moderate hypoxic vasoconstrictory capacity compared with other species. Severe hypoxic complications can develop with this technique. When a one-lung ventilation technique is used, close monitoring of arterial blood gases is an absolute necessity. Having the lung region of interest collapsed makes surgical procedures much easier to perform because visibility is greatly enhanced. However, the average exploration and biopsy procedure in veterinary patients does not require this technique.

### Preoperative Staging

A plan is essential for any thoracoscopic exploration. Approaching thoracoscopy without a plan can be disastrous! Several questions should be asked before a thoracoscopy procedure is started: Why is the procedure being performed? Depending on the findings, what will be done next (open thoracotomy, biopsy, etc.)? Has the approach been adequately planned? Which intercostal space will be entered? Where is the lesion of interest? Have preparations been made to convert to an open procedure if it becomes necessary? Preoperative staging allows the clinician to avoid the common serious complications of thoracoscopy, which include "kebab" lung (spearing the lung with the trocar), entering the wrong side or location, penetrating viscera of a large diaphragmatic hernia, and entering a clotted hemothorax. Risk limitation is key to successful thoracoscopy. A *complete* patient evaluation, including thoracic radiographs obtained within 24 hours of performing the procedure, can limit costly mistakes.

### Approaches to the Thoracic Cavity

Before trocars are placed in the thorax, the patient should be draped in the same way as for a standard thoracotomy. The sterilized telescope should be immersed in warm sterile saline or distilled water to prevent fogging of the lens. Application of a sterile antifogging solution further decreases optical fogging of the telescope. The light cable is attached to the telescope, and the surgical video camera is placed in a sterile camera bag with the assistance of a surgery room technician unless the camera has already been sterilized using etylene oxide gas or cold sterilization solutions. The video camera should be color balanced according to the manufacturer's instructions. The assembly is then ready for insertion when the cannulas are placed (Figure 20-9).

At my hospital we have developed three basic approaches to the thorax: the *paraxyphoid transdiaphragmatic* approach, the *intercostal* approach, and the *thoracic inlet* approach. Each approach has a particular application based on the locations to be accessed (Table 20-1).

### Paraxyphoid Transdiaphragmatic Approach

The paraxyphoid approach is useful for most applications and facilitates excellent evaluation of the ventral aspects of both hemi-thoraces. It is also the easiest ap-

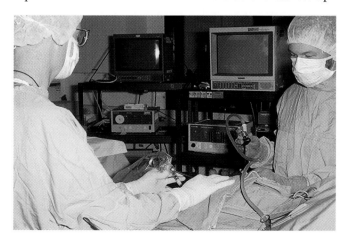

**Figure 20-9** Telescope equipped with a surgical video camera. The camera and cables are within a sterile camera bag. The telescope and camera are shown inserted into a multifunctional trocar placed in the paraxyphoid position.

**Table 20-1    Trocar Insertion Approaches and Visualization of Major Anatomic Features**

| Major anatomic feature | Paraxyphoid approach | Intercostal approach | Thoracic inlet approach |
|---|---|---|---|
| **GENERAL DIAPHRAGM** | + | + + + | + + + * |
| Aortic hiatus | − | + + + * | + + * |
| Caval foramen | − | + + + * | + + * |
| Esophageal hiatus | − | + + + * | + + * |
| Diaphragmatic reflection | + | + + | + + + * |
| Central tendon | − | + + + | + + + * |
| Pars sternalis | − | + + + | + + + * |
| Pars costalis | + | + + + | + + + * |
| Esophagus | + + | + + + | + |
| **HEART** | | | |
| Pericardium | + + + | + + * | + |
| Base | + * | + + + * | + + * |
| Ductus arteriosus/ligament | − | + + + * | + * |
| Apex | + + + | + | − |
| **HILUS OF THE LUNG** | | | |
| General | − | + + + * | + + * |
| Lymph nodes | − | + + + * | + * |
| Neurovascular components | + * | + + + * | + * |
| **LUNG LOBES** | | | |
| Right and left cranial | + + | + + + | + + + |
| Right and left caudal | + + | + + + | + |
| Accessory lobe | + | + + + | − |
| Middle lobe | + + | + + + | + |
| Dorsal aspect | − | + + + | + + |
| Ventral aspect | + + + | + + | + |
| Cardiac notch | + + | + + + | + |
| Trachea | + * | + + + * | + + * |
| Bronchi | + * | + + + * | + * |
| **MEDIASTINUM** | | | |
| Cranial | + + | + + + | + + |
| Lymph nodes | + | + + + | + + + * |
| Thymus | + | + + + | + + + * |
| Caudal | + + + | + + + | + |
| **NERVOUS SYSTEM** | | | |
| Vagus nerve | + + | + + + | + |
| Phrenic nerve | + + + | + + + | + |
| **STERNUM** | | | |
| Sternebrae | + + + | + + * | + + + |
| Sternal lymph nodes | + + + | + + * | + + + |
| **VASCULAR SYSTEM** | | | |
| Aorta | + + | + + + | + + * |
| Azygos vein | + + | + + + | − |
| Carotid artery | + | + + + * | + + * |
| Cranial vena cava | + | + + + | + + |
| Caudal vena cava | + + + | + + + | + |
| Internal thoracic artery and vein | + + + | + + + | + + |
| Lateral thoracic artery and vein | + + + | + + | + |
| **PULMONARY VESSELS** | | | |
| Arteries | + + | + + + * | + * |
| Veins | + + | + + + * | + * |

+ + +, Excellent visualization; + +, good visualization; +, fair to poor visualization; −, no visualization.
*Manipulation of overlying structures using additional trocars and a standard palpation probe was required to visualize these structures.

proach for the beginning thoracoscopist to master. The insertion technique is performed using a typical laparoscopic 6-mm-diameter multifunctional-valve or trumpet-valve trocar. For the examination the patient is positioned in a dorsal recumbent position and is clipped and prepared as for a standard median thoracotomy. A small stab incision is made to the right or left of the xyphoid. Then the trocar is inserted, with the diaphragm penetrated along a preplanned path. The trocar is grasped to control penetration depth to a region just inside the thoracic cavity. After penetrating the ventral abdominal musculature and the abdominal surface of the ventromedial portion of the pars sternalis (diaphragm), I usually move the sharp tip of the trocar in a cranial ventral direction (i.e., toward the sternum). After the pleural surface of the diaphragm is penetrated, the sharp trocar is withdrawn. The telescope assembly is then inserted into the cannula valve, and the scope is advanced until the ventral thoracic cavity is visualized. The thoracic cavity is examined by advancing the scope cranially.

The paraxyphoid transdiaphragmatic approach is useful for evaluating the ventral aspects of both hemithoraces. When the scope moves through the diaphragm, a long-axis view of the thorax is obtained (see Plate 20-1). The ventral and lateral aspects of the pericardium and phrenic nerve are easily visualized. The telescope is gently advanced until the caudal mediastinum is penetrated. The scope can then be moved along the ventrolateral aspects of the right and left hemithoraces to the thoracic inlet. The internal thoracic artery and vein are prominent landmarks as the thoracic inlet is approached (see Plate 20-2). Exploration of cranial thoracic structures and the cranial mediastinum is limited only by the length of the scope. The ventral aspects of each lung lobe can be accessed using the paraxyphoid transdiaphragmatic approach. The vascular structures of the ventral aspect of the pulmonary hilus can also be visualized and approached. However, the dorsal aspects of the lobes and vessels cannot be visualized. The esophagus, aorta, and caudal vena cava are easily located, allowing rapid anatomic orientation.

By directing the scope in a steep dorsal direction, the operator can view the dorsal aspect of the costal diaphragmatic reflection. With steep direction of the scope ventrally, the sternebrae can be evaluated and sternal lymph nodes can be seen if they are enlarged. With maximal ventral lateral deflection, the sternal diaphragmatic recesses can be seen in some patients.

Additional trocars can be placed in the intercostal spaces cranially, and a palpation probe can be inserted to gently retract the lung lobes away. With this technique the scope can be directed between the lobar fissures. This allows excellent visualization of visceral pleural surface and the pulmonary vessels. With the insertion of a for-

ceps and scissors, the pericardium can be easily grasped and incised from this position (see Plates 20-3 and 20-15). The phrenic nerve is a distinct landmark to the limitation of incision on the pericardium (see Plates 20-16, 20-17, and 20-18).

## Intercostal Approach

The intercostal approach is the most common approach described in the literature. The patient can be positioned in a right lateral, left lateral, or dorsal recumbent position, or even in an oblique position, depending on the structures that are to be evaluated. The typical trocar insertion site is in the seventh intercostal space midway between the costochondral junction and ventral border of the epaxial muscles. Intercostal insertion in the caudal location of the seventh intercostal space or cranially in the fourth intercostal space allows access to most anatomic structures in each hemithorax. The trocar typically used for this location is a short (6- to 8-cm) cannula or a flexible cannula that can be trimmed to a desired length. A one-way valve may or may not be attached. Trocar insertion at the seventh intercostal space allows wide exploration and visualization of the entire lateral thorax.

Care must be exercised in entering the thoracic cavity via the intercostal approach. After a small (6- to 7-mm) skin incision is made, the subcutaneous tissue and underlying musculature are split with a hemostat to enter the pleural space. Once atmospheric communication with the pleural space is achieved, the lung falls away from the chest wall slightly unless significant adhesions exist. The trocar can be gently and safely inserted with this technique. With the placement of an additional trocar in the fourth intercostal space, a palpation probe can be used to manipulate and move adjacent lung lobes and can also facilitate the visualization of peribronchial tissues, pulmonary arteries and veins, hilar lymph nodes, and all aspects of the pleural surface of the diaphragm (see Plates 20-5 through 20-10).

The diaphragm can be visualized when the scope is rotated maximally toward the thoracic wall and then directed caudally. Cranial telescope insertion (fourth intercostal space) allows better visualization of cranial mediastinal structures. When the scope is directed caudally, a superior long-axis examination of the diaphragm is possible (see Plate 20-7).

## Thoracic Inlet Approach

The thoracic inlet approach is reserved for evaluation of the most cranial structures in the mediastinum, which cannot be reached via a cranial intercostal approach. For this approach the patient is positioned in a dorsal recumbent position. The trocar insertion sites are on the right and left sides of the thoracic inlet between the cranial medial edge of the first rib and the lateral aspect of the trachea. A small (6- to 7-mm) skin incision is made on the right or left side of the thoracic inlet. The trocar is inserted under the skin and advanced in a caudal lateral direction toward the medial surface of the second rib. With this approach both the right and left hemithoraces can be examined, and the cranial aspect of the left and right cranial lung lobes and the cranial thoracic lymph nodes can be well visualized. A long axis view of the entire hemithorax can be obtained once the mediastinal structures and cranial lung lobes are passed by gently pushing the scope caudally. The membranous nature of the cranial mediastinum makes initial anatomic orientation difficult with this approach. An end-on cranial-to-caudal view of each hemithorax is possible. This approach is limited by the size of the dog being examined. It is difficult to visualize the entire hemithorax in long or deep-chested breeds. By directing the scope medially as the diaphragm is approached, the operator can see the vena cava, aorta, and esophagus entering the diaphragm.

Additional trocar placement can be easily visualized from inside the thorax in both the cranial and caudal locations. *Blind* trocar insertion must be *avoided* because it involves passing the instrument close to the internal thoracic artery, brachiocephalic trunk, subclavian arteries and veins, common carotid arteries, and vagus and phrenic nerves. Without direct visualization the risk of injuring one of these structures is too great.

The thoracic inlet approach is seldom indicated. Maneuvering the scope with the redundant nature of the cranial mediastinum can make orientation frustrating and difficult. Most structures can be visualized via the considerably safer cranial intercostal technique.

## Additional Instrument Trocar Insertion

Insertion sites are planned in a triangular fashion relative to the telescope. This allows instruments to be brought into the field of view and easily oriented by the operator. Additional trocar insertion sites can be visualized thoracoscopically in each of the three approaches by applying digital pressure on the external thoracic wall. Inward deflection of the medial thoracic wall is visualized through the telescope to determine the adequacy of the penetration site.

A skin incision 6 or 7 mm in length is made in the region of digital manipulation. The sharp tip of the trocar is inserted through the skin and advanced into the chest cavity. The penetration should be limited and observed internally with the scope (Figure 20-10). The sharp trocar is quickly removed, leaving a nearly airtight cannula

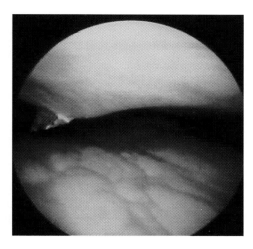

**Figure 20-10** Sharp tip of an ancillary instrument trocar penetrating the pleural surface (9 o'clock position in the field of view). Lung tissue is ventral.

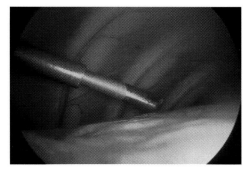

**Figure 20-11** Palpation probe inserted through an instrument cannula. The ribs can be clearly seen just beyond the cannula and palpation probe.

sleeve in place through which ancillary instruments can be introduced (Figure 20-11).

## Biopsy Procedures

Biopsy sample procurement is one of the most common procedures conducted during thoracoscopy. Specimens from a variety of pathologic conditions can be obtained. A number of biopsy instruments are available, including the grasping, crushing, and cutting types (see Figure 14-10) or needle instruments such as a Tru-Cut biopsy instrument. These instrument types all work well. The larger specimens obtained with the cup instruments make the pathologist's evaluation easier because more tissue is provided for microscopic evaluation. Hemorrhage associated with biopsy depends on the vascularity of the structure involved. Surface clamping and electrocautery can be performed if hemorrhage is extensive.

The operator should be able to *visualize* the structure adequately before a biopsy is taken. The jaws of the instrument should *not* be closed unless the margins of the biopsy site are clearly visible.

Lung biopsy specimens may be obtained in three ways: First, small lesions can be sampled with a standard grasping biopsy (Figure 20-12) or Tru-Cut instrument. Second, a wedge resection of the peripheral lung can be performed. With this method an endoscopic stapling device (see Figure 20-7) is inserted through a 12- to 15-mm-diameter trocar-cannula unit, and a wedge of lung tissue is removed (Figure 20-13). The wedge resection technique is the preferred method in human medicine. In the third method a pretied ligature (Endoloop) is passed onto the shaft of a grasping forceps. The lung is then grasped and elevated with the forceps, and the ligature is pushed down the shaft and over the lesion of interest. The knot is secured, and the tissue above the ligature is transected and removed from the thorax.

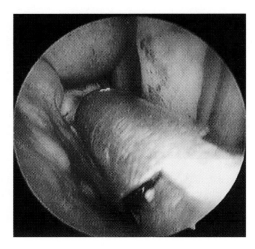

**Figure 20-12** SEMM biopsy forceps instrument (Karl Storz Veterinary Endoscopy–America, Inc.). A biopsy is being obtained from a cranial thoracic mass.

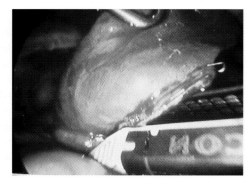

**Figure 20-13** A surgical stapling device being used to procure a lung biopsy specimen. (Courtesy Laura Potter, Ethicon Endo-Surgery Inc.).

An alternative method for evaluating deep pulmonary lesions is needle aspiration or Tru-Cut biopsy. We have obtained biopsy specimens in patients with a number of pathologic conditions (see Plates 20-9 through 20-14). Several of our patients have been spared unnecessary thoracotomy procedures by the demonstration of disseminated and unresectable disease.

## Operative Procedures

The human thoracic surgery literature contains a vast number of descriptions of new surgical procedures related to thoracoscopy. In veterinary medicine these procedures have been limited to subtotal pericardectomies and the formation of pericardial windows. To date, experimental techniques such as thoracic intravertebral discectomies, esophagomyotomy, and partial lobectomies have not been routinely used in clinical veterinary patients.

Pericardial surgery can be performed from an intercostal or a paraxyphoid approach. The latter approach can be used to make a simple pericardial window at the apex of the pericardium. The paraxyphoid approach allows excellent visualization of the pericardium and full visualization of the phrenic nerves. With this approach the telescope cannula penetrates the diaphragm, giving the operator a full view of the ventral aspect of the thorax. The caudal mediastinal tissue can be incised away from the sternal attachments so that the operator has an unobstructed view of the entire apex of the pericardium. Two additional instrument ports are required to insert a grasping forceps and scissors into the field of view. As previously described, instruments should be triangulated into the operator's field of view. The apex of the pericardium is grasped with the forceps (see Plate 20-15), and the telescope is positioned to ensure adequate visualization of the phrenic nerves (see Plate 20-16). The operator moves the scissors under the grasping forceps and makes a small incision in the pericardial sac (see Plate 20-17). Electrocautery is used to facilitate hemostasis because a thickened pathologic pericardium has a great propensity to hemorrhage when incised. A suction tip and operative suction are often required to drain the pericardial sac. The pericardium is then further incised ventral to the phrenic nerves (see Plate 20-18).

Alternatively, an intercostal approach with selective bronchial intubation and one-lung ventilation techniques may be used. A lateral pericardial window can be established, and occasionally a subtotal pericardectomy can be performed from one side. Often the patient must be rotated to allow visualization of the contralateral side of the heart in order to complete the pericardectomy. Usually only one side of the pericardium can be removed from an intercostal approach. The patient must also be repositioned, and selective intubation of the opposite lung must be performed. The additional placement of instrument ports is also required. In my experience, damage to the phrenic nerve is more likely to occur with the intercostal approach than with the paraxyphoid technique. With the intercostal technique the phrenic nerve is often difficult to visualize on the lateral surface of the pathologic pericardium. Furthermore, the intercostal technique requires much more time to complete because of the need for selective intubation and one-lung ventilation.

## Postoperative Care

To as great a degree as is possible, the air that has been introduced into the thoracic space should be withdrawn before the end of the procedure. Standard suction can be applied to the stopcock valve on the insertion cannula to evacuate the thorax at the conclusion of the examination.

A thoracic drain should be placed after the completion of each procedure, and the patient should be closely evaluated in the early postoperative period to ensure that the thoracic cavity remains evacuated. Adequate placement of the tube should be confirmed before the telescope is withdrawn (Figure 20-14). A standard thoracic drain should be used (Argyle Trocar Thoracic Catheter). These drains are manufactured in a variety of sizes (12 to 20 French). I typically use a 20-French thoracic drain in medium- to large-sized dogs and a 12- to 16-French drain in small dogs and in cats. Although the drain can be placed directly through an instrument port, leakage around the tube is apt to occur with this technique. The best method is to tunnel the thoracic drain from a distant site and to observe penetration and placement thoracoscopically. Red rubber feeding tubes can also be

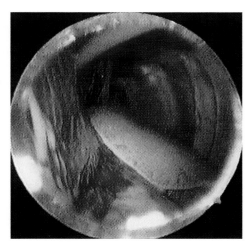

**Figure 20-14** Thoracic drain (12 o'clock position) placed before the evacuation of free air from the thorax.

used, but they may induce more pleural effusion and inflammation than Argyle tubes, which are definitely preferred for thoracic drainage.

Intermittent or continuous suction should be applied to the drain during the recovery period until the lungs are fully expanded. A postoperative thoracic radiograph may be used to confirm the resolution of a pneumothorax. In many patients the thoracic drain can be removed early in the recovery period. However, the length of time the thoracic drain is maintained depends on the individual pathologic process. I typically leave the thoracic drain in place for 12 to 24 hours in routine thoracoscopy procedures. A general rule of thumb is to leave the drain in pace until normal negative intrathoracic pressures have been reestablished.

The degree of evacuation and the placement of the thoracic drain can be observed before the last telescope cannula is removed. After removal of the cannulas, the wounds are sutured closed. A standard two-layer closure is adequate.

## Complications

Severe hemorrhage is the most common reported complication of thoracoscopy. Potential complications include puncture of the pulmonary parenchyma during trocar insertion and laceration of a vessel or nerve during biopsy or pericardectomy. Although the complication rate associated with thoracoscopy is low, the clinician should be prepared to perform an emergency thoracotomy in the event of severe hemorrhage. Most mild to moderate hemorrhage resolves with conservative management and the use of a thoracic drain.

Removal of biopsy specimens directly through small holes in the thoracic wall or cannulas may cause malignant or infected material to contaminate the pleural or abdominal space. Specimen retrieval bags (Endobag; Dexide, Fort Worth, Tex.) have been developed to prevent this complication (Figure 20-15). Unfortunately these bags are quite expensive. A simple alternative is to use a surgical glove. The specimen can be maneuvered into the glove and retrieved via a small intercostal incision.

Mild to moderate and persistent pneumothoraces are the most common postoperative complications of thoracoscopy. These problems are more likely to occur when biopsy or other surgical procedures are performed.

## CONCLUSION

If carefully planned, thoracoscopy is a safe and effective method for evaluating intrathoracic pathology without the expense and morbidity of open thoracotomy. The view obtained via thoracoscopy is often superior to that obtained via open thoracotomy because the telescope

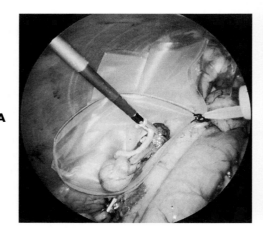
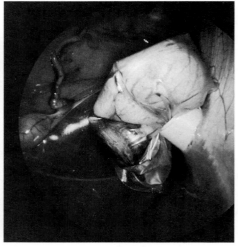

**Figure 20-15** Specimen retrieval bag (Endobag; Dexide, Fort Worth, Tex.) used for specimen retrieval. The bag is made of polyurethane foil. These photographs demonstrate the use of the retrieval sack in a human abdominal procedure. **A,** The bag is open, and the resected tissue is being nudged into it. **B,** The bag is pulled closed with the tissue to be removed contained completely within it.

can be placed directly on the lesion in question, providing the operator with a magnified, well-illuminated view. Thoracoscopic techniques are not intended to replace traditional surgical techniques, but they can be used to help evaluate patients in a less invasive manner before a decision is made to perform an open thoracotomy procedure.

## SUGGESTED ADDITIONAL READINGS

Allen MS et al: Video assisted thoracic surgical procedures: the Mayo experience, *Mayo Clin Proc* 71:351, 1996.

Bauer T, Thomas WP: Pulmonary diagnostic techniques, *Vet Clin North Am Small Anim Pract* 13:273, 1983.

Braimbridge MV: The history of thoracoscopic surgery, *Ann Thorac Surg* 56:610, 1993.

Daniel TM: Diagnostic thoracoscopy for pleural disease, *Ann Thorac Surg* 56:639, 1993.

Horswell JL: Anesthetic techniques for thoracoscopy, *Ann Thorac Surg* 56:624, 1993.

Kadukura M: Pathologic comparisons of video-assisted thoracoscopic lung biopsy with traditional lung biopsy, *J Thorac Cardiovasc Surg* 109:494, 1995.

Kaiser LR, Bavaria JE: Complications of thoracoscopy, *Ann Thorac Surg* 56:796, 1993.

McCarthy TC, McDermaid SL: Thoracoscopy, *Vet Clin North Am Small Anim Pract* 20:1341, 1990.

Naruke T et al: Thoracoscopy for staging of lung cancer, *Ann Thorac Surg* 56:661, 1993.

Potter LA: Video-assisted thoracic surgery (VATS). In *ACVS Forum Proceedings*, San Francisco, 1996.

**COLOR PLATES    PAGES 483-488**

## NORMAL CANINE THORAX: VARIOUS APPEARANCES

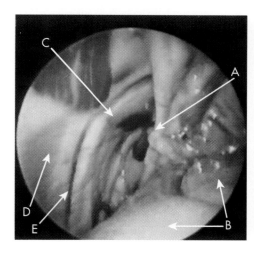

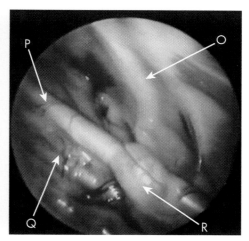

**Plate 20-1** View of a normal ventral thorax obtained via the paraxyphoid approach. The internal thoracic artery and vein are prominent landmarks in the cranial thorax. In this view the lung is ventral and the sternum is dorsal. The mediastinal tissue is easily breached, allowing passage to the right or left hemithorax. (*A*, Internal thoracic artery and vein; *B*, lung; *C*, rib; *D*, chest wall; *E*, intercostal artery.)

**Plate 20-2** Normal internal thoracic artery and vein in the cranial thorax as visualized from a paraxyphoid approach. (*O*, Rib; *P*, internal thoracic artery; *Q*, internal thoracic vein; *R*, mediastinal fat.)

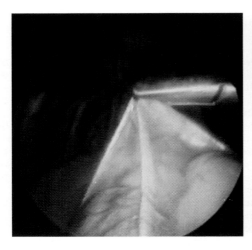

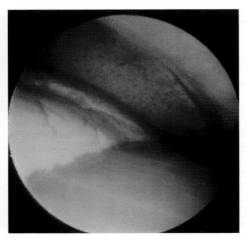

**Plate 20-3** Normal pericardium. The pericardium has been grasped with a forceps. Note that the epicardial surface can be seen through the normal pericardium.

**Plate 20-4** View from a caudal intercostal approach with only a minimal pneumothorax. The lung *(middle left)*, chest wall *(upper)*, and diaphragm *(lower)* are easily observed from this position.

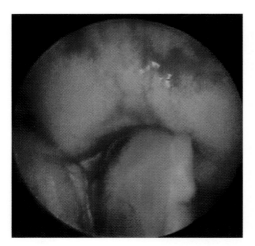

**Plate 20-5** Normal pulmonary vessels with the right middle lung lobe retracted dorsal from an intercostal scope insertion.

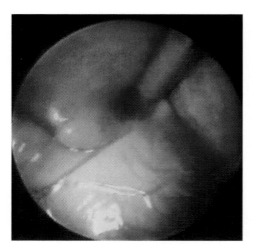

**Plate 20-6** Pericardium (heart base) with the right cranial lung lobe retracted dorsally from an intercostal scope insertion. The right auricle can be seen through the translucent pericardium.

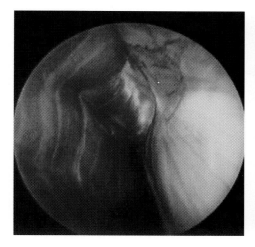

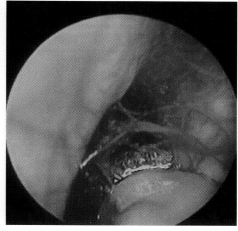

**Plate 20-7** Normal diaphragm and esophagus (light colored structure on right side) from a fourth intercostal approach.

**Plate 20-8** Normal right cranial lung lobe and proliferative cranial-mediastinal tissue viewed from a thoracic inlet approach.

## THORACIC CAVITY NEOPLASIA

Thoracoscopy is a very useful technique for examining the thoracic cavity structures for evidence of neoplasia and for procuring samples for biopsy. In some cases the decision on whether or not to proceed to open thoracotomy for a more definitive procedure is based on the thoracoscopic findings. Some patients can be spared major surgery as a result of a diagnostic thoracoscopy procedure.

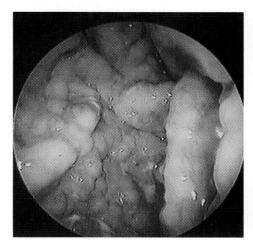

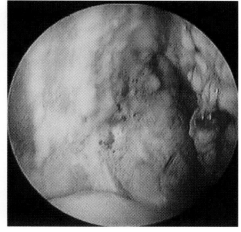

**Plate 20-9** Severe disseminated pulmonary carcinomatosis in a 12-year-old male castrated German shepherd. Frozen sections were obtained, and the diagnosis was made at the time of the examination.

**Plate 20-10** Generalized pulmonary histiocytoma. Note the proliferative lesions on the thoracic wall.

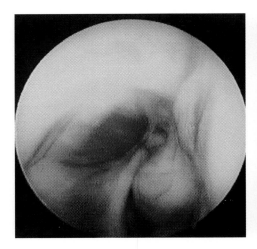

**Plate 20-11** Cranial thoracic lymph node enlargement. Percutaneous attempts at aspiration and biopsy were unsuccessful. The mass was easily biopsied via thoracoscopy.

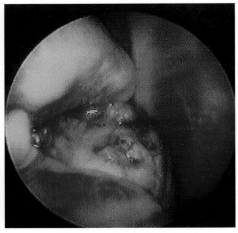

**Plate 20-12** Cranial thoracic mass (thymoma). A biopsy instrument was used to procure a biopsy specimen for frozen section before open thoracotomy was performed.

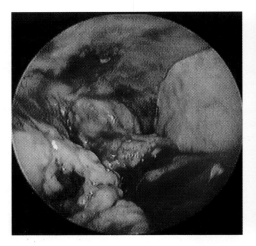

**Plate 20-13** Diffuse, poorly differentiated mesenchymal lesion in a 9-year-old male castrated Labrador retriever.

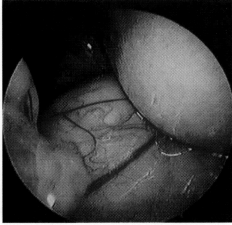

**Plate 20-14** Large hilar lymph node. The diagnosis was bronchogenic adenocarcinoma metastasis.

# PERICARDIAL WINDOW TECHNIQUE

Subtotal pericardectomy is a useful technique for managing recurrent pericardial effusion. The technique is described in the text. A paraxyphoid approach is preferred.

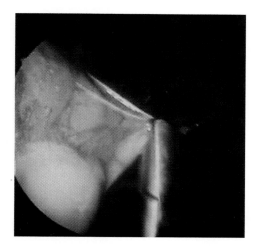

**Plate 20-15** Forceps are used to grasp the pericardium.

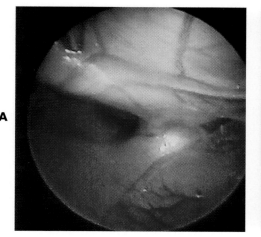

A

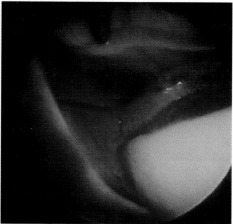

B

**Plate 20-16** Phrenic nerve on the lateral surface of the pericardium. **A,** Location of the phrenic nerve. **B,** Phrenic nerve is in the upper field, coursing left to right. An instrument is touching the nerve.

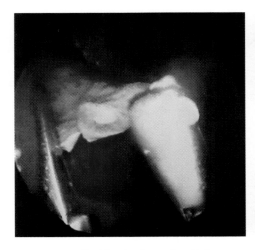

**Plate 20-17** Incision in the pericardial sac. Scissors are on left, and grasping forceps are on right.

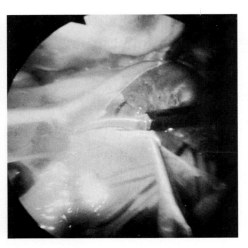

**Plate 20-18** Close-up of a pericardial incision below the phrenic nerve. The cutting instrument is in the center, and the phrenic nerve is indicated by the arrow.

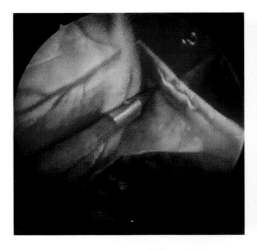

**Plate 20-19** Open pericardial sac.

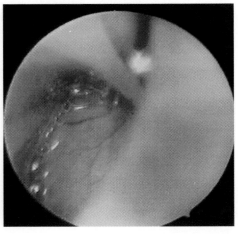

**Plate 20-20** The scope is within the pericardial sac, and the right auricle is in view at the bottom of the field of view.

## LUNG BIOPSY

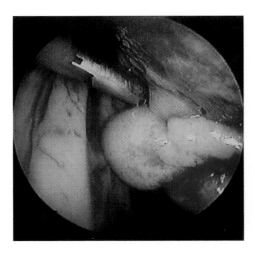

**Plate 20-21** SEMM biopsy instrument procuring a surface biopsy specimen of the lung

# Index

Page numbers in *italics* indicate illustrations; *t* indicate tables; *b* indicates boxes.